Encyclopedia of Neurodegeneration

Encyclopedia of Neurodegeneration

Edited by **Natalie Theresa**

hayle medical

New York

Published by Hayle Medical,
30 West, 37th Street, Suite 612,
New York, NY 10018, USA
www.haylemedical.com

Encyclopedia of Neurodegeneration
Edited by Natalie Theresa

International Standard Book Number: 978-1-63241-175-4 (Hardback)

Printed in China.

Contents

Preface

This book aims to highlight the current researches and provides a platform to further the scope of innovations in this area. This book is a product of the combined efforts of many researchers and scientists, after going through thorough studies and analysis from different parts of the world. The objective of this book is to provide the readers with the latest information of the field.

This book is designed to serve as a companion for the readers to help them comprehend the concept of neurodegeneration. At present, the human population is on a course to collision in terms of social and economic troubles. As a result of varying demographics and growth in human population over the age of 60, age-related neurodegenerative complications are prone to become more common. Therefore, it becomes necessary to attain a better perception of such neurodegenerative disorders so that these diseases can be managed more pro-actively with new processes. The purpose of this book is to present a picture of current developments in the understanding of essential biological processes that can modify the onset and continuum of neurodegenerative processes. This issue is dealt with at the molecular, cellular and whole organism level. We are hopeful that some of the latest findings depicted in this book will aid in better defining of the fundamental biological mechanisms underlying neurodegenerative processes and help in the development of new therapeutic pathways in the longer run.

I would like to express my sincere thanks to the authors for their dedicated efforts in the completion of this book. I acknowledge the efforts of the publisher for providing constant support. Lastly, I would like to thank my family for their support in all academic endeavors.

Editor

1

SIRT2 (Sirtuin2) – An Emerging Regulator of Neuronal Degeneration

Tatsuro Koike*, Kazuhiko Suzuki and Tomohiro Kawahata
Hokkaido University Graduate School of Life Science, Sapporo, Japan

1. Introduction

SIRT2(sirtuin 2) is one of the mammalian orthologs (sirtuins) of yeast silent information regulator 2 (Sir2) proteins that regulate cell differentiation and calorie restriction (Gan and Mucke, 2008; Nakagawa and Guarente, 2011 for review). In contrast to other family members of sirtuins, SIRT2 is mostly localized in the cytoplasm, and regulates post-translational modifications of proteins such as microtubules via tubulin deacetylation (North et al., 2003)(Fig. 1). The enzyme catalyzes the hydrolysis of NAD^+ and transfer of the acetyl moiety of acetylated alpha-tubulin to the resultant ADP-ribose, thus yielding free alpha-tubulin, 2'-O-acetylated ADP-ribose, and niconinamide. This stoichiometry indicates that its activities are modulated by the status of energy metabolism, and nicotinamide serves as an inhibitor. It has well been appreciated that SIRT2 plays a crucial role in cellular functions including oligodendrocyte differentiation (Li et al., 2007; Ji et al., 2011) and cell cycle (Dryden et al., 2003; Inoue et al., 2007) in non-neuronal cells. So far very few studies have ever addressed the question as to whether its expression in neurons shows any functional significance. We will briefly summarize our results on its functional involvement in axon degeneration, and discuss some of recent findings, highlighting an emerging role of SIRT2 in the regulation of neuronal degeneration and plasticity.

2. Tubulin acetylation and axon stability

2.1 Acetylation and deactylation of tubulin

With long axons and elaborated dendrites, neurons establish the circuitry that receives, stores and transmits information to perform neuronal functions (Horton and Ehlers, 2003). The establishment and maintenance of this circuitry requires a coordinated and widespread regulation of the cytoskeleton and membrane trafficking system. Microtubles, whose building block is a heterodimer of alpha- and beta- tublins, play a pivotal role in this function (Fig. 1). There are multiple pathways through which microtubules are stabilized. For instance, acetylation is mostly observed in stable microtubules in neurons as revealed by their low sensitivity to drug-induced depolymerization (Black and Greene, 1982) or upregulation of acetylated alpha-tubulin in response to trophic factor (Black and Keyser,

---

*Corresponding Author

1987). These findings support a correlate between axon stability and acetylation of alpha-tubulin, but still pose a yet unresolved question regarding the causal relationship between the two (Westermann and Weber, 2003). Acetylation, the major post-translational modification of alpha-tubulin, occurs at the epsilon-amino moiety of Lys40 in the amino terminal region of alpha-tubulin (MacRae,1997). The level of acetylation will be regulated by a balance of tubulin acetyltransferase and tubulin deacetylase activities (Laurent and Fleury, 1996). Although tubulin acetyltransferase (alpha-TAT/MEC-17) has recently been into focus, its regulation is still unknown. Both microtubles and, to a lesser extent, tublins may serve as the substrate for this enzyme (Maruta et al., 1986). The mechanism by which this enzyme works in the lumenal space of the microtubules remains a mystery. Recently, histone deacetylase 6 (HDAC6) (Hubbert et al., 2002; Matsuyama, 2002) and SIRT2 (North et al., 2003) have been identified as an enzyme that catalyzes deacetylation of acetylated alpha-tubulin (Fig. 1). Each enzyme is likely to play an independent role in each compartment of axons.

2.2 The *Wld*^{s} gene and axon stability

In a mutant mouse strain (*Wld*^{S} :Wallerian degeneration resistance) axon degeneration, but not cell somal death, is delayed (Coleman, 2005 for review). Researchers found that transected axons from *Wld*^{S} mice are morphologically indistinguishable from intact axons and capable of conducting action potentials for more than 2 weeks, whereas transected axons from wild-type mice rapidly degenerate within 2 days (Lunn et al., 1989), suggesting that the axonal cytoskeleton is highly stabilized in these mutant *Wld*^{S} mice. This model provides evidence that axonal degeneration is an active process intrinsic to axon itself, which is consistent with the notion that axons often undergo degeneration, independently of cell somal apoptosis during development (Koike et al., 2008, for review). The responsible gene for this phenotype has been demonstrated to encode a chimeric protein (Wld^{S}) of the full-length of Nmnat1 and N-terminal 70 amino acids of Ufd2a (Conforti et al., 2000). Researchers have shown that the overexpression of the chimeric protein or Nmnat1, or NAD treatment delays axonal degeneration (Mack et al., 2001; Araki et al., 2004; Wang et al., 2005). Nmnat1 is a key enzyme for NAD biosynthesis, and hence it has been postulated that NAD-dependent pathways are involved in the mechanisms underlying Wld^{S}-mediated axonal protection (Araki et al., 2004; Sasaki et al., 2006). However, both Wld^{S} and Nmnat1 are localized in the nucleus, and NAD level remains unchanged irrespective of Wld^{S} or Nmnat1 overexpression (Mack et al., 2001; Araki et al., 2004). The precise mechanism of this neuroprotection is still not yet clear, but these findings suggest the involvement of putative downstream target(s) responding to *Wld*^{S} expression in cell soma. Moreover, *Wld*^{S} phenotype shows a substantial resistance to microtubule depolymerizing drugs (Wang et al., 2000; Ikegami and Koike, 2003), suggesting that this system provides a model to examine the correlation between axon stability and microtubule acetylation.

2.3 Involvement of SIRT2 in axon stability

2.3.1 Evidence for SIRT2 involvement in the axon stability in the *Wlds* model

Based on our preliminary finding on the presence of SIRT2 in cerebellar granule neurons (CGNs), we have put forward our hypothesis that SIRT2 may be involved in microtubule stability by regulating the level of tubulin acetylation. If our hypothesis is correct, the level of acetylated alpha-tubulin of CGN axons from *Wld^S* mice should be higher than those from wild-type mice, and lowering the levels should ameliorate the resistance of these mutant axons to degenerative stimuli including colchicine. Westernblot analysis showed that the basal levels of both acetyl microtubule and acetyl alpha-tubulin were indeed higher in cultured CGNs from *Wld^S* mice than those from wild-type mice (Suzuki, 2007; Suzuki and Koike, 2007a). This is also the case for in vivo; Fig. 2 shows that the level of acetylated alpha-tubulin per total alpha-tubulin is significantly higher in the *Wld^S* cerebellum compared to the wild-type cerebellum at postnatal 21 days (P21).

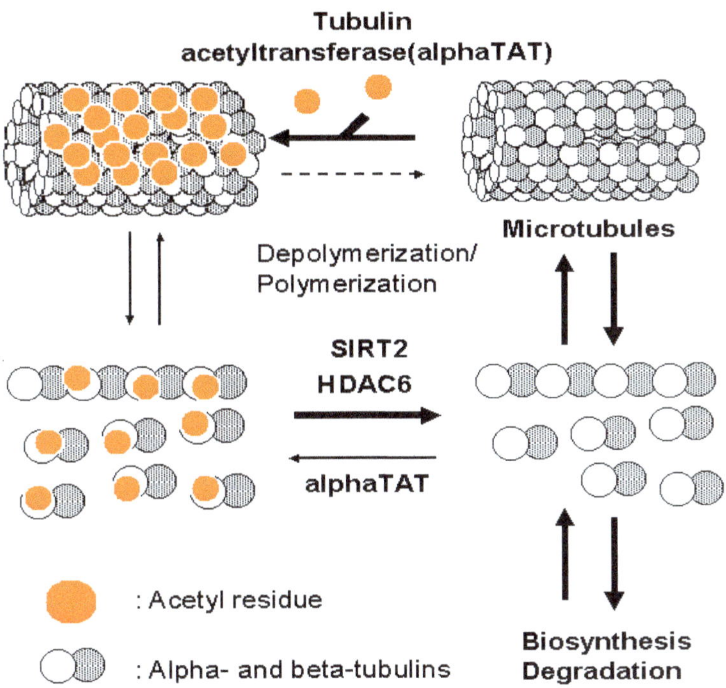

Fig. 1. Acetylation and microtubule dynamics of assembly and disassembly. Microtubules, whose building block is a heterodimer of alpha- and beta- tubulins, are in a dynamic equilibrium of assembly and disassembly. Major acetylation site is at Lys40 of alpha-tubulin. Both microtubles and tublins may serve as the substrate for acetyltransferase (Maruta et al., 1986). Both SIRT2 (North et al., 2003) and histone deacetylase 6 (HDAC6) (Hubbert et al., 2002; Matsuyama, 2002) are known to catalyze the deacetylation of acetylated alpha-tubulin. The level of acetylation will be regulated by a balance of tubulin acetyltransferase and tubulin deacetylase activities.

To further test our hypothesis, CGNs from *Wld^S* mice were transfected with the expression vector for GFP or GFP-*sirt2*, and then immunostained with anti-acetylated alpha-tubulin (Suzuki, 2007; Suzuki and Koike, 2007a). The proximal region of the axons was clearly stained in CGNs expressing GFP alone, consistent with the previous reports (Baas and Black, 1990; Shea, 1999), whereas it was markedly reduced in those expressing active GFP-

SIRT2. The results suggest that SIRT2 overexpression is sufficient to substantially reduce the hyperacetylation of CGN axons from *Wld^S* mice. Morphologically, changes in the number and length of CGN axons expressing GFP or GFP-*sirt2* were measured overtime after treatment with colchicine: 50% of axons per GFP-positive CGNs from *Wld^S* mice still remained alive, whereas in *Wld^S* CGNs expressing active *sirt2*, only 10% of axons per GFP-positive cell remained alive at 24 h after colchicine treatment. These results clearly indicate that SIRT2 overexpression downregulated the elevated level of tubulin aceylation and amiliorated the resistance of CGN axons from *Wld^S* mice to the degenerative stimulus (Suzuki and Koike, 2007a).

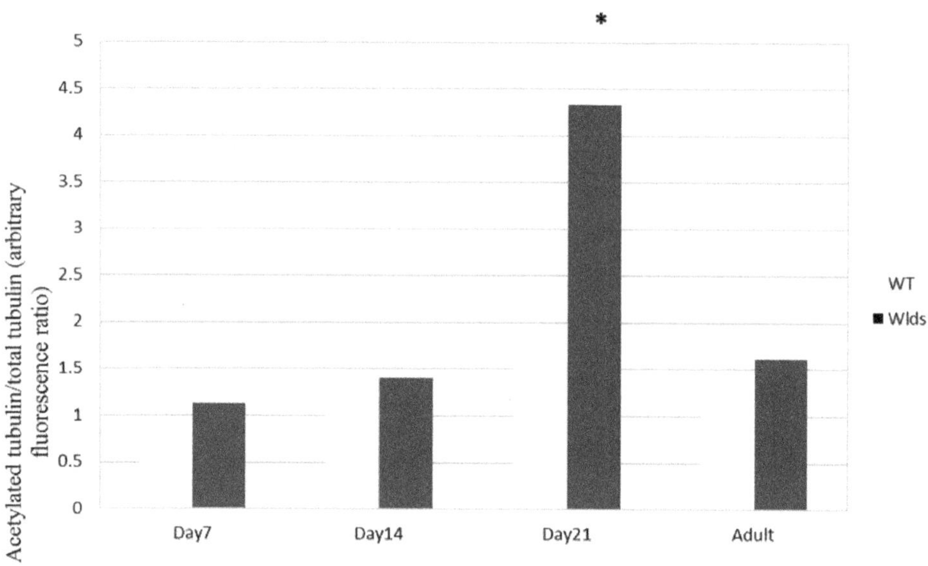

Fig. 2. The level of alpha-tubulin acetylation in the molecular layer of the cerebellum from wild-type (WT) and Wld^S mice during postnatal development. Details of the procedures are previously described (Suzuki and Koike, 2007a). Staining intensities on the sections were measured by using Scion Image software. Relative intensities of total and acetylated alpha-tubulins were calculated by normalizing staining intensities of total and acetylated alpha-tubulins to those of phalloidin, respectively. Tubulin acetylation was determined as a ratio of the intensities of acetylated alpha-tubulin to those of total alpha-tubulin in adjacent sections. The data are shown as mean ± S.D. (n = 3 animals). Statistical significance was detected by Student's t-test (*$p < 0.05$ between groups at wild-type and Wld^S). Data from Suzuki (2007).

2.3.2 Functional correlate between SIRT2 levels and axon resistance against degenerative stimuli

If microtubule hyperacetylation is involved in acquiring resistance of CGN axons from mutant mice to degenerative stimuli, then similar resistance would be attainable for wild-type CGN axons by the use of SIRT2 inhibitors or *sirt2* silencing technology. By exposing wild-type CGNs from wild-type mice to nicotinamide, the inhibitor of SIRT2, prior to colchicine application, we obtained evidence for enhanced tubulin acetylation and increased resistance to colchicine (Suzuki and Koike, 2007a). Immunoblot analysis shows that the level of alpha-tubulin acetylation increased following treatment with nicotinamide in a concentration- and time-dependent manner (Suzuki, 2007). However, treatment with 3-aminobenzamide(3-AB), an inhibitor for PARP, failed to elevate the level, suggesting that the effect of nicotinamide on tubulin deacetylation is mediated by SIRT2 but not by PARP. On the other hand, trichostatin A (TSA), a specific inhibitor for HDAC6 tubulin deacetylase (Matsuyama et al., 2002), failed to enhance tubulin acetylation. Morphologically, more than 70% of axons were viable, whereas 90% of cell somata were dead when CGNs were treated with 10 mM nicotinamide and then with colchicine for a further 24h. However, it should be noted that nicotinamide was neuroprotective only after its exposure to CGNs for more than 2 days, and that this agent elevated the level of alpha-tubulin acetylation, but not the level of microtubule acetylation.

To eliminate the possibility that nicotinamide acted through other pathways, CGNs were transfected with a lentiviral vector expressing SIRT2 small interfering RNA (siRNA). SIRT2 silencing indeed caused an increase in the level of acetylated alpha-tubulin (Fig. 3). Morphologically, more than 50 % of axons were viable as revealed by calcein-AM staining, whereas more than 90% of cell bodies were dead as revealed by PI staining, after colchicine treatment for 48hr (Suzuki, 2007). These results show that CGN axons form wild-type mice acquired resistance to degenerative stimuli by downregulating *sirt2* expression.

2.3.3 Resveratrol-mediated modulation of axon degeneration

Resveratrol, a natural polyphenol, shows a wide range of interesting biological and pharmacological activities. Besides acting as a general inhibitor against oxidative stress, this agent is known to activate SIRT1, thus providing a potential effect for longevity (Fulda and Debatin, 2006; Buer, 2010 for review). To asses the effect of resveratrol on SIRT2 HEK293 cells were transfected with GFP alone, active GFP-SIRT2, or GFP-SIRT2 N168A, a catalytically inactive mutant (North et al., 2003), and then the cellular lysates were immunoprecipitated by anti-GFP antibody. The resultant immunoprecipitates were used as SIRT2 enzymes for tubulin deacetylation assay. We found that resveratrol decreased the level of acetylated alpha-tubulin in the immunoprecipitates from CGNs transfected with active GFP-SIRT2, but not inactive GFP-SIRT2 or GFP alone, suggesting that resveratrol indeed activates SIRT2 (Suzuki, 2007).

Westernblot analysis showed that resveratrol decreased the level of acetylated alpha-tubulin in the CGN lysates from wild-type mice in a time- and dose-dependent manner (Suzuki, 2007; Suzuki and Koike, 2007b). Moreover, resveratrol decreased the level of tubulin acetylation, and, as a result, reduced the resistance of CGN axons from *Wld^S* mice to the degenerative stimulus. The effect of resveratrol on cell body degeneration appeared to be minimal, which is consistent with the previous report (De Ruvo et al., 2000). These results suggest that resveratrol amiliorated the resistance of CGN axons from *Wld^S* mice to colchicine by enhancing tubulin deacetylation. However, it should be noted that resveratrol was neuroprotective after its treatment for more than 2days, suggesting that it may acts indirectly on SIRT2 or other targets including nuclear transcriptional factors that regulate the expression of a variety of genes (Fulda and Debatin, 2006).

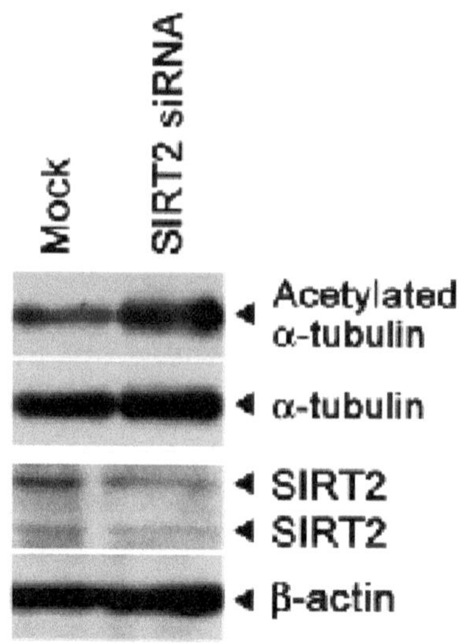

Fig. 3. The enhancement of the level of acetylated alpha-tubulin in wild-type CGNs by silencing of *sirt2*. CGNs from wild-type mice were mock infected or infected with lentivirus expressing SIRT2 siRNA at 1 moi, and cultured for a further 48 h. Five micrograms of total proteins from the cytoskeletal fraction (microtubules fraction) of both cultures were applied on a gel, and analyzed by immunoblotting with anti-acetylated alpha-tubulin antibody. Equal loading was confirmed by reprobing the same blot with anti-alpha-tubulin antibody (upper 2 blots). For immunoblotting with anti-SIRT2 antibody, twenty micrograms of total proteins from the total cellular fraction were analyzed. Equal loading was confirmed by the same blot with anti-beta-actin antibody (lower 2 blots). Each experiment was repeated three times with similar results. Note that both long (43kDa) and short (39kDa) forms of the SIRT2 proteins are detected. Data from Suzuki (2007).

3. Evidence for neuronal distribution of acetyl alpha-tubulin and SIRT2: An immunoreactivity study during postnatal development of mouse cerebellum

In the mouse brain, the expression of alpha-tubulin is high during early postnatal days, and subsequently decrease upon maturation (Burgoyne and Cambray-Deakin, 1988), whereas tubulin acetylation in vivo is known to occur concomitantly with maturation (Black and Keyser, 1987), indicative of its association with microtubule stability (Westermann and Weber, 2003). Immunohistochemistry using the monoclonal antibody specific for acetylated alpha-tubulin showed intense particulate staining in the molecular layer of postnatally developing and adult mouse cerebellum (Suzuki, 2007; Kawahara, 2007). Bergmann glial fibers and Purkinje cell dendrites were not stained, whereas Purkinje cell bodies were intensely stained in developing mouse cerebellum (Suzuki, 2007; Kawahara, 2007), consistent with the previous findings (Cambray-Deakin and Burgoyne, 1987). During postnatal development the external granular layer becomes thinner, while the molecular layer becomes enlarged (Burgoyne and Cambray-Deakin, 1988). Along with this, intense staining was observed in the molecular layer from wild-type and *Wld*^{S} mice. The level of microtubule acetylation in *Wld*^{S} cerebellum was increased at P14-21 (Suzuki, 2007; Kawahara, 2007), which corresponds to the stage when granule cells migrate into the internal granule layer (IGL) along extending parallel fiber axons, and form short dendrites (Burgoyne and Cambray-Deakin, 1988). These findings suggest that microtubule acetylation occurs in a manner that depends on developmental stages. In vitro, Wallerian degeneration of transected axons is further delayed by extending culture period of time prior to axotomy in cerebellar explant cultures from Wld^S mice (Buckmaster et al., 1995).

Fig. 4 shows the immunostaining patterns of SIRT2 of wild-type and *Wld*^{S} mouse cerebella during development; intense immunostaining was observed in the EGL, the IGL and the Purkinje cell layer at P1, and the EGL and the Purkinje cell layer at P7, and then gradually declined in both cerebella, although the intensity was lower in the *Wld*^{S} cerebellum. At P21 and, to a lesser extent, in adult, clear and distinct staining was observed for the Purkinje cell layer. Fig. 4 clearly shows that SIRT2 immunoreactivity is localized in the cytoplasm of Purkinje cells; though less clearly, the staining of CGNs were rather uniform. In the molecular layer of both adult wild-type and *Wld*^{S} cerebella immunostaining was far less intense, consistent with the recent report (Li et al., 2007). Our findings clearly show that both CGNs and Purkinje neurons are positively stained with the antibodies against SIRT2 at the critical period of time when these neurons are undergoing differentiation and migration (Suzuki and Koike, 1997; Powell et al., 1997). SIRT2 immostaining clearly showed the localization of SIRT2 in developing CGNs and Purkinje neurons in contrast to the previous finding on its distribution in non-neuronal cells. Recent study has revealed a widespread distribution of SIRT2 in CNS neurons (Maxsell et al., 2011).

4. Possible roles of SIRT2 in neurodegeneration

4.1 Acetylated alpha-tubulin as a marker of stable microtubules

We have showed that alpha-tubulins and microtubules are hyperacetylated in CGNs from wld^s mutant mice, and the resistance of these CGN axons to degenerative stimuli is ameliorated by downregulating the level of acetylation by multiple methods including silencing of *sirt2*. Similarly, CGN axons from wild-type mice acquired resistance to colchicine by *sirt2* silencing, which was associated with reduced levels of tubulin deacetylation, but not enhanced levels of microtubule acetylation. The reason for this is unclear, since both acetylated and non-acetylated alpha-tubulins are known to be a good substrate for tubulin acetylatransferase in vitro. It is likely that the degeneration pathway may play a role in the regulation of axon stability given the fact that deacetylated tublin is rapidly degradated (Black et al., 1989; Ren et al., 2003) as shown in Fig. 5, and therefore, if this step is blocked, acetylated microtubules are metabolically stabilized (but not accumulated). Consistently, the level of acetylated alpha-tubulin is a signal for fine-tuning microtubule dynamics by modulating alpha-tubulin turnover (Solinger et. al., 2010). It has been shown that microtubules were stabilized and the level of acetylated alpha-tubulin was elevated in the cells transfected with microtubule-associated proteins tau or other associated proteins (Takemura et al., 1998), suggesting these microtubule associated proteins influence microtubule stability by modulating tubulin acetylase activities; Fig. 5 shows that the association of alpha-tubulin with tau stabilizes microtubules via a yet unknown mechanism.

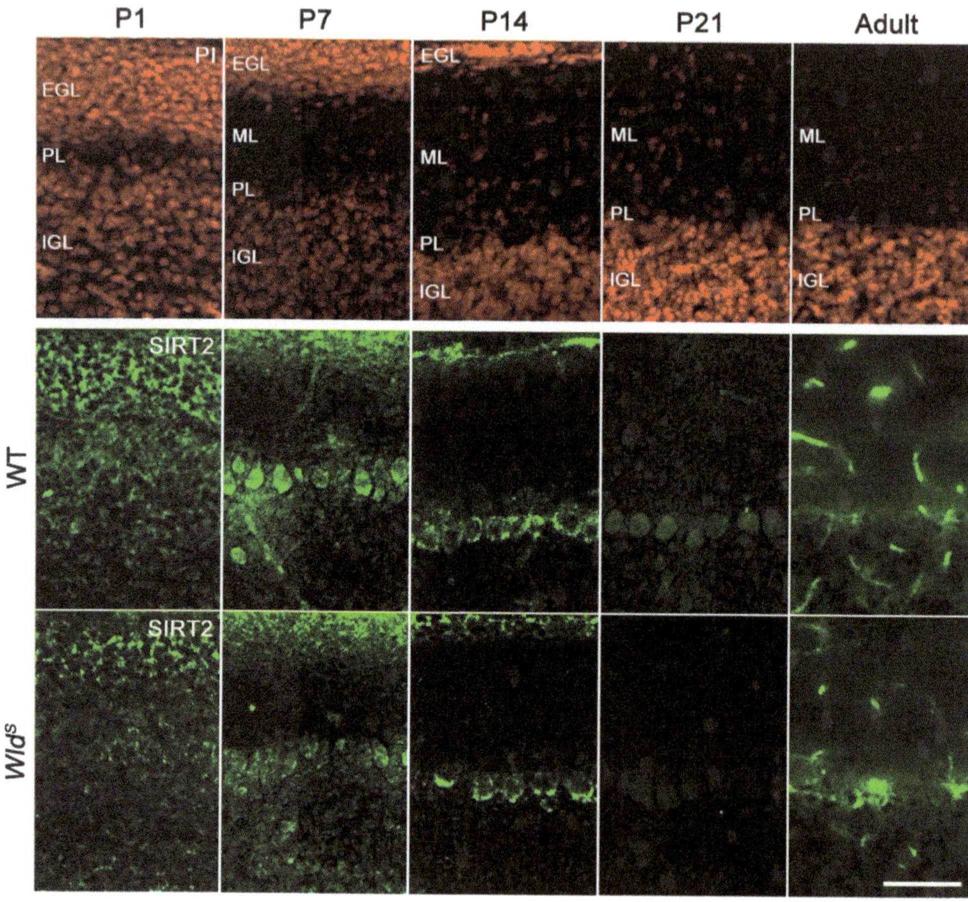

Fig. 4. Immunohistochemical staining patterns of SIRT2 during postnatal development of the cerebellum from wild-type and WldS mutant mice. Coronal crysections from cerebella from each mouse were immunostained with anti-SIRT2 antibody (green). As a reference, nuclear stainings with PI (red) in wild-type cerebellum are shown. Details of this method have been described (Suzuki and Koike, 2007a). Note that oligodendrosites are intensely stained in the adult cerebellum (Li et al., 2007). EGL, the external granular layer; ML, the molecular layer; PL, the Purkinje cell layer; the IGL, internal granular layer. Scale bar represents 25 microm. Data from Suzuki (2007) and Kawahara (2007).

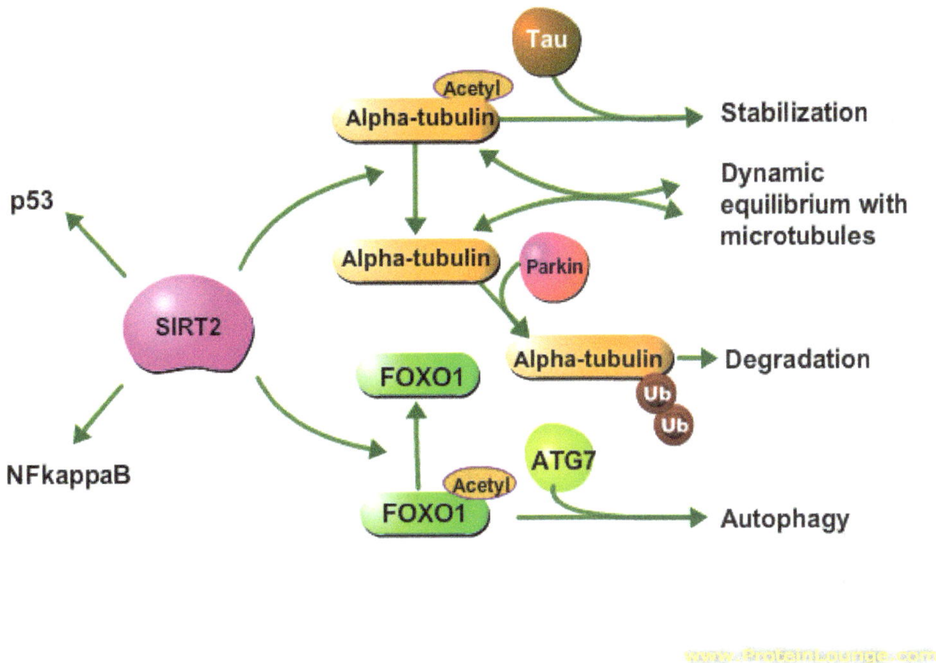

Fig. 5. SIRT2 targets and its functions. Targets of SIRT2 include a number of transcription factors including p.53, p.300, 14-3-3, p.65, Foxo's, NFkappaB, SREBP-2 and others, only two of which are shown in this figure. Besides these transcription factors, SIRT2 is known to act on FOXO1 and tubulins. FOXO-1 in the cytoplasm plays a crucial role in autophagic mechanisms, although its neuronal distribution is not currently available. Alpha-tubulin is shown to bind to Parkin, and is thereby ubiquitinated and quickly degradated. On the other hand, acetylated-tubulin is able to bind to tau and is involved in microtubule stabilization. The plus ends of Microtubules are in a dynamic equilibrium of assembly and disassembly and their minus ends with extensive acetylation and association with tau are relatively stable.

4.2 Multiforms of SIRT2

Previous reports have shown that SIRT2 is localized mainly in the cytoplasm (North et al., 2003; Dryden et al., 2003). For CGNs, SIRT2 immunoreactivity was observed throughout the cells. Westernblot analysis shows two different isoforms of SIRT2 proteins. Interestingly, the long isoform (43 kDa) was barely detectable in the cytoplasmic fraction in both WT and *Wld*^{S} granule cells (Suzuki, 2007). The short form (39 kDa) lacks the corresponding N-terminal 37 amino acids in the long isoform (Voelter-Mahlknecht et al., 2005) and may be located in the cytoplasm and the nucleus. Recent study shows that there is a *sirt2* transcript expressed preferentially in aging CNS (Maxsell et al., 2011). Further experiments should be needed to delineate the precise roles of these nuclear, cytoplasmic, age-specific forms of the *Sirt2* transcripts.

4.3 Degradation pathways of SIRT2

Dryden et al. (2003) reported that SIRT2 is dephosphorylated by the phosphatase CDC14B and then degradated via the ubiquitin-proteasome pathway. This finding suggests that the level of SIRT2 proteins could be regulated by phosphorylation in the nucleus where this phosphatase is located, and ubiquitination in the cytoplasm. CDC14B overexpression promotes microtubule acetylation and stabilization, indicative of the involvement of the nucleo-cytoplasmic shuttling in the degadation pathway of SIRT2 (Cho et al., 2005). Parkin, an ubiquitin E3 ligase linked to Parkinson's disease, is also shown to bind to alpha- and beta-tubulins and enhance their ubiquitination and degradation (Ren et al., 2003)(Fig. 5). Regulation by phosphorylation has also been shown for HDAC6, another tubulin deacetylase.

Recently, researchers have shown that FOXO (Forkhead box, class O) transcription factors are clearly involved in the degradation pathway in a number of important ways. SIRT2 facilitates FOXO3 deacetylation, promotes its ubiquitination and subsequent proteosomal degradation (Wang et al., 2011). Fig. 5 shows various targets of SIRT2 in which there are number of transcription factors. including NFkappaB (Rothgieser at al., 2010). On the other hand, cytosolic FOXO1 acts independently of its capability as being a transcription factor and is shown to be essential for the induction of autophagy in response to stress (Zhao et al., 2010). Fig. 5 shows that FOXO1 is acetylated by dissociation from SIRT2, and the acetylated FOXO1 forms a complex with Atg7, an E1-like protein, in the autophagy signaling pathway (Zhao et al., 2010). As shown previously, autophagic degradation processes play a key role in the survival and degeneration of axons and dendrites (Koike et al., 2008).

4.4 SIRT2 versus HDAC6

SIRT2 is shown to be localized in the proximal region of CGN axons (Suzuki, 2007), whereas HDAC6 tubulin deacetylate distributes in the distal region of axons of Hipocampal neurons (Black et al., 1998), suggesting each tubulin acetylase may have different regulatory roles in microtubule stability and the protein-protein interaction along axons. Previous studies have shown that HDAC6 inhibition or suppression regulates the interaction of ankyrinG or similar axonal domain-interacting proteins with voltage gated sodium channels that diffuse along the axon (Black et al., 1998). Thus, the distribution of SIRT2 in the proximal region of the axon and its absence from the distal region of the axon may regulate the formation of different microtubules domains in the axon. HDAC6 regulated activity at the distal axon can promote axonal growth (Tapia et al., 2010), while microtubules at the proximal region of the axon can be more acetylated and allow the maintenance of the axon initial segment, necessary for polarized axonal transport, tethering of ankyrin proteins and generation of neuronal action potentials. It is interesting to point out that both the protein-protein interactions along axons and the protein degradation pathway are regulated through the acetylation/deacetylation pathway. Therefore, its switching is a key event for the regulation of microtubule degradation and hence stability of various axonal domains. Further experiments will be necessary to understand how SIRT2 or HDAC6 deacetylase activities are locally regulated and involved in the axon stability and degeneration.

5. Conclusion & future issues

SIRT2, a NAD-dependent protein deacetylase, is mostly localized in the cytoplasm and regulates post-translational modifications of proteins such as microtubules via tubulin deacetylation. We have shown evidence that SIRT2 could modulate hyperacetylation of alpha-tubulin in cerebellar granule axons and thereby abrogate their resistance to degenerative stimuli in a mutant mouse strain where axon degeneration, but not cell somal death, is markedly delayed. We have provided evidence for its functional involvement in axon stability, and discuss some of recent findings, highlighting the emergence of SIRT2 as a novel regulator of neuronal degeneration and plasticity.

Recently, the suppression of SIRT2 effectively ameliorates neurotoxicity in a variety of neuronal disease models including Drosophila model of Huntington disease (Pallos et al., 2008), mutant huntingtin neurotoxicity (Luthi-Cortea et al., 2010), alpha-synuclein-mediated toxicity in models of Parkinson's disease (Outeiro et al., 2007). It has been proposed that the SIRT2 inhibitors or SIRT2 suppression may function by promoting the formation of enlarged inclusion bodies, and thereby provide neuroprotection. Nicotinamide is also shown to increase the level of acetylated alpha-tubulin, tau stability, and restore memory loss in a transgenic mouse model of Alzheimer's disease (Green et al., 2008). The mechanisms of neuroprotection found in these disease models are still unknown. These findings should be discussed in the light of the functional diversity of SIRT2 subtypes and their localization in axonal domains.

6. References

Araki T., Sasaki Y., and Milbrandt J. (2004) Increased nuclear NAD biosynthesis and SIRT1 activation prevent axonal degeneration. Science 305, 1010-1013.

Baas P.W., and Black M.M. (1990) Individual microtubules in the axon consist of domains that differ in both composition and stability. J. Cell Biol. 111, 495-509.

Baur JA.(2010) Biochemical effects of SIRT1 activators. Biochim Bio phys Acts. 1804:1626-1634.

Black M.M., Baas P.W., and Humphrey S. (1989) Dynamics of alpha-tubulin deacetylation in intact neurons. J. Neuroscience. 9, 358-368.

Black M.M., and Greene L.A. (1982) Changes in the colchicine susceptibility of microtubules associated with neurite outgrowth: studies with nerve growth factor-responsive PC12 pheochromocytoma cells. J. Cell Biol. 95, 379-386.

Black M.M., and Keyser P. (1987) Acetylation of alpha-tubulin in cultured neurons and the induction of alpha-tubulin acetylation in PC12 cells by treatment with nerve growth factor. J. Neurosci. 7, 1833-1842.

Buckmaster E.A., Perry V.H., and Brown M.C. (1995) The rate of Wallerian degeneration in cultured neurons from wild type and C57BL/WldS mice depends on time in culture and may be extended in the presence of elevated K^+ levels. Eur. J. Neurosci. 7, 1596-1602.

Burgoyne R.D., and Cambray-Deakin M.A. (1988) The cellular neurobiology of neuronal development: the cerebellar granule cell. Brain Res. 472, 77-101.

Cambray-Deakin M.A., and Burgoyne R.D. (1987) Posttranslational modifications of alpha-tubulin: acetylated and detyrosinated forms in axons of rat cerebellum. J. Cell Biol. 104, 1569-1574.

Cho H.P., Liu Y., Gomez M., Dunlap J., Tyers M., and Wang Y. (2005) The dual-specificity phosphatase CDC14B bundles and stabilizes microtubules. Mol. Cell Biol. 25, 4541-4551.

Coleman M. (2005) Axon degeneration mechanisms: commonality and diversity. Nat. Rev. Neurosci. 6, 889-898.

Conforti L., Tarlton A., Mack T.G., Mi W., Buckmaster E.A., Wagner D., Perry V.H., and Coleman M.P. (2000) A Ufd2/D4Cole1e chimeric protein and overexpression of Rbp7 in the slow Wallerian degeneration (WldS) mouse. Proc. Natl Acad. Sci. USA 97, 11377-11382.

De Ruvo C., Amodio R., Algeri S., Martelli N., Intilangelo A., D'Ancona G.M., Esposito E. (2000) Nutritional antioxidants as antidegenerative agents. Int. J. Dev. Neurosci. 18, 359-366.

Dryden S.C., Nahhas F.A., Nowak J.E., Goustin A.S., and Tainsky M.A. (2003) Role for human SIRT2 NAD-dependent deacetylase activity in control of mitotic exit in the cell cycle. Mol. Cell Biol. 23, 3173-3185.

Fulda S., and Debatin K.M. (2006) Resveratrol modulation of signal transduction in apoptosis and cell survival: a mini-review. Cancer Detect. Prev. 30, 217-223.

Gan L and Mucke L (2008) Paths of convergence: Sirtuins in aging and neurodegeneration. Neuron 58:10-14.

Green KN, Steffan JS, Martinez-Coria H, Sun X, Schreiber SS, Thompson LM, LaFerla FM. (2008) Nicotinamide restores cognition in Alzheimer's disease transgenic mice via a mechanism involving sirtuin inhibition and selective reduction of Thr231-phosphotau.Neurosci. 28:11500-10.

Horton A.C., and Ehlers M.D. (2003) Neuronal polarity and trafficking. Neuron 40, 277-295.

Hubbert C., Guardiola A., Shao R., Kawaguchi Y., Ito A., Nixon A., Yoshida M., Wang X.F., and Yao T.P. (2002) HDAC6 is a microtubule-associated deacetylase. Nature 417, 455-458.

Ikegami K., and Koike T. (2003) Non-apoptotic neurite degeneration in apoptotic neuronal death: pivotal role of mitochondrial function in neurites. Neuroscience 122, 617-626

Inoue T., Hiratsuka M., Osaki M., Yamada H., Kishimoto I., Yamaguchi S., Nakano S., Katoh M., Ito H., and Oshimura M. (2007) SIRT2, a tubulin deacetylase, acts to block the entry to chromosome condensation in response to mitotic stress. Oncogene 26, 945-957.

Ji S, Doucette JR, Nazarali AJ.(2011) Sirt2 is a novel in vivo downstream target of Nkx2.2 and enhances oligodendroglial cell differentiation. J Mol Cell Biol., 3:351-359

Kawahara T (2007) Immunohistochemical study of tubulin acetylation during cerebellar development: comparison between wild-typw and Wlds mutant mouse. Dissertation for a BA, Hokkaido University, p.1-16.

Koike T, Yang Y, Suzuki K, Zheng X. (2008) Axon & dendrite degeneration: its mechanisms and protective experimental paradigms. Neurochem Int. 52:751-760.

Laurent M., and Fleury A. (1996) Hysteretic behavior and differential apparent stability properties of microtubule species emerge from the regulation of post-translational modifications of microtubules. J. Cell Sci. 109, 419-428.

Li W., Zhang B., Tang J., Cao Q., Wu Y., Wu C., Guo J., Ling E.A., and Liang F. (2007) Sirtuin 2, a mammalian homolog of yeast silent information regulator-2 longevity regulator, is an oligodendroglial protein that decelerates cell differentiation through deacetylating alpha-tubulin. J. Neurosci. 27, 2606-2616.

Lunn E.R., Perry V.H., Brown M.C., Rosen H., and Gordon S. (1989) Absence of Wallerian degeneration does not hinder regeneration in peripheral nerve. Eur. J. Neurosci. 1, 27-33.

Luthi-Carter R, Taylor DM, Pallos J, Lambert E, Amore A, Parker A, Moffitt H, Smith DL, Runne H, Gokce O, Kuhn A, Xiang Z, Maxwell MM, Reeves SA, Bates GP, Neri C, Thompson LM, Marsh JL, Kazantsev AG.(2010) SIRT2 inhibition achieves neuroprotection by decreasing sterol biosynthesis. Proc Natl Acad Sci U S A. 107, 7927-7932.

Mack T.G., Reiner M., Beirowski B. Mi W., Emanuelli M., Wagner D., Thomson D., Gillingwater T., Court F., Conforti L., Fernando F.S., Tarlton A., Andressen C., Addicks K., Magni G., Ribchester R.R., Perry V.H., and Coleman M.P. (2001) Wallerian degeneration of injured axons and synapses is delayed by a Ube4b/Nmnat chimeric gene. Nat. Neurosci. 4, 1199-1206.

MacRae T.H. (1997) Tubulin post-translational modifications - enzymes and their mechanisms of action. Eur. J. Biochem. 244, 265-278.

Maruta H., Greer K., and Rosenbaum J.L. (1986) The acetylation of alpha-tubulin and its relationship to the assembly and disassembly of microtubules. J. Cell Biol. 103, 571-579.

Matsuyama A., Shimazu T., Sumida Y., Saito A., Yoshimatsu Y., Seigneurin-Berny D., Osada H., Komatsu Y., Nishino N., Khochbin S., Horinouchi S., and Yoshida M. (2002) In vivo destabilization of dynamic microtubules by HDAC6-mediated deacetylation. EMBO J. 21, 6820-6831.

Maxwell MM, Tomkinson EM, Nobles J, Wizeman JW, Amore AM, Quinti L, Chopra V, Hersch SM, Kazantsev AG (2011) The Sirtuin 2 microtubule deacetylase is an abundant neuronal protein that accumulates in the aging CNS. Hum Mol Genet. 20, 3986-3996.

Nakagawa T and Guarente L (2011) Sirtuins at glance. J Cell Sci124,833-838

North B.J., Marshall B.L., Borra M.T., Denu J.M., and Verdin E. (2003) The human Sir2 ortholog, SIRT2, is an NAD^+-dependent tubulin deacetylase. Mol. Cell 11, 437-444.

Outeiro TF, Kontopoulos E, Altmann SM, Kufareva I, Strathearn KE, Amore AM, Volk CB, Maxwell MM, Rochet JC, McLean PJ, Young AB, Abagyan R, Feany MB, Hyman BT, Kazantsev AG.(2007) Sirtuin 2 inhibitors rescue alpha-synuclein-mediated toxicity in models of Parkinson's disease. Science 317, 516-519.

Pallos J, Bodai L, Lukacsovich T, Purcell JM, Steffan JS, Thompson LM, Marsh JL. (2008) Inhibition of specific HDACs and sirtuins suppresses pathogenesis in a Drosophila model of Huntington's disease. Hum Mol Genet. 17, 3767-3775.

Powell S.K., Rivas R.J., Rodriguez-Boulan E., and Hatten M.E. (1997) Development of polarity in cerebellar granule neurons. J. Neurobiol. 32, 223-236.

Ren Y., Zhao J., and Feng J. (2003) Parkin binds to alpha/beta tubulin and increases their ubiquitination and degradation. J. Neurosci. 23, 3316-3324.

Rothgiesser KM, Erener S, Waibel S, Lüscher B, Hottiger MO.(2010)SIRT2 regulates NF-κB dependent gene expression through deacetylation of p65 Lys310. J Cell Sci. 123, 4251-4258.

Sasaki Y., Araki T., and Milbrandt J. (2006) Stimulation of nicotinamide adenine dinucleotide biosynthetic pathways delays axonal degeneration after axotomy. J. Neurosci. 26, 8484-8491.

Shea T.B. (1999) Selective stabilization of microtubules within the proximal region of developing axonal neurites. Brain Res. Bull. 48, 255-261.

Solinger JA, Paolinelli R, Klöss H, Scorza FB, Marchesi S, Sauder U, Mitsushima D, Capuani F, Stürzenbaum SR, Cassata G. (2010) The Caenorhabditis elegans Elongator complex regulates neuronal alpha-tubulin acetylation. PLoS Genet. 6(1):e1000820.

Suzuki K (2007) The role of microtubule acetylation in resistance to axon degeneration. Dissertation for a Ph.D., Hokkaido University, p.1-95.

Suzuki K., and Koike T. (1997) Brain-derived neurotrophic factor suppresses programmed death of cerebellar granule cells through a posttranslational mechanism. Mol. Chem. Neuropathol. 30, 101-124.

Suzuki K., and Koike T. (2007a) SIRT2-mediated modulation of resistance to axonal degeneration in slow Wallerian degeneration (WldS) mice: a crucial role of tubulin deacetylation. Neuroscience147, 599-612.

Suzuki K., and Koike T. (2007b) Resveratrol abolishes resistance to axonal degeneration in slow Wallerian degeneration (WldS) mice: activation of SIRT2, an NAD-dependent tubulin deacetylase. Biochem. Biophys. Res. Commun.359:665-671

Takemura R., Okabe S., Umeyama T., Kanai Y., Cowan N.J., and Hirokawa N. (1992) Increased microtubule stability and alpha tubulin acetylation in cells transfected with microtubule-associated proteins MAP1B, MAP2 or tau. J. Cell Sci. 103, 953-964.

Tapia M, Wandosell F, Garrido JJ.(2010) Impaired function of HDAC6 slows down axonal growth and interferes with axon initial segment development. PLoS One. 5(9):e12908

Voelter-Mahlknecht S., Ho A.D., and Mahlknecht U. (2005) FISH-mapping and genomic organization of the NAD-dependent histone deacetylase gene, Sirtuin 2 (Sirt2). Int. J. Oncol. 27, 1187-1196.

Wang F, Chan CH, Chen K, Guan X, Lin HK, Tong Q. (2011) Deacetylation of FOXO3 by SIRT1 or SIRT2 leads to Skp2-mediated FOXO3 ubiquitination and degradation. Oncogene. Doi:10.1038/onc.2011.347.

Wang J., Zhai Q., Chenhg Y., Lin E., Gu W., McBurney M.W., and He Z. (2005) A local mechanism mediates NAD-dependent protection of axon degeneration. J. Cell Biol. 170, 349-355.

Wang M., Wu Y., Culver D.G., and Glass J.D. (2000) Pathogenesis of axonal degeneration: parallels between Wallerian degeneration and vincristine neuropathy. J. Neuropathol. Exp. Neurol. 59, 599-606.

Westermann S., and Weber K. (2003) Post-translational modifications regulate microtubule function. Nat. Rev. Mol. Cell Biol. 4, 938-947.

Zhao Y, Yang J, Liao W, Liu X, Zhang H, Wang S, Wang D, Feng J, Yu L, Zhu WG. (2010) Cytosolic FoxO1 is essential for the induction of autophagy and tumour suppressor activity. Nat Cell Biol. 12, 665-675.

2

Neuroprotective Effects of Neuropeptide Y and Y2 and Y5 Receptor Agonists *In Vitro* and *In Vivo*

Maria Śmialowska and Helena Domin
Institute of Pharmacology, Department of Neurobiology, Polish Academy of Sciences, Krakow, Poland

1. Introduction

Neuropeptide Y (NPY) is a 36 amino acid peptide, widely distributed in the nervous system where it plays the role of a neurotransmitter and neuromodulator (Chronwall et al., 1985; Gray & Morley, 1986). It belongs to the pancreatic polypeptide family (PP family) together with peptide YY (PYY) and pancreatic polypeptide (PP), which are mainly gut and endocrine regulatory peptides (Tatemoto et al., 1982). All these peptides have a common hairpin-like tertiary structure, consisting of an N-terminal poly-proline helix and a long alpha-helix connected by a beta turn (Allen et al., 1987; Glower et al., 1984). NPY contains 5 tyrosine residues in its primary structure, (Fig.1) therefore, it is named neuropeptide Y or neuropeptide tyrosine, as "Y" is an abbreviation of tyrosine.

Tyr^{1}-Pro-Ser-Lys-Pro-Asp-Asn-Pro-Gly-Glu^{10}-Asp-Ala-Pro-Ala-Glu-Asp-Met-Ala-Arg-**Tyr**^{20}-

Tyr-Ser-Ala-Leu-Arg-His-**Tyr**-Ile-Asn-Leu^{30}-Ile-Thr-Arg-Gln-Arg-**Tyr**^{36}-NH_2

Fig. 1. Primary structure of NPY (human, rat).

NPY is present in the central and peripheral neurons and is described as one of the most abundant peptides in the brain (Chronwall, 1989). In the brainstem, it often coexists with noradrenaline (NA) and adrenaline (A) in some projecting catecholaminergic neurons, and with serotonin in human and rabbit, (but not rat) medullary neurons (Everitt & Hökfelt, 1989). In the forebrain NPY is present mainly in local inhibitory interneurons, where it coexists with GABA and often with somatostatin (Everitt & Hökfelt, 1989). Besides the central nervous system (CNS), NPY occurs also in the periphery: in chromaffin cells of the adrenal medulla (coexisting with A and NA), in sympathetic neurons (coexisting with NA) and in some (few) parasympathetic neurons. NPY was also found in blood cells, spleen, bone marrow, magakaryocytes and thrombocytes (Ericsson et al., 1987; Persson et al., 1989).

NPY is involved in many physiological functions, such as: regulation of blood pressure (in the periphery NPY is a potent vasoconstrictor), cardiorespiratory parameters and body temperature, control of the release of luteinizing hormone releasing hormone (LHRH) and corticotropin releasing factor (CRF), and modulation of feeding, sexual behavior, pain,

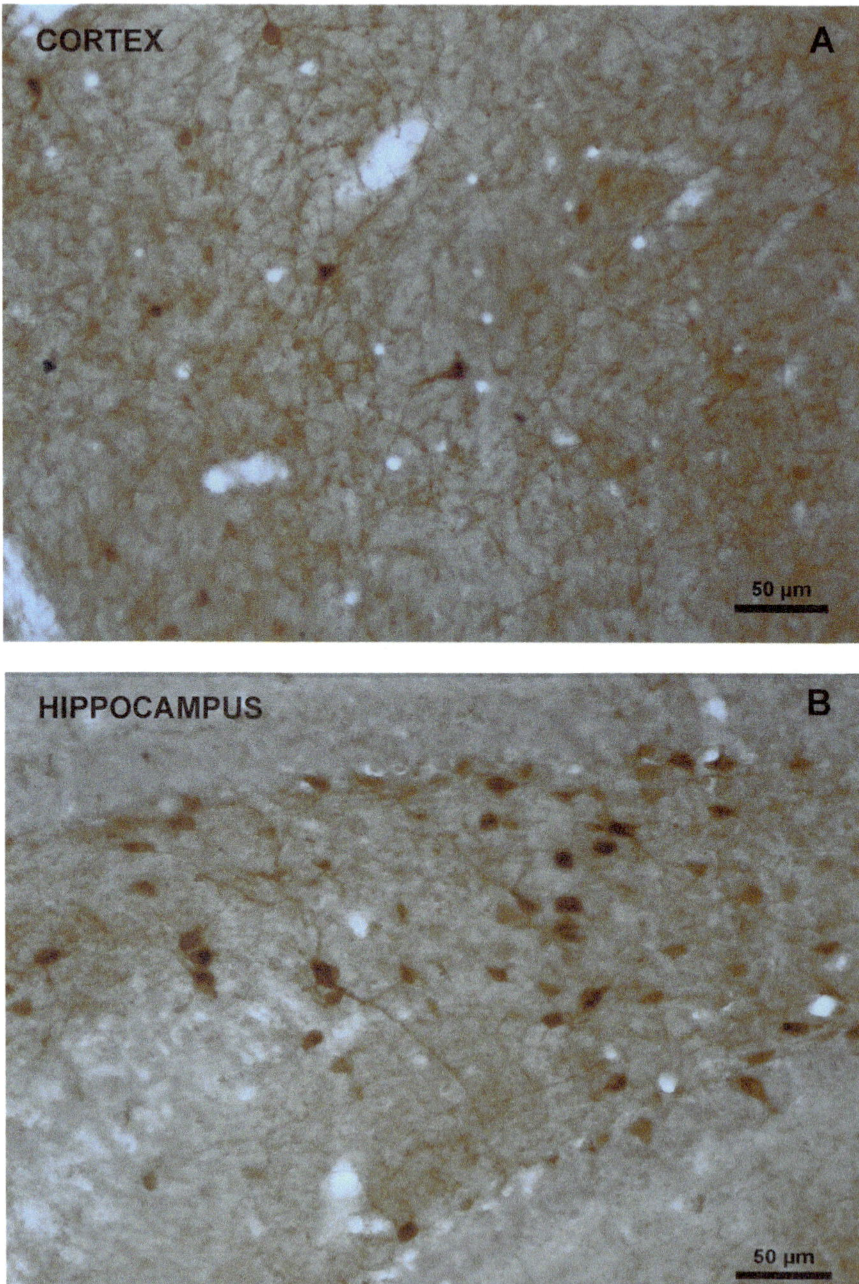

Fig. 2. Microphotographs showing NPY-immunoreactive neurons in the frontal sections of the mouse brain. A: the cerebral cortex; B: the hilar region of the hippocampus. Nerve cell bodies and varicose fibres can be seen. ABC staining.

anxiety (NPY has a strong antianxiety effect), circadian rhythms, memory processing, inhibition of the release of other neurotransmitters (Colmers et al., 1990; Danger et al., 1990; Gray & Morley, 1986; Greber et al., 1994; Wettstein, et al., 1995). NPY plays an important role in the regulation of neuronal activity, it reduces epileptiform activity in the hippocampus (Woldbye et al., 1997) by inhibition of glutamate release (Colmers & Bleakman, 1994; Greber et al., 1994; Silva et al., 2005b; Vezzani et al., 1999).

The numerous and diverse actions of NPY are mediated by specific, G-protein coupled heptahelical receptors, called Y receptors. Six Y receptors have been identified (Y1, Y2, Y3, Y4, Y5, and y6) based on different pharmacological profiles (Dumont et al., 1992). Five of them, except for Y3, have been cloned. The Y1, Y2 and Y5 receptors preferentially bind NPY and PYY, whereas Y4 is activated preferentially by PP. The Y3 receptor has not been cloned till now and was only pharmacologically characterized as having a very low affinity for PYY (ten times weaker than for NPY). In the brain, it was found only in the nucleus of the solitary tract. The y6 receptor functions only in the mouse and the rabbit and is absent in the rat, human and other primates (Michel et al., 1998; Silva et al., 2002, 2005a). Activation of all Y receptor types inhibits adenylate cyclase and in most of cells, that effect is abolished by botulin toxin, which indicates that Gi/Go proteins participate in the signal transduction from Y receptors to adenylate cyclase. The Y receptor activation influences also ion channels but the final effects depend on the type of target cell. It was best characterized for Y1 and Y2 receptors. In neurons, Y1 receptor activation enhanced Ca++ availability via inositol triphosphate (IP3)-mediated mobilization of intracellular Ca++ stores or by enhancing calcium ion entry through L-type channels, causing neuronal excitation. Inhibition of K+ channels after Y1 stimulation has also been described. On the other hand, Y2 receptor activation reduced Ca++ availability (via N-type channels) and inhibited neuronal function. Much evidence supports the excitatory role of Y1 receptors but opposite effects have also been noted, e.g. small neurons of dorsal root ganglia are inhibited by Y1 receptor activation by their hyperpolarization. The Y5 receptors have inhibitory properties and such effects have also been postulated for other Y receptors but were much less studied.

NPY activates all Y receptors with similar potency as PYY except for Y3 which is characterized by a higher affinity for NPY than for PYY and Y4 receptor which binds PP with high affinity, but PYY and NPY with very low affinity. If we want to study a role of particular Y receptor types, a more specific ligands are needed. Agonistic ligands are still only peptides (no smaller non-peptide molecules have been introduced). Y1 receptors are selectively activated by peptides NPY or PYY modified at the C-terminal end i.e. [Pro^{34}]-NPY, [Leu^{31},Pro^{34}]-NPY, [Leu^{31},Pro^{34}]-PYY. Such modification induces a loss of Y2 receptor affinity. It indicates that N-terminal part of the peptide is essential for Y1 receptor binding. In contrast, the binding to Y2 receptors does not require N-terminal sequence but C-terminal part of the peptide is crucial. Thus, the selective agonists of Y2 receptors include NPY (13-36) and some cyclic analogs of NPY. Receptors of Y5 type are activated by NPY(2-36), PYY(3-36), but the peptides stimulate also Y2 receptors. Selective Y5 receptor agonists were synthesized during the last 10 years, and one of them, a chimeric peptide of PP with changed NPY fragment, [cPP^{1-7},NPY^{19-23},Ala^{31},Aib^{32},Gln^{34}]-hPancreatic Polypeptide was described as a very selective Y5 agonist (Cabrele et al., 2000). A better situation is with the availability of non-peptide antagonists of Y receptors. There are several non-peptide Y1 receptor antagonists and one of them BIBO3304 has a good selectivity profile and high affinity (Brothers & Wahlestedt, 2010; Dumont et al., 2000). Y2 receptors are successfully and specifically blocked by BIIE0246 (Doods et al., 1999) but submicromollar affinities for opioid and alpha1 adrenergic receptors were also noted. Y5 receptors can be antagonized by the compounds called MK-0557, S-2367, L152,804 or 2-36[K4,RYYSA(19-23)]PP, and a very selective compound, CGP 71683 synthesized in the last years showed more than 1000-fold higher selectivity for Y5 over Y1, Y2 and Y4 receptors (Brothers & Wahlestedt, 2010).

Receptor	Agonists	Antagonists
Y1R	NPY = PYY = $Leu^{31},Pro^{34}NPY$ >> NPY13-36 > PP	BIBP3226 BIBO3304 BMS193885
Y2R	NPY = PYY ≥ NPY13-36 >> $Leu^{31},Pro^{34}NPY$ > PP PYY3-36	BIIE0246 SF 11 JNJ 5207787 JNJ 31020028
Y5R	NPY ≥ PYY ≥ PP $[cPP^{1-7},NPY^{19-23},Ala^{31}Aib^{32}, Gln^{34}]$-hPP BWX 46	CGP 71683 MK-0557 S-2367 L-152,804
NPY - neuropeptide Y, PYY - peptide YY, PP- pancreatic polypeptide		

Table 1. Representative NPY receptor ligands for Y1, Y2 and Y5 receptors

2. Modulation of an excitatory glutamatergic transmission by NPY

Glutamate is the most abundant excitatory neurotransmitter in the mammalian brain and participates in the changes of synaptic transmission underlying learning and memory (Bliss & Collingridge, 1993), but on the other hand, an overactivation of glutamatergic transmission may lead to excitotoxic cell death (Ankarcrona et al., 1995; Choi, 1985; Conn & Pin, 1997). It is generally assumed that excitotoxicity is a common pathological condition to a variety of neuronal degenerations. It comprises supraphysiological stimulation of ionotropic glutamate receptors and an increase in intracellular Ca++ which triggers downstream processes resulting in neuronal death (acc. to Silva et. al., 2005a). Thus, control of extracellular glutamate concentration seems to be critical for both neuronal signaling and survival. One of the important functions of NPY is related to the inhibition of glutamate release and reduction of glutamatergic excitatory activity which may result in neuroprotection. It was found that NPY reduced epileptiform activity in the hippocampus and cortex (Bijak, 1999; Bijak & Śmiałowska, 1995; Klapstein & Colmers, 1997), inhibited glutamate release (Colmers, 1990; Greber et al., 1994; Silva et al., 2001) and reduced kainic acid (KA)-induced seizures (Madsen et al., 1999; Woldbye et al., 1997). Moreover, increases in the synthesis and content of NPY in the limbic structures were found after seizures of different origin (Bellmann et al., 1991; Bendotti et al., 1991; Marksteiner et al., 1990; Schwarzer et al., 1996; Silva et al., 2005a; Śmiałowska et al., 2003) which may indicate a possibility of neuroprotective role of endogenous NPY.

Our earlier studies showed the neuroprotective effects of NPY against KA-induced neurotoxicity both *in vivo* in the rat hippocampus (Śmialowska et al., 2003) and *in vitro* in the hippocampal and cortical neuronal cultures (Domin et al., 2006). Results of other authors were controversial showing both protective and toxic effects of NPY (Chen & Cheung, 2002; Cheung & Cechetto, 2000). The cause of such a discrepancy may be connected with differentiation of Y receptors.

2.1 The role of particular Y receptors in neuroprotection

Among NPY receptors, Y1R, Y2R and Y5R were postulated to play the most important role in the regulation of neurotoxicity and neuroprotection. Since specific agonists and antagonists of those receptors have been synthesized (Aguirre et al., 1990; Cabrele et al., 2000; Doods et al., 1999; Dumont et al., 2000; Fuhlendorff et al., 1990; Rudolf et al., 1994; Wieland et al., 1998) the studies on the role of particular receptors in neuroprotection became possible. Most of evidences demonstrated neuroprotective effects after Y2 and Y5 receptor agonists (Silva et al., 2003b, 2005a; Śmialowska et al., 2009; Wu & Li, 2005). Neuroprotective role of Y2 and Y5 receptor stimulation was also suggested by electrophysiological and behavioral studies in which the activation of these receptors suppressed epileptiform bursting or seizures (Bijak, 1999; Klapstein & Colmers, 1997; Marsh et al., 1999; Woldbye et al., 1997; Vezzani et al., 1999). The role of Y1R in neuroprotection is ambiguous. The activation of Y1 receptors produced neuroprotective effects in kainate excitotoxicity model of rat organotypic hippocampal slice cultures (Xapelli et al., 2007) and in methamphetamine neurotoxicity model in the mouse striatum (Thieriet et al., 2005), but in both models Y1R had a little weaker effect than Y2R agonists. Excitotoxicity induced by AMPA in organotypic mouse hippocampal slice cultures showed that AMPA-induced degenerations of CA1 and CA3 pyramidal neurons were strongly inhibited by Y2 but not Y1 or Y5 receptor agonists (Xapelli et al., 2008). More detailed studies in hippocampal slices have shown that neuroprotective properties of a particular Y receptor may depend on the region where the receptor is located. Thus Y1, Y2 and Y5 receptor agonists were neuroprotective against AMPA or kainate excitotoxicity in dentate granule cells and CA3 region, while CA1 pyramidal neurons were protected only by Y2 agonist (Silva et al., 2003a, 2005a). On the contrary, the excitotoxic effects of Y1 receptor activation in the rat hippocampus were suggested by the results of Gariboldi et al. (1998) in which Y1R stimulation potentiated convulsions, while administration of Y1R antagonist inhibited kainate-induced seizures. Moreover, studies in an ischemic model both in vitro and in vivo, have demonstrated that Y1 receptor activation enhances neurodegeneration, while Y1R antagonists produced neuroprotective effects (Chen & Cheung, 2003, 2004). No protection after a Y1 receptor agonist was also found in our studies both in vitro and in vivo (Śmialowska et al., 2009).

2.1.1 Neuroprotective effect of Y receptor agonists in kainic acid-induced excitotoxicity

The model of kainic acid (KA)-induced excitotoxicity was described as a good and validated simulation of different excitotoxic neurodegenerations, connected with the secondary release of endogenous glutamate (Coyle, 1983; Ferkany & Coyle, 1983; Malva et al., 1998;

Wang et al., 2005). The KA activates kainate receptors, which belong to ionotropic glutamate receptors, but effects after KA develop progressively and endogenous glutamate release enhances degeneration. Therefore, the KA-model seems to be especially suitable for studying the delayed neuroprotection.

The main goal of our studies was to explore a possibility of neuroprotection induced by NPY or specific Y receptor ligands. We focused our attention on Y1, Y2 and Y5 receptors, as it is generally assumed that these receptors play the most important role in the regulation of neurodegeneration and neuroprotection. Moreover, we investigated the efficacy of the treatment delayed even by a few hours while in the majority of other studies NPY and its ligands were applied before or simultaneously with a neurotoxic damage, however, the delayed treatment resembles more closely the situation of patients, who are usually treated some time after an injury.

We performed studies both in vitro and in vivo (Śmialowska et al., 2009). In *in vitro* experiments primary cultures of mouse cortical and hippocampal neurons were used. The cultures were exposed to KA for 24 or 48 h and then Y receptor ligands were added 30 min, 1, 3 or 6 h after starting the KA exposure. Cell death was quantified by measurements of lactate dehydrogenase (LDH) release from damaged cells into the cell culture media. Apoptosis was evaluated by measurements of caspase-3 activation and additionally by fluorescent Hoechst 33342 staining which visualized condensed DNA fragments, characteristic for apoptotic cells. A huge increase in the LDH release and caspase-3 activation was found after the KA and these increases were strongly attenuated by both Y2 receptor agonist (NPY13-36) and Y5 receptor agonist ([cPP$^{1-7}$,NPY$^{19-23}$,Ala^{31},Aib^{32}Gln^{34}]hPP), added as late as 3 hours after starting KA intoxication. The results indicated neuroprotective and antiapoptotic effects of these peptides. Receptor specificity was confirmed by experiments with antagonists which prevented the neuroprotection. No neuroprotective effects were observed after Y1 receptor agonist [Leu^{31}, Pro^{34}]-NPY given after the KA (for details see Śmialowska et al., 2009). Our *in vitro* results are in line with the studies of other authors showing the protective effect of Y2 and Y5 receptors, but not Y1 in the KA-induced excitotoxicity (Silva et al., 2001, 2003b; Woldbye & Kokaia, 2004; Xapelli et al., 2007).

The same picture of Y receptor efficacy in neuroprotection emerges also from the *in vivo* experiments. Wu and Li (2005) found that NPY and specific Y2 and Y5 receptor agonists rescued mouse hippocampal pyramidal neurons from KA-induced apoptosis (visualized by the TUNEL staining) when the peptides were intracerebroventricularly (icv) injected as late as 2 or 8 h after intraperitoneal KA injection. Also in our *in vivo* studies the neuroprotective effects were found after treatment of the peptides delayed by 30 min or 1 h, but not 3 h, after the KA injection. Our model was different than that of the above-mentioned authors as we used rats and injected KA into the CA1 hippocampal region in a dose and manner which did not induce seizures. The peptides were also microinjected intrahippocampally. Brains were removed and fixed 7 days after the treatment and degeneration and protection were evaluated by stereological counting of neurons in the CA pyramidal layer in the dorsal hippocampus. The results showed the protective effects of Y2 and Y5, but not Y1 receptor agonists (for details see Śmialowska et al., 2009).

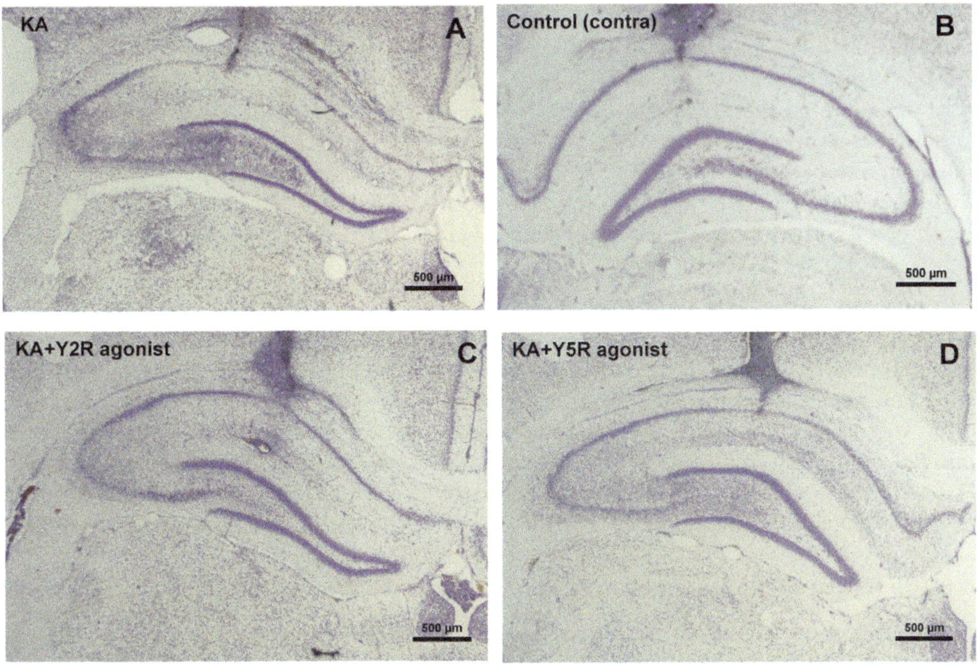

Fig. 3. Microphotographs of frontal sections of the rat brain hippocampi, stained with cresyl violet for visualization of nerve cell bodies. A: The hippocampus after KA injection into the CA1 region. Strong degeneration of pyramidal neurons and extensive gliosis are seen. B: non-degenerated, contralateral hippocampus microinjected with a phosphate buffer used as a control side. C: Neuroprotective effect of Y2 receptor agonist injected 30 min after the KA. The lesion is much smaller. D: A similar neuroprotective effect is seen after Y5 receptor agonist microinjected 30 min after the KA. After Y2 (C) and Y5 (D) receptor agonists pyramidal neurons are much more numerous than after KA alone (A).

2.1.2 The role of NPY and Y receptors in ischemic neurodegeneration

Much less is known about the neuroprotective role of NPY in ischemic degenerations. A possibility of such function of endogenous NPY was postulated on the basis of the observations that NPY-immunoreactivity increased locally in the cerebral cortex around the site of infarct following middle cerebral artery occlusion (MCAO) in rats (Allen et al., 1995, Cheung & Cechetto, 1997; Cheung et al., 1995). On the other hand, an increase in the infarct volume in a similar MCAO model was observed after intravenous or central NPY administration into the rat (Chen & Cheung, 2002). The effect was suggested to be connected with a vasoconstrictive action of NPY, via Y1 receptors, as these authors reported a reduction of the cerebral blood flow after NPY injection. The possibility of neuroprotective function of endogenous NPY was also suggested by the experiments in which ischemic preconditioning induced an increase in NPY-immunoreactivity in the gerbils' hippocampus (Duszczyk et al., 2009). Quite different results were obtained when antisense oligonucleotide to Y1 receptors was given to rats prior to MCAO. Such treatment strongly reduced cortical

Y1 receptor density and evoked a huge increase in the infarct volume (Cheung & Cechetto, 2000). The result suggested a positive role of Y1 receptors in the protection against ischemia as the lack of Y1 receptors resulted in an increased degeneration. However, other studies have demonstrated that Y1 receptor activation enhanced ischemic degenerations. Again in MCAO model in rats intracerebroventricular injection of Y1 agonist increased, while antagonist reduced the infarct volume (Chen & Cheung, 2003). Similarly in *in vitro* model in which neuronal cultures were deprived of oxygen and glucose (OGD model) Y1 receptor agonist worsened while antagonist improved survival of neurons (Chen & Cheung, 2004).

Therefore, the results of studies on the role of NPY and Y receptors in ischemic neurodegenerations obtained so far were divergent and insufficient. Our group also examined this problem. We found that Y2 receptor agonist (NPY13-36) given intracerebroventricularly 30 min after the onset of ischemia significantly diminished the infarct volume in the rat transient MCAO model (Śmialowska et al., 2009). Our preliminary *in vitro* studies on primary cultures of mouse cortical neurons indicated also that in cultures subjected to oxygen and glucose deprivation (OGD model) Y2 receptor agonist induced neuroprotection and moreover, similar protective effect was observed after Y5 receptor agonist but not after Y1 receptor agonist (data in preparation).

2.1.3 The role of NPY and Y receptors in chronic neurodegenerative diseases

An involvement of NPY in chronic neurodegenerations has been postulated on the basis of clinical studies and animal or in vitro experiments.

Huntington's disease

Patients with Huntington's disease (HD) have pathological changes mainly in the striatum and cerebral cortex and show characteristic abnormal motor activity (chorea movements), cognitive impairment and emotional disturbances (Colton & Vitek, 2006). HD is one of neurodegenerative diseases in which a pathological protein is expressed in the cells. The hallmark of HD is the protein huntingtin with pathological repeat length and the most affected neurons are medium spiny neurons in the striatum. Loss of these neurons, projecting to the globus pallidus and substantia nigra is the main reason of the motor abnormalities in HD. In contrast, NPY interneurons in the striatum are relatively resistant to degenerations in HD. Many cortical and striatal interneurons contain NPY, usually coexisting with somatostatin (SOM), and it was found that the level of both NPY and SOM increased 3-5 fold in the caudate, putamen, nucleus accumbens and cortex in HD in comparison to control brains (Beal et al., 1988; Dawbarn et al., 1985; Mazurek et al., 1997). The analysis of transgenic mouse models of HD displayed divergent results, both decreases or increases in NPY and SOM and their mRNAs were reported (Figueredo-Cardenas et al., 1994; Kumar, 2004; Luthi-Carter et al., 2000). The degeneration of the striatal medium spiny neurons in HD may be connected with their abundant glutamatergic innervation from the cortex and high density of glutamate receptors (Kumar et al., 1997; Sieradzan & Mann, 2001; Zeron et al., 2002), so excitotoxic cell death is supposed to occur in HD. Therefore, NPY could be neuroprotective but till now a possible role of NPY in HD is unclear. Experiments with transgenic mouse model of HD (R6/2 strain) showed that a single intraventricular injection of NPY improved motor function, increased survival time and diminished cerebral and striatal atrophy. The positive effects were proposed to be connected with an increased neurogenesis in the subventricular zone (Decressac et al., 2010) induced by NPY and migration of new cells into the striatum, where they differentiate to GABAergic interneurons. On the other hand, the development of the disease in HD patients proceeded in spite of NPY increase, therefore, it may be supposed that protective action of NPY, if happened, is insufficient for preventing the progression of the disease.

Alzheimer's disease

Alzheimer's disease (AD) is a chronic brain neurodegeneration with progressive memory loss, cognitive dysfunction, various neuro-psychiatric and behavioural disturbances that seriously interfere with daily life activity and eventually lead to death. The neuropathological hallmarks of AD are senile plaques (containing a pathological form of amyloid beta) and neurofibrillary tangles (containing hyperphosphorylated tau protein). Advanced stages of AD are characterized by an extensive neuronal loss especially in the hippocampus, cortex and nucleus basalis of Meynert. The damage in the hippocampal and cortical regions was postulated to be associated with dementia. NPY is present in some hippocampal and cortical interneurons and seems to have a role in learning and memory thus the possible involvement of this peptide in AD pathogenesis and/or symptoms has been studied but results are divergent. A number of clinical studies showed a reduced or unchanged level of NPY in the cerebrospinal fluid (Atack et al., 1988; Edvinsson et al., 1993; Heilig et al., 1995; Martignoni et al., 1992; Minthon et al., 1990; Nilsson et al., 2001) or plasma (Koide et al., 1995) of AD patients. Losses of cortical receptor sites for NPY (Nordberg, 1992) and decrease in NPY receptor density in the hippocampus and temporal cortex but not in the putamen have also been reported (Martel et al., 1990). Immunohistochemistry of brain sections evidenced a strong reduction in the number of NPY-immunoreactive neurons in the hippocampal formation and enthorinal cortex and alternation of the morphology of the remaining neurons (Kowall & Beal, 1988). The results obtained from studies of a transgenic mouse model of AD, overexpressing amyloid precursor protein and demonstrating amyloid plaques showed quite different changes in NPY, namely an increased NPY immunoreactivity in the hippocampus and enthorinal cortex (Diez et al., 2000, 2003). However, other models that co-express amyloid plaques and neurofibrillary tangles have altered NPY levels and more resemble changes in human AD (Oddo et al., 2003, 2004).

A possibility of neuroprotective effects of NPY in AD neurodegeneration arises from the neuroprotective potential of NPY in excitotoxicity and its ability to decrease the calcium ion influx into neurons, that is one of the mechanism of this protection. Since amyloid beta (Abeta) peptides were found to disrupt calcium ion homeostasis and increased intraneuronal Ca++ (Fedrizzi & Carafoli, 2011; Pereira et al., 2005; Shirvany et al., 2007), NPY may inhibit this damaging process. Moreover, it was found that NPY increased the production of neurotrophins and protected SY5Y neuroblastoma cells against beta amyloid toxicity with concomitant increase in neurotrophin production (Croce et al., 2011). Additional mechanisms of therapeutic action of NPY in AD might be related to the activation of neurogenesis in the hippocampus (Howell et al., 2005, 2007) as well as to neurogenesis and cell proliferation in other structures (see above in the chapter about HD). A new possibility of neuroprotection based on NPY has also been postulated by Rose et al. (2009), who found protective effects of neuropeptide fragments (mainly NPY 21-36 and 31-36) derived from neprilysin processing in a transgenic mouse model of AD. No studies of the role of specific Y receptors were performed yet.

Parkinson's disease

Parkinson's disease (PD) is a chronic neurodegeneration characterized mainly by progressive degeneration of dopaminergic neurons in the substantia nigra pars compacta with disappearance of their projections into the striatum. It leads to development of motor symptoms such as bradykinesia, rigidity and tremor. Therapies used in PD can temporarily alleviate motor symptoms but do not prevent progression of the disease as the mechanism of PD development is still unclear. There are only a few studies concerning NPY in human PD. A decrease in NPY level in the cerebrospinal fluid (Martignoni et al., 1992), no changes in the cortex and hippocampus (Allen et al., 1985) or decrease in adrenal medulla (Stoddard et al., 1991) were described in PD patients. Besides, it has been postulated that NPY may play some role in the pathogenesis and/or symptoms of PD as both nerve cell bodies and terminals containing NPY are quite abundant in extrapyramidal structures engaged in the disease and, moreover, a reciprocal interactions were found between dopaminergic and NPY neurons. In animal experiments, a decrease or disappearance of dopaminergic innervation in the striatum (such situation occurs in PD) induced a significant increase in NPY synthesis and content in the striatal interneurons (Engber et al., 1992; Kerkerian et al., 1986, 1988; Midgley et al., 1994; Śmialowska, 1995). In situ hybridization immunohistochemical studies of postmortem human brain structures showed an increase in NPYmRNA in the striatum especially in the ventral caudate nucleus and the nucleus accumbens (Cannizzaro et al., 2003) in PD.

A regulatory function of NPY in DA transmission was demonstrated in rats, as an NPY injection into the striatum increased the DA turnover in that structure (Beal et al., 1986). More detailed studies on the role of particular Y receptors in the rat striatum have shown that Y2 receptor activation enhanced dopamine synthesis while Y1 and Y5 receptor stimulation attenuated the DA synthesis (Adewale et al., 2005). Since no genetic mouse model of PD currently exists, studies have focused primarily on the models with lesioned nigro-striatal dopaminergic systems. The lesions were performed by means of dopaminergic toxins 6-hydroxydopamine or MPTP. Recently, Decressac et al., (2011a) described a neuroprotective effect of NPY in PD models. They found that NPY protected dopaminergic neuroblastoma cells (SH-SY5Y) from 6-hydroxydopamine induced toxicity. The neuroprotective effect of NPY was also confirmed in vivo, in the rat and mouse model of PD in which striatal NPY injection inhibited dopaminergic degenerations induced by the toxins and improved motor performance. Moreover, detailed studies using Y receptor ligands evidenced a protective action of Y2 but not Y1 receptors both on dopamine neurons and the behavioral impairments (Decressac et al., 2011a). Therefore, the authors suggested a possibility of therapeutic use of NPY ligands in the future.

2.2 How does NPY modulate neurodegenation and neuroprotection?

NPY appears to be particularly promising for neuroprotection, since it has a significant modulating effect on excitatory neurotransmission. As mentioned above, many studies have shown that NPY inhibits glutamatergic transmission (Bijak, 2000; Colmers et al., 1987; Greber et al., 1994; Klapstein & Colmers, 1992; McQuiston & Colmers 1996; Śmialowska et al., 1996;) through presynaptic inhibition of glutamate release from nerve terminals (Greber et al., 1994; Silva et al., 2003a). It is assumed that such inhibition is associated with the inhibition of N-type calcium channels (Qian et al., 1997; Silva et al., 2001; Silva et al., 2003a). Since NPY receptors activate signaling pathways involved in the regulation of intracellular Ca^{2+} homeostasis (Silva et al., 2002), one of the possible mechanism of neuroprotective action of NPY consists in the inhibition of calcium channels thereby inhibiting the influx of calcium ions into the cell (Thiert et al., 2005; Xapelli et al., 2007). In our studies, NPY as well as Y2R and Y5R agonists inhibited the toxic effects of KA, decreased the KA-induced caspase-3 activation and the number of apoptotic bodies (Śmialowska et al., 2009). It is known that KA disturbs the homeostasis of calcium ions in cells, cytochrome c release and caspase-3 activation, which leads to cell death (Wang et al., 2005). Therefore, it has been proposed that the antiexcitatory and antiapoptotic properties of the peptides under study are connected with a decrease in the input of calcium ions into neurons and a decrease in glutamate release.

As mentioned above, the role of Y1 receptors in neuroprotection is unclear. It is supposed that the neurotoxic effect of Y1R activation observed in our and other studies may be due to the fact that these receptors are situated mainly postsynaptically, and their activation induces calcium influx and inhibition of potassium channels, which increases neuronal excitability (Dumont et al., 1992; Gobbi et al., 1996). Stimulation of calcium release from the endoplasmic reticulum (Aakerlund et al., 1990) and enhancement of nitric oxide production (Bitran et al., 1999; Chen et al., 2002) have also been proposed as possible mechanisms of neurotoxicity after Y1R activation. On the other hand, it has been found in the brain that some Y1 receptors are located presynaptically (Kopp et al., 2002) and the putative neuroprotective mechanism of action Y1R agonist in some models might be due to the presynaptic inhibition of glutamate release by inhibition of Ca++ entry (McQuiston et al., 1996; Silva et al., 2001; Silva et al., 2003a, 2003b). Such presynaptic inhibitory Y1 receptors were found, for instance, in the hippocampal dentate region (McQuiston et al., 1996; Silva et al., 2001, 2003b), rat cerebral cortex (Wang, 2005) or arcuate nucleus (Sun & Miller, 1999). The Y1 receptor stimulation may have also positive effects in neurodegenerations by quite different mechanism. It has been shown that NPY promotes neurogenesis and proliferation of progenitor cells in the rat dentate gyrus of the hippocampal formation and the effects are mediated by Y1 receptors as they were also observed after Y1R but not after Y2R agonists (Descressac et al., 2011b; Howell et al., 2005; Kopp et al., 2002; Xapelli et al., 2006). Moreover, the proliferation was reduced in Y1 receptor knockout mice, or after co-administration of Y1 antagonist. Similarly, Y1 receptor-mediated stimulation of neurogenesis and proliferation by NPY was also found in the mouse olfactory epitelium (Hansel et al., 2001). As mentioned above, NPY increased neurogenesis in the telencephalic subventricular zone (Decressac et al., 2010) but no receptor specificity was studied. In rat retinal cell cultures, NPY stimulated neural cell proliferation mainly via Y2 and Y5 receptors but some role of Y1R was also postulated as Y1 antagonist decreased the cell proliferation induced by NPY (Alvaro et al., 2008).

Neurogenesis, proliferation and differentiation of neurons may be also regulated by neurotrophic factors, and a cross-talk between NPY and brain derived neurotrophic factor (BDNF) in the mammalian brains has been suggested. Seizures and excitotoxicity induced a significant increase in BDNF in the injured region (Ballarin et al., 1991; Dugich-Djordjevic et al., 1992; Humpel et al., 1993). As the increase in BDNF always precedes the NPY expression

(Reibel et al., 2000) the BDNF overexpression after excitotoxicity may be neuroprotective by inducing NPY production. Many studies have shown that BDNF enhanced an expression of NPY in the striatum, cortex and the hippocampus (Barnea & Roberts, 2001; Barnea et al., 2004; Nawa et al., 1994; Reibel et al., 2000; Takei et al., 1996; Wirth et al., 2005; Yoshimura et al., 2009). In the mouse organotypic hippocampal slice cultures exposed to glutamate receptor agonist, degeneration of CA1 and CA3 pyramidal neurons was diminished by Y2 receptor agonist and such protection strongly inhibited the stimulating effect of AMPA on the BDNF level (Xapelli et al., 2008). It was also found that NPY treatment decreased BDNF and increased nerve growth factor production in the rat hypothalamus (Gelfo et al., 2011). All these results indicate mutual relations between NPY and BDNF (or maybe other trophic factors).

Nitric oxide (NO) a reactive free radical, gas produced enzymatically from L-arginine by NO synthases is a very important molecule connected with the NPY role in excitotoxicity and neuroprotection. In normal physiological state, NO concentration in the brain amounts to less than 10 nM and NO plays an important role in vascular tone, blood pressure and neuronal signaling (Garthwaite, 1991) but during cerebral ischemia NO production increased which is an important factor inducing ischemic damage, as NO quickly forms highly toxic radicals (Matsui et al., 1999). It was found that in the rat MCAO model of ischemia, the brain NO concentration increased and intracerebroventricular injection of NPY or Y1R agonist enhanced this increase, while, in contrast, a Y1R antagonist strongly inhibited the NO formation. The results indicated harmful effect of Y1R stimulation via an increase in toxic NO formation. On the other hand a possibility of neuroprotection in ischemia by agents blocking Y1 receptors may be suggested.

3. Conclusions

Neuropeptide Y (NPY) reveals many important regulatory function in the brain both under physiological and pathological conditions. The present paper reviews the data on the role of NPY and its receptors in neuroprotection. The peptide counteracts neuronal glutamatergic excitation, inhibits seizures and has significant neuroprotective effects which are produced mainly via Y2 and Y5 receptors. The activation of Y1 receptors gives ambiguous results, usually induces harmful effects but in some situations and some brain regions may also be protective via both inhibition of glutamate release and the induction of repair mechanisms (cell proliferation, trophic factors or others). The results obtained by our group and by a few other authors suggest that NPY and Y2 or Y5 receptor agonists may reveal their protective activity not only when they are given before or simultaneously with a traumatic event but also as the delayed treatment, 30 min or even few hours after the onset of the damaging action. A possible role of NPY in some chronic neurodegenerative disorders is also discussed.

4. Acknowledgment

The study was partially supported by grants No. 2P05A 114 28 and No. N N401 091037 from the Ministry of Science and Higher Education, Poland and partially by statutory founds of the Institute of Pharmacology, Polish Academy of Sciences, Krakow, Poland.

5. References

Aakerlund, L., Gether, U., Fuhlendorff, J., Schwartz, T.W. & Thastrup, O. (1990). Y1 receptors for neuropeptide Y are coupled to mobilization of intracellular calcium and inhibition of adenylate cyclase. *FEBS Lett.*, 260(1), 73-78.

Adewale, A.S., Macarthur, H. & Westfall, T.C. (2005). Neuropeptide Y induced modulation of dopamine synthesis in the striatum. *Regul Pept.*, 129(1-3), 73-78.

Aguirre, J.A., Fuxe, K., Agnati, L.F. & von Euler, G. (1990). Centrally injected neuropeptide Y (13-36) produces vasopressor effects and antagonizes the vasodepressor action of neuropeptide Y (1-36) in the awake male rat. *Neurosci Lett.*, 118(1), 5-8.

Allen, G.V., Cheung, R.T. & Cechetto, D.F. (1995). Neurochemical changes following occlusion of the middle cerebral artery in rats. *Neuroscience*, 68(4), 1037-1050.

Allen, J., Novotný, J., Martin, J. & Heinrich, G. (1987). Molecular structure of mammalian neuropeptide Y: analysis by molecular cloning and computer-aided comparison with crystal structure of avian homologue. *Proc Natl Acad Sci U S A.*, 84(8), 2532-2536.

Allen, J.M., Cross, A.J., Crow, T.J., Javoy-Agid, F., Agid, Y. & Bloom, S.R. (1985). Dissociation of neuropeptide Y and somatostatin in Parkinson's disease. *Brain Res.*, 337(1), 197-200.

Alvaro, A.R., Martins, J., Araújo, I.M., Rosmaninho-Salgado, J., Ambrósio, A.F. & Cavadas, C. (2008). Neuropeptide Y stimulates retinal neural cell proliferation--involvement of nitric oxide. *J Neurochem.*, 105(6), 2501-2510.

Ankarcrona, M., Dypbukt, J.M., Bonfoco, E., Zhivotovsky, B., Orrenius, S., Lipton, S.A. & Nicotera, P. (1995). Glutamate-induced neuronal death: a succession of necrosis or apoptosis depending on mitochondrial function. *Neuron*, 15(4), 961-973.

Atack, J.R., Beal, M.F., May, C., Kaye, J.A., Mazurek, M.F., Kay, A.D. & Rapoport, S.I. (1988). Cerebrospinal fluid somatostatin and neuropeptide Y. Concentrations in aging and in dementia of the Alzheimer type with and without extrapyramidal signs. *Arch Neurol.*, 45(3), 269-274.

Ballarín, M., Ernfors, P., Lindefors, N. & Persson, H. (1991). Hippocampal damage and kainic acid injection induce a rapid increase in mRNA for BDNF and NGF in the rat brain. *Exp Neurol.*, 114(1), 35-43.

Barnea, A. & Roberts, J. (2001). Induction of functional and morphological expression of neuropeptide Y (NPY) in cortical cultures by brain-derived neurotrophic factor (BDNF): evidence for a requirement for extracellular-regulated kinase (ERK)-dependent and ERK-independent mechanisms. *Brain Res.*, 919(1), 57-69.

Barnea, A., Roberts, J. & Croll, S.D. (2004). Continuous exposure to brain-derived neurotrophic factor is required for persistent activation of TrkB receptor, the ERK signaling pathway, and the induction of neuropeptide Y production in cortical cultures. *Brain Res.*, 1020(1-2), 106-117.

Beal, M.F., Frank, R.C., Ellison, D.W. & Martin, J.B. (1986). The effect of neuropeptide Y on striatal catecholamines. *Neurosci Lett.*, 71(1), 118-123.

Beal, M.F., Mazurek, M.F., Ellison, D.W., Swartz, K.J., McGarvey, U., Bird, E.D. & Martin, J.B. (1988). Somatostatin and neuropeptide Y concentrations in pathologically graded cases of Huntington's disease. *Ann Neurol.*, 23(6), 562-569.

Bellmann, R., Widmann, R., Olenik, C., Meyer, D.K., Maas, D., Marksteiner, J. & Sperk G. (1991). Enhanced rate of expression and biosynthesis of neuropeptide Y after kainic acid-induced seizures. *J Neurochem.*, 56(2), 525-530.

Bendotti, C., Vezzani, A., Serafini, R., Servadio, A., Rivolta, R. & Samanin, R. (1991). Increased prepronenropeptide Y mRNA in the rat hippocampus during the development of hippocampal kindling: comparison with the expression of preprosomatostatin mRNA. *Neurosci Lett.*, 132, (2), 175-178.

Bijak, M. (1999). Neuropeptide Y suppresses epileptiform activity in rat frontal cortex and hippocampus in vitro via different NPY receptor subtypes. *Neurosci Lett.*, 268(3), 115-118.

Bijak, M. (2000). Neuropeptide Y reduces epileptiform discharges and excitatory synaptic transmission in rat frontal cortex in vitro. *Neuroscience*, 96(3), 487-494.

Bijak, M. & Smiałowska, M. (1995). Effects of neuropeptide Y on evoked potentials in the CA1 region and the dentate gyrus of the rat hippocampal slice. *Pol J Pharmacol.*, 47(4), 333-338.

Bitran, M., Tapia, W., Eugenín, E., Orio, P. & Boric, M.P. (1999). Neuropeptide Y induced inhibition of noradrenaline release in rat hypothalamus: role of receptor subtype and nitric oxide. *Brain Res.*, 851(1-2), 87-93.

Bliss, T.V. & Collingridge, G.L. (1993). A synaptic model of memory: long-term potentiation in the hippocampus. *Nature*, 361(6407), 31-39. Review.

Brothers, S.P. & Wahlestedt, C. (2010). Therapeutic potential of neuropeptide Y (NPY) receptor ligands. *EMBO Mol Med.*, 2(11), 429-439. Review.

Cabrele, C., Langer, M., Bader, R., Wieland, H.A., Doods, H.N., Zerbe, O. & Beck-Sickinger, A.G. (2000). The first selective agonist for the neuropeptide Y Y5 receptor increases food intake in rats. *J Biol Chem.*, 275(46), 36043-36048.

Cannizzaro, C., Tel, B.C., Rose, S., Zeng, B.Y. & Jenner, P. (2003). Increased neuropeptide Y mRNA expression in striatum in Parkinson's disease. *Brain Res Mol Brain Res.*, 110(2), 169-176.

Chen, S.H. & Cheung, R.T. (2002). Peripheral and central administration of neuropeptide Y in a rat middle cerebral artery occlusion stroke model reduces cerebral blood flow and increases infarct volume. *Brain Res.*, 927(2), 138-143.

Chen, S.H. & Cheung, R.T. (2003). Intracerebroventricular injection of a neuropeptide Y-Y1 receptor agonist increases while BIBP3226, a Y1 antagonist, reduces the infarct volume following transient middle cerebral artery occlusion in rats. *Neuroscience*, 116(1), 119-126.

Chen, S.H. & Cheung, R.T. (2004). Neuropeptide Y-Y1 receptor agonist worsens while antagonist improves survival of cultured Y1-expressing neuronal cells following oxygen and glucose deprivation. *J Biomed Sci.*, 11(6), 781-788.

Chen, S.H., Fung, P.C. & Cheung, R.T. (2002). Neuropeptide Y-Y1 receptor modulates nitric oxide level during stroke in the rat. *Free Radic Biol Med.*, 32(8), 776-784.

Cheung, R.T. & Cechetto, D.F. (1997). Colchicine affects cortical and amygdalar neurochemical changes differentially after middle cerebral artery occlusion in rats. *J Comp Neurol.*, 387(1), 27-41.

Cheung, R.T. & Cechetto, D.F. (2000). Neuropeptide Y-Y1 receptor antisense oligodeoxynucleotide increases the infarct volume after middle cerebral artery occlusion in rats. *Neuroscience*, 98(4), 771-777.

Cheung, R.T., Diab, T. & Cechetto, D.F. (1995). Time-course of neuropeptide changes in peri-ischemic zone and amygdala following focal ischemia in rats. *J Comp Neurol.*, 360(1), 101-120.

Choi, D.W. (1985). Glutamate neurotoxicity in cortical cell culture is calcium dependent. *Neurosci Lett.*, 58(3), 293-297.

Chronwall, B.M. (1989). Anatomical distribution of NPY and NPY messenger RNA in rat brain., In: *Neuropeptide Y,* Mutt, V., Hokfelt, T., Fuxe, K. & Lundberg, J.M. (Ed.), pp. 51-59, ISBN 0-88167-556-3, Raven Press, New York.

Chronwall, B.M., DiMaggio, D.A., Massari, V.J., Pickel, V.M., Ruggiero, D.A. & O'Donohue, T.L. (1985). The anatomy of neuropeptide-Y-containing neurons in rat brain. *Neuroscience,* 15(4), 1159-1181.

Colmers, W.F. & Bleakman, D. (1994). Effects of neuropeptide Y on the electrical properties of neurons. *Trends Neurosci.,* 17(9), 373-379. Review.

Colmers, W.F. (1990). Modulation of synaptic transmission in hippocampus by neuropeptide Y: presynaptic actions. *Ann N Y Acad Sci.,* 611, 206-218.

Colmers, W.F., Lukowiak, K. & Pittman Q.J. (1987). Presynaptic action of neuropeptide Y in area CA1 of the rat hippocampal slice. *J Physiol.,* 383, 285-299.

Colton, C.A. & Vitek, M.P. (2006). NPY and chronic neurodegenerative disease, In: *NPY family of peptides in neurobiology, cardiovascular and metabolic disorders: from genes to therapeutics.* Zukowska, Z. & Feuerstein, G.Z. (Ed.), pp. 223-244, ISBN 3-7643-7155-2, Birkhauser Verlag, Basel - Boston - Berlin.

Conn, P.J. & Pin, J.P. (1997). Pharmacology and functions of metabotropic glutamate receptors. *Annu Rev Pharmacol Toxicol.,* 37, 205-237.

Coyle, J.T. (1983). Neurotoxic action of kainic acid. *J Neurochem.,* 41(1), 1-11. Review.

Croce, N., Dinallo, V., Ricci, V., Federici, G., Caltagirone, C., Bernardini, S. & Angelucci, F. (2011). Neuroprotective effect of neuropeptide Y against beta-amyloid 25-35 toxicity in SH-SY5Y neuroblastoma cells is associated with increased neurotrophin production. *Neurodegener Dis.,* 8(5), 300-309.

Danger, J.M., Tonon, M.C., Jenks, B.G., Saint-Pierre, S., Martel, J.C., Fasolo, A., Breton, B., Quirion, R., Pelletier, G. & Vaudry, H. (1990). Neropeptide Y: localization in the central nervous system and neuroendocrine functions. *Fundam Clin Pharmacol.,* 4(3), 307-340. Review

Dawbarn, D., De Quidt, M.E. & Emson, P.C. (1985). Survival of basal ganglia neuropeptide Y-somatostatin neurones in Huntington's disease. *Brain Res.,* 340(2), 251-260.

Decressac, M., Pain, S., Chabeauti, P.Y., Frangeul, L., Thiriet, N., Herzog, H., Vergote, J., Chalon, S., Jaber, M. & Gaillard, A. (2011a). Neuroprotection by neuropeptide Y in cell and animal models of Parkinson's disease. *Neurobiol Aging.* [Epub ahead of print]

Decressac, M., Wright, B., David, B., Tyers, P., Jaber, M., Barker, R.A. & Gaillard, A. (2011b). Exogenous neuropeptide Y promotes in vivo hippocampal neurogenesis. *Hippocampus,* 21(3), 233-238. doi: 10.1002/hipo.20765.

Decressac, M., Wright, B., Tyers, P., Gaillard, A. & Barker, R.A. (2010). Neuropeptide Y modifies the disease course in the R6/2 transgenic model of Huntington's disease. *Exp Neurol.,* 226(1), 24-32.

Diez, M., Danner, S., Frey, P., Sommer, B., Staufenbiel, M., Wiederhold, K.H. & Hökfelt, T. (2003). Neuropeptide alterations in the hippocampal formation and cortex of transgenic mice overexpressing beta-amyloid precursor protein (APP) with the Swedish double mutation (APP23). *Neurobiol Dis.,* 14(3), 579-594.

Diez, M., Koistinaho, J., Kahn, K., Games, D. & Hökfelt, T. (2000). Neuropeptides in hippocampus and cortex in transgenic mice overexpressing V717F beta-amyloid precursor protein--initial observations. *Neuroscience,* 100(2), 259-286.

Domin, H., Kajta, M. & Śmiałowska, M. (2006). Neuroprotective effects of MTEP, a selective mGluR5 antagonists and neuropeptide Y on the kainate-induced toxicity in primary neuronal cultures. *Pharmacol Rep.,* 58(6), 846-858.

Doods, H., Gaida, W., Wieland, H.A., Dollinger, H., Schnorrenberg, G., Esser, F., Engel, W., Eberlein, W. & Rudolf K. (1999). BIIE0246: a selective and high affinity neuropeptide Y Y(2) receptor antagonist. *Eur J Pharmacol.,* 384(2-3), R3-5.

Dugich-Djordjevic, M.M., Tocco, G., Lapchak, P.A., Pasinetti, G.M., Najm, I., Baudry, M. & Hefti, F. (1992). Regionally specific and rapid increases in brain-derived neurotrophic factor messenger RNA in the adult rat brain following seizures induced by systemic administration of kainic acid. *Neuroscience,* 47(2), 303-315.

Dumont, Y., Cadieux A., Doods H., Fournier A. & Quirion R. (2000). Potent and selective tools to investigate neuropeptide Y receptors in the central and peripheral nervous systems: BIB03304 (Y1) and CGP71683A (Y5). *Can J Physiol Pharmacol.,* 78(2), 116-125.

Dumont, Y., Martel, J.C., Fournier, A., St-Pierre, S. & Quirion, R. (1992). Neuropeptide Y and neuropeptide Y receptor subtypes in brain and peripheral tissues. *Prog Neurobiol.,* 38(2), 125-167. Review.

Duszczyk, M., Ziembowicz, A., Gadamski, R., Wieronska, J.M., Smialowska, M.& Lazarewicz, J.W. (2009). Changes in the NPY immunoreactivity in gerbil hippocampus after hypoxic and ischemic preconditioning. *Neuropeptides,* 43(1), 31-39.

Edvinsson, L., Minthon, L., Ekman, R. & Gustafson, L. (1993). Neuropeptides in cerebrospinal fluid of patients with Alzheimer's disease and dementia with frontotemporal lobe degeneration. *Dementia,* 4(3-4), 167-171.

Engber, T.M., Boldry, R.C., Kuo, S. & Chase, T.N. (1992). Dopaminergic modulation of striatal neuropeptides: differential effects of D1 and D2 receptor stimulation on somatostatin, neuropeptide Y, neurotensin, dynorphin and enkephalin. *Brain Res.,* 581(2), 261-268.

Ericsson, A., Schalling, M., McIntyre, K.R., Lundberg, J.M., Larhammar, D., Seroogy, K., Hökfelt, T. & Persson, H. (1987). Detection of neuropeptide Y and its mRNA in megakaryocytes: enhanced levels in certain autoimmune mice. *Proc Natl Acad Sci U S A.,* 84(16), 5585-5589.

Everitt, B.J. & Hökfelt, T. (1989). The coexistence of neuropeptide Y with other peptides and amines in the central nervous system, In: *Neuropeptide Y,* Mutt, V., Hokfelt, T., Fuxe, K. & Lundberg, J.M. (Ed.), pp. 61-71, Raven Press, New York.

Fedrizzi, L. & Carafoli, E. (2011). Ca2+ dysfunction in neurodegenerative disorders: Alzheimer's disease. *Biofactors.,* 37(3), 189-96. doi: 10.1002/biof.157. Review.

Ferkany, J.W. & Coyle, J.T. (1983). Kainic acid selectively stimulates the release of endogenous excitatory acidic amino acids. *J Pharmacol Exp Ther.,* 225(2), 399-406.

Figueredo-Cardenas, G., Anderson, K.D., Chen, Q., Veenman, C.L. & Reiner, A. (1994). Relative survival of striatal projection neurons and interneurons after intrastriatal injection of quinolinic acid in rats. *Exp Neurol.,* 129(1), 37-56.

Fuhlendorff, J., Gether, U., Aakerlund, L., Langeland-Johansen, N., Thøgersen, H., Melberg, S.G., Olsen, U.B., Thastrup, O. & Schwartz T.W. (1990). [Leu31, Pro34]neuropeptide Y: a specific Y1 receptor agonist. *Proc Natl Acad Sci U S A.*, 87(1), 182-186.

Gariboldi, M., Conti, M., Cavaleri, D., Samanin, R. & Vezzani, A. (1998). Anticonvulsant properties of BIBP3226, a non-peptide selective antagonist at neuropeptide Y Y1 receptors. *Eur J Neurosci.*, 10(2), 757-759.

Garthwaite, J. (1991). Glutamate, nitric oxide and cell-cell signalling in the nervous system. *Trends Neurosci.*, 14(2), 60-67. Review.

Gelfo, F., De Bartolo, P., Tirassa, P., Croce, N., Caltagirone, C., Petrosini, L. (2011). Angelucci, F. Intraperitoneal injection of neuropeptide Y (NPY) alters neurotrophin rat hypothalamic levels: Implications for NPY potential role in stress-related disorders. *Peptides,* 32(6), 1320-1323.

Gobbi, M., Monhemius, R., Samanin, R., Mennini, T. & Vezzani, A. (1996). Cellular localization of neuropeptide-Y receptors in the rat hippocampus: long-term effects of limbic seizures. *Neuroreport,* 7(9), 1475-1480.

Glover, I.D., Barlow, D.J., Pitts, J.E., Wood, S.P., Tickle, I.J., Blundell, T.L., Tatemoto, K., Kimmel, J.R., Wollmer, A., Strassburger, W. & et al. (1984). Conformational studies on the pancreatic polypeptide hormone family. *Eur J Biochem.*, 142(2), 379-385.

Gray, T.S. & Morley, J.E. (1986). Neuropeptide Y: anatomical distribution and possible function in mammalian nervous system. *Life Sci.*, 38(5), 389-401.

Greber, S., Schwarzer, C. & Sperk, G. (1994). Neuropeptide Y inhibits potassium-stimulated glutamate release through Y2 receptors in rat hippocampal slices in vitro. *Br J Pharmacol.,*113(3), 737-740.

Hansel, D.E., Eipper, B.A. & Ronnett, G.V. (2001). Neuropeptide Y functions as a neuroproliferative factor. *Nature,* 410(6831), 940-944.

Heilig, M., Sjögren, M., Blennow, K., Ekman, R. & Wallin, A. (1995). Cerebrospinal fluid neuropeptides in Alzheimer's disease and vascular dementia. *Biol Psychiatry,* 38(4), 210-216.

Howell, O.W., Doyle, K., Goodman, J.H., Scharfman, H.E., Herzog, H., Pringle, A., Beck-Sickinger, A.G. & Gray, W.P. (2005). Neuropeptide Y stimulates neuronal precursor proliferation in the post-natal and adult dentate gyrus. *J Neurochem.,* 93(3), 560-570.

Howell, O.W., Silva, S., Scharfman, H.E., Sosunov, A.A., Zaben, M., Shatya, A., McKhann, G. 2nd, Herzog, H., Laskowski, A. & Gray, W.P. (2007). Neuropeptide Y is important for basal and seizure-induced precursor cell proliferation in the hippocampus. *Neurobiol Dis.,* 26(1), 174-188.

Humpel, C., Wetmore, C. & Olson, L. (1993). Regulation of brain-derived neurotrophic factor messenger RNA and protein at the cellular level in pentylenetetrazol-induced epileptic seizures. *Neuroscience,* 53(4), 909-918.

Kerkerian, L., Bosler, O., Pelletier, G. & Nieoullon, A (1986). Striatal neuropeptide Y neurones are under the influence of the nigrostriatal dopaminergic pathway: immunohistochemical evidence. *Neurosci Lett.,* 66(1), 106-112.

Kerkerian, L., Salin, P. & Nieoullon, A (1988). Pharmacological characterization of dopaminergic influence on expression of neuropeptide Y immunoreactivity by rat striatal neurons. *Neuroscience,* 26(3), 809-817.

Klapstein, G.J. & Colmers, W.F. (1992). 4-Aminopyridine and low Ca2+ differentiate presynaptic inhibition mediated by neuropeptide Y, baclofen and 2-chloroadenosine in rat hippocampal CA1 in vitro. *Br J Pharmacol.*, 105(2), 470-474.

Klapstein, G.J. & Colmers, W.F. (1997). Neuropeptide Y suppresses epileptiform activity in rat hippocampus in vitro. *J Neurophysiol.*, 78(3), 1651-1661.

Koide, S., Onishi, H., Hashimoto, H., Kai, T. & Yamagami, S.(1995). Plasma neuropeptide Y is reduced in patients with Alzheimer's disease. *Neurosci Lett.*, 198(2), 149-151.

Kopp, J., Xu, Z.Q., Zhang, X., Pedrazzini, T., Herzog, H., Kresse, A., Wong, H., Walsh, J.H. & Hökfelt, T. (2002). Expression of the neuropeptide Y Y1 receptor in the CNS of rat and of wild-type and Y1 receptor knock-out mice. Focus on immunohistochemical localization. *Neuroscience*, 111(3), 443-532.

Kowall, N.W. & Beal, M.F. (1988). Cortical somatostatin, neuropeptide Y, and NADPH diaphorase neurons: normal anatomy and alterations in Alzheimer's disease. *Ann Neurol.*, 23(2), 105-114.

Kumar, U. (2004). Differential expression of Huntington's disease gene (IT15) mRNA in developing rat brain. *Brain Res Mol Brain Res.*, 128(1), 39-47.

Kumar, U., Asotra, K., Patel, S.C. & Patel, Y.C. (1997). Expression of NMDA receptor-1 (NR1) and huntingtin in striatal neurons which colocalize somatostatin, neuropeptide Y, and NADPH diaphorase: a double-label histochemical and immunohistochemical study. *Exp Neurol.*, 145(2 Pt 1), 412-424.

Luthi-Carter, R., Strand, A., Peters, N.L., Solano, S.M., Hollingsworth, Z.R., Menon, A.S., Frey, A.S., Spektor, B,S., Penney, E.B., Schilling ,G., Ross, C.A., Borchelt, D.R., Tapscott, S.J., Young, A.B., Cha, J.H. & Olson, J.M. (2000). Decreased expression of striatal signaling genes in a mouse model of Huntington's disease. *Hum Mol Genet.*, 9(9), 1259-1271.

Madsen, T.M., Woldbye, D.P., Bolwig, T.G. & Mikkelsen, J.D. (1999). Kainic acid seizure suppression by neuropeptide Y is not correlated to immediate early gene mRNA levels in rats. *Neurosci Lett.*, 271(1), 21-24.

Malva, J.O., Carvalho, A.P. & Carvalho, C.M. (1998). Kainate receptors in hippocampal CA3 subregion: evidence for a role in regulating neurotransmitter release. *Neurochem Int.*, 32(1), 1-6. Review.

Marksteiner, J., Lassmann, H., Saria, A., Humpel, C., Meyer, D.K. & Sperk, G. (1990). Neuropeptide Levels after Pentylenetetrazol Kindling in the Rat. *Eur J Neurosci.*,2(1), 98-103.

Marsh, D.J., Baraban, S.C., Hollopeter, G. & Palmiter, R.D. (1999). Role of the Y5 neuropeptide Y receptor in limbic seizures. *Proc Natl Acad Sci U S A.*, 96(23), 13518-13523.

Martel, J.C., Alagar, R., Robitaille, Y. & Quirion, R. (1990). Neuropeptide Y receptor binding sites in human brain. Possible alteration in Alzheimer's disease. *Brain Res.*, 519(1-2), 228-235.

Martignoni, E., Blandini, F., Petraglia, F., Pacchetti, C., Bono, G. & Nappi, G. (1992). Cerebrospinal fluid norepinephrine, 3-methoxy-4-hydroxyphenylglycol and neuropeptide Y levels in Parkinson's disease, multiple system atrophy and dementia of the Alzheimer type. *J Neural Transm Park Dis Dement Sect.*, 4(3), 191-205.

Matsui, T., Nagafuji, T., Kumanishi, T. & Asano, T. (1999). Role of nitric oxide in pathogenesis underlying ischemic cerebral damage. *Cell Mol Neurobiol.*, 19(1), 177-189. Review.

Mazurek, M.F, Garside, S. & Beal, M.F. (1997). Cortical peptide changes in Huntington's disease may be independent of striatal degeneration. *Ann Neurol.*, 41(4), 540-547.

McQuiston, A.R. & Colmers W.F. (1996). Neuropeptide Y2 receptors inhibit the frequency of spontaneous but not miniature EPSCs in CA3 pyramidal cells of rat hippocampus. *J Neurophysiol.*, 76(5), 3159-3168.

McQuiston, A.R., Petrozzino, J.J., Connor, J.A. & Colmers, W.F. (1996). Neuropeptide Y1 receptors inhibit N-type calcium currents and reduce transient calcium increases in rat dentate granule cells. *J Neurosci.*, 16(4), 1422-1429.

Michel, M.C., Beck-Sickinger, A., Cox, H., Doods, H.N., Herzog, H., Larhammar, D., Quirion, R., Schwartz, T. & Westfall, T. (1998). XVI. International Union of Pharmacology recommendations for the nomenclature of neuropeptide Y, peptide YY, and pancreatic polypeptide receptors. *Pharmacol Rev.*, 50(1), 143-150. Review.

Midgley, L.P., Wagstaff, J.D., Singh, N.A., Bush, L.G., Gibb, J.W. & Hanson, G.R. (1994). Dynamic dopaminergic regulation of neuropeptide Y systems in discrete striatal and accumbens regions. *Eur J Pharmacol.*, 251(2-3), 191-199.

Minthon, L., Edvinsson, L., Ekman, R. & Gustafson, L. (1990). Neuropeptide levels in Alzheimer's disease and dementia with frontotemporal degeneration. *J Neural Transm Suppl.*, 30, 57-67.

Nawa, H., Pelleymounter, M.A. & Carnahan, J. (1994). Intraventricular administration of BDNF increases neuropeptide expression in newborn rat brain. *J Neurosci.*, 14(6), 3751-3765.

Nilsson, C.L., Brinkmalm, A., Minthon, L., Blennow, K. & Ekman, R. (2001). Processing of neuropeptide Y, galanin, and somatostatin in the cerebrospinal fluid of patients with Alzheimer's disease and frontotemporal dementia. *Peptides,* 22(12), 2105-2112.

Nordberg, A. (1992). Neuroreceptor changes in Alzheimer disease. *Cerebrovasc Brain Metab Rev.*, 4(4), 303-328. Review

Pereira, C., Agostinho, P., Moreira, P.I., Cardoso, S.M. & Oliveira, C.R. (2005). Alzheimer's disease-associated neurotoxic mechanisms and neuroprotective strategies. *Curr Drug Targets CNS Neurol Disord.*, 4(4), 383-403. Review.

Persson, H., Ericsson, A., Hemsen, A., Hokfelt, T., Larhammar, D., Lundberg, J.M., McIntyre, K.R. & Schalling, M. (1989). Expression of neuropeptide tyrosine (NPY) messenger RNA and peptide in non-neuronal cells, In: *Neuropeptide Y,* Mutt, V., Hokfelt, T., Fuxe, K. & Lundberg, J.M. (Ed.), pp. 43-50, ISBN 0-88167-556-3, Raven Press, New York.

Oddo, S., Billings, L., Kesslak, J.P., Cribbs, D.H. & LaFerla, F.M. (2004). Abeta immunotherapy leads to clearance of early, but not late, hyperphosphorylated tau aggregates via the proteasome. *Neuron,* 43(3), 321-332.

Oddo, S., Caccamo, A., Kitazawa, M., Tseng, B.P. & LaFerla, F.M. (2003). Amyloid deposition precedes tangle formation in a triple transgenic model of Alzheimer's disease. *Neurobiol Aging.*, 24(8), 1063-1070.

Qian, J., Colmers, W.F. & Saggau, P. (1997). Inhibition of synaptic transmission by neuropeptide Y in rat hippocampal area CA1: modulation of presynaptic Ca2+ entry. *J Neurosci.*, 17(21), 8169-8177.

Reibel, S., Vivien-Roels, B., Lê, B.T., Larmet, Y., Carnahan, J., Marescaux, C. & Depaulis, A. (2000). Overexpression of neuropeptide Y induced by brain-derived neurotrophic factor in the rat hippocampus is long lasting. *Eur J Neurosci.*, 12(2), 595-605.

Rose, J.B., Crews, L., Rockenstein, E., Adame, A., Mante, M., Hersh, L.B., Gage, F.H., Spencer, B., Potkar, R., Marr, R.A. & Masliah, E. (2009). Neuropeptide Y fragments derived from neprilysin processing are neuroprotective in a transgenic model of Alzheimer's disease. *J Neurosci.*, 29(4), 1115-1125.

Rudolf K., Eberlein W., Engel W., Wieland H.A., Willim K.D., Entzeroth M., Wienen W., Beck-Sickinger A.G. & Doods H.N. (1994). The first highly potent and selective non-peptide neuropeptide Y Y1 receptor antagonist: BIBP3226. *Eur J Pharmacol.*, 271(2-3), R11-13.

Schwarzer, C., Sperk, G., Samanin, R., Rizzi, M., Gariboldi, M. & Vezzani, A. (1996). Neuropeptides-immunoreactivity and their mRNA expression in kindling: functional implications for limbic epileptogenesis. *Brain Res Brain Res Rev.*, 22(1), 27-50. Review.

Sieradzan, K.A. & Mann, D.M. (2001). The selective vulnerability of nerve cells in Huntington's disease. *Neuropathol Appl Neurobiol.*, 27(1), 1-21

Silva, A.P., Carvalho, A.P., Carvalho, C.M. & Malva, J.O. (2001). Modulation of intracellular calcium changes and glutamate release by neuropeptide Y1 and Y2 receptors in the rat hippocampus: differential effects in CA1, CA3 and dentate gyrus. *J Neurochem.*, 79(2), 286-296.

Silva, A.P., Carvalho, A.P., Carvalho, C.M. & Malva, J.O. (2003a). Functional interaction between neuropeptide Y receptors and modulation of calcium channels in the rat hippocampus. *Neuropharmacology*, 44(2), 282-292.

Silva, A.P., Cavadas, C. & Grouzmann, E. (2002). Neuropeptide Y and its receptors as potential therapeutic drug targets. *Clin Chim Acta.*, 326(1-2), 3-25. Review.

Silva, A.P., Pinheiro, P.S., Carvalho, A.P., Carvalho, C.M., Jakobsen, B., Zimmer, J. & Malva, J.O. (2003b). Activation of neuropeptide Y receptors is neuroprotective against excitotoxicity in organotypic hippocampal slice cultures. *FASEB J.*, 17(9), 1118-1120.

Silva, A.P., Xapelli, S., Grouzmann, E. & Cavadas, C. (2005a). The putative neuroprotective role of neuropeptide Y in the central nervous system. *Curr Drug Targets CNS Neurol Disord.*, 4(4), 331-347. Review.

Silva, A.P., Xapelli, S., Pinheiro, P.S., Ferreira, R., Lourenço, J., Cristóvão, A., Grouzmann, E., Cavadas, C., Oliveira, C.R. & Malva, J.O. (2005b). Up-regulation of neuropeptide Y levels and modulation of glutamate release through neuropeptide Y receptors in the hippocampus of kainate-induced epileptic rats. *J Neurochem.*, 93(1), 163-170.

Shirwany, N.A., Payette, D., Xie, J. & Guo, Q. (2007). The amyloid beta ion channel hypothesis of Alzheimer's disease. *Neuropsychiatr Dis Treat.*, 3(5), 597-612.

Śmialowska, M. (1995). An inhibitory dopaminergic regulation of the neuropeptide Y immunoreactivity expression in the rat cerebral cortex neurons. *Neuroscience*, 66(3), 589-595.

Śmialowska, M., Bijak, M., Sopala, M. & Tokarski K. (1996). Inhibitory effect of NPY on the picrotoxin-induced activity in the hippocampus: a behavioural and electrophysiological study. *Neuropeptides*, 30(1), 7-12.

Śmialowska, M., Domin, H., Zieba, B., Koźniewska, E., Michalik, R., Piotrowski, P. & Kajta, M. (2009). Neuroprotective effects of neuropeptide Y-Y2 and Y5 receptor agonists in vitro and in vivo. *Neuropeptides.*, 43(3), 235-249.

Śmiałowska, M., Wierońska, J.M. & Szewczyk B. (2003). Neuroprotective effect of NPY on kainate neurotoxicity in the hippocampus. *Pol J Pharmacol.*, 55(6), 979-986.

Stoddard, S.L., Tyce, G.M., Ahlskog, J.E., Zinsmeister, A.R., Nelson, D.K. & Carmichael, S.W. (1991). Decreased levels of [Met]enkephalin, neuropeptide Y, substance P, and vasoactive intestinal peptide in parkinsonian adrenal medulla. *Exp Neurol.*, 114(1), 23-27.

Sun, L. & Miller, R.J. (1999). Multiple neuropeptide Y receptors regulate K+ and Ca2+ channels in acutely isolated neurons from the rat arcuate nucleus. *J Neurophysiol.*, 81(3), 1391-1403.

Takei, N., Sasaoka, K., Higuchi, H., Endo, Y. & Hatanaka, H. (1996). BDNF increases the expression of neuropeptide Y mRNA and promotes differentiation/maturation of neuropeptide Y-positive cultured cortical neurons from embryonic and postnatal rats. *Brain Res Mol Brain Res.*, 37(1-2), 283-289.

Tatemoto, K. (1982). Neuropeptide Y: complete amino acid sequence of the brain peptide. *Proc Natl Acad Sci U S A.*, 79(18), 5485-5489.

Thiriet, N., Deng, X., Solinas, M., Ladenheim, B., Curtis, W., Goldberg, S.R., Palmiter, R.D. & Cadet, J.L. (2005). Neuropeptide Y protects against methamphetamine-induced neuronal apoptosis in the mouse striatum. *J Neurosci.*, 25(22), 5273-5279.

Vezzani, A., Sperk, G. & Colmers, W.F. (1999). Neuropeptide Y: emerging evidence for a functional role in seizure modulation. *Trends Neurosci.*, 22(1), 25-30. Review.

Wang, Q., Yu, S., Simonyi, A., Sun, G.Y. & Sun, A.Y. (2005). Kainic acid-mediated excitotoxicity as a model for neurodegeneration. *Mol Neurobiol.*, 31(1-3), 3-16. Review.

Wang, S.J. (2005). Activation of neuropeptide Y Y1 receptors inhibits glutamate release through reduction of voltage-dependent Ca2+ entry in the rat cerebral cortex nerve terminals: suppression of this inhibitory effect by the protein kinase C-dependent facilitatory pathway. *Neuroscience*, 134(3), 987-1000.

Wettstein, J.G., Earley, B. & Junien, J.L. (1995). Central nervous system pharmacology of neuropeptide Y. *Pharmacol Ther.*, 65(3), 397-414. Review.

Wieland, H.A., Engel, W., Eberlein, W., Rudolf, K. & Doods, H.N. (1998). Subtype selectivity of the novel nonpeptide neuropeptide Y Y1 receptor antagonist BIBO 3304 and its effect on feeding in rodents. *Br J Pharmacol.*, 125(3), 549-555.

Wirth, M.J., Patz, S. & Wahle, P. (2005). Transcellular induction of neuropeptide Y expression by NT4 and BDNF. *Proc Natl Acad Sci U S A.*, 102(8), 3064-3069.

Woldbye, D.P., Larsen, P.J., Mikkelsen, J.D., Klemp, K., Madsen, T.M. & Bolwig, T.G. (1997). Powerful inhibition of kainic acid seizures by neuropeptide Y via Y5-like receptors. *Nat Med.*, 3(7), 761-764.

Woldbye, D.P. & Kokaia, M. (2004). Neuropeptide Y and seizures: effects of exogenously applied ligands. *Neuropeptides*, 38(4), 253-260. Review.

Wu, Y.F. & Li, S.B. (2005). Neuropeptide Y expression in mouse hippocampus and its role in neuronal excitotoxicity. *Acta Pharmacol Sin.*, 26(1), 63-68.

Xapelli, S., Agasse, F., Ferreira, R., Silva, A.P. & Malva, J.O. (2006). Neuropeptide Y as an endogenous antiepileptic, neuroprotective and pro-neurogenic peptide. *Recent Pat CNS Drug Discov.*, 1(3), 315-324. Review.

Xapelli, S., Bernardino, L., Ferreira, R., Grade, S., Silva, A.P., Salgado, J.R., Cavadas, C., Grouzmann, E., Poulsen, F.R., Jakobsen, B., Oliveira, C.R., Zimmer, J. & Malva, J.O. (2008). Interaction between neuropeptide Y (NPY) and brain-derived neurotrophic factor in NPY-mediated neuroprotection against excitotoxicity: a role for microglia. *Eur J Neurosci.*, 27(8), 2089-2102.

Xapelli, S., Silva, A.P., Ferreira, R. & Malva, J.O (2007). Neuropeptide Y can rescue neurons from cell death following the application of an excitotoxic insult with kainate in rat organotypic hippocampal slice cultures. *Peptides*, 28(2), 288-294.

Yoshimura, R., Ito, K. & Endo, Y. (2009). Differentiation/maturation of neuropeptide Y neurons in the corpus callosum is promoted by brain-derived neurotrophic factor in mouse brain slice cultures. *Neurosci Lett.*, 450(3), 262-265.

Zeron, M.M., Hansson, O., Chen, N., Wellington, C.L., Leavitt, B.R., Brundin, P., Hayden, M.R. & Raymond, L.A. (2002). Increased sensitivity to N-methyl-D-aspartate receptor-mediated excitotoxicity in a mouse model of Huntington's disease. *Neuron*, 33(6), 849-860.

3

Structural and Computational Studies of Interactions of Metals with Amyloid Beta

V. Chandana Epa
CSIRO Materials Science & Engineering,
Preventative Health Flagship and the CRC for Mental Health,
Parkville, Victoria,
Australia

1. Introduction

With rapidly ageing populations, dementia caused by neurodegenerative diseases has become a global socioeconomic issue. Globally, more than 24 million people were suffering from dementia in 2005 (C. Ferri et al.,2005). Alzheimer's disease (AD) is the most common cause of dementia. While characterized by the presence of Amyloid-beta (Aβ) peptide plaques in the brain (Masters and Beyreuther, 2006), a major source of the neurotoxicity in AD is now believed to be due to the action of soluble Aβ oligomers (Crouch et al., 2008). Aβ is generated from the amyloid precursor protein (APP) by the action of β- and γ- secretases, and yields peptides 39-43 amino acid residues long, with Aβ(1-40) and Aβ(1-42) the most common. Aβ(1-42) has the primary sequence $D_1AEFRH_6DSGY_{10}E_{11}VH_{13}H_{14}QK_{16}LVFFAEDVGSNK_{28}GAIIGLM_{35}VGGVVIA_{42}$). Structural characterization of the formation of the Aβ oligomers is currently the subject of intensive research. Among the possible mechanisms are those mediated by the interaction of Aβ with metal ions. This includes both redox-active metals such as Copper, and Iron, as well as redox-inactive metals such as Zinc. For example, interaction of Cu(II) (i.e. Cu^{2+}) with Aβ in the presence of reducing agents leads to the production of reactive oxygen species (ROS). This in turn can generate toxic soluble Aβ oligomers via the formation of di-tyrosine cross-linked Aβ dimers (Barnham et al., 2004). The Copper-chelating compound PBT2 has shown efficacy and safety in Phase IIa clinical trials (Adlard et al., 2008). More recently, Platinum and Ruthenium compounds have been synthesized and shown to ablate Aβ-mediated neurotoxicity. Clearly, interaction of metals with Aβ plays an important role in the aetiology of AD and is very relevant to the design of effective therapeutics. Knowledge of the atomic structure of metals bound to the Aβ peptide would greatly facilitate the design of such chemical entities and assist in the elucidation of the mechanisms of neurotoxicity.

This chapter will review important recent developments in determination of the structure of Aβ bound to transition metals (in different oxidation states) and organometallic compounds. While X-ray crystallography has so far been unsuccessful in determining the structure of any metal-Aβ complexes, methods such as NMR (nuclear magnetic resonance), EPR (electron paramagnetic resonance), and XAS (X-ray Absorption Spectroscopy) have been used, with varying degrees of success, in the structural determinations of metal binding sites and interactions of Aβ. These experiments have been carried out on human and rat or murine Aβ, mutants of Aβ, and on constructs of different lengths, for example 1-16, 1-40, and 1-42. In a number of instances, these experiments have been supplemented by computational studies, usually *ab initio* quantum mechanical calculations. Computational simulations have also been instrumental in shedding light on how redox-active metals may initiate mechanisms of toxicity via binding to Aβ. This review will also discuss how recent computational studies have helped in the elucidation of metal interactions of Aβ and the interplay between theory/computation and experiment in furthering our understanding of the atomic structures of metal-Aβ complexes. The following sections of this chapter will consider, in turn, the interactions of amyloid beta with the transition metals copper, iron, and zinc. This will be followed by a section of the interaction of Aβ with organometallic compounds containing Pt, Ru, Rh, and Ir, before concluding the chapter.

2. Copper and amyloid beta

Copper interaction with amyloid-beta has been the subject of more experimental and computational investigations than any other metal. This is not only because plaques in AD brains are significantly enriched in copper, and Cu(II) binding facilitates aggregation of Aβ in vitro (Atwood et al., 1998), but also because as a very redox-active metal it plays a direct role in the generation of toxic reactive oxygen species (ROS).

Cu(II) concentration in the synaptic cleft can reach as much as 15 μM following post-synaptic release (Duce and Bush, 2010). Lovell et al. (1998) found that senile plaques in AD brains are enriched in copper almost five times compared with normal neuropils. AD brains also typically exhibit signs of oxidative stress such as enhanced levels of dityrosine species, 4-hydroxy nonenal, 8-hydroxy guanosine, protein carbonyl, and lipid peroxidation species (Sayre et al., 1997, Hensley et al., 1998). Cu(II) bound to Aβ can, in the presence of reducing agents such as ascorbate and glutathione, abundant in the brain, activate and reduce molecular O_2 to produce H_2O_2. During this redox cycle, Cu(II) bound to Aβ first gets reduced to Cu(I) by the reducing agent, and then gets oxidized back to Cu(II). This H_2O_2 produced can then lead to a cascade of ROS being generated through Fenton-like and Haber-Weiss chemistry (Smith et al., 2007). Attack by these very reactive free radicals on proteins, nucleic acids, and lipids would lead to the formation of the oxidatively modified products isolated from AD brain tissue. The amyloid beta peptide is itself modified by the ROS, leading for example, hydroxylation of the histidine side-chains and the oxidation of the methionine side-chain (Nadal et al. 2008). The most important modification of Aβ may be at the Tyrosine 10 position. The tyrosyl radicals produced may combine, leading to covalently cross-linked Aβ dimers. Barnham et al. (2004) showed that the Y10A mutant of Aβ was not toxic in neuronal cell assays. This was the case despite Y10A mutant producing H_2O_2 at half the rate of that by the wild-type peptide. Cappai and Barnham (2008) proposed that the covalently cross-linked Aβ oligomers produced by this Cu(II) catalyzed redox process is the genesis of Aβ-induced neurotoxicity. Hence, it is possible that the Cu(II)/Aβ redox chemistry initiates the generation of toxic soluble Aβ oligomers (which are toxic by mechanisms as of yet undetermined) rather than the neurodegeneration in AD being directly the result of the ROS generation.

Early reports (Huang et al., 1999a, 1999b) of Cu(II)/Aβ generation of H_2O_2 appeared to indicate that this process could occur in the absence of any external reducing agents, presumably via the involvement of Met 35 residue of the peptide itself. They also reported a rather high reduction potential (E^0) of +0.74-0.79 V versus the Normal Hydrogen Electrode (NHE) for the Cu(II)/Aβ system. However, later cyclic voltammetry experiments by Jiang et al. (2007) established this value to be +0.28 V. The latter also point out that the measured oxidation potential value for Met 35 makes it unlikely to act as a reductant in vitro. Likewise, the standard reduction potential values of 0.370 V, 0.372 V, and 0.384 V vs. NHE for dopamine, epinephrine, and norepinephrine, respectively, render them incapable of acting as external reducing agents in the generation of H_2O_2 by Cu(II)/Aβ. X-ray Absorption spectroscopy (XAS) studies performed on the Cu(II)/Aβ(1-16)/dopamine system by Streltsov and Varghese (2008) confirmed this when they did not observe the characteristic Cu(I) XANES (X-ray Absorption Near Edge Spectroscopy) spectra. On the other hand, the reduction potential for ascorbic acid, 0.051-0.058 V vs. NHE allows the oxidation of ascorbate by Cu(II)/Aβ to be thermodynamically favourable. Finally, Nadal et al. (2008) observed that the Cu(II)/Aβ/Ascorbate system generated the same amount of H_2O_2 as Cu(II) /Ascorbate (in the absence of Aβ) and inferred that Aβ acts as an antioxidant or free radical scavenger by quenching the hydroxyl ions produced by Cu(II)/Ascorbate. Their ^{1}H NMR spectra showed that the imidazoles of the histidine residues of Aβ had been oxidized to 2-oxo imidazoles, and also that Met 35 sulfur atom had been oxidized. It should be noted, however, that they did not investigate the kinetics of H_2O_2 production, i.e. did not compare the relative rates of H_2O_2 formation by Cu(II)/Ascorbate versus that of Cu(II)/Aβ/Ascorbate. This group also states that reduction of Cu(II) to Cu(I) by Aβ occurs in the absence of ascorbate using an bathocuproinedisulfonic acid assay. This is contrary to the conclusions drawn from the reduction potential measurements of Jiang et al. (2007) as discussed above. Moreover, the XAS experiments by Streltsov et al. (2008) did not show any evidence for the reduction of Cu(II) by Aβ alone in the absence of any addition of a reducing agent. The effect on the binding of Cu(II) and the neurotoxicity of such oxidative modifications of Aβ is also of some interest.

2.1 Cu(II) structural and modelling studies

With the critical role Cu(II) plays in the properties of Aβ when it is bound to the peptide, considerable effort has gone into the structural determination of the Cu(II) binding site on Aβ. While there have been a number of reports of widely varying values for the binding affinity of Cu(II) for Aβ, one of the more reliable was the study by Hatcher et al. (2008). Their isothermal calorimetry (ITC) experiments for Aβ(1-40) at 37 C gave values of 1.1×10^9 M^{-1} and 2.4×10^9 M^{-1} at pH 7.2 and pH 7.4, respectively. Under the same conditions Aβ(1-16) gave similar binding constants, indicating that the metal ion binding site is located in this N-terminal fragment. The stoichiometry between Cu(II) and Aβ was 1:1. This is likely the binding at the higher affinity site since there are also several findings in the literature of Aβ binding more than 1 mole equivalent of Cu(II). For example, Caine et al. (2007) found that their maltose binding protein (MBP) - Aβ(1-42) fusion protein bound Cu(II) with a stoichiometry of 1:2. There has been some speculation as to the location of the second, weaker affinity binding site of Cu(II), (which is most likely an intermolecular site), but the major effort, as discussed below, has been on the high affinity binding site.

Streltsov et al. (2008) used a combined extended X-ray Absorption Fine Structure - Density Functional Theory (EXAFS-DFT) approach in their study of the Cu(II) binding site in Aβ(1-16) where the experimental data was collected at 16.5 K with a metal:peptide ratio of 1:1 buffered to a pH of 7.4. As the initial data analysis indicated a first shell coordination number of 6, they computed with Density Functional Theory (DFT) (at B3LYP/LANL2DZ level) two different optimized geometries with 3N3O coordination: in each case the nitrogen coordination was via three histidine imidazoles while the oxygen coordination was with a glutamate carboxylate (bidentate) and a water molecule in one case, and with a tyrosine hydroxyl oxygen and two water molecules in the other case. Using these two models in the EXAFS spectra fitting and refinement they found that the fit was significantly better with the octahedral Cu(II)/Glu/3His/Wat geometry, where the three histidine N atoms (at distances of 1.9-2.1 Å from the Cu ion) and one of the Glu carboxylate O atoms (1.9 Å distant from the Cu) are in approximately square planar equatorial arrangement while the other carboxylate O atom (2.3 Å distant from the Cu) and the water O (2.0 Å distant from the Cu) are in an axial arrangement. Figure 1 shows the arrangement of Aβ residues at the Cu(II) binding site for a molecular mechanics (MM) model developed for Cu(II)/Aβ(1-16) using the EXAFS determined coordination distances as constraints. (No constraints were applied to the peptide termini.) In analogy with the NMR solution structure for Zn(II)/Aβ(1-16) by Zirah et al. (2006) (discussed in Section 4), the glutamate is taken as Glu 11. Streltsov et al. also found that their fit could be further improved by placing two more oxygen atoms (assumed as coming from the Asp 1 carboxylate) 4.4 Å distant from the Cu(II) and hydrogen-bonded to the axially placed water.

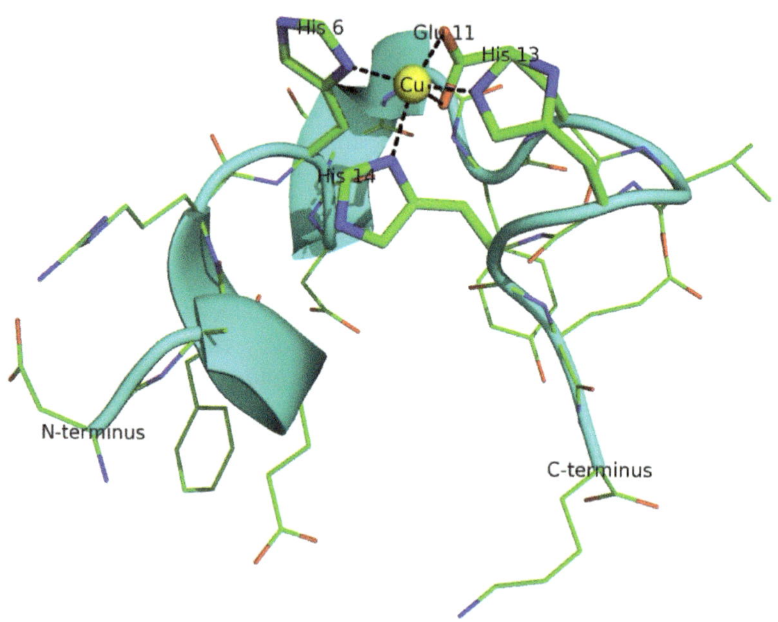

Fig. 1. Molecular model of Cu(II) bound to Aβ(1-16) from EXAFS-DFT studies of Streltsov et al. (2008).

Numerous experiments in the past have shown the importance of the histidine residues of Aβ to copper binding. Smith et al. (2006) reported the loss of Cu/Aβ-induced toxicity when the histidine imidazole δ or ε N atom is methylated. They reported the observation of a histidine -bridged Cu(II)/Aβ dimer by EPR spectroscopy at Cu:peptide ratios greater than 0.6:1. From the same laboratory, Smith et al. (2010) showed that the Aβ mutant H14A had no toxicity in primary neuronal cell cultures. Histidine-bridged Cu(II)/Aβ dimers were not seen in the EXAFS experiments of Streltsov et al.; however, as mentioned earlier this was at a Cu:peptide concentration ratio of 1:1. There is less evidence for the participation of Glu 11 in the Cu(II) binding. It is interesting to note that the x-ray crystal structure of quercetin 2,3-dioxygenase (Fusetti et al., 2002) contains a Cu(II) ion liganded by three histidines and a glutamate in a trigonal bipyramidal geometry. Furthermore, Hureau et al. (2011) very recently solved the x-ray crystal structure of Cu(II) bound to the peptide Gly-His-Lys, where Cu(II) displays a 3N1O coordination in the equatorial plane and a carboxylate O atom coordinating axially. Hence, the type of Cu(II) coordinating geometry proposed by Streltsov et al. has been seen in other contexts. However, the model would need to be validated by the results from EXAFS studies on Aβ mutants such as E11A.

EXAFS and X-ray crystallography result in structures that are mostly static. However, there is ample evidence that the binding of metal ions to Aβ is a dynamical process, and is exquisitely sensitive to the experimental conditions such as pH and type of buffer. Drew et al. (2009a, 2009b) in a series of experiments involving continuous wave electron paramagnetic spectroscopy (CW-EPR) and hyperfine sublevel correlation spectroscopy (HYSCORE) showed that Cu(II) binding to Aβ is pleomorphic in nature. Using a number of ^{15}N labelled and ^{13}C labelled Aβ(1-16) analogues, they found that the nature of the Cu(II) coordination shell was dependent on the pH. With these methodologies they conclude that at both pH 6.3 ("low pH") and at pH 8.0 ("high pH"), the equatorial coordination of Cu(II) is 3N1O. At low pH, two binding modes predominate ("component Ia" and "component Ib"): the imidazole N of His 6 and N-terminal Asp 1 NH_2 and carbonyl O coordinate in both modes while the imidazole N of His 13 in one mode and the imidazole N of His 14 in the other mode constitute the fourth ligand. Drew et al. model (2009b) for the binding mode at high pH ("component II") has the three histidine imidazole N atoms and the backbone carbonyl O atom of Ala 2 as the Cu(II) binding partners. They propose that this binding mode results in the polarization of the carbonyl C=O bond and facilitates the hydrolytic cleavage of the amide peptide bond between Ala 2 and Glu 3. This may be the possible source of Aβ(pyroglutamate 3-40 or 3-42) found in significant quantities in AD plaques. (Presumably glutaminyl cyclase in the brain cyclizes Glu 3 in the truncated N-terminal Aβ(3-40 or 3-42).) Moreover, ^{13}C, ^{15}N, and ^{17}O isotopic labelling provided no evidence of the involvement of the O atoms of the amino acid residues Glu 3, Asp 7, Glu 11 and Tyr 10. On the other hand, after performing both EPR and NMR experiments on isotopically labelled Aβ species, the Peter Faller group (Dorlet et al. 2009, Eury et al. 2011) proposed that the equatorial coordination of component II consists of one histidine imidazole N, N-terminal Asp 1 NH2, Ala 2 carbonyl O, and finally the deprotonated Asp1-Ala2 peptide backbone amide N atom. They also proposed that the carboxylate O atom of Asp 1 binds in an axial position. However, it should be noted that EPR measurements are less sensitive to axially coordinating ligands and the interpretation of data is not straightforward (Sarell et al., 2009, Faller and Hureau, 2009).

Binding of Cu(II) to rat or murine Aβ is also of some interest as rats do not display amyloid plaque deposits (Shivers et al., 1998). Compared to the human Aβ peptide, the rat or mouse sequence contains the mutations R5G, H13R, and Y10F. Again using isotopically labelled EPR and NMR studies, Eury et al. (2011) propose that the component II binding mode of Cu(II)/murine Aβ(1-16) is characterized by hexa-coordination, with the 3N1O equatorial binding via His 6 imidazole N, N-terminal Asp 1 NH2 and carbonyl O, and the (deprotonated) Gly 5-His 6 backbone amidyl N atom. The axial ligands proposed are the His 14 imidazole N atom and a carboxylate O atom from one of the acidic residues.

Recently, Streltsov et al. (2011) solved the x-ray crystal structure of Aβ(18-41) within the framework of the CDR3 loop of shark IgNAR (Ig New Antigen Receptor) single variable domain antibody. The Aβ(18-41) portion of the structure that is observed in the crystal structure is tetrameric. By constructing oligomeric models with these tetramer units (see Figure 2), they noticed that the neighbouring tetramers align Glu 22 and Asp 23 on the same face and speculate that these acidic side chains, along with contributions from solvent exposed backbone N and O atoms, may constitute the second, weaker affinity intermolecular Cu(II) binding site.

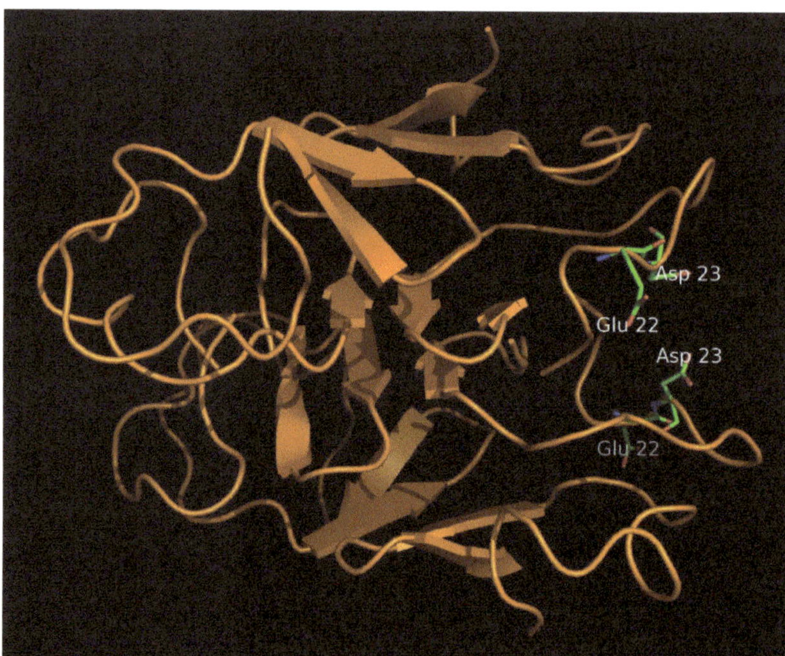

Fig. 2. Putative second binding site of Cu(II) from the Aβ(18-41) tetramer crystal structure of Streltsov et al. (2011)

2.2 Cu(I) structural and modelling studies

During the production of H_2O_2 by Copper/Abeta in the presence of a reducing agent, the oxidation state of copper continually cycles between the +2 and +1 states. Hence, the structure of Cu(I) bound to Aβ is also of interest. XAS and EPR experiments by Shearer and Szalai (2008) on Cu(II)/Aβ(1-16) reduced with ascorbate showed the disappearance of the characteristic near-edge (XANES) spectral peaks of Cu(II) and the appearance of the peaks characteristic of Cu(I). The EXAFS data could be best fit with a linear imidazole-Cu(I)-imidazole geometry with Cu-N distance of 1.9 Å. They hypothesize that these imidazoles belong to His 13 and His 14. Large basis set DFT calculations (B2-PLYP hybrid functional of Grimme, Ahlrichs' def2-aug-TZVP basis for Cu and ligating N atoms, Ahlrichs' TZVP basis set for other atoms) resulted in an optimized geometry with parameters similar to those measured by EXAFS. Figure 3 depicts their DFT-optimized geometry. In contrast, the XAS and NMR studies done by Hureau et al. (2009) indicate pleotropy in Cu(I) binding to Aβ , showing that all three histidines contribute in a dynamical process. They propose a model where Cu(I) moves between binding to a histidine dyad (His 13 and His 14) and binding to a histidine triad (all three His). An alternative model would be an equilibrium between three histidine dyads: (His 13, His 14), (His 13, His 6), and (His 6, His 14).

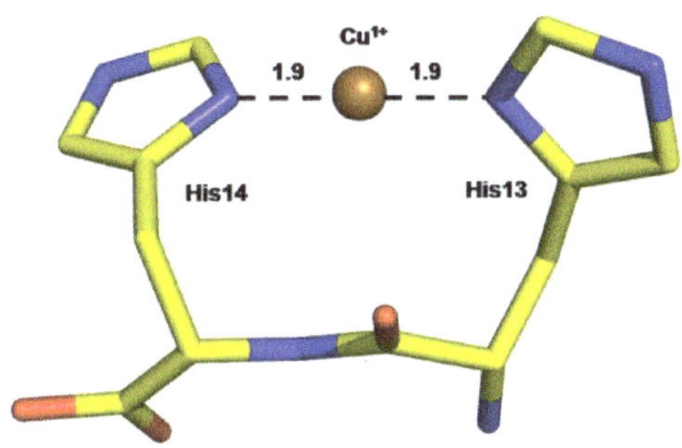

Fig. 3. Structural model of His 13 - Cu(I) - His 14 from DFT studies of Shearer & Szalai (2008), Reprinted from http://www.publish.csiro.au/nid/51/paper/CH09454.htm.

2.3 Cu(II)/Cu(I) ROS chemistry modeling

As mentioned above, quantum mechanical (QM) and molecular mechanical (MM) calculations have played important roles in the structural elucidation of Cu binding to Aβ. Structural models of DFT optimized geometries were an integral part of the EXAFS high-affinity Cu(II) binding site determination by Streltsov et al. (2008).

Computational chemistry, in particular *ab initio* QM calculations also have a major role to play in the elucidation of the mechanisms of ROS chemistry that occur as the result of Cu(II) binding to the N-terminus of Aβ. The laboratory of Rauk has carried out a number of *ab initio* computational studies of Cu binding to Aβ and the resultant H_2O_2 production (Raffa et al., 2005; Raffa et al., 2007; Hewitt and Rauk, 2009). Hewitt and Rauk (2009) examined the mechanism of H_2O_2 generation by Cu(II)/Aβ model system in the presence of an unspecified external reducing agent. The model system that they selected was two imidazoles linked by a peptide backbone, representing the His 13 - His 14 fragment of Aβ. The geometry optimizations were done with DFT calculations at B3LYP/6-31+G(d) level while enthalpy calculations were done with single point energy calculations at B3LYP/6-311+(2df, 2p) level. The reaction pathway or redox cycle computed in this study is depicted schematically in Figure 4. In the first step, the most stable (according to their calculations) Cu(II) species is reduced to the most stable Cu(I) species. The former species has 2N2O coordination, with the N ligands being His 13 and His 14 imidazole N atoms while the O ligands are the backbone carbonyl O and a water molecule. The most stable Cu(I) species has a linear geometry, with the Cu(I) coordinated by His 13 and His 14 imidazole N atoms.

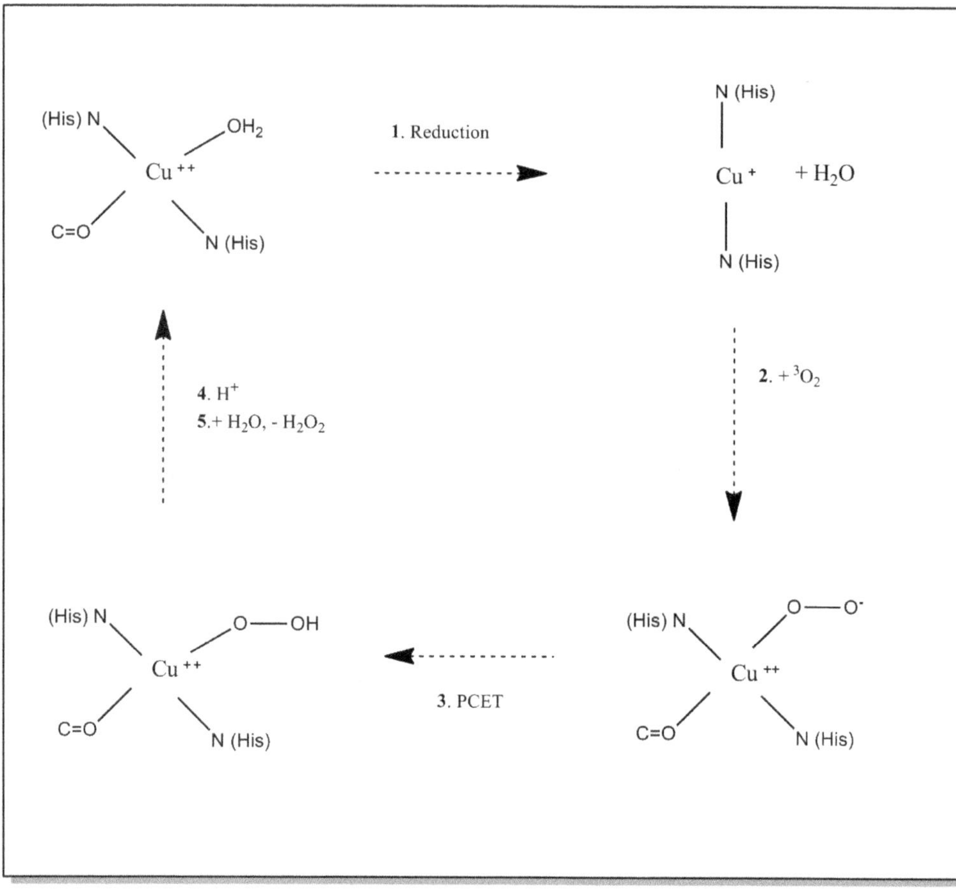

Fig. 4. Simplified reaction scheme of Hewitt and Rauk for the generation of H_2O_2 by Cu(II)/Aβ. Adapted with permission from Hewitt and Rauk (2009). Copyright (2009) American Chemical Society.

In the next step, this Cu(I) species forms a loose adduct with molecular O_2 (in its triplet spin state). This species then takes part in a proton coupled electron transfer (PCET) reaction due to the participation by some external reducing agent (such as ascorbate or glutathione). In the final step, protonation followed by associative substitution by a water molecule leads to the production of H_2O_2 and the regeneration of the original Cu(II) species. Among their findings is that the generation of superoxide to be energetically unfavourable, consistent with the non-observation of superoxide by Huang et al. (1999b) during the Cu(II)/Aβ generation of H_2O_2. However, their starting structural model for Cu(II)/Aβ, i.e. 2N2O coordination, is at variance with most experimental studies on the Cu(II) binding site as discussed in the previous section. Hewitt and Rauk state that at the level of theory that they employed, axial ligands to Cu(II) dissociate in water. They computed a reduction potential of 0.52 V (vs. the NHE) for the first step. This is significantly higher than the value of 0.28 V measured by Jiang et al. (2007) for Cu(II)/Cu(I) couple when bound to Aβ.

A few years previous to the work of Hewitt and Rauk, Barnham et al. (2004) also used *ab initio* DFT calculations to propose a reaction mechanism for the production of H_2O_2 by Cu(II)/Aβ in the presence of (excess of) ascorbate. Their computation (at the B3LYP/LANL2DZ level) starts the redox cycle with Cu(II) coordinated by three histidines and tyrosine. Cu(II) is reduced to Cu(I) by ascorbate in a PCET step, dissociating the tyrosine. Molecular O_2 coordinates the Cu(I) and oxidizes it back to Cu(II). Hydrogen atom transfer from the tyrosine and simultaneous abstraction of a proton from the medium leads to the formation of H_2O_2 and a tyrosyl radical. Tyrosyl radicals from Aβ molecules close to each other can then lead to the formation of experimentally observed dityrosine-linked Aβ dimer. The presence of transient radicals was shown by the use of the radical trapping agent 2-methyl-2-nitrosopropane. Such radicals were absent in the case of the Aβ mutant Y10A, which was also not toxic in neuronal cell assays. On the other hand, subsequent structural work on the Cu(II) binding site (discussed above) have now ruled out the participation of tyrosine 10 in the binding of Cu(II). Furthermore, Barnham et al. (2004) also reported that the Y10A mutant still produced H_2O_2, albeit at half the rate of wild-type Aβ. Obviously, other mechanisms, not involving binding of Tyr 10 to Cu(II), can lead to the generation of H_2O_2 by Cu(II)/Aβ in the presence of ascorbate.

It is by now quite apparent that Cu binding to Aβ is a pleotropic, dynamical phenomenon, although at a given set of conditions such as pH and buffer a particular species may predominate over others. Molecular dynamics (MD) calculations would be the preferred computational tool to investigate such dynamical processes. Classical MD employing empirical force fields cannot deal with breaking and formation of bonds, so techniques such as CPMD and QM/MM-MD are advantageous in this regard. Furlan et al. (2010) have used *ab initio* (or Car-Parrinello) molecular dynamics (CPMD) calculations to investigate the Cu(I) binding to Aβ. Starting from a number of different Cu(I)/Aβ geometries (employing either two histidine or three histidine topologies), the simulations of Furlan et al. showed that a linear His 13 - Cu(I) - His 14 arrangement was the most stable, although certain interactions between the peptide and the metal ion may lead to the approach and binding of His 6. It must be noted that because of the highly compute-intensive nature of CPMD, their simulation was quite short at 1 ps. It is known that the linear imidazole-Cu(I)-imidazole geometry is particularly stable (Le Clainche et al., 2000), and it is interesting to speculate whether a transient formation of a triply coordinated Cu(I) species might be necessary for its reactivity towards molecular dioxygen.

Concurrent with the studies described above on elucidating the nature of Cu interaction with Aβ and the effects on toxicity, there have been work designing novel chemical entities to ablate the neurotoxicity by interfering with the Cu binding to Aβ. As mentioned in the introduction, successful results of phase IIa clinical trials of a copper ligand PBT2 have been announced (Adlard et al., 2008; Lannfelt et al., 2008). This compound is the second-generation version of another copper ligand, Clioquinol (Figure 5). These two compounds were shown to be capable of significantly reducing the amount of Aβ aggregation, H_2O_2 generation, and dityrosine-linked Aβ production. They significantly improved the level of cognition in AD patients. Adlard et al. (2008) hypothesized that these compounds act more as ionophores, i.e. removing the copper bound to Aβ and transporting it inside the neuronal cells, leading to upregulation of matrix metalloproteases and subsequently to the degradation of Aβ.

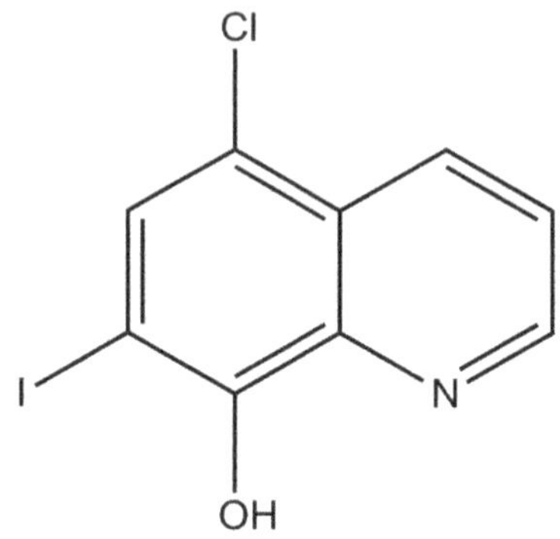

Fig. 5. Chemical structure of Clioquinol

3. Iron and amyloid beta

Iron, like copper, is a redox-active metal and plays a critical role in the human body, being an essential component of haemoglobin and a number of enzymes. After the liver, the organ with the richest concentration of iron is the brain, normally containing in the order of 60 mg of non-haeme iron in the adult brain (Duce & Bush, 2010). However, being redox-active, it is also capable of participating in Fenton and Haber-Weiss type reactions and generating hydroxyl radicals, superoxide, and other reactive oxygen species, and is a potential source of oxidative stress in the brain. The Fe(III)/Fe(II) system has a standard reduction potential of 0.77 V, i.e. greater than that of the Cu(II)/Cu(I) system. Maintaining strict homeostasis of the iron levels and the oxidation state it is in is essential for maintaining the health of the body. This occurs in the healthy body with the activities of ferroxidases such as ceruloplasmin, iron transport proteins like transferrin, and iron strorage proteins such as ferritin. Recently, Duce et al. (2010) proposed that the amyloid precursor protein, APP, also has ferroxidase activity, converting Fe(II) to Fe(III). They found this function was located in the E2 domain (residues 365-495) of APP, associated with the motif REXXE, and to be inhibited by Zn(II). With normal ageing, the iron content in the brain has been found to increase. Iron also has been found to be concentrated in senile plaques of AD brains. Lovell et al. (1998) found AD neuropils to contain more than twice the amount of iron found in control neuropils.

Despite this importance of iron, there has not been much published work on the interaction of iron with amyloid beta. Liu et al. (2010) have proposed that iron promoted the toxicity of Aβ by actually delaying the formation of well-ordered aggregates of Aβ such as the fibrils found in AD. The easy oxidation of Fe(II) to Fe(III) and the hydrolysis and precipitation of

Fe(III) at physiological pH are some of the reasons hindering experimental studies. To get around the latter problem, Jiang et al. (2009) used the complex between Fe(III) and nitrilotriacetic acid (NTA) in their work on the interaction with Aβ and redox properties. They found that Fe(III)-NTA bound to Aβ extremely strongly, with a measured dissociation constant of $6.3x10^{-21}$ M. In comparison, that for Fe(II)-NTA was $5.0x10^{-12}$ M. Furthermore, using cyclic voltametry they determined that the redox potential for Fe(II)-NTA to be 0.23 V when complexed to Aβ.

Just as in the case of Cu(II), there have been contradictory reports on the amino acid residues of Aβ involved in coordinating Fe. An early Raman spectroscopic study by Miura et al. (2001) concluded that while Tyr 10 was central to the binding of Fe(III), the three histidines in the N-terminal Aβ region were not involved. On the other hand, Nakamura et al. (2007) in their study of the redox activity of Cu and Fe in association with Aβ, conclude that, just like for Cu, the three histidines are necessary of the binding of Fe. Most recently, the group of Faller and Hureau used NMR, including ^{1}H, ^{13}C, and 2D studies in an attempt to determine the coordination shell of Fe(II) in binding to Aβ (Bousejra-El Garah et al., 2011). Analyzing the line broadening in the NMR spectra induced by Fe(II) binding to Aβ(1-16), Aβ(1-28), and Aβ(1-4) peptides, they concluded that firstly, neither Tyr 10 nor Met 35 had any role in Fe(II) coordination. Secondly, they identified Asp 1, Glu 3, His 6, His 13, and His 14 as the residues involved in binding Fe(II). Assuming hexa-coordination of Fe(II), they propose a 3N3O first coordination shell for Fe(II). i.e. The equatorial ligands are the imidazoles of His 6 and His 13 or His 14 as well as the N-terminus of Asp1 and the backbone carbonyl oxygen from Asp1 or His 6. The axial ligands consist of the carboxylate oxygens of Asp 1 and Glu 3. This is schematically depicted in Figure 6. More precise determination of the 3D structure of the binding site awaits future work. No EXAFS studies on Fe binding to Aβ have been reported yet. Notably, Bousejra-El Garah et al. did not find any pH dependence for the Fe(II) binding to Aβ near physiological pH.

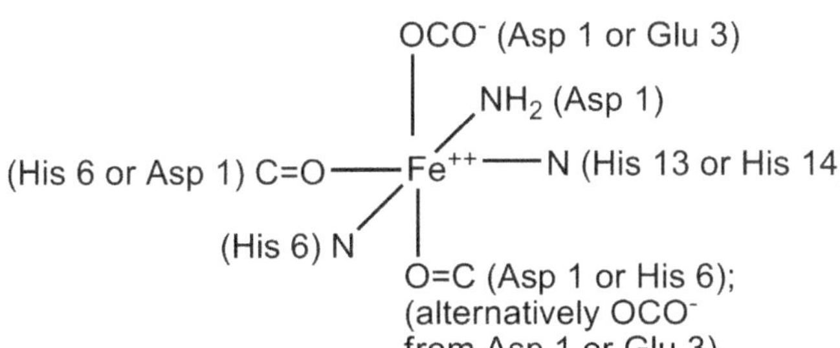

Fig. 6. Model for Fe(II)/Aβ coordination by Bousejra-El Garah et al. (2011). Adapted with permission from Bousejrah-El Garah et al. (2011). Copyright (2011) American Chemical Society.

Also very recent is an *ab initio* study by Rauk and co-workers on the structures and stabilities of Fe(II) and Fe(III) complexes with Aβ fragments (Ali-Torres et al., 2011). Their calculations consisted of single point energies calculated at MP2 level with a large 6-311+G(2df,2p) basis set at geometries optimized with the DFT functional B3LYP with a small 6-31G(d) basis set. Solvent effects were included with an IEFPCM (polarisable continuum model with the integral equation formalism variant). They determined that the most stable complexes containing His-His (i.e. His 13 - His 14) and phenolate (derived from Tyr 10) are the two penta-coordinated species $[Fe(II)(O\text{-}HisHis)(PhO^-)(H_2O)]^+$ and $[Fe(III)(N\text{-}HisHis)(PhO^-)(H_2O)]^+$. These structures are shown in Figure 7. They concluded that the simultaneous coordination of Tyr10 and His 13 - His 14 to Fe(II) and to Fe(III) is thermodynamically favourable. However, as we saw from the NMR results by Bousejra-ElGarah et al., it is unlikely that Aβ utilizes Tyr 10 in coordination to Fe(II). Ali-Torres et al. computing the standard reduction potentials, determined that this coordination by Tyr and His-His reduces Fe(III)/Fe(II) reduction by about 0.5 V (compared to aqueous Fe(III)/Fe(II)) to 0.20 V. We note that this value is quite close to the value of 0.23 V experimentally determined by Jiang et al. (2009) for the Fe(III)-NTA system complexed to Aβ.

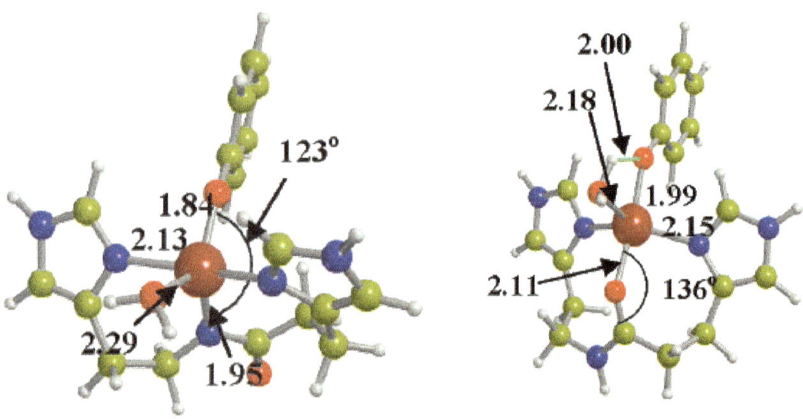

Fig. 7. The most stable Fe(II) (left) and Fe(III) (right) structural models by Ali Torres et al. (2011). Reprinted with permission from Ali Torres et al. (2011). Copyright (2011) American Chemical Society.

Finally, it should be mentioned that some Fe(III) chelating compounds have been tested as possible therapeutics for AD. Two such compounds are desferrioxamine and deferiprone (Figure 8). While they are used as iron chelators to treat iron overload conditions, their efficacy as AD therapeutics is doubtful, and they also bind other metal ions such as Cu(II) and Zn(II).

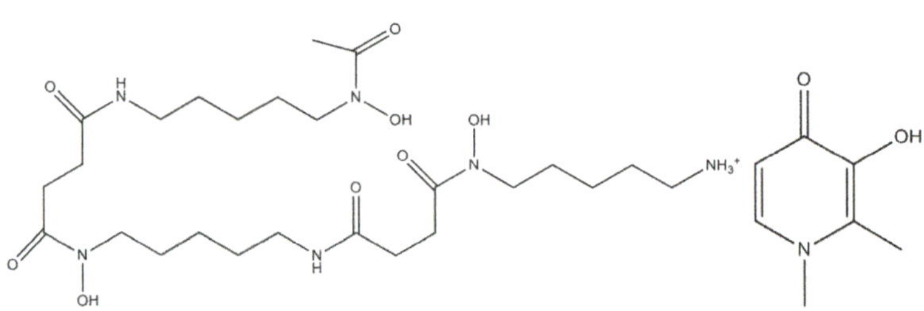

Fig. 8. Chemical structures of desferrioxamine (left) and deferiprone (right)

4. Zinc and amyloid beta

Zinc, like Copper, is known to play a major role in Alzheimer's Disease pathogenesis. However, unlike copper (and iron), zinc, normally found only in the Zn(II) state, is not redox-active. While Zn is an essential component in a number of enzymes, its role is probably mostly structural rather than reactive chemically. The brain is a rich source of Zn(II). During neuronal activity, the concentration of Zn(II) released into the synaptic cleft can be as high as 1mM (Duce & Bush, 2010). The zinc transporter ZnT3 activity is key during this process. With age, hippocampal Zn as well as ZnT3 levels have been found to decrease (Adlard, 2010). Zn(II) binding to Aβ facilitates the amyloid aggregation. AD brain plaques are highly enriched in zinc, reaching millimolar concentrations (Lovell, 1998). The metal ionophores, Clioquinol and PBT2, discussed earlier, show moderate binding of Zn(II), and Adlard et al. (2008) observed the dissolution of Zn-induced Aβ(1-42) aggregates upon treatment with these compounds. Faller and Hureau (2009) concluded that Zn(II) had a binding affinity to Aβ of 1-20 μM, which is weaker than that shown by Cu(II). However, this value is highly dependent on the assay conditions and probably on the aggregation state of Aβ.

The structure of the Zn(II) binding site in Aβ has been the subject of a number of studies. While most experiments appear to agree that the triad of histidines, His 6, His 13, and His 14 coordinate the Zn(II) ion, there is some disagreement on the identity of the fourth coordinating amino acid residue. In 2006, Zirah et al. (2006) determined the solution structure of Zn(II) bound to Aβ(1-16) in aqueous solution at pH 6.5 using ^{1}H and ^{13}C 1- and 2-dimensional NMR experiments. Here, Zn(II) displays a flattened tetrahedral geometry with the N^{δ} atoms of His 6 and His 14, and the N^{ε} atom of His 13 at the 'base' and the carboxylate O atoms of the bidentate Glu 11 at the apex. Notably, the two O atoms of Glu 11 are equidistant from the Zn at 2.1 Å. His 6 and His 13 are also 2.1 Å distant from the metal while His 14 is at 2.3 Å. It is noteworthy that the peptide used in these studies was N-acetylated at the N-terminus, thus hindering any potential involvement of Asp 1 in the Zn coordination. The geometry of the Zn(II) binding site is depicted below in Figure 9 (PDB id: 1ZE9).

When the N-terminal of Aβ is not acetylated, NMR studies point to the involvement of Asp 1 in the coordination of Zinc. For example, using high resolution NMR ^{1}H-^{13}C and ^{1}H-^{15}N heterocorrelation experiments on Aβ(1-40), Danielsson et al. (2007) propose that the three histidines and most likely the N-terminal NH2 of Asp 1 coordinate Zn(II). However, they do not rule out the possibility of the carboxylate oxygen atom of Asp 1 as a Zn(II) ligand. On the other hand, Minicozzi et al. (2008) observed that at pH 7, the EXAFS spectrum of Aβ(5-23) looked very similar to those of Aβ(1-16), Aβ(1-28), and Aβ(1-40). They determine that the best fit to the data is with 4 histidines and a oxygen atom, and hence conclude that what they observe is best explained by Zn(II) cross-linking 2 Aβ chains, each chain contributing 2 histidines to the first coordination shell. Finally, comparative ^{1}H NMR studies on human and rat Aβ(1-28) in water/sodium dodecyl sulphate (SDS) micelles were carried out at pH 7.5 by Gaggelli et al. (2008). The chemical shift variations and line broadening led them to a penta-coordinated structural model for Zn(II)/Aβ(1-28) where the Zn(II) is liganded by Asp 1 (N-terminal NH2 group), His 6, His 13, His 14, and the carboxylate oxygen atom of Glu 11. The last ligand was strongly evidenced by the down field ^{1}H chemical shifts for Glu 11 upon the addition of Zn(II). Notably, large downfield shifts were also observed for Tyr 10, which were ascribed to conformational changes brought about by Zn(II) binding rather than direct involvement of Tyrosine as a ligand. They also determined the Zn(II) coordination shell when bound to the rat Aβ(1-28). The rat Aβ differs from the human peptide in three important mutations: Arg 5 → Gly, Tyr 10 → Phe, and His 13 → Arg. Their structural model for Zn(II) with rat Aβ(1-28) has the metal ion tetrahedrally coordinated with the ligands Asp 1 NH_2 group, His 6 and His 14 imidazoles, and Glu 11 carboxylate. Thus there is very little change in the mode of binding in going from the human to rat sequence, resulting only in the loss of His 13 as a ligand.

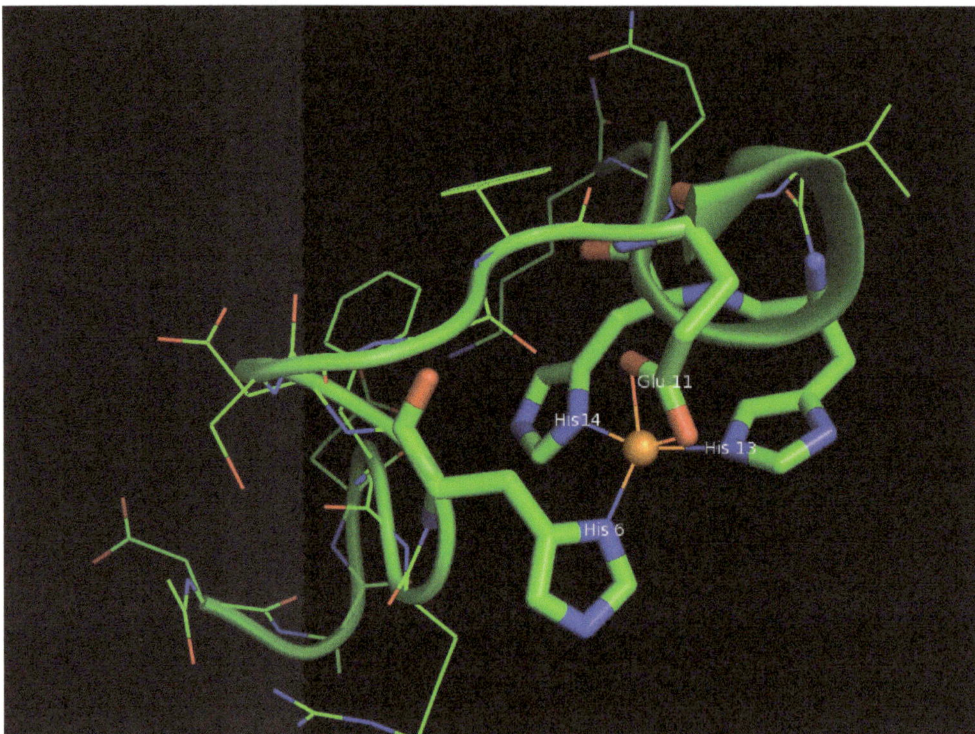

Fig. 9. Zn(II)/Aβ(1-16) NMR solution structure of Zirah et al. (2006).

The minimal Zn(II) binding fragment of Aβ has been the subject of QM/MM (hybrid quantum mechanics / molecular mechanics) simulations and ITC (isothermal calorimetry) experiments (Tsvetkov et al., 2010). The QM/MM calculations (performed combining the Car-Parinello molecular dynamics code CPMD with the MM package GROMACS) used the NMR solution structure of Zirah et al. (2006) as the initial geometry and included the metal ion and the side-chains of His6, His 13, His 14 and Glu 11 in the QM region. These calculations (run for a maximum of 8 ps) on Zn(II) complexed to Aβ(1-16) and Aβ(6-14) showed stable structures when Zn(II) was liganded by the three histidines and Glu 11. ITC on different sized Aβ fragments as well as H6R and E11A mutants of Aβ(1-16) at pH 7.3 all indicated that (6-14) contained the minimal binding region of Aβ. They proposed Zn(II) is first coordinated by $E^{11}VH^{13}H^{14}$, followed by His 6 binding. *Ab initio* molecular dynamics was also the computational methodology of choice used by Furlan and La Penna (2009) to investigate the stability of Zn(II) binding by different Aβ(1-16) residues (this time using an implementation of CPMD in the Quantum Espresso package). Simulations *in vacuo* at 300 K of 1-2 ps length supported the structural model of coordination by the three histidines and Glu 11. On the other hand, involvement of Asp1 in the binding resulted in the expulsion of a histidine from the coordination shell. Finally, Tyr 10 liganding the metal ion in competition with Glu 11 or Asp1 appeared to be possible only when the tyrosine is first deprotonated. It should also be noted that in these theoretical models discussed above, Glu 11 displays monodentate, not bidentate binding to Zn(II). Miller et al. (2010) performed replica exchange molecular dynamics simulations with Zn(II)/Aβ models found that the zinc ions can simultaneously coordinate Aβ both intramolecularly as well as intermolecularly, and hence facilitate Aβ aggregation. Their simulations, commenced from structural models constructed using the Zirah et al. Zn(II)/Aβ(1-16) structure discussed above and the Aβ(17-42) fibril structure of Luhrs et al. (2005), ran for 20 ns. They observed that the Zn(II) coordination decreased the solvation energy of Zn(II)/Aβ oligomers, again facilitating the amyloid aggregation.

Finally, it is also interesting that the high resolution NMR studies by Danielsson et al. (2007) also appeared to suggest the presence of a second, weaker, Zn(II) binding site in the central region of Aβ, involving residues 23, 24, 26, and 28. The putative second Cu(II) binding site mentioned in section 2.1, suggested by the p3-IgNAR tetrameric crystal structure of Strelsov et al. (2011) has the potential also to be a second Zn(II) binding site. Confirmation of this as a second Zn(II) binding site awaits future experiments.

5. Platinum, Ruthenium, Rhodium, and Iridium metals and amyloid beta

While the major body of work of on the interactions of metals with Amyloid beta (Aβ) has been of those metals with biological significance and found in the brain, i.e. Cu, Zn, and Fe, more recently there has been interest in the study of the interaction of Aβ with organometallic compounds involving transition metals Platinum (Pt), Ruthenium (Ru), Rhodium (Rh), and Iridium (Ir). While there is no evidence that the interaction of these metals with Aβ is of any biological significance, and indeed that such interactions occur at all in the human brain, they do have significance as prototypes or templates for potential therapeutics in order to ablate the neurotoxicity induced by Aβ.

The first study in this area was that by Barnham et al. (2008) on the effects of binding of Aβ to Cisplatin and Cisplatin-derived compounds. The Pt compounds involved in this study were cisplatin, Pt(1,10-phenanthroline)Cl_2, Pt(4,7-diphenyl-[1,10]-phenanthroline)Cl_2 and Pt(4,7-diphenyl-[1,10]-phenanthroline disulfonate)Cl_2, (i.e. compounds 1, 2, 3, and 4 in this study), and are depicted in Figure 10. The impetus behind this work was the knowledge that the N-terminal residues, and in particular the histidines at positions 6-, 13-, and 14- were important in the toxicity induced by Aβ(Atwood et al., 2000), and that aromatic compounds appeared to bind to Aβ and, at the least, affect its fibril forming tendency. In particular, 1,10-phenanthroline compounds (in the absence of any metals) appear to have a weak affinity to the N-terminal residues Phe 4, Tyr 10, and Phe 19 (Yao et al., 2004). The three histidines, His 6, His 13, and His 14, of course, are included in this segment of Aβ.

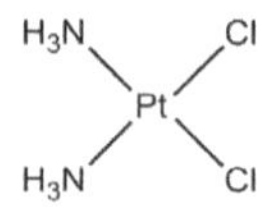

1

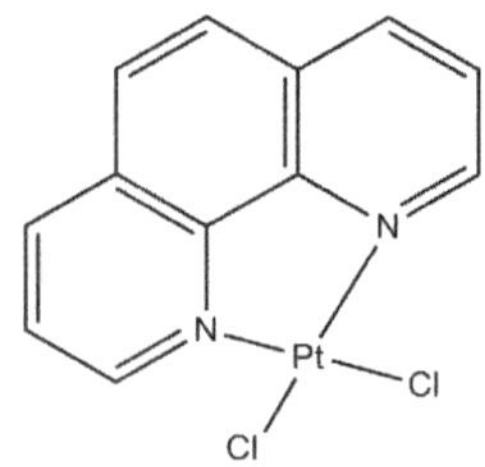

2

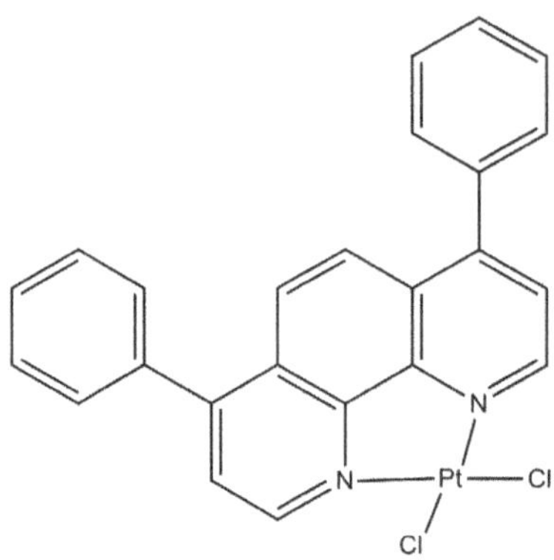

3

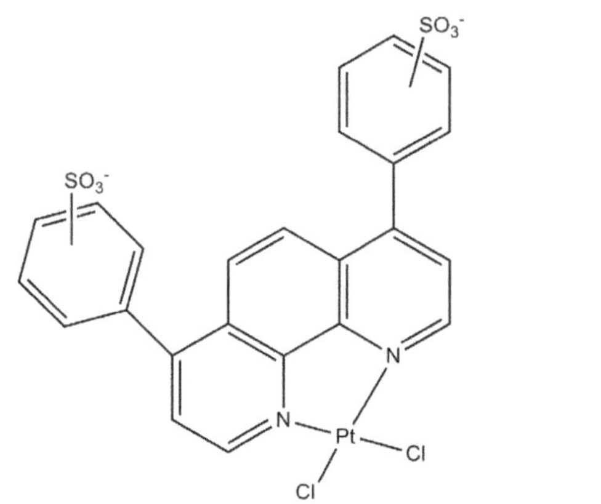

4

Fig. 10. Platinum compounds used for binding to Aβ by Burnham et al. (2008)

Barnham et al. found that while all four compounds bound to Aβ(1-40), only compounds 2, 3, and 4, and not 1, (i.e. cisplatin), had significant effects on the behaviour of the peptide. Compounds 2, 3, 4 inhibited the aggregation of Aβ(1-40), with EM showing the absence of fibrils. They significantly inhibited the Cu(II) induced generation of H_2O_2, with the measured IC_{50} values in the nanomolar range. This is comparable to the inhibition of ROS generation by clioquinol as discussed earlier. Furthermore, these compounds significantly inhibited the Aβ induced neurotoxicity, increasing the cell viability of primary mouse cortical neurons in cell cultures. Finally, they rescued the Aβ induced inhibition of long-term potentiation (LTP) in mouse hippocampal slices. How do these compounds have such beneficial effects on Aβ biological properties while cisplatin does not? The ^1H NMR experiments of Barnham et al. appear to show that while compounds 2-4 bind the N-terminal histidines of Aβ, cisplatin binds the C-terminal Met 35. At a first glance, this appears to explain why compounds 2-4 and not cisplatin inhibits H_2O_2 generation. (And incidentally, is further confirmation that Met 35 is not involved in the ROS generating activity of Aβ.) However, determination of all the coordinating residues of Aβ has not been done, and more extensive and definitive structural studies on the complexes of Aβ with these Pt compounds are necessary. Such studies, both experimental as well as computational, are now underway at our laboratory (CSIRO). These would, hopefully, provide complete 3-dimensional structural models of the Aβ-Pt compound complexes. Such structures would not only explain the differences in the chemical properties of the different compound complexes, but also be templates or leads for the development of effective therapeutics for AD. Among the qualities effective neuroprotective agents should have are good blood-brain barrier crossing properties. It should be noted that cisplatin has been used for some time as a cytotoxic drug in anti-cancer therapy. However, Barnham et al. did not notice toxicity to cells of these Pt compounds at the concentrations that were used in their experiments, i.e. 5 μM and 10 μM.

Following this work, Valensin et al. (2009) published their study of the interaction of Aβ(1-28) with the Ruthenium compound *fac*-[$Ru(CO)_3Cl_2$-N^1-1,3-thiazole] (where Ru has a +2 charge). Given the fact that Ru compounds are in general far less cytotoxic than Pt compounds, and the fact that Ru compounds prefer coordination to imidazole nitrogen atoms, they strongly suggest Ru compounds such as theirs be considered as potential therapeutics for Alzheimer's Disease. The ^1H NMR experiments they carried out appear to indicate that the chlorines in the compound are substituted by the histidine imidazoles of the Aβ peptide. In addition to the histidines, Tyr 10 also appears to be implicated. Supporting their conclusions, rat Aβ(1-28) (which differs in the mutations R5G, Y10F, and H13R) was significantly less affected by the Ru compound. Once again, definitive structural determinations remain to be done. The circular dichroism experiment carried out by Valensin showed that the peptide underwent conformational changes upon binding to the Ru compound. However, they did not perform any peptide aggregation, ROS generation, cell viability, or LTP studies with their compound.

More recently, Man et al. (2011) have investigated the use of Group 9 transition metal Rhodium (Rh(III)) and Iridium (Ir(III)) compounds to inhibit Aβ aggregation via these metals' coordination to the N-terminal histidines. Their Rh and Ir solvato-complexes contain 2-phenyl pyridine, benzoquinoline, or phenyl quinoline ligands. Presumably, the labile solvent (H_2O) molecules are displaced by the histidine imidazoles upon binding to Aβ. Man et al. found that the Rh(III) compound with phenyl pyridine as ligand was the most effective in the inhibition of fibril formation by Aβ(1-40).

6. Conclusion

Diverse experimental techniques have been utilized over the past few years in elucidating the nature of the interactions of transition metal ions with the amyloid beta peptide. Much of it has concerned copper, in both its oxidation states, due to its redox activity and biological relevance. It is clear that the interactions are complex, and very sensitive to ambient conditions. This makes it quite challenging to discern the interactions that are occurring in the brain. As of yet there is no x-ray crystallographic structure of a metal ion complexed with Aβ. The pleotropic nature of the binding as well as the lack of definite (secondary) structure in the N-terminal region of Aβ makes obtaining such a crystal structure an arduous task. On the other hand, crystal structures of metal ions with Aβ as suitable fusion protein constructs or within stable protein scaffolds or ternary complexes with Aβ and antibody fragments are worthy goals. Also of great interest would be the structural determination of complexes of any of the organometallic compounds with Aβ. Such structures could provide templates for the design of therapeutics and diagnostics for AD. Computational studies, particularly when done in conjunction with experiments, also have contributed considerably to our current understanding of metal interaction with Aβ. *Ab initio* MD and hybrid QM/MM-MD methodologies hold great promise in providing insight into the dynamical processes and the ROS chemistry resulting from the metal-peptide interactions. In performing these simulations carrying them out in biologically relevant time scales will be a challenge that will need to be met. It will also be of use to tie in the calculations as close as possible to the experiments, for example commencing simulations from reliable and relevant experimental structural models. Finally, we note that two fundamental questions in the study of the aetiology of AD are yet to be answered satisfactorily: what is the toxic species and what is the mechanism of toxicity.

7. References

Adlard, P.A., Cherny, R.A., Finkelstein, D.I., Gautier, E., Robb. E., Cortes, M., Volitakis, I., Liu, X., Smith, J.P., Perez, K., Laughton, K., Li, Q.-X., Charman, S.A., Nicolazzo, J.A., Wilkins, S., Deleva, K., Lynch, T., Kok, G., Ritchie, C.W., Tanzi, R.E., Cappai, R., Masters, C.L., Barnham, K.J., & Bush, A.I., (2008). Rapid restoration of cognition in Alzheimer's transgenic mice with 8-hydroxy quinoline analogs is associated with decreased interstitial Aβ, *Neuron*, 59, pp. 43-55.

Adlard, P.A., Parncutt, J.M., Finkelstein, D.I., & Bush, A.I. (2010). Cognitive Loss in Zinc Transporter-3 Knock-Out Mice: A Phenocopy for the Synaptic and Memory Deficits of Alzheimer's Disease? *Journal of Neuroscience*, 30, pp. 1631-1636.

Ali-Torres, J., Rodriguez-Santiago, L., Sodupe, M. & Rauk, A. (2011). Structures and Stabilities of $Fe^{2+/3+}$ Complexes Relevant to Alzheimer's Disease: An Ab Initio Study, *J. Phys. Chem. A*, on-line, dx.doi.org/10.1021/jp2026626

Atwood, C.S., Moir, R.D., Huang X., Scarpa, R.C., Bacarra, N.M.E., Romano, D.M., Hartshorn, M.E., Tanzi, R.E., & Bush, A.I. (1998). Dramatic Aggregation of Alzheimer Aβ by Cu(II) Is Induced by Conditions Representing Physiological Acidosis, *Journal of Biological Chemistry*, 273, pp. 12817-12826.

Atwood, C.S., Scarpa, R.C., Huang, X., Moir, R.D., Jones, W.D., Fairlie, P., Tanzi, R.E., & Bush, A.I. (2000). Characterization of Copper Interactions with Alzheimer Amyloid β Peptides: Identification of an Attomolar-Affinity Copper Binding Site on Amyloid β 1–42, *Journal of Neurochemistry*, 75, pp. 1219-1233.

Barnham, K.J, Haeffner, F, Ciccotosto, G.D., Curtain, C.C., Tew, D Mavros, C., Beyreuther, K., Carrington, D., Masters, C.L., Cherny, R.A., Cappai, R.,& Bush, A.I., (2004). Tyrosine gated electron transfer is key to the toxic mechanism of Alzheimer's disease β-amyloid, *FASEB Journal*, 18, pp. 1427-1429.

Barnham, K.J., Kenche, V.B., Ciccotosto, G.D., Smith, D.P., Tew, D.J., Liu, X., Perez, K., Cranston, G.A., Johanssen, T.J., Volitakis, Bush, A.I., Masters, C.L., White, A.R., Smith, J.P., Cherny, R.A., & Cappai, R. (2008). Platinum-based inhibitors of amyloid-β as therapeutic agents for Alzheimer's disease, *Proc. Nat. Acad. Sci. USA*, 105, pp. 6813-6818.

Bousejra-ElGarah, F., Bijani, C., Coppel, Y. Faller, P. & Hureau, C. (2011). Iron(II) Binding to Amyloid-β, the Alzheimer's Peptide, *Inorganic Chemistry*, 50, pp. 9024-9030.

Cappai, R., & Barnham, K.J. (2008). Delineating the Mechanism of Alzheimer's Disease Aβ Peptide Neurotoxicity, *Neurochemical Research.*, 33, pp. 526-532.

Crouch, P.J., Harding, S.M., White, A.R., Camakaris, J., Bush, A.I., & Masters, C.L., (2008). Mechanisms of Aβ-mediated neurodegeneration in Alzheimer's disease, *International Journal of Biochemstry & Cell Biology*, 40, pp. 181-198.

Danielsson, J., Pierattelli, R., Banci, L.& Graslund, A. (2007). High-resolution NMR studies of the zinc-binding site of the Alzheimer's amyloid β-peptide, *FEBS Journal*, 274, pp. 46-59.

Dorlet, P., Gambarelli, S., Faller, P. & Hureau, C., (2009). Pulse EPR Spectroscopy Reveals the Coordination Sphere of Copper(II) Ions in the 1–16 Amyloid-β Peptide: A Key Role of the First Two N-Terminus Residues, *Angew. Chem. Int. Ed.* 48, pp. 9273 - 9276

Drew, S. C., Noble, C. J., Masters, C.L., Hanson,G. R.& Barnham, K. J. (2009). Pleomorphic Copper Coordination by Alzheimer's Disease Amyloid-β Peptide,. *J. Am. Chem. Soc.* , 131, pp. 1195–1207.

Drew, S.C., Masters, C.L., & Barnham, K.J. (2009), Alanine-2 Carbonyl is an Oxygen Ligand in Cu^{2+} Coordination of Alzheimer's Disease Amyloid-β Peptide - Relevance to N-Terminally Truncated Forms, *J. Am. Chem. Soc.*, 131, pp. 8760–8761.

Duce, J.A. & Bush A.I., (2010). Biological metals and Alzheimer's Disease: implications for therapeutics and diagnosis, *Progress in Neurobiology*, 92, pp. 1-18.

Duce, J.A., Tsatsanis, A., Cater, M.A., James, S.A., Robb, E., Wikhe, K., Leong, S.L., Perez, K., Johanssen, T., Greenough, M.A., Cho, H.-H., Galatis, D., Moir, R.D., Masters, C.L., McLean, C., Tanzi, R.E., Cappai, R., Barnham, K.J, Ciccotosto, G.D., Rogers, J.T., & Bush, A.I., (2010), Iron export ferroxidase activity of β-amyloid precursor protein is inhibited by zinc in Alzheimer's Disease, *Cell*, 142, pp. 857-867.

Eury, H., Bijani, C., Faller, P. & Hureau, C. (2011). Copper(II) Coordination to Amyloid β: Murine versus Human Peptide, *Angew. Chem. Int. Ed.*, 50, pp. 901-905.

Faller, P. & Hureau, C. (2009). Bioinorganic chemistry of copper and zinc ions coordinated to amyloid-β peptide, *Dalton Transactions*, 2009, pp. 1080-1094.

Ferri, C., Prince, M., Brayne, C., Brodaty, H., Fratigliani, L., Ganguli, M., Hall, K., Hasegawa, K., Hendrie, H., Huang, Y., Jorm, A., Mathers, C., Menzes, P.R., Rimmer, E. & Scazufca, M., (2005). Global Prevalence of Dementia: A Delphi consensus study, *Lancet*, 366, pp. 2112-2117.

Furlan, S, Hureau, C. Faller, P., & La Penna, G. (2010). Modeling the Cu+ Binding in the 1-16 Region of the Amyloid-β Peptide Involved in Alzheimer's Disease, *Journal of Physical Chemistry B*, 114, pp. 15119-15133.

Furlan, S. & La Penna, G. (2009). Modeling of the Zn^{2+} binding in the 1–16 region of the amyloid β peptide involved in Alzheimer's disease, *Physical Chemistry Chemical Physics*, 11, pp. 6468-6481.

Fusetti, F., Schroeter, K.H., Steiner, R.A., van Noort, P.I., Pijning, T., Rozeboom, H.J., Kalk, K.H., Egmond, M.R. & Dijkstra, B.W. (2002). Crystal Structure of the Copper-Containing Quercetin 2,3-Dioxygenase from Aspergillus japonicas, *Structure*, 10, pp. 259-268.

Gaggelli,E., Janicka-Klos, A., Jankowska, E., Kozlowski, H., Migliorini, C., Molteni, E., Valensin, D., Valensin, G., & Wieczerzak, E. (2008). NMR Studies of the Zn^{2+} Interactions with Rat and Human β-Amyloid (1-28) Peptides in Water-Micelle Environment, *Journal of Physical Chemistry B*, 112, pp. 100-109.

Hensley, K., Maidt, M.L. Yu, Z. Sang, H., Markesbery, W.R.,& Floyd, R.A. (1998). Electrochemical Analysis of Protein Nitrotyrosine and Dityrosine in the Alzheimer Brain Indicates Region-Specific Accumulation, *Journal of Neuroscience*, 18, pp. 8126–8132.

Hewitt, N. & Rauk, A. (2009). Mechanism of Hydrogen Peroxide Production by Copper-Bound Amyloid Beta Peptide: A Theoretical Study, *Journal of Physical Chemistry B*, 113, pp. 1202-1209.

Huang, X., Cuajungco, M.P., Atwood, C.S., Hartshorn, M.A., Tyndall, J.D.A., Hanson, G.R., Stokes, K.C., Leopold, M., Multhaup, G., Goldstein, L.E., Scarpa, R.C., Saunders, A.J., Lim, J., Moir, R.D., Glabe, C., Bowden, E.F., Masters, C.L., Fairlie, D.P., Tanzi,R.E. & Bush, A.I., (1999b). Cu(II) Potentiation of Alzheimer Aβ neurotoxicity correlation with cell-free hydrogen peroxide production and metal reduction, *Journal of Biological Chemistry*, 274, pp. 37111-37116.

Huang, X., Atwood, C.S., Hartshorn, M.A., Multhaup, G., Goldstein, L.E., Scarpa, R.C., Cuajungco, M.P., Gray, D.N., Lim, J., Moir, R.D., Tanzi, R.E.&, Bush, A.I. (1999a). The Aβ Peptide of Alzheimer's Disease Directly Produces Hydrogen Peroxide through Metal Ion Reduction, *Biochemistry*, 38, pp. 7609-7616.

Hureau , C., Eury, H., Guillot, R., Bijani, C., Sayen, S., Solari, P.-L., Guillon, E., Faller, P.,& Dorlet, P. (2011). X-ray and Solution Structures of Cu^{II}GHK and Cu^{II}DAHK Complexes: Influence on Their Redox Properties, *Chemistry A European Journal*, 17, pp. 10151-10160.

Hureau, C., Balland, V.,Coppel, Y. Solari , P.L., Fonda, E. & Faller, P. (2009). Importance of dynamical processes in the coordination chemistry and redox conversion of copper amyloid-β complexes, *Journal of Biological Inorganic Chemstry*, 14, pp. 995–1000.

Jiang, D., Li, X., Williams, R., Patel, S., Men, L., Wang, Y. & Zhou, F. (2009). Ternary Complexes of Iron, Amyloid-β, and Nitrilotriacetic Acid: Binding Affinities, Redox Properties, and Relevance to Iron-Induced Oxidative Stress in Alzheimer's Disease, *Biochemistry*, 48, pp. 7939–7947 7939.

Jiang, D., Men, L., Wang, J., Zhang, Y., Chickenyen, S., Wang, Y. & Zhou, F. (2007). Redox Reactions of Copper Complexes Formed with Different β-Amyloid Peptides and Their Neuropathological Relevance, *Biochemistry*, 46, pp. 9270-9282.

Lannfelt, L., Blennow, K., Zetterberg, H., Batsman, S., Ames, D., Harrison, J., Masters, C.L., Targum, S., Bush, A.I., Murdoch, R., Wilson, J. & Ritchie, C.W. (2008). Safety, effi cacy, and biomarker fi ndings of PBT2 in targeting A *β* as a modifying therapy for Alzheimer's disease: a phase IIa, double-blind, randomised, placebo-controlled trial, *Lancet Neurology*, 7, pp. 779-786.

Le Clainche, L., Giorgi, M. & Reinaud O. (2000). Synthesis and Characterization of a Novel Calix[4]arene-Based Two-Coordinate Copper(I) Complex That Is Unusually Resistant to Dioxygen, *European Journal of Inorganic Chemistry*, 2000, pp. 1931-1933.

Liu, B., Molone, A., Meehan, S., Morris, K., Thomas, S.E., Serpell, L.C., Hider, R., Marciniak, S.J., Lomas, D.A & Crowther, D.C. (2010). Iron Promotes the Toxicity of Amyloid β Peptide by Impeding Its Ordered Aggregation, *Journal of Biological Chemistry*, 286, pp. 4248-4256.

Lovell, M.A., Robertson, J.D., Teesdale, W.J., Campbell, J.L., Markesbery, W.R. (1998). Copper, iron and zinc in Alzheimer's disease senile plaques, *Journal of the Neurological Sciences*, 158, pp. 47–52.

Luhrs, T., Ritter, C., Adrian, M., Riek-Loher, D., Bohrmann, B., Doebeli, H., Schubert, D., & Riek, R. (2005). 3D structure of Alzheimer's amyloid-beta(1-42) fibrils, *Proc. Natl. Acad. Sci. USA*, 102, pp. 17342-17347.

Man, B. Y.-W., Chan, H.-M., Leung,C.-H., Chan, D.S.-H., Bai, L.-P., Jiang, Z.-H., Li, H.-W. & Ma, D.-L. (2011). Group 9 metal-based inhibitors of β-amyloid (1–40) fibrillation as potential therapeutic agents for Alzheimer's disease, *Chemical Science*, 2, pp. 917-921.

Masters, C.L. & Beyreuther, K., (2006). Alzheimer's centennial legacy: prospects for rational therapeutic intervention targeting the Aβ amyloid pathway, *Brain*, 129, pp. 2823-2839.

Minicozzi, V., Stellato, F., Comai, M., Dalla Serra, M., Potrich, C., Meyer-Klaucke, W., & Morante, S. (2008). Identifying the Minimal Copper- and Zinc-binding Site Sequence in Amyloid-β Peptides, *Journal of Biological Chemistry*, 283, pp. 10784-10792.

Miura, T., Suzuki, K. & Takeuchi, H. (2001). Binding of iron(III) to the single tyrosine residue of an amyloid-β peptide probed by Raman spectroscopy, *Journal of Molecular Structure*, 598, pp. 79-84.

Nadal, R.C., Rigby, S.E.J. & Viles, J. H. (2008). Amyloid β-Cu^{2+} Complexes in Both Monomeric and Fibrillar Forms Do Not Generate H_2O_2 Catalytically but Quench Hydroxyl Radicals, *Biochemistry*, 47, pp. 11653-11664.

Nakamura, M., Shishido, N., Nunomura, A., Smith, M.A., Perry, G., Hayashi, Y., Nakayama, K. &. Hayashi, T. (2007). Three Histidine Residues of Amyloid-β Peptide Control the Redox Activity of Copper and Iron, *Biochemistry*, 46, pp. 12737-12743

Raffa, D.F., Go´mez-Balderas, R., Brunelle, P. Rickard , G.A. & Rauk, A. (2005). Ab initio model studies of copper binding to peptides containing a His–His sequence: relevance to the β-amyloid peptide of Alzheimer's disease, *Journal of Biological Inorganic Chemistry*, 10, pp. 887-902.

Raffa, D.F., Rickard , G.A. & Rauk, A. (2007). Ab initio modelling of the structure and redox behaviour of copper(I) bound to a His–His model peptide: relevance to the β-amyloid peptide of Alzheimer's disease, *Journal of Biological Inorganic Chemistry*, 12, pp. 147-164.

Sarell, C.J., Syme, C.D., Rigby, S.E.J. & Viles, J.H. (2009). Copper(II) Binding to Amyloid-β Fibrils of Alzheimer's Disease Reveals a Picomolar Affinity: Stoichiometry and Coordination Geometry Are Independent of Aβ Oligomeric Form, *Biochemistry*, 48, pp. 4388- 4402.

Sayre, L.M., Zelasko, D.A., Harris, P.L.R., Perry, G., Salomon, R.G. & Smith, M.A. (1997). 4-Hydroxy Nonenal-derived Advanced Lipid Peroxidation End Products Are Increased in Alzheimer's Disease, *Journal of Neurochemistry*, 68, pp. 2092-2097.

Shearer, J. & Szalai, V.A. (2008). The Amyloid-β Peptide of Alzheimer's Disease Binds Cu^{I} in a Linear Bis-His Coordination Environment: Insight into a Possible Neuroprotective Mechanism for the Amyloid-β Peptide, *J. Am. Chem. Soc.*, 130, pp. 17826-17835.

Shivers, B.D., Hilbich, C., Multhaup, G., Salbaum, M., Beyreuther, K. & Seeburg, P.H. (1988). Alzheimer's disease amyloidogenic glycoprotein expression pattern in rat brain suggests a role in cell contact, *EMBO Journal*, 7, pp. 1365- 1370.

Smith D.G., Ciccotosto, G.D., Tew, D.J., Perez, K., Curtain, C.C., Boas, J.F., Masters, C.L., Cappai, R., Barnham K.J. (2010). Histidine 14 modulates membrane binding and neurotoxicity of the Alxzheimer's Disease amyloid-beta peptide, *Journal of Alzheimer's Disease*, 19, pp. 1387-1400.

Smith, D.G, Cappai, R.& Barnham, K.J., (2007). The redox chemistry of the Alzheimer's disease amyloid β peptide, *Biochimica et Biophysica Acta,* 1768, pp. 1976–1990.

Smith, D.P, Smith, D.G., Curtain, C.C., Boas, J.F., Pilbrow, J.R., Ciccotosto, G.D., Lau, T.-L., Tew, D. J., Perez, K., Wade, J.D., Bush, A.I., Drew, S.C., Separovic, F., Masters, C.L., Cappai, R.,& Barnham, K.J. (2006). Copper-mediated Amyloid-_ Toxicity Is Associated with an Intermolecular Histidine Bridge, *Journal of Biological Chemistry,* 281, pp. 15145-15154.

Streltsov, V.A. & Varghese, J.N. (2008). Substrate mediated reduction of copper-amyloid-β complex in Alzheimer's disease, *Chemical Communications*, 2008, pp. 3169-3171.

Streltsov, V.A., Titmuss, S.J., Epa, V.C., Barnham, K.J., Masters, C.L. & Varghese, J.N. (2008). The Structure of the Amyloid-β Peptide High-Affinity Copper II Binding Site in Alzheimer's Disease, *Biophysical Journal*, 95, pp. 3447-3456.

Streltsov, V.A., Varghese, J.N., Masters, C.L., & Nuttall, S.N. (2011). Crystal Structure of the Amyloid-β p3 Fragment Provides a Model for Oligomer Formation in Alzheimer's Disease, *Journal of Neuroscience*, 31, pp. 1419 -1426.

Tsvetkov, P.O., Kulikova, A.A., Golovin, A.V., Tkachev, Y.V., Archakov, A.I., Kozin, S.A., & Makarov, A.A. (2010). Minimal Zn^{2+} Binding Site of Amyloid-β, *Biophysical Journal,* 99, pp. L84–L86.

Valensin,D., Anzini, P., Gaggelli,E., Gaggelli,N., Tamasi, G., Cini, R., Gabbiani, C., Michelucci, E., Messori, L., Kozlowski, H., & Valensin, G. (2010). fac-$\{Ru(CO)_3\}^{2+}$ Selectively Targets the Histidine Residues of the β-Amyloid Peptide 1-28. Implications for New Alzheimer's Disease Treatments Based on Ruthenium Complexes, *Inorganic Chemistry*, 49, pp. 4720–4722.

Yao S, Cherny RA, Bush AI, Masters CL, & Barnham K.J. (2004). Characterizing bathocuproine self-association and subsequent binding to Alzheimer's disease amyloid beta peptide by NMR,. *Journal of Peptide Science*, 10, 210–217.

Zirah, S., Kozin, S.A., Mazur, A.K., Blond, A., Cheminant, M., Se´galas-Milazzo, I., Debey, P. & Rebuffat, S., (2006). Structural Changes of Region 1–16 of the Alzheimer Disease Amyloid β-Peptide upon Zinc Binding and in Vitro Aging, *Journal of Biological Chemistry*, 281, pp. 2151–2161.

4

Chronic Formaldehyde-Mediated Impairments and Age-Related Dementia

Junye Miao and Rongqiao He*
State Key Laboratory of Brain and Cognitive Sciences, Institute of Biophysics, Chinese Academy of Sciences, Beijing
China

1. Introduction

1.1 Formaldehyde (FA) in the human environment

FA (H_2CO), the simplest aldehyde (Kilburn, 1994), existed in the pre-biological atmosphere of the primordial earth (Canuto et al., 1983) and is also present in the outer galaxies (Blair et al., 2008). FA is believed to have been the first organic molecule, being derived from photochemical reactions between simple gas elements in the primeval earth's atmosphere (Reaction 1) (Pinto et al., 1980; Canuto et al., 1983).

$$CO_2 + 2H_2 \rightarrow H_2CO + H_2O\ (h\nu) \qquad (1)$$

FA is also a basic biological building block, and participates in the synthesis of amino acids such as glycine and alanine in aqueous medium (Miller, 1953; Sokolskaya, 1976; Sakurai&Yanagawa, 1984). It is involved in the generation of carbohydrates via the formose cycle in bacteria (Kalapos, 1999). FA is believed to form complex organic molecules (Canuto et al., 1983) and play a key role in the process of evolution (Kalapos, 1999).

As reported by the U.S. Environmental Protection Agency (June 18, 2010), FA is present in products such as abrasive materials, plywood adhesives, insecticides, insulation and embalming fluids. Anthropogenic production of FA is mainly from power plants, petroleum refineries, coking operations, incineration, motor vehicle exhaust, and tobacco smoke (He et al., 2010). This simplest aldehyde has become one of the highest risk factors in the pollution of the human environment.

1.2 Toxicity of exogenous formaldehyde and cognitive impairments

Due to its high reactivity, FA leads to the formation of stable methylene bridges between nucleic acids and the amines of proteins (Conaway et al., 1996), resulting in crosslinking between nucleic acids and/or proteins and their subsequent polymerization (Kast et al., 2008). Both the amino-terminals of proteins and residues containing ε-amino and thiol groups, such as lysine, arginine, histidine, cysteine, tyrosine and tryptophan, are modifiable

---

*Corresponding Author

targets of FA, and form methylol groups or Schiff-bases after modification (Metz et al., 2004). A number of reports have indicated that FA usually acts as a chemical crosslinker for biomacromolecules in cells. Exposure to FA at a concentration of 0.21 mM for 6 h reduces the growth rate of human bronchial epithelial cells to 50% that of controls due to FA depression of RNA synthesis and the formation of both DNA single-strand breaks and DNA-protein crosslinks (DPCs) (Saladino et al., 1985). When cultured with FA at concentrations of 0.1-0.3 mM, human lung A549 cells, primary human nasal epithelial cells and DT40 cells undergo the process of DPC formation (Nakamura et al., 2007; Speit et al., 2008). Treatment of rat aorta endothelial cells with FA at 0.01-2.00 mM promotes the formation of DPC, a potential risk factor in atherosclerosis (Yu&Deng, 1998; Zhang et al., 2006). FA has also been shown to induce chromosomal aberrations (CAs) and sister chromatid exchanges (SCEs) in cultured cells (Conaway et al., 1996). It is worth noting that FA has biphasic effects on cell lines depending on its concentration: enhancing apoptosis, necrosis and even causing cell death at high concentrations (>1 mM), while promoting cell proliferation at low dose (0.1 mM) (Tyihak et al., 2001).

Excess exposure to exogenous FA can induce carcinogenesis and cardiovascular dysfunction, possibly due to the formation of DPC (Shaham et al., 2003). Inhalation of FA vapor at concentration of up to 0.50 mM can cause rhinitis, epithelial dysplasia, squamous metaplasia, and even squamous cell carcinomas in rodents (Swenberg et al., 1980). Similar results have also been observed in a study on monkeys exposed to FA at 0.20 mM (Conaway et al., 1996). Tumor generation has been observed in humans when excess FA has been inhaled over a long period (Soffritti et al., 2002). In addition, oral administration of FA in drinking water at concentrations of 33.3 mM and 166.5 mM can cause hyperplasia, hyperkeratosis, erosion and/or ulcers in the alimentary system of rats (Conaway et al., 1996). Exposure to FA vapor also induces myocardical ischemia (Rety&Marin, 1957), while rats infused with 0.12 mM FA suffer cardiovascular attacks (Strubelt et al., 1990).

Studies on the relationship between exogenous FA and the immune system have indicated that exposure to FA promotes the response of cultured mast cells (Fujimaki et al., 1992), activates the immune system, and increases related antibodies in human sera (Patterson et al., 1986; Thrasher et al., 1990).

An overload of exogenous FA induces damage to the nervous system including changes in neurofilament proteins and demyelination (Perna et al., 2001). When exposed to FA, rats perform poorly at finding food in a maze, compared with controls (Pitten et al., 2000) and are also deficient in locomotor and explorative behavior (Malek et al., 2003). Hsp70 is upregulated in neonatal rats which have inhaled 0.40 mM FA for 30 days, leading to damage to the hippocampus, such as the loss of neurons and granule cells, and reduction in the volume of the dentate gyrus (DG) and cornu ammonis (CA) (Sarsilmaz et al., 2003; Petushok et al., 2005; Aslan et al., 2006; Sarsilmaz et al., 2007). Inhalation of FA at a concentration of 13.3 μM alters the expression of mouse genes, such as N-methyl-D-aspartate (NMDA) receptor subunits (NR2A and NR2B), cyclic AMP responsive element-binding protein (CREB)-1, CREB-2, FosB/ΔFosB, dopamine receptor subtypes (D1 and D2) and transient receptor potential vanilloid receptor (TRPV1), affecting synaptic plasticity (Ahmed et al., 2007; Lu et al., 2008). Epidemiological studies on the exposure of pathologists, embalmers, and chemical workers, have shown that increased hours of exposure to FA per day are associated with reduced performance in memory, equilibrium, and dexterity, and even result in damage to the central nervous system (Kilburn et al., 1987; Perna et al., 2001; Yu et al., 2007) and headache, eye irritation and asthma-like symptoms of wheezing and bronchoconstriction (Conaway et al., 1996).

1.3 Endogenous formaldehyde

1.3.1 Source of endogenous formaldehyde

FA is present in living organisms in three states, that is, the free-state, or reversibly or irreversibly bound to macromolecules (Zhiqian Tong, 2008). FA is involved in one-carbon metabolism and plays a role in physiological processes (Abeles R.H., 1992). Increased levels of endogenous FA are believed to be a potential risk factor for health and an indicator of either pathological processes, malnutrition or environmental contamination (Kalasz, 2003).

There are several sources of endogenous FA in living organisms, arising from enzymatic or nonenzymatic reactions (Zhiqian Tong, 2008). In plants, FA is produced as a byproduct of photosynthesis and is present at a level of 0.5-1.0 mM. After its generation, the aldehyde moiety immediately combines with L-arginine to form N(G)-trihydroxymethyl-L-arginine (TriHMA) through a series of enyzmic reactions (Trezl et al., 1998).

In animals, oxidative deamination is considered to be the major source of endogenous FA (Yu et al., 2003a). One important enzyme involved in FA generation by deamination is semicarbazide-sensitive amine oxidase (SSAO). SSAO, a copper-containing enzyme, is located primarily in cardiovascular smooth muscle, cartilage and other organs including the lung, liver, duodenum, kidney, and adrenal gland, and is circulated in the blood (Morrison et al., 1996; Yu et al., 1997; Mahy et al., 2001). The main substrates of SSAO are aromatic and aliphatic amines, which are deaminated into ammonia, hydrogen peroxide and FA as final products (Mahy et al., 2001; Conklin et al., 2004). In addition, monoamine oxidase (MAO) A and B, enzymes which have a similar function of that of SSAO, also generate FA (Ramonet et al., 2003). Adrenaline, whose excretion is enhanced by stress, is deaminated by monoamine oxidase (MAO) A and forms methylamine as a product. This product can be further deaminated by SSAO, yielding FA in vivo (Yu et al., 1997). In the rat liver microsome, N-nitrosodimethylamine can be metabolized into FA via oxidative deamination (Keefer et al., 1990).

FA is also generated in the demethylation step of methionine-homocysteine cycles. For example, demethylation of S-adenosyl-L-methionine, a methyl donor in enzymatic transmethylation reactions, generates FA (Kalasz, 2003). In addition, Generation of FA can also be achieved via demethylation of other substrates. For example, liver mitochondria produce FA by the oxidation of sarcosine methyl carbons (Abeles&Mackenzie, 1956). In normal and leukemic human leukocytes, N^5-methyltetrahydrofolate undergoes an oxidative reaction catalyzed by a reductase to form N^5,N^{10}-methylenetetrahydrofolate which then spontaneously releases FA. Moreover, production of FA is higher in the lymphocytes of chronic lymphocytic leukemia patients than in those of healthy individuals (Thorndike&Beck, 1977).

Histone demethylation is another way of generating FA in vivo (Kalasz, 2003; Ehrlich, 2009). Histone demethylases catalyze the removal of histone methyl groups at lysine or arginine residues, generating FA as a byproduct (Fang&Tian, 2007). There are two kinds of histone demethylases, namely lysine specific demethylase 1 (LSD 1) and Jumonji C (JmjC) domain family proteins (Fang&Tian, 2007). LSD1, a nuclear homolog of amine oxidases, functions as a histone demethylase and transcriptional co-repressor, catalyzing the demethylation of histone H3 at lysine 4 and the generation of FA (Shi et al., 2004). JHDM1 (JmjC domain-containing histone demethylase 1), an enzyme which plays a role in the demethylation of histone H3 at lysine 36, also releases FA as a product (Zhang et al., 2006).

Demethylation of DNA and RNA is also believed to involve FA generation. Fat mass and obesity associated enzyme (FTO), a Fe(II)-and-2-oxoglutarate-dependent oxygenase, is able to demethylate 3-methylthymine in single-stranded DNA, leading to the formation of FA (Gerken et al., 2007). In addition, human ABH2 and ABH3, homologues of *E. coli* AlkB, are non-Fe(II)-mediated oxidative demethylases. They are involved in catalysis, releasing the methyl carbon of DNA and RNA as FA (He et al., 2009).

Microsomal cytochrome P-450 dependent oxidation of xenobiotics such as drugs, is another demethylation reaction which results in the production of endogenous FA. In addition, endogenous FA can also come from food, such as milk, ham, sausage, potato, grape and cauliflower (Trezl et al., 1997).

1.3.2 Analysis of endogenous formaldehyde

A variety of methods have been established for the analysis of endogenous FA. According with the universal principle, measurements by different methods result in different values for the concentration of endogenous FA. Dimedone-^{14}C, a reagent for radiometric analysis, can be used to estimate the FA concentration in human blood and urine. Using this method, FA levels in blood and urine have been shown to vary between 0.01-0.02 mM and 0.08-0.13 mM, respectively (Szarvas et al., 1986). Gas chromatography (GC) has been used to compare the concentration of FA in the expired air of tumor-bearing mice (1.43-2.98 μM) and control mice (0.77-1.01 μM) (Shibamoto et al., 1997). The concentration of FA in urine from healthy individuals ranges from 1.89-4.81 μM, as determined by gas chromatography (Takigawa et al., 2007). The level of FA in the rat brain is reported to be 0.33-30.0 μM, as determined by GC-MS (P. Maboudou, 2002). Using selected ion flow tube mass spectrometry (SIFT-MS), the mean values of urine FA concentrations in patients with prostate cancer and bladder cancer was shown to be 0.83 μM and 2.83 μM, respectively, compared with 0.37 μM in healthy controls (Smith et al., 1999). In another study, preconcentration of the body fluid samples rendered FA more detectable by SIFT-MS. FA concentrations in Hela S3 cervical cancer, K562 leukemia and MCF-7 breast cancer cell lines range from 1.5 to 4.0 μM (Bierbaum et al., 2001). The use of high performance liquid chromatography (HPLC) combined with an electrochemical procedure is an established method for the measurement of FA in vivo (Su et al., 2011). An adduct between FA and other reagents can be selectively separated by HPLC, and then quantified by an electrochemical approach. Using this method, the FA concentration of rabbit urine was found to be about 18 nM and that of mouse liver, kidney and brain tissues to be 63, 51 and 11 nmol/g tissue, respectively (Yu et al., 2003a). Another method to determine FA in blood samples by HPLC utilizes a fluorescence assay. Derivatization of human plasma with ampicillin leads to a fluorescent adduct which can be measured with a fluorescence spectrophotometer. The FA level in human blood as determined by Fluo-HPLC is 0.04 mM (Luo et al., 2001). Thin-layer chromatography can also be used to estimate the level of FA (Kalasz, 2003). In addition, the FA level in solid tissues such as teeth can be measured by HPLC-OPLC-MS. Results show an increase in FA level in carietic teeth in comparison to healthy teeth (Rozylo et al., 2000).

1.3.3 Degradation of endogenous formaldehyde

The degradation of endogenous FA mainly occurs via enzymatic catalysis. Aldehyde dehydrogenase I, and III (ADH I, ADH III), and alcohol dehydrogenase II (ALDH II) are three important enzymes involved in these reactions (Iborra et al., 1992; Zhiqian Tong, 2008). There are five classes (I-V) of alcohol dehydrogenase located in human tissues. Transcripts of class II (ALDH II) are abundant in the liver, but low in the stomach, pancreas and small intestine (Estonius et al., 1996). It has been reported that ADH III is also present in the human brain, being distributed mainly in the dendrites and cytoplasm of cerebellar Purkinje cells. The location of ADH III in the brain contributes to defending the brain against degeneration (Mori et al., 2000; Olson et al., 2003). In addition, S-formylglutathione hydrolase, glyoxalase II and catalase also function in the degradation of FA (Zhiqian Tong, 2008).

2. In vitro investigations

2.1 Low concentrations of formaldehyde promote Tau aggregation

Neuronal Tau, an important microtubule-associated protein, functions in facilitating the assembly of microtubules and maintaining their stability (Weingarten et al., 1975; Drechsel et al., 1992). Aberrant modifications of Tau protein, such as hyperphosphorylation which induces misfolding and aggregation, lead to microtubule system damage and subsequent disturbance of axonal transport and neuronal morphogenesis (Cuenda et al., 2005; Terwel et al., 2008). Hyperphosphorylated Tau is the major component of paired helical filaments (PHFs) in neurofibrillary tangles (NFTs), an important characteristic of tauopathies which include neurodegenerative conditions such as Alzheimer's disease (Goedert et al., 1996; Hardy, 2006).

The focus of research in our group is on the relationship between FA-meditated impairments and age-related dementia. Our results showed that native Tau exhibited globules with a diameter of 9±2 nm, while FA-treated Tau had a significantly increased diameter of 18±3 nm in the presence of 18.0 mM FA. The increased diameter of Tau globules was dependent on FA concentration. The rapid onset of aggregation (within 10 min) was followed by a marked increase in particle size. These results were confirmed by SDS-PAGE, where an increase in the polymer bands and a decrease in the monomer bands was seen with increasing FA concentration or time. In addition, light-scattering data (at 480 nm) showed that the intensity of FA-treated Tau was considerably enhanced compared with the control, further confirming that FA induced the aggregation of Tau (Nie et al., 2005). Thus, we proposed a putative mechanism of FA-induced Tau aggregation. A formaldehyde molecule first interacts with a Tau monomer. As additional FA molecules interact with other Tau monomers, the FA molecules polymerise, finally resulting in the cross-linking of the Tau molecules (Nie et al., 2007).

The wormlike conformation of Tau at room temperature, as determined by circular dichroism (CD), is reported to have a minimal content of secondary structures (Schweers et al., 1994). It was observed that the probability of the collision of KI with Tyr residues became smaller after the aggregation of Tau, and suggesting that Tyr residues may shift to the interior of the Tau molecule during aggregation, leading to the lower availability of Tyr residues for KI. The fluorescence of 8-Anilino-1-naphthalene-sulfonic acid (ANS), a fluorescent probe which binds to the hydrophobic regions of proteins, was enhanced as Tau was treated with FA, demonstrating the formation of a hydrophobic core during Tau aggregation. Protease rapidly cleaved native Tau to produce fragments with an apparent molecular mass of 36-37 kDa. However, no digested fragments were observed after Tau was incubated with FA, suggesting that the cleavage sites recognized by the protease were buried in the aggregates of Tau (Nie et al., 2005). In conclusion, these reports indicate that FA is able to induce neuronal Tau to misfold, resulting in aggregation and conformational changes.

2.2 Tau aggregates induced by formaldehyde are molten globules

Though protein misfolding is believed to induce cellular metabolic dysfunction and even cell death, the mechanism of this phenomenon remains unclear. A number of pathological mechanisms have been proposed and can be divided into two categories: one which suggests that the products of protein misfolding initiate the "death pathway" (Lipton&Nakamura, 2009; Gu et al., 2010), and the other which proposes that "aspecific amyloid ion channels" composed of misfolded proteins cause damage to membrane permeability and result in the disturbance of ion metabolism (Lin et al., 2001; Lal et al., 2005; Lal et al., 2007). ThT fluorescence (λ_{ex} = 450 nm) and Congo Red staining (measured by light absorbance at 400 nm - 600 nm) increased markedly, indicating that Tau aggregates had features of amyloid-like protein. Using atomic force microscopy, we observed that FA-induced Tau aggregates appeared to have a "pore-like" structure with a diameter of 8.94 ± 1.62 nm in the middle of the aggregate. In addition, when Tau was incubated without FA, it formed fibril-like or amorphous aggregates instead of "pore-like" aggregates. It should be noted that these "pore-like" aggregates were observed at a high FA concentration under the experimental conditions, and whether they exist in vivo need to be further investigated. This might provide insights into the mechanism of tauopathies which result from protein misfolding and aggregation (Naqvi et al., 2010).

2.3 Formaldehyde-induced aggregation interferes with Tau's protection of DNA

Many studies have shown that Tau protein is located in axons and neuronal soma and has important functions in the microtubule system as a microtubule-associated protein (Binder et al., 1985). Recent findings have demonstrated that Tau is also present in the nucleus (Loomis et al., 1990; Johnson&Davis, 1999) and functions in the protection of DNA (Galas et al., 2011). Heat stress and oxidative stress induce the accumulation of nonphosphorylated Tau in the nuclei of neurons. These nuclear Tau accumulations display an enhanced capacity for interacting with DNA and protect DNA from damage by stress (Galas et al., 2011). Other studies have reported that nuclear Tau binds preferentially to polynucleotides of ~13 bp in length, while further research has indicated that Tau binds to the minor groove of the DNA double helix and that both its proline-rich domain (PRD) and microtubule-binding domain (MTBD) contribute to its interaction with DNA. This binding protects DNA from both digestion by DNase I and damage by peroxidation (Wei et al., 2008).

Electrophoretic mobility shift assays (EMSA) showed that native Tau retarded the mobility of DNA while no retardation was observed when DNA was incubated with either Tau aggregates induced by FA, or with BSA, indicating that Tau binding to DNA is suppressed by aggregation. That is, the aggregation of Tau induced by FA inhibits its ability to bind to DNA and may result in the loss of Tau's protection of DNA (Hua&He, 2002; Lu et al., 2011). These observations suggest a novel mechanism of cell death during the pathological progress of tauopathies, such as neurodegenerative conditions.

3. In vivo investigations

3.1 Formaldehyde-induced aggregation of Tau can be observed in vivo

FA induced significant aggregates in cells. Tau-1 (an antibody which recognizes Tau protein) signals confirmed that Tau forms aggregates in the presence of FA. In addition, apoptosis of HEK 293 cells transfected with *tau* increased, while cells transfected with a control vector showed no increase in apoptosis (Nie et al., 2007). In another study we found that FA-induced Tau aggregates promoted apoptosis in both the SH-SY5Y cell line and rat hippocampal primary cells (Nie et al., 2006). These reports indicate that Tau aggregates induced by FA lead to apoptosis.

3.2 Formaldehyde treated mice perform abnormally in spatial reference memory tests

Test of mice by Morris water maze showed that the latency to platform of FA-treated mice was twice as long as controls and the length of time they spent in the target quadrant was nearly half that of controls, indicating that significant impairment of spatial reference memory function occurred when mice were treated with FA for 30 days. When resveratrol (0.5 mM), a natural FA scavenger, was administrated to mice along with FA, the FA-induced effects on learning memory were attenuated. That is, FA-administrated mice act in abnormal performance in spatial reference memory tests.

3.3 Excess endogenous formaldehyde is positively correlated with memory decline and cognitive impairment in animals

Since FA can pass through the blood brain barrier (Grönvall et al, 1998; Shcherbakova et al., 1986), it is necessary to detect the level of FA in the brain in order to determine the influence of FA on the central nervous system (CNS). The FA level in the brain of three types of Alzheimer's disease mouse model, 5 month-old senescence accelerated mice (SAMP8), 3 month-old APP/PS1-transgenic mice, and 6-month old APP-transgenic mice, was estimated by Fluo-HPLC to be about 0.33, 0.46 and 0.56 mM/g, respectively. Concentrations of FA in the brains of these AD models were all significantly higher than their respective controls (Tong et al., 2011). In addition, FA levels in the brains of rats were inversely correlated to their behavioral performance in the Morris water maze (Tong et al., 2011). In summary, endogenous FA concentrations in the brains of AD animal models (SAMP8, APP/PS1 and APP transgenic mice) are significantly higher than their respective controls, and excess endogenous FA can induce memory decline and cognitive impairment in animals.

In addition, β-amyloid deposits, the other main characteristic of AD in addition to neurofibrillary tangles, increase on treatment with FA in vitro (Yu et al., 2006) and excess endogenous FA also promotes the deposition of Aβ (Yu et al., 2007). Elevated levels of FA have also been detected in patients with multiple sclerosis (Khokhlov et al., 1989).

4. Clinical trials

4.1 Urine formaldehyde levels in AD patients are correlated with the degree of dementia

The study on the relationship between urine FA level and the degree of dementia showed that the percentage of patients with mild cognitive impairment (MCI), and medium and severe dementia in which concentrations of urine FA increased compared with that of age-matched healthy controls was 42% (21/50), 82.05% (32/39) and 88.46% (46/52), respectively (Tong et al., 2011) (Weishan Wang, 2010).

These results indicate that cognitive impairments of patients with age-related dementia are probably related to endogenous FA levels, and suggest that measuring urine FA levels together with mini mental state examination (MMSE) may be a useful non-invasive method for the investigation and diagnosis of age-related dementia.

4.2 High levels of formaldehyde are observed in the brains of AD patients

In addition to urine samples, we also measured the FA levels in homogenates from autopsy hippocampus tissues of AD patients by Fluo-HPLC. We found significant increases in the FA concentrations in AD patients (about 0.081 mM/g; n = 4) compared with normal controls (about 0.047 mM/g; n = 4) (Tong et al., 2011), indicating once again that endogenous FA level in AD patients is correlated with the progress of dementia.

5. Formaldehyde stress

Though the concept of "formaldehyde stress" has been mentioned in studies on *Methylobacterium extorquens* AMI (Miller, 2009) and tuberculosis (Bottiglioni&Sturani, 1955), the definition of "formaldehyde stress" in neural cells was first proposed by our group. Abnormal accumulation of endogenous FA can cause abnormal modifications and misfolding of proteins, resulting in neural cell responses such as DNA damage, and even cell death (Figure 1). These may lead to dysfunction of related nervous system and cognitive impairments (He et al., 2010).

5.1 Endogenous formaldehyde overload can induce chronic impairment and sporadic age-related dementia

Studies indicate that the level of endogenous FA in humans is maintained homeostatically (around 0.083 mM in urine), but increases with aging. Endogenous FA levels in AD patients and AD mouse models are notably higher than their respective normal controls. Stress induced by excess endogenous FA leads to chronic impairments of the CNS and may contribute to age-related dementia (He et al., 2010; Hao et al., 2011).

5.2 Putative mechanism of formaldehyde accumulation and formaldehyde stress

As mentioned above, generation and degradation of endogenous FA mainly depends on enzymatic reactions. With aging, dysfunction of these enzymes may cause abnormalities in the formaldehyde cycle and aberrant enzymatic production of FA from endogenous and exogenous substrates results in the accumulation of FA, leading to stress and subsequent pathogenic neurodegeneration (Morrison et al., 1996; Tyihak et al., 1998; Kamino et al., 2000; Yu et al., 2003b; Unzeta et al., 2005; Unzeta et al., 2007). Other factors in aging can also produce excess endogenous FA. Decreased levels of glutathione (GSH) induced by oxidative stress lead to higher levels of endogenous FA (Tyihak et al., 1998; Ling et al., 2006). β-amyloid peptide, a biomarker of Alzheimer's disease, is believed to enhance ROS production and cause a decline in the activity of ALDH2, leading to the production of excess FA (Ohta&Ohsawa, 2006). APOE ε4, considered to be a risk factor of AD, can act synergistically with the deficiency of ALDH 2 to result in accumulation of FA (Ohta et al., 2008). In addition, lipid peroxidation (LPO) (Lemeshko&Nikitchenko Iu, 1982b, a; Dahl&Hadley, 1983; Fokin et al., 1989; Halliwell&Chirico, 1993), abuse of drugs (for example, nicotine and cocaine) (Dahl&Hadley, 1983), and air pollutants (for example, endrin) (Bagchi et al., 1992) can also lead to the accumulation of FA. Polymorphisms in aldehyde dehydrogenase may be correlated with the metabolism and accumulation of FA (Thomasson et al., 1991; Wang et al., 2002; Li Hai-han 2006; Yang et al., 2008). *Adh3* mutant mice are more vulnerable to FA, indicating that dysfunction of this gene is related to abnormal metabolism of FA and causes severe toxicity (Duester et al., 1999).

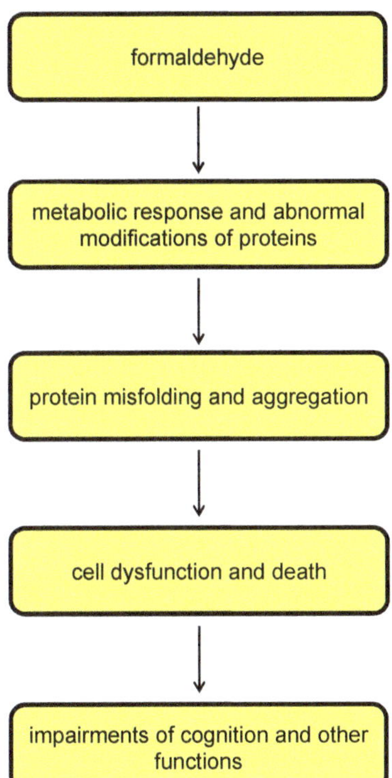

Fig. 1. A putative scheme for formaldehyde stress. Formaldehyde stress is defined as a cellular response which occurs when there is an overload of formaldehyde. Under formaldehyde stress, abnormal modifications of proteins, such as hydroxymethylation and hyperphosphorylation, is present, leading to protein misfolding and aggregation and even to cell death.

6. Perspective

Since FA level is related to cognitive impairments, eliminating excess endogenous FA may become a novel therapy for age-related dementia. Trans-resveratrol (trans-3,5,4'-trihydroxystilbene, Res), a phytoalexin, is a natural ingredient in grapes and various medicinal plants. Res, as a scavenger of FA, can eliminate excess FA and may prevent cells from formaldehyde stress (Tyihak et al., 1998; Marcsek et al., 2007; Marambaud et al., 2008; Gibson et al., 2009; Sun et al., 2010). Antioxidant drugs, such as vitamin E and C, can inhibit lipid peroxidation and the resultant generation of FA (Arlt S, 2001; Yu et al., 2007; Jin-xia., 2009). In addition, iron chelators can enhance the ability of cells to resist the cytotoxicity of FA (O'Brien et al., 2001).

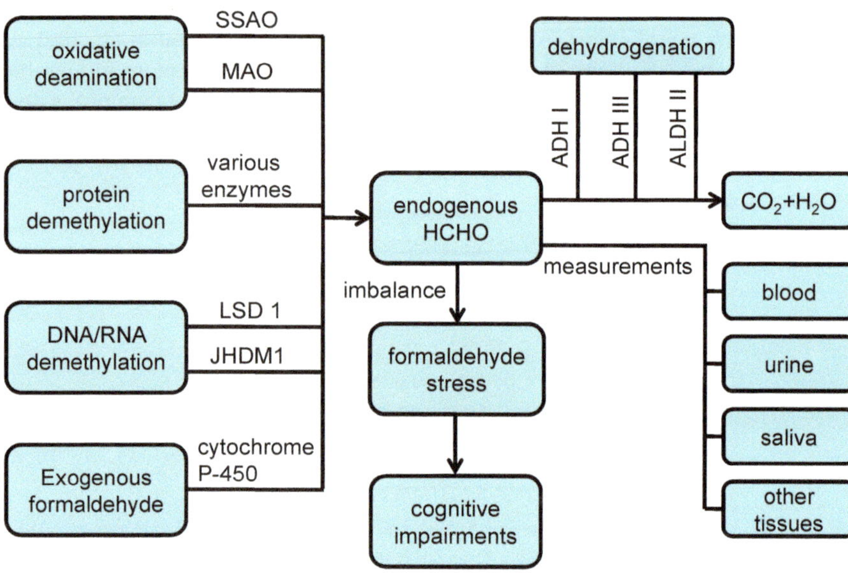

Fig. 2. Formaldehyde stress and the metabolism of endogenous formaldehyde. Endogenous formaldehyde is generated by a variety of enzymes via deamination, demethylation and other reactions. Aldehyde (alcohol) dehydrogenases are the main enzymes involved in the degradation of formaldehyde. Endogenous formaldehyde exists in all tissues such as blood, urine, saliva and brain. Aberrant metabolism causes an increase in endogenous formaldehyde and induces formaldehyde stress, resulting in the dysfunction of organs, especially cognitive impairments.

In summary, excess endogenous FA leads to "formaldehyde stress", which causes aberrant modification of protein and subsequent protein misfolding and aggregation. The aggregated protein loses its normal physiological function and initiates cell death, organ dysfunction, cognitive impairments and even age-related dementia. Elimination of excess endogenous FA may provide an approach to the therapy of dementia (Figure 2).

Though the relationship between endogenous FA and neurodegeneration has recently received considerable attention, the molecular events involved in FA-induced dementia are still unclear. Since the pathological factors in neurodegenerative diseases including

Alzheimer's disease are complicated and synergistic, further studies should be carried out to reveal the mechanism by which FA contributes to the induction of age-related dementia.

7. Fundings

This work was supported by grants from the 973-Projects (2012CB911004; 2010CB912303), the Natural Scientific Foundation of China (NSFC 30970695), CAS-KSCX2-YW-R-119, KSCX2-YW-R-256 and QCAS Biotechnology Fund (GJHZ1131). The funders had no role in study design, data collection and analysis, decision to publish, or preparation of the manuscript.

8. References

Abeles& Mackenzie (1956) Production of active formaldehyde in the mitochondrial oxidation of sarcosine-CD3. *J Biol Chem*,Vol.222,No.1,pp. 145-150,0021-9258

Abeles R.H. (1992) Chapter 25. Biochemistry, In: *One Carbon Metabolism*, pp. 675

Ahmed, Tsukahara, Tin Tin Win, Yamamoto, Kunugita, Arashidani& Fujimaki (2007) Effects of low-level formaldehyde exposure on synaptic plasticity-related gene expression in the hippocampus of immunized mice. *J Neuroimmunol*,Vol.186,No.1-2,pp. 104-111,0165-5728

Arlt S (2001) Lipid peroxidation as a common pathomechanism in coronary heart disease and Alzheimer disease. *Z Gerontol Geriatr*,Vol.34,No.6,pp. 461-465

Aslan, Songur, Tunc, Ozen, Bas, Yagmurca, Turgut, Sarsilmaz& Kaplan (2006) Effects of formaldehyde exposure on granule cell number and volume of dentate gyrus: a histopathological and stereological study. *Brain Res*,Vol.1122,No.1,pp. 191-200,0006-8993

Bagchi, Bagchi, Hassoun& Stohs (1992) Endrin-Induced Urinary-Excretion of Formaldehyde, Acetaldehyde, Malondialdehyde and Acetone in Rats. *Toxicology*,Vol.75,No.1,pp. 81-89,0300-483X

Bierbaum, Kato, Burke& Koch (2001) Formaldehyde in human cancer cells: Detection by preconcentration-chemical ionization mass spectrometry. *Analytical Chemistry*, Vol.73, No.13, pp. 2992-2997,0003-2700

Binder, Frankfurter& Rebhun (1985) The distribution of tau in the mammalian central nervous system. *J Cell Biol*,Vol.101,No.4,pp. 1371-1378,0021-9525

Blair, Magnani, Brand& Wouterloot (2008) Formaldehyde in the far outer galaxy: constraining the outer boundary of the galactic habitable zone. *Astrobiology*, Vol.8, No.1, pp. 59-73,1531-1074

Bottiglioni& Sturani (1955) [Formaldehyde stress and experimental tuberculosis. II. Modifications of ground substance of the connective tissue in the skin, in the specific granuloma and in the kidneys]. *Arch Patol Clin Med*,Vol.32,No.3,pp. 210-219,0004-0142

Canuto, Levine, Augustsson, Imhoff& Giampapa (1983) The Young Sun and the Atmosphere and Photochemistry of the Early Earth. *Nature*,Vol.305,No.5932,pp. 281-286,0028-0836

Conaway, Whysner, Verna& Williams (1996) Formaldehyde mechanistic data and risk assessment: endogenous protection from DNA adduct formation. *Pharmacol Ther*,Vol.71,No.1-2,pp. 29-55,0163-7258

Conklin, Cowley, Wiechmann, Johnson, Trent& Boor (2004) Vasoactive effects of methylamine in isolated human blood vessels: role of semicarbazide-sensitive amine oxidase, formaldehyde, and hydrogen peroxide. *American Journal of Physiology-Heart and Circulatory Physiology*,Vol.286,No.2,pp. H667-H676,0363-6135

Cuenda, Feijoo, Campbell, Jakes& Goedert (2005) Evidence that phosphorylation of the microtubule-associated protein Tau by SAPK4/p38 delta at Thr50 promotes microtubule assembly. *Journal of Cell Science*,Vol.118,No.2,pp. 397-408,0021-9533

Dahl& Hadley (1983) Formaldehyde Production Promoted by Rat Nasal Cytochrome P-450-Dependent Monooxygenases with Nasal Decongestants, Essences, Solvents, Air-Pollutants, Nicotine, and Cocaine as Substrates. *Toxicology and Applied Pharmacology*,Vol.67,No.2,pp. 200-205,0041-008X

Drechsel, Hyman, Cobb& Kirschner (1992) Modulation of the Dynamic Instability of Tubulin Assembly by the Microtubule-Associated Protein Tau. *Molecular Biology of the Cell*,Vol.3,No.10,pp. 1141-1154,1059-1524

Duester, Deltour& Foglio (1999) Metabolic deficiencies in alcohol dehydrogenase Adh1, Adh3, and Adh4 null mutant mice - Overlapping roles of Adh1 and Adh4 in ethanol clearance and metabolism of retinol to retinoic acid. *Journal of Biological Chemistry*,Vol.274,No.24,pp. 16796-16801,0021-9258

Ehrlich (2009) DNA hypomethylation in cancer cells. *Epigenomics*,Vol.1,No.2,pp. 239-259,1750-1911

Estonius, Svensson& Hoog (1996) Alcohol dehydrogenase in human tissues: localisation of transcripts coding for five classes of the enzyme. *FEBS Lett*,Vol.397,No.2-3,pp. 338-342,0014-5793

Fang& Tian (2007) Current perspectives on histone demethylases. *Acta Biochimica Et Biophysica Sinica*,Vol.39,No.2,pp. 81-88,1672-9145

Fokin, Ponomareva, Orlov, Liderman& Erin (1989) [The relationship of the electrical reactions of the brain to lipid peroxidation processes in pathological aging]. *Biull Eksp Biol Med*,Vol.107,No.6,pp. 682-684,0365-9615

Fujimaki, Kawagoe, Bissonnette& Befus (1992) Mast cell response to formaldehyde. 1. Modulation of mediator release. *Int Arch Allergy Immunol*,Vol.98,No.4,pp. 324-331,1018-2438

Galas, Sultan, Nesslany, Violet, Begard, Loyens, Talahari, Mansuroglu, Marzin, Sergeant, Humez, Colin, Bonnefoy& Buee (2011) Nuclear Tau, a Key Player in Neuronal DNA Protection. *Journal of Biological Chemistry*,Vol.286,No.6,pp. 4566-4575,0021-9258

Gerken, Girard, Tung, Webby, Saudek, Hewitson, Yeo, McDonough, Cunliffe, McNeill, Galvanovskis, Rorsman, Robins, Prieur, Coll, Ma, Jovanovic, Farooqi, Sedgwick, Barroso, Lindahl, Ponting, Ashcroft, O'Rahilly& Schofield (2007) The obesity-associated FTO gene encodes a 2-oxoglutarate-dependent nucleic acid demethylase. *Science*,Vol.318,No.5855,pp. 1469-1472,1095-9203

Gibson, Karuppagounder, Pinto, Xu, Chen& Beal (2009) Dietary supplementation with resveratrol reduces plaque pathology in a transgenic model of Alzheimer's disease. *Neurochemistry International*,Vol.54,No.2,pp. 111-118,0197-0186

Grönvall , Garpenstrand, Oreland, Ekblom. (1998). Autoradiographic imaging of formaldehyde adducts in mice: possible relevance for vascular damage in diabetes. Life Sci. No.63, pp. 759-768.

Goedert, Jakes, Spillantini, Hasegawa, Smith& Crowther (1996) Assembly of microtubule-associated protein tau into Alzheimer-like filaments induced by sulphated glycosaminoglycans. *Nature*,Vol.383,No.6600,pp. 550-553,0028-0836

Gu, Nakamura& Lipton (2010) Redox Reactions Induced by Nitrosative Stress Mediate Protein Misfolding and Mitochondrial Dysfunction in Neurodegenerative Diseases. *Molecular Neurobiology*,Vol.41,No.2-3,pp. 55-72,0893-7648

Halliwell& Chirico (1993) Lipid peroxidation: its mechanism, measurement, and significance. *Am J Clin Nutr*,Vol.57,No.5 Suppl,pp. 715S-724S; discussion 724S-725S, 0002-9165

Hao, Li, Cui, Li, Li, Wang & He. Correlation of urine formaldehyde levels and mini mental state examination scores in Alzheimer's disease. Chinese Journal of Gerontology, 2011, Vol.31, No.18, pp.3442-3444, 1005-9202

Hardy (2006) A hundred years of Alzheimer's disease research. *Neuron*,Vol.52,No.1,pp. 3-13,0896-6273

He, Yi& Yang (2009) A Non-Heme Iron-Mediated Chemical Demethylation in DNA and RNA. *Accounts of Chemical Research*,Vol.42,No.4,pp. 519-529,0001-4842

He, Lu& Miao (2010) Formaldehyde stress. *Sci China Life Sci*,Vol.53,No.12,pp. 1399-1404,1869-1889

Naqvi, Wang, Miao & He (2010) Pore-like Aggregates of Tau Protein Induced by Formaldehyde. *Progress in Biochemistry and Biophysics*,Vol.37, No.11, pp. 1195-1203, 1000-3282

Nie, Wang, Liu, Perrett & He (2006) Amyloid-like aggregates of neuronal tau are induced by formaldehyde exposure and promote apoptosis of neuronal cells. BMC Neurosci, Vol.8, No.9

Nie, Wei, Chen, Liu, Dui, Liu, Davies, Tendler & He (2007) Formaldehyde at Low Concentration Induces Protein Tau into Globular Amyloid-Like Aggregates In Vitro and In Vivo. *Plos One*,Vol.2,No.7,pp.,1932-6203

Tong, Zhang, Luo, Wang, Li, Li, Luo, Lu, Zhou, Wan & He (2011) Urine formaldehyde level is inversely correlated to mini mental state examination scores in senile dementia. *Neurobiology of Aging*,Vol.32,No.1,pp. 31-41,0197-4580

Hua& He (2002) Effect of phosphorylation and aggregation on tau binding to DNA. *Protein and Peptide Letters*,Vol.9,No.4,pp. 349-357,0929-8665

Iborra, Renau-Piqueras, Portoles, Boleda, Guerri& Pares (1992) Immunocytochemical and biochemical demonstration of formaldhyde dehydrogenase (class III alcohol dehydrogenase) in the nucleus. *Journal of Histochemistry & Cytochemistry*, Vol.40, No.12, pp. 1865-1878,0022-1554

Jin-xia. (2009) Effect of vitamin E against impairment on learning and memory ability. *Modern Preventive Medicine*,Vol.36,No.10,pp. 1833-1835

Johnson& Davis (1999) The microtubule binding of tau and high molecular weight tau in apoptotic PC12 cells is impaired because of altered phosphorylation. *Journal of Biological Chemistry*,Vol.274,No.50,pp. 35686-35692,0021-9258

Kalapos (1999) A possible evolutionary role of formaldehyde. *Exp Mol Med*,Vol.31,No.1,pp. 1-4,1226-3613

Kalasz (2003) Biological role of formaldehyde, and cycles related to methylation, demethylation, and formaldehyde production. *Mini Rev Med Chem*,Vol.3,No.3,pp. 175-192,1389-5575

Kamino, Nagasaka, Imagawa, Yamamoto, Yoneda, Ueki, Kitamura, Namekata, Miki& Ohta (2000) Deficiency in mitochondrial aldehyde dehydrogenase increases the risk for late-onset Alzheimer's disease in the Japanese population. *Biochem Biophys Res Commun*,Vol.273,No.1,pp. 192-196,0006-291X

Kast, Toews, Rogalski& Clark (2008) Mass spectrometric identification of formaldehyde-induced peptide modifications under in vivo protein cross-linking conditions. *Analytica Chimica Acta*,Vol.618,No.2,pp. 168-183,0003-2670

Keefer, Kroeger-Koepke, Ishizaki, Michejda, Saavedra, Hrabie, Yang& Roller (1990) Stereoselectivity in the microsomal conversion of N-nitrosodimethylamine to formaldehyde. *Chem Res Toxicol*,Vol.3,No.6,pp. 540-544,0893-228X

Khokhlov, Zavalishin, Savchenko Iu& Dziuba (1989) [Disorders of formaldehyde metabolism and its metabolic precursors in patients with multiple sclerosis]. *Zh Nevropatol Psikhiatr Im S S Korsakova*,Vol.89,No.2,pp. 45-48,0044-4588

Kilburn (1994) Neurobehavioral impairment and seizures from formaldehyde. *Arch Environ Health*,Vol.49,No.1,pp. 37-44,0003-9896

Kilburn, Warshaw& Thornton (1987) Formaldehyde impairs memory, equilibrium, and dexterity in histology technicians: effects which persist for days after exposure. *Arch Environ Health*,Vol.42,No.2,pp. 117-120,0003-9896

Lal, Lin& Quist (2007) Amyloid beta ion channel: 3D structure and relevance to amyloid channel paradigm. *Biochim Biophys Acta*,Vol.1768,No.8,pp. 1966-1975,0006-3002

Lal, Quist, Doudevski, Lin, Azimova, Ng, Frangione, Kagan& Ghiso (2005) Amyloid ion channels: A common structural link for protein-misfolding disease. *Proceedings of the National Academy of Sciences of the United States of America*,Vol.102,No.30,pp. 10427-10432,0027-8424

Lemeshko& Nikitchenko Iu (1982a) [Lipid peroxidation of myocardial membranes and its regulation during aging]. *Biull Eksp Biol Med*,Vol.94,No.11,pp. 12-14,0365-9615

Lemeshko& Nikitchenko Iu (1982b) [Lipid peroxidation in rat liver mitochondria in aging and in hyperthyroidism]. *Biokhimiia*,Vol.47,No.5,pp. 752-759,0320-9725

Li Hai-han (2006) Polymorphisms of aldehyde and alcohol dehydrogenase genes associated with susceptibility to trichloroethylene-induced medicamentosa-like dermatitis. *Journal of Hygiene Research*,Vol.35,No.2,pp. 149-151

Lin, Bhatia& Lal (2001) Amyloid beta protein forms ion channels: implications for Alzheimer's disease pathophysiology. *FASEB J*,Vol.15,No.13,pp. 2433-2444,1530-6860

Ling, Zhu& Carvey (2006) Age-related changes in glutathione and glutathione-related enzymes in rat brain. *Brain Research*,Vol.1090,No.35-44,0006-8993

Lipton& Nakamura (2009) Cell death: protein misfolding and neurodegenerative diseases. *Apoptosis*,Vol.14,No.4,pp. 455-468,1360-8185

Loomis, Howard, Castleberry& Binder (1990) Identification of Nuclear Tau-Isoforms in Human Neuroblastoma-Cells. *Proceedings of the National Academy of Sciences of the United States of America*,Vol.87,No.21,pp. 8422-8426,0027-8424

Lu, Miao, Pan & He. Formaldehyde-mediated hyperphosphorylation disturbs the interaction between Tau protein and DNA. Prog Biochem Biophys, 2011. doi: 10.3724/SP.J.1206.2011.00451

Lu, Li, Qiao, Yan& Yang (2008) Effect of inhaled formaldehyde on learning and memory of mice. *Indoor Air*,Vol.18,No.2,pp. 77-83,1600-0668

Luo, Li, Zhang& Ang (2001) Determination of formaldehyde in blood plasma by high-performance liquid chromatography with fluorescence detection. *Journal of Chromatography B*,Vol.753,No.2,pp. 253-257,0378-4347

Mahy, Andres, Lizcano, Rodriguez, Romera& Unzeta (2001) Tissue activity and cellular localization of human semicarbazide-sensitive amine oxidase. *Journal of Histochemistry & Cytochemistry*,Vol.49,No.2,pp. 209-217,0022-1554

Malek, Moritz& Fanghanel (2003) Formaldehyde inhalation & open field behaviour in rats. *Indian J Med Res*,Vol.118,No.90-96,0971-5916

Marambaud, Vingtdeux, Dreses-Werringloer, Zhao& Davies (2008) Therapeutic potential of resveratrol in Alzheimer's disease. *Bmc Neuroscience*,Vol.9,No.,1471-2202

Marcsek, Kocsis, Szende& Tompa (2007) Effect of formaldehyde and resveratrol on the viability of Vero, HepG2 and MCF-7 cells. *Cell Biology International*,Vol.31,No.10,pp. 1214-1219,1065-6995

Metz, Kersten, Hoogerhout, Brugghe, Timmermans, de Jong, Meiring, ten Hove, Hennink, Crommelin& Jiskoot (2004) Identification of formaldehyde-induced modifications in proteins: reactions with model peptides. *J Biol Chem*,Vol.279,No.8,pp. 6235-6243,0021-9258

Miller (1953) A production of amino acids under possible primitive earth conditions. *Science*,Vol.117,No.3046,pp. 528-529,0036-8075

Miller (2009) Formaldehyde Stress Response in Methylobacterium extorquens AMI. *A dissertation submitted in partial fulfillment of the requirements for the degree of Doctor of Philosophy*

Mori, Haseba, Kameyama, Shimizu, Kudoh, Ohaki, Arai, Yamazaki& Asano (2000) Histological distribution of class III alcohol dehydrogenase in human brain. *Brain Research*,Vol.852,No.1,pp. 186-190,0006-8993

Morrison, Smith& Kish (1996) Brain S-Adenosylmethionine levels are severely decreased in Alzheimer's disease. *Journal of Neurochemistry*,Vol.67,No.3,pp. 1328-1331,0022-3042

Nakamura, Ridpath, Nakamura, Tano, Luke, Sonoda, Arakawa, Buerstedde, Gillespie, Sale, Yamazoe, Bishop, Takata, Takeda, Watanabe& Swenberg (2007) Cells deficient in the FANC/BRCA pathway are hypersensitive to plasma levels of formaldehyde. *Cancer Research*,Vol.67,No.23,pp. 11117-11122,0008-5472

Nie, Zhang, Zhang& He (2005) Changes in conformation of human neuronal tau during denaturation in formaldehyde solution. *Protein Pept Lett*,Vol.12,No.1,pp. 75-78,0929-8665

O'Brien, Teng, Beard, Pourahmad, Moridani, Easson& Poon (2001) The formaldehyde metabolic detoxification enzyme systems and molecular cytotoxic mechanism in isolated rat hepatocytes. *Chemico-Biological Interactions*,Vol.130,No.1-3,pp. 285-296,0009-2797

Ohta& Ohsawa (2006) Dysfunction of mitochondria and oxidative stress in the pathogenesis of Alzheimer's disease: on defects in the cytochrome c oxidase complex and aldehyde detoxification. *J Alzheimers Dis*,Vol.9,No.2,pp. 155-166,1387-2877

Ohta, Ohsawa, Nishimaki, Murakami, Suzuki& Ishikawa (2008) Age-dependent neurodegeneration accompanying memory loss in transgenic mice defective in mitochondrial aldehyde dehydrogenase 2 activity. *Journal of Neuroscience*, Vol.28, No.24, pp. 6239-6249,0270-6474

Olson, Galter, Carmine, Buervenich& Duester (2003) Distribution of class I, III and IV alcohol dehydrogenase mRNAs in the adult rat, mouse and human brain. *European Journal of Biochemistry*,Vol.270,No.6,pp. 1316-1326,0014-2956

P. Maboudou (2002) Detection of oxidative stress. Interest of GC-MS for malondialdehyde and formaldehyde monitoring. *Biomedical Chromatography*,Vol.16,No.199-202

Patterson, Pateras, Grammer& Harris (1986) Human antibodies against formaldehyde-human serum albumin conjugates or human serum albumin in individuals exposed to formaldehyde. *Int Arch Allergy Appl Immunol*,Vol.79,No.1,pp. 53-59,0020-5915

Perna, Bordini& Deinzer-Lifrak (2001) A case of claimed persistent neuropsychological sequelae of chronic formaldehyde exposure: clinical, psychometric, and functional findings. *Arch Clin Neuropsychol*,Vol.16,No.1,pp. 33-44,0887-6177

Petushok, Petushok, El'chaninova, Ban'kovskii& Trebukhina (2005) [Functional activity of blood and liver cells under formaldehyde intoxication via inhalation]. *Biomed Khim*,Vol.51,No.1,pp. 76-80

Pinto, Gladstone& Yung (1980) Photochemical Production of Formaldehyde in Earth's Primitive Atmosphere. *Science*,Vol.210,No.4466,pp. 183-185,0036-8075

Pitten, Kramer, Herrmann, Bremer& Koch (2000) Formaldehyde neurotoxicity in animal experiments. *Pathol Res Pract*,Vol.196,No.3,pp. 193-198,0344-0338

Ramonet, Rodriguez, Saura, Lizcano, Romera, Unzeta, Finch, Billett& Mahy (2003) Localization of monoamine oxidase A and B and semicarbazide-sensitive amine oxidase in human peripheral tissues. *Inflammopharmacology*,Vol.11,No.2,pp. 111-117,0925-4692

Rety& Marin (1957) [Coronary manifestations with myocardial ischemia after inhalation of formaldehyde vapors]. *Arch Mal Prof*,Vol.18,No.3,pp. 314-315,0003-9691

Rozylo, Siembida, Nemeth, Albert& Tyihak (2000) HPLC-OPLC-MS investigation of change of formaldehyde and its generators in human teeth of different physiological stage. *Biomedical Chromatography*,Vol.14,No.3,pp. 173-179,0269-3879

Sakurai& Yanagawa (1984) Prebiotic synthesis of amino acids from formaldehyde and hydroxylamine in a modified sea medium. *Orig Life*,Vol.14,No.1-4,pp. 171-176,0302-1688

Saladino, Willey, Lechner, Grafstrom, LaVeck& Harris (1985) Effects of formaldehyde, acetaldehyde, benzoyl peroxide, and hydrogen peroxide on cultured normal human bronchial epithelial cells. *Cancer Res*,Vol.45,No.6,pp. 2522-2526,0008-5472

Sarsilmaz, Songur, Akpolat, Kus, Ozen& Zararsiz (2003) The effects of the inhaled formaldehyde during the early postnatal period in the hippocampus of rats: A morphological and immunohistochemical study. *Neuroscience Research Communications*,Vol.33,No.3,pp. 168-178,0893-6609

Sarsilmaz, Kaplan, Songur, Colakoglu, Aslan, Tunc, Ozen, Turgut& Bas (2007) Effects of postnatal formaldehyde exposure on pyramidal cell number, volume of cell layer in hippocampus and hemisphere in the rat: a stereological study. *Brain Res*,Vol.1145,No.157-167,0006-8993

Schweers, Schonbrunnhanebeck, Marx& Mandelkow (1994) Structural Studies of Tau-Protein and Alzheimer Paired Helical Filaments Show No Evidence for Beta-Structure. *Journal of Biological Chemistry*,Vol.269,No.39,pp. 24290-24297,0021-9258

Shaham, Bomstein, Gurvich, Rashkovsky& Kaufman (2003) DNA-protein crosslinks and p53 protein expression in relation to occupational exposure to formaldehyde. *Occup Environ Med*,Vol.60,No.6,pp. 403-409,1351-0711

Shcherbakova, Telpukhov, Trenin, Bashikov& Lapkina (1986) Permeability of the Blood-Brain-Barrier for Intravascular Formaldehyde. *Bulletin of Experimental Biology and Medicine*,Vol.102,No.11,pp. 1553-1554,0007-4888

Shi, Lan, Matson, Mulligan, Whetstine, Cole& Casero (2004) Histone demethylation mediated by the nuclear amine oxidase homolog LSD1. *Cell*,Vol.119,No.7,pp. 941-953,0092-8674

Shibamoto, Ebeler& Clifford (1997) Quantitative analysis by gas chromatography of volatile carbonyl compounds in expired air from mice and human. *Journal of Chromatography B*,Vol.702,No.1-2,pp. 211-215,0378-4347

Smith, Spanel, Holland, Al Singary& Elder (1999) Analysis of formaldehyde in the headspace of urine from bladder and prostate cancer patients using selected ion flow tube mass spectrometry. *Rapid Communications in Mass Spectrometry*,Vol.13,No.14,pp. 1354-1359,0951-4198

Soffritti, Belpoggi, Lambertin, Lauriola, Padovani& Maltoni (2002) Results of long-term experimental studies on the carcinogenicity of formaldehyde and acetaldehyde in rats. *Ann N Y Acad Sci*,Vol.982,No.87-105,0077-8923
Sokolskaya (1976) Glycine and alanine synthesis from formaldehyde and hydroxylamine in the field of ultrasound waves. *Orig Life*,Vol.7,No.3,pp. 183-185,0302-1688
Speit, Schmid, Neuss& Schutz (2008) Genotoxic effects of formaldehyde in the human lung cell line A549 and in primary human nasal epithelial cells. *Environ Mol Mutagen*,Vol.49,No.4,pp. 300-307,0893-6692
Strubelt, Brasch, Pentz& Younes (1990) Experimental studies on the acute cardiovascular toxicity of formalin and its antidotal treatment. *J Toxicol Clin Toxicol*,Vol.28,No.2,pp. 221-233,0731-3810
Su, Wei & He. Assay of brain endogenous formaldehyde with 2,4-dinitrophenylhydrazine through UV-HPLC. Prog Biochem Biophys, 2011. doi: 10.3724/SP.J.1206.2011.00407
Sun, Wang, Simonyi& Sun (2010) Resveratrol as a Therapeutic Agent for Neurodegenerative Diseases. *Molecular Neurobiology*,Vol.41,No.2-3,pp. 375-383,0893-7648
Swenberg, Kerns, Mitchell, Gralla& Pavkov (1980) Induction of squamous cell carcinomas of the rat nasal cavity by inhalation exposure to formaldehyde vapor. *Cancer Res*,Vol.40,No.9,pp. 3398-3402,0008-5472
Szarvas, Szatloczky, Volford, Trezl, Tyihak& Rusznak (1986) Determination of Endogenous Formaldehyde Level in Human-Blood and Urine by Dimedone-C-14 Radiometric Method. *Journal of Radioanalytical and Nuclear Chemistry-Letters*,Vol.106,No.6,pp. 357-367,0236-5731
Takigawa, Takeuchi, Abe, Kawai, Endo, Yasugi, Endo& Ogino (2007) Determination of formaldehyde in urine by headspace gas chromatography. *Bulletin of Environmental Contamination and Toxicology*,Vol.79,No.1,pp. 1-4,0007-4861
Terwel, Muyllaert, Dewachter, Borghgraef, Croes, Devijver& Van Leuven (2008) Amyloid activates GSK-3beta to aggravate neuronal tauopathy in bigenic mice. *Am J Pathol*,Vol.172,No.3,pp. 786-798,0002-9440
Thomasson, Edenberg, Crabb, Mai, Jerome, Li, Wang, Lin, Lu& Yin (1991) Alcohol and aldehyde dehydrogenase genotypes and alcoholism in Chinese men. *Am J Hum Genet*,Vol.48,No.4,pp. 677-681,0002-9297
Thorndike& Beck (1977) Production of formaldehyde from N5-methyltetrahydrofolate by normal and leukemic leukocytes. *Cancer Res*,Vol.37,No.4,pp. 1125-1132,0008-5472
Thrasher, Broughton& Madison (1990) Immune activation and autoantibodies in humans with long-term inhalation exposure to formaldehyde. *Arch Environ Health*,Vol.45,No.4,pp. 217-223,0003-9896
Trezl, Hullan, Szarvas, Csiba& Szende (1998) Determination of endogenous formaldehyde in plants (fruits) bound to L-arginine and its relation to the folate cycle, photosynthesis and apoptosis. *Acta Biologica Hungarica*,Vol.49,No.2-4,pp. 253-263,0236-5383
Trezl, Csiba, Juhasz, Szentgyorgyi, Lombai& Hullan (1997) Endogenous formaldehyde level of foods and its biological significance. *Zeitschrift Fur Lebensmittel-Untersuchung Und-Forschung a-Food Research and Technology*,Vol.205,No.4,pp. 300-304,1431-4630
Tyihak, Bocsi, Timar, Racz& Szende (2001) Formaldehyde promotes and inhibits the proliferation of cultured tumour and endothelial cells. *Cell Prolif*,Vol.34,No.3,pp. 135-141,0960-7722
Tyihak, Albert, Nemeth, Katay, Kiraly-Veghely& Szende (1998) Formaldehyde cycle and the natural formaldehyde generators and capturers. *Acta Biologica Hungarica*,Vol.49,No.2-4,pp. 225-238,0236-5383

Unzeta, Sole, Boada& Hernandez (2007) Semicarbazide-sensitive amine oxidase (SSAO) and its possible contribution to vascular damage in Alzheimer's disease. *J Neural Transm*,Vol.114,No.6,pp. 857-862,0300-9564

Unzeta, Hernandez, Esteban, Szabo& Boada (2005) Human plasma semicarbazide sensitive amine oxidase (SSAO), beta-amyloid protein and aging. *Neuroscience Letters*,Vol.384,No.1-2,pp. 183-187,0304-3940

Wang, Nakajima, Kawamoto& Honma (2002) Effects of aldehyde dehydrogenase-2 genetic polymorphisms on metabolism of structurally different aldehydes in human liver. *Drug Metabolism and Disposition*,Vol.30,No.1,pp. 69-73,0090-9556

Wei, Qu, Wang, Chen, Wang, Liu, Hua& He (2008) Binding to the Minor Groove of the Double-Strand, Tau Protein Prevents DNA from Damage by Peroxidation. *Plos One*,Vol.3,No.7,pp.,1932-6203

Weingarten, Lockwood, Hwo& Kirschner (1975) A protein factor essential for microtubule assembly. *Proc Natl Acad Sci U S A*,Vol.72,No.5,pp. 1858-1862,0027-8424

Weishan Wang (2010) Research on urine formaldehyde concentration in Alzheimer's disease elderly and mormal elderly. *Chin J Geriatr Heart Brain Vessel Dis*,Vol.12,No.721-722

Yang, Wang, Wang, Zhou, Tan, He, Xie, Li, Zheng& Ma (2008) The association of mitochondrial aldehyde dehydrogenase gene (ALDH2) polymorphism with susceptibility to late-onset Alzheimer's disease in Chinese. *Journal of the Neurological Sciences*,Vol.268,No.1-2,pp. 172-175,0022-510X

Yu& Deng (1998) Endogenous formaldehyde as a potential factor of vulnerability of atherosclerosis: involvement of semicarbazide-sensitive amine oxidase-mediated methylamine turnover. *Atherosclerosis*,Vol.140,No.2,pp. 357-363,0021-9150

Yu, Lai& Zuo (1997) Formation of formaldehyde from adrenaline in vivo; A potential risk factor for stress-related angiopathy. *Neurochemical Research*,Vol.22,No.5,pp. 615-620,0364-3190

Yu, Chen& Maley (2006) Potential implications of endogenous aldehydes in beta-amyloid misfolding, oligomerization and fibrillogenesis. *Journal of Neurochemistry*, Vol.99, No.5, pp. 1413-1424,0022-3042

Yu, Chen& Kazachkov (2007) Effect of aldehydes derived from oxidative deamination and oxidative stress on beta-amyloid aggregation; pathological implications to Alzheimer's disease. *Journal of Neural Transmission*,Vol.114,No.6,pp. 835-839,0300-9564

Yu, Cauglin, Wempe& Gubisne-Haberle (2003a) A novel sensitive high-performance liquid chromatography/electrochemical procedure for measuring formaldehyde produced from oxidative deamination of methylamine and in biological samples. *Analytical Biochemistry*,Vol.318,No.2,pp. 285-290,0003-2697

Yu, Wright, Fan, Lun& Gubisne-Harberle (2003b) Physiological and pathological implications of semicarbazide-sensitive amine oxidase. *Biochimica Et Biophysica Acta-Proteins and Proteomics*,Vol.1647,No.1-2,pp. 193-199,1570-9639

Zhang, Tsukada, Fang, Erdjument-Bromage, Warren, Borchers& Tempst (2006) Histone demethylation by a family of JmjC domain-containing proteins. *Nature*, Vol.439, No.7078,pp. 811-816,0028-0836

Zhiqian Tong (2008) Endogenous formaldehyde and related diseases in human. *Progress in Natural Science*,Vol.18,No.11,pp. 1202-1210

5

An Overview of Target Specific Neuro-Protective and Neuro-Restorative Strategies

Ahmad Al Mutairy[1], Khalaf Al Moutaery[2], Abdulrahman Al Asmari[2], Mohammed Arshaduddin[2] and Mohammad Tariq[2]

[1]*University of Dammam,*
[2]*Riyadh Military Hospital, Riyadh,*
Saudi Arabia

1. Introduction

The cellular mechanisms underlying neuronal loss and neurodegeneration have been an area of great interest for neuroscientists throughout the world. The development of animal models that simulate critical components of clinical neurodegenerative diseases have provided tremendous insight into the pathophysiological pathways and have facilitated the application of targeted pharmacotherapy. Although neurodegenerative diseases (ND), such as Alzheimer's disease (AD), Parkinson's disease (PD), amyotrophic lateral sclerosis (ALS), Huntington's disease (HD), and multiple sclerosis (MS) each have distinct clinical symptoms and pathologies, they also share common mechanisms such as intra- and/or extracellular accumulation of misfolded proteins; apoptosis; neuroinflammation; mitochondrial injury, oxidative stress and excitotoxic insult (Tarawneh and Galvin, 2010). No one mechanism appears to be primary in all cases of a particular ND, and these pathogenic most mechanisms most likely act synergistically through complex interactions to promote neurodegeneration. Discussion of these mechanisms is briefly reviewed here in reference to their implications for the development of novel neuroprotective /neuro-restorative agents targeting one or more of these pathways.

2. Misfolding of protein: An important target of treatment for neurodegenerative diseases

Protein misfolding is the physical process by which a polypeptide folds into its characteristic and functional three dimensional structures. Failure to fold into native structure results in inactive protein which is referred to as misfolded protein (Soto, 2003). Neuronal tissues are exquisitely sensitive to defective protein folding, and the accumulation of misfolded proteins is proteotoxic due to dominant effects of insolubility, inappropriate intermolecular interactions, and long half-lives (Neef et al., 2010). Protein misfolding and improper processing by the cellular quality-control system causes many highly debilitating disorders, ranging from heritable diseases, such as cystic fibrosis (CF) and α1-antitrypsin deficiency as well as several other several neurodegenerative disorders (Soto, 2003; Singh, 2010). Hereditary protein conformational disorders are characterized by coding region trinucleotide expansions resulting in the insertion of poly-glutamine (polyQ) tracts that adopt β-sheet structures and that are prone to incorrect folding and aggregation (Neef et al., 2010; Soto, 2003). Expansion of poly Q tracts has been associated with at least nine neurodegenerative diseases (Khare et al., 2005). There are currently no cure for any of the polyQ diseases, but researchers hypothesize that if the abnormal polyQ proteins could be stabilized into their correct conformation, the neurotoxicity associated with protein misfolding in neuronal tissues might be prevented, leading to arrest of the disease process (Heller, 2010).

2.1 Alzheimer's disease (AD)

Alzheimer's disease is characterized by the aggregation and accumulation of two proteins: amyloid beta-peptide (A) which is deposited in extracellular senile plaques and the microtubule-associated protein tau which accumulates in a highly phosphorylated form as paired helical filaments that comprise the intraneuronal neurofibrillary tangles (NFTs) and neuropil threads (Hanger et al., 2009). In AD, tau appears to become hyperphosphorylated, which may contribute to destabilization of microtubules and may be incorporated into neuro-fibrillary tangles. One approach used with transgenic mice has involved NAP (Asn-Ala-Pro- Val-Ser-Ile-Pro-Gln; NAPVSIPQ), an octapeptide that prevents disruption of microtubules by binding to tubulin. Administration of this compound decreased hyperphosphorylation of tau and improved cognitive function in mice (Matsuoka et al., 2008), recently this drug has entered a clinical trial (Potter, 2010). Another approach focuses on enzymes involved in phosphorylating tau. Glycogen synthase kinase-3 (GSK-3), has been shown to cause hyperphosphorylation of tau when over expressed in transgenic mice, and inhibition of this enzyme decreases levels of β-amyloid (Phiel et al., 2003). Lithium chloride by inhibiting GSK-3, decreases hyperphosphorylation of tau and improves cognition (Noble et al., 2005).

One of the approaches to decrease the levels of β-amyloid is passive immunization with antibodies targeting portions of the β-amyloid molecule. Bapineuzumab (AAB-001) is a humanized monoclonal antibody to the N-terminus of β -amyloid. Two phase 2 trials have been conducted with this drug. In one trial, cortical β-amyloid load was significantly decreased (Rinne et al., 2010). In the other trial, no statistically significant difference in cognitive function was found (Salloway et al., 2009). Interestingly, bapineuzumab appeared to produce some beneficial cognitive effects in individuals who did not have the e4 allelle of the apolipoprotein E (ApoE) gene, but those results were not statistically significant (Rinne et al., 2010). Treatment with bapineuzumab has also been found to reduce tau levels in patients with AD in two clinical trials (Kerchner & Boxer, 2010). A phase 3 clinical trial is currently being conducted with bapineuzumab. Ponezumab (PF- 04360365), an antibody targeted to the free carboxy terminus of β-amyloid 1-40, has undergone preliminary human trials and has been shown to increase CSF β-amyloid (Zhao et al., 2010). It seems likely that drugs targeting β-amyloid would need to be given to patients early in the course of disease—before neurodegeneration becomes severe enough to impair cognitive function (Potter, 2010).

The most common pathogenesis of familial AD involves misprocessing of amyloid precursor protein (APP) by enzyme gamma secretase. Targeting of gamma-secretase is another area of drug development for AD (Tomita, 2009). One of these gamma-secretase inhibitors, begacestat (GSI- 953), decreased plasma levels, but not CSF levels, of β-amyloid in humans (Jacobsen et al., 2009; Martone et al., 2009). Another gamma-secretase inhibitor, BMS- 708163, decreased CSF levels of β-amyloid in humans (Ereshfksy et al., 2009). A third gamma- secretase inhibitor, PF-3084014 ([(S)-2-((S)-5,7- difluoro-1,2,3,4-tetrahydronaphthalen-3-ylamino)-N-(1-(2-methyl-1-(neopentylamino) propan-2-yl)-1H-imidazol-4-yl), pentanamide]), decreased plasma and CSF levels of β-amyloid in animals, but only plasma levels in humans (Soares et al., 2009). Stimulation of ά-secretase leads to non-amyloidogenic processing of amyloid processing protein (APP). Some of the muscarinic agonists have been shown to increase ά-secretase activity, and a number of other drugs are being investigated for their ability to inhibit gamma secretase (Mangliasche et al., 2010).

Inhibition of tau aggregation is yet another approach. Immunotherapy with antibodies directed at tau decreased tangles in the Tg P301L mouse model (Asuni et al., 2007). Another avenue that has currently passed a phase 2 trial is blocking tau aggregation with methylene blue (Staff et al., 2008). Methylene blue has also been shown to enhance mitochondrial function (Pandey et al., 2008), and decrease the levels of β-amyloid, and cognitive deficits in 3xTg-AD transgenic mice (Medina et al., 2011). A larger phase 3 trial has been planned. Other such inhibitors which are being studied as potential therapeutic agents for AD include phenothiazines, porphyrins and polyphenols (Brunden et al., 2009).

Heat shock protein 90 (Hsp90) is a member of a large family of molecules that help in regulating pathogenic transformation, and the stability of abnormally folded neuronal proteins, allowing the accumulation of toxic aggregates (Lu et al., 2009; Luo et al., 2010). Inhibition of Hsp 90 activates heat shock factor I (HSF- I) to induce production of Hsp 70 and Hsp40 as well as other chaperones may be promising treatment for AD and other neurodegenerative diseases (Luo et al., 2010). A new Hsp90 inhibitor novobiocin provided excellent neuroprotection, with little or no toxicity in a cell culture model of beta-amyloid (Lu et al., 2009).

2.2 Parkinson's disease (PD)

PD is characterized mainly by progressive and selective loss of dopaminergic neurons in the substantia nigra pars compacta, with subsequent dopamine (DA) decline in the nigrostriatal pathway, and by the presence of intracytoplasmic fibrillar α-Synuclein (*α*-Syn) protein aggregates (Lewy Bodies, LB) in the remaining nigral neurons (Turturici et al., 2011). α-Syn is a 140- amino acid neuronal protein probably involved in regulating cell differentiation, synaptic plasticity, and dopaminergic neurotransmission. The presence of large amounts of α-syn aggregates in the presynaptic nerve terminals has been reported. It is plausible that either misfolded α-Syn, or increased amounts of normal α-syn, contribute to neurotoxicity in PD (Kramer & Schaeffer, 2007). The formation of an N-methylated derivative of α-Syn, by the replacement of the Gly73 with sarcosine, resulted in reduced fibril formation and markedly reduces toxicity (Paleologou et al., 2005). α-Syn peptide fragments that bind to full length α-syn have also been studied as potential targets for inhibiting α-syn aggregation. Peptides derived from the N-terminal of the non-amyloidogenic component (NAC) region of α-syn can bind to the full length α-syn and block the assembly of α-syn into both early oligomers and mature amyloid-like fibrils. Furthermore, the addition of a polyarginine-peptide delivery system has allowed the development of a cell permeable inhibitor of aggregation, the peptide RGGAVVTGRRRRR-amide, that inhibits iron-induced DNA damage in cells transfected with α-synuclein (A53T) (Paleologou et al., 2005). The other compounds which have been shown to inhibit α- synuclein aggregation include melatonin (Sae-Ung et al., 2011), and statins (Bar-On et al., 2008).

2.3 Huntington's disease (HD)

Inclusion bodies of aggregated mutant huntingtin protein (htt) fragments are a neuropathological hallmark of HD. The disease is caused by expansion of a CAG repeat in the Huntington's gene coding for polyQ which leads to the formation of fibrillar protein aggregates and neuronal cell death. Preventing misfolding steps and thereby aggregation of the polyQ containing protein htt may represent an attractive therapeutic strategy to postpone the onset and progression of HD (Wyttenbach et al., 2002). Moreover expression of several molecular chaperones such as Hsp70, Hsp40, Hsp27, Hsp84, and Hsp105 have been shown to increase the solubility of polyQ proteins in Drosophila and mouse models of HD (Tarawneh & Galvin, 2010).

Intracellular antibodies (intrabodies) which target polyQ protein and prevent its aggregation have been identified. Clumps of htt have also been seen in neuronal nucleus and cytoplasm in mice and monkey model of HD. Intrabodies created by injecting the virus into mice brain have been shown to mop up mutant proteins that drive neurodegeneration in HD (Wang et al., 2008). One of the first detectable signs of cellular dysfunction in strial medium spiny neurons in HD is the loss of cannibinoid G protein coupled receptors (GPCRs) (Glass et al., 2000). Activation of cannabinoid receptor 1 (CB1), in an invitro model of HD has been recently observed to confer significant level of protection against mutant htt induced cell death, (Scotter et al., 2010). Endocannabinoids act as neuromodulatory and neuroprotective cues by engaging type 1 cannabinoid receptors (CB1). Drugs that can activate CB1 receptor are expected to attenuate disease progression (Blazquez et al., 2011). It has been suggested that the htt, aggregates may be cleared by autophagy (Rubinsztein et al., 2005). In addition, administration of small molecules that promote autophagy has improved phenotypes in cell and animal models of HD (Ravikumar et al., 2004).

Enhancing autophagy with rapamycin accelerated mutant htt clearance and improved cell viability. The levels of wild-type htt were not affected by these compounds, suggesting that autophagy plays a specific role in the clearance of aggregate-prone htt (Krainc, 2010). Recent studies have identified microtubule-associated protein light chain 3 proteins (LC3), interacting proteins, such as p62, that play a role in the autophagic clearance of protein aggregates (Komatsu et al., 2007). A multifunctional protein, p62 has been shown to bind ubiquitin and LC3; possibly providing a molecular shuttle for misfolded aggregated proteins to promote their clearance by autophagy (Bjorkoy et al., 2005). This data supports the idea that P62 induced autophagy may have significant potential for treating HD. Studies have also demonstrated that mutant htt interacts directly with the histone acetyltransferase (HAT) domain of the cyclic AMP response element binding protein (CBP) (Steffan et al., 2001). Depletion of CBP enhances toxicity whereas over expression of CBP suppresses toxicity by mutant htt. Jeong et al. (2009) showed that acetylation of mutant htt by CBP leads to neuroprotection by improving clearance of the mutant protein.

The green tea polyphenol (−) - epigallocatechin-3-gallate (EGCG), can potently inhibit htt aggregation in vitro and in a Drosophila model of HD (Ehrnhoefer et al., 2006). The agents that can stabilize native conformation such as dimethyl sulfoxide (DMSO), glycerol, trimethylamine N-oxide (TMAO), and trehalose offer utility in preventing aggregation (Nagai and Popiel, 2008).

2.4 Amyotrophic lateral sclerosis (ALS)

Abnormal protein aggregates are seen in brain and spinal cord samples from patients with sporadic ALS, which suggests that protein misfolding and aggregation contribute to the pathogenesis of ALS, although a causative role remains controversial (Bosco et al., 2010; Kerman et al., 2010; Liu et al., 2009). The development of a vaccine or immunoglobulins to remove misfolded protein in ALS is a novel therapeutic strategy. There is emerging evidence for the existence of secretory pathways for superoxide dismutase (SOD1) mutant linked to ALS. Vaccination with SOD1 mutant protein in the ALS SOD1 transgenic mouse model delayed disease onset and significantly extended survival suggesting that immunization strategies should be considered as potential for treatment of familial ALS (Takeuchi et al., 2010).

Arimoclomol an amplifier of heat shock protein expression is involved in cellular stress response, and has emerged as a potential therapeutic candidate in ALS in recent years. Treatment with arimoclomol was reported to improve survival and muscle function in a mouse model of motor neuron disease. Several single and multiple dose safety studies have been completed in healthy control subjects. A 3 month Phase IIa study in people with ALS demonstrated safety at dosages up to 300mg/day and another study is currently recruiting participants with familial ALS (Lanka et al., 2009). Up-regulation of endoplasmic reticulum chaperones and eukaryotic initiation factor 2 (eIF2) (Ilieva et al., 2007), activation of unfolded protein response cascades (Atkin et al., 2006) and ribosomal detachment resulting in endoplasmic reticulum distention and motor neuron shrinkage have all been demonstrated in pathological studies of sporadic ALS (Oyanagi et al., 2008). Increased levels of protein disulfide isomerase (PDI), an endoplasmic reticulum-localized chaperone molecule that promotes protein folding, have been found in cerebrospinal fluid of ALS (Atkin et al., 2006).

These findings indicate an important role for endoplasmic reticulum stress and unfolded protein response dysregulation in the pathogenesis of ALS. Interestingly, lithium and valproic acid induce BiP and other endoplasmic reticulum chaperone proteins and reduce endoplasmic reticulum stress. Both of these drugs have been investigated in human studies without benefit (Aggarwal et al., 2010).

3. Mitochondrial dysfunction

Mitochondrial dysfunction has long been associated with neurodegenerative diseases (Burchell et al., 2010). Several lines of research suggest that mitochondrial abnormalities, including defects in oxidative phosphorylation, increased accumulation of mitochondrial DNA defects, impaired calcium influx, and accumulation of mutant proteins in mitochondria, are important cellular changes in both early and late-onset neurodegenerative diseases (Burchell et al., 2010). Therefore, one would predict that agents that alleviate mitochondrial dysfunction could be beneficial and exert neuroprotective effects (Burchell et al., 2010).

3.1 Alzheimer's disease (AD)

There is accumulating evidence suggesting that mitochondrial dysfunction occurs prior to the onset of symptoms in AD (Su et al., 2009). Mitochondria are exceptionally poised to play a crucial role in neuronal cell survival or neurodegeneration because they are regulators of both energy metabolism and apoptotic pathways (Su et al., 2009). In a recent study the mitochondria-targeted antioxidants (MTAs) MitoQ and SS31 and the anti-aging agent resveratrol were found to have a protective effect on neurons in a mouse model of AD (Manczak et al., 2010). In primary neurons from AβPP transgenic mice, which were treated with MitoQ and SS31, neurite outgrowth significantly increased and cyclophilin D expression significantly decreased indicating potential of these drugs to treat AD (Manczak et al., 2010).

Mitochondrial antioxidants acetyl-L-carnitine (ALCAR) and R-α-lipoic acid (LA) reduced oxidative stress and mitochondrial abnormalities in cellular mouse models of AD and restored cognitive functions in aged rats (Aliev et al., 2009). A meta analysis of 21 double blind randomized, placebo controlled studies showed that ALCAR either improved cognitive deficits or delayed the progression of cognitive decline in AD (Montgomery et al., 2003).

Coenzyme Q10 (CoQ10) is essential for mitochondrial energy production. CoQ10 was observed to reduce oxidative stress and tau pathology in mice (Dumont et al., 2011), and inhibited β-amyloid (βA) formation (Ono et al., 2005). CoQ10 treatment has also been shown to decrease brain oxidative stress, reduce βA plaque load, and improve cognitive performance in a transgenic mouse model of Alzheimer's disease (Dumont et al., 2011). In a recent study dietary supplementation of carnosine an endogenous peptide with metal chelating and free radical scavenging properties was observed to completely rescue AD and aging related mitochondrial dysfunction and was suggested as a potential candidate for a combined therapeutic approach for the treatment of AD (Corona et al., 2011).

3.2 Parkinson's disease (PD)

The most convincing evidence for the role of mitochondrial damage in PD comes from studies of rare familial forms of PD, in which genetic mutations linked to PD result in mitochondrial impairments and increased susceptibility to oxidative stress (Martin et al., 2011). Parkin knockout mouse model demonstrate impaired mitochondrial activity and altered oxidative stress proteins in PD (Palacino et al., 2004). Further studies in this direction are likely to provide elaborate knowledge about mitochondrial dysfunction pathways in PD and help in developing new therapeutic strategies.

A significant reduction in CoQ10 levels in mitochondria has been reported in the platelets of patients with PD, which directly correlates with a decrease in complex-I activity. CoQ10 provides significant protection against MPTP-induced dopaminergic neuronal degeneration (Faust et al., 2009). The oral administration of CoQ10 in PD patients resulted in reduction of Unified Parkinson's Disease Rating Scale (UPDRS) scores (Shults et al., 2004). The mitochondrial targeted antioxidant MitoQ has been shown to help in preservation of mitochondrial function after glutathione depletion, this drug is currently in a phase II clinical trial for Parkinson's disease (http://www.parkinsons.org.nz/news/protectstudy.asp). The other compounds which have shown promise in ameliorating the mitochondrial dysfunction in experimental PD studies include creatine, lanosterol, melatonin, edaravone and trolox (Shim et al., 2011). However further studies are warranted before the clinical use of these drugs.

3.3 Huntington's disease (HD)

Abnormal mitochondrial function, decreased respiratory enzyme complex activities, increased electron leakage, and increased Ca^{2+} entry have all been shown to play a significant role in the pathophysiology of many neurodegenerative disorders including HD. Current evidence from genetic models of HD including mutation of the Huntington gene (mhtt), supports the mitochondrial dysfunction as major cause of the disease, with respiratory chain impairment relegated to a late secondary event . HD is associated with significant defects in mitochondrial respiratory enzymes, including mitochondrial succinate dehydrogenase (SDH, complex II) and aconitase a transglutaminase substrate. Protein aggregates interfere with mitochondrial function, mitochondrial trafficking in axons, and result in mitochondrial fragmentation and inhibition of mitochondrial fusion. SDH inhibitors including 3-nitropropionic acid and malonate cause medium spiny neuronal loss and clinical and pathological features reminiscent of HD in rodents and non-human primates (Chaturvedi and Beal, 2008).

High dose of CoQ10 significantly extends survival, improves motor performance and grip strength, and reduces brain atrophy in R6/2 HD mice. The combination of CoQ10 and minocycline in R6/2 mouse model of HD resulted in significantly improved behavioral measures, reduced neuropathological deficits, extended survival, and attenuated striatal neuron atrophy, as compared to either agent alone. Similarly, the combination of CoQ10 and remacemide resulted in significantly improved motor performance and increased survival in the R6/2 and the N-171-82Q transgenic mouse models of HD (Ferrante, 2002). These two compounds have been clinically tested separately and in combination in 340 patients with HD. Administration of CoQ10 resulted in a 14% decrease in disease progression while remacemide demonstrated no efficacy (Huntington Study Group, 2001). Creatine significantly improves survival, improves motor performance, increases brain ATP levels, and delays atrophy of striatal neurons and the formation of htt-positive aggregates in transgenic mice (Andreassen, 2001). Sirtuins (silent information regulators SIRT) are members of the NAD+-dependent histone deacetylase family of proteins in yeast, and play an important role in regulating mitochondrial function. Inhibition of sirtuins has been shown to suppress disease pathogenesis in Drosophila models of HD (Pallos, 2008).

Reduced levels of peroxisome proliferator activated receptor gamma co activator alpha (PGC-1α), a transcriptional regulator of several enzymes has been shown in the striatum of R6/2 HD mice. The PGC-1α pathway plays an important role in regulating cellular energy metabolism. PGC-1α induces mitochondrial biogenesis and respiration in muscle cells and regulates several aspects of adaptive thermogenesis by increasing expression of nuclear-encoded electron transport chain components, metabolic enzymes, and uncoupling proteins. Increasing PGC-1α levels dramatically protect neural cells in culture from oxidative stress-mediated death (St -Pierre et al., 2006). Thus activity of PGC-1α pathways promises to be an effective therapeutic approach for mitochondrial disorders. Metformin can enhance the PGC-1α expression and mitochondrial biogenesis possibly at least in part via AMPK phosphorylation in the skeletal muscle (Suwa et al., 2006). The therapeutic effects of metformin on HD warrants further studies. A recent study demonstrated that transcription factor peroxisome proliferator activated receptor γ (PPARγ) plays a major role in energy homeostatis of HD. Rosiglitazone a potent agonist of PPAR γ has been shown to prevent mitochondrial dysfunction in mutant htt expressing cells and in R6/2 HD mice (Chiang et al., 2010; Quintanilla et al., 2008). These findings support the view that upregulation of PPARγ plays a major role in HD.

3.4 Amyotrophic lateral sclerosis (ALS)

Mitochondrial and bioenergetic defects have been claimed to play vital role in ALS pathogenesis. Altered respiratory chain enzyme activities and CNS energy hypometabolism in spinal cord and motor cortex are the hallmark of ALS (Sasaki et al 2005). Swelling and vacuolar degeneration of mitochondria is a prominent finding prior to the onset of clinical deficits in experimental HD mice. Mutant SOD1 is found in the mitochondrial inter-membrane space and binds to the inner mitochondrial membrane in the SOD1G93A mouse (Ahtoniemi et al., 2008) causing peroxidation of cardiolipin and alteration of anchor cytochrome c to the inner mitochondrial membrane which activates programmed cell death (Kirkinezos et al., 2004).

Pramipexole a lipophilic cation that concentrates into brain and mitochondria significantly lowers oxidative stress, maintains mitochondrial function, and has neuroprotective effects independent of dopamine-receptor agonism. R+ pramipexole, prolonged survival of ALS SOD1 transgenic mice, and in a phase 2 study of 102 patients with ALS it was found to be safe and well tolerated (Cudkowicz et al., 2010). Motor decline seemed to lessen with increasing doses (Cudkowicz et al., 2010). These encouraging results in Phase II studies warrant further studies. Olesoxime (previously TRO19622) is a mitochondrial pore modulator that was discovered after screening about 40,000 compounds in an in-vitro motor neuron cell death assay (Bordet et al., 2007). In SOD1 transgenic mouse model, olesoxime showed a delayed onset and prolonged survival (Bordet et al., 2007). A phase 2/3 study of olesoxime is underway in Europe (NCT00868166).

3.5 Multiple sclerosis (MS)

There is increasing evidence implicating mitochondria in the pathogenesis of multiple sclerosis. Mitochondrial respiratory chain complex I and complex III activity is reduced in non-lesional motor cortex, where a number of nuclear DNA-encoded transcripts of mitochondrial proteins are decreased (Dutta et al., 2006). Interestingly, complex IV activity and mitochondrial DNA copy number are increased in chronic active lesion homogenates and within normal appearing grey matter neurons, respectively, possibly as a compensatory mechanism (Blokhin et al., 2008). Defects of mitochondrial respiratory chain complexes and depletion of mitochondria not only cause an energy deficit but may increase the susceptibility of axons to excitotoxic injury through impaired calcium handling capacity (Blokhin et al., 2008). The detoxification of mitochondrial superoxide by transfecting adeno associated virus containing manganese super oxide dismutase (SOD), led to a reduction in degeneration of mitochondrial structure (Qi et al., 2007). The Carboxyfullerene a fullerene compound that increased survival of mice lacking mitochondrial MnSOD (SOD-1) localized to mitochondria and reduced superoxide production. When combined with N-methyl D-aspartate (NMDA) receptor antagonist a fullerene derivative (ABS75) reduced axonal degeneration and disease progression. The mitochondrial permeability transition pore which allows calcium efflux from mitochondria, when opened and is modulated during hypoxic preconditioning has been identified as a potential therapeutic target in MS (Forte et al., 2007)

Polyunsaturated fatty acid (PUFA) and antioxidant deficiencies along with decreased cellular antioxidant defense mechanisms have been observed in MS patients. Both dietary antioxidants and PUFAs have the potential to diminish disease symptoms by targeting specific pathomechanisms and supporting recovery in MS (van Meeteren et al., 2005). Supplementation with long chain omega-3 PUFAs in MS patients and healthy controls decreased the secretion of the pro-inflammatory cytokines, IL-1b, TNF-α, IL-2, and IFN-γ by stimulated peripheral blood mononuclear cells as well as reduced secretion of the inflammatory eicosanoids such as, prostaglandin E2, and leukotriene B4 (LTB4), which are known to be increased in MS patients (Weinstock–Guttman et al., 2005). Thus dietary supplements which can modulate these eicosanoids help to reduce the severity of the disease and prevent recurrence, and in particular fish oil supplementation given together with vitamins C and E. can improve clinical outcome in patients with newly diagnosed MS. Although a few antioxidants showed some efficacy in animal models, there is limited and conflicting evidence of potential therapeutic effects of antioxidants such as vitamins C and E in treating MS.

4. Inflammation

Brain inflammation is a typical feature of neurodegenerative diseases and acute forms of brain injury. A large number of neurodegenerative diseases are associated with chronic inflammation, including Alzheimer's disease, Parkinson's disease, amyotrophic lateral sclerosis, multiple sclerosis and all of the tauopathies, and age-related macular degeneration (Tansey and Goldberg, 2010). Considering the involvement of inflammatory processes in mechanism of neurodegeneration, and keeping in mind that activated microglia and astrocytes are a rich source of oxygen radicals, nitric oxide and neurotoxic and proinflammatory cytokines; anti-inflammatory drugs acting on these targets have the potential to exert beneficial effects in experimental and clinical neurodegenerative disorders.

4.1 Alzheimer's disease (AD)

The brains of AD patients have increased concentrations of acute phase reactants, cytokines, and complement protein as compared to age-matched controls (Heng et al., 2007). In a prospective cohort study of subjects with AD, high baseline levels of tumor necrosis factor (TNF) alpha were also found to be associated with a 4-fold increase in the rate of cognitive decline (Holmes et al., 2009).

Earlier studies have suggested a beneficial effect from non steroidal anti-inflammatory drugs (NSAIDs) in decreasing the risk of AD· Treatment with NSAIDs has been shown to decrease β-amyloid and tau levels in animal models of AD (Yoshiyama et al., 2007). These effects of NSAID's have been attributed to the inhibition of APP-associated γ-secretase (Sastre and Gentleman, 2010). It has been proposed that NSAIDs cause a delay in the onset or slow down progression of AD, through the inhibition of cyclooxygenase (COX) and lipooxygenases, leading to a decrease in prostaglandin synthesis and reactive oxygen species formation (Leoutsakos et al., 2011). On the other hand, some other studies have suggested a possible deleterious effect of NSAIDs on cognition and an increase in neuronal damage (Breitner et al., 2011). The neurohormone melatonin was observed to exert inhibitory effects on β-amyloid aggregation, oxidation, and inflammation in vitro, and showed behavioral improvement in animal model of AD. Although melatonin can improve mild cognition impairment, it is not a cure for AD (Olcese, 2009). Combination of ibuprofen with glutathione and lipoic acid has proven to be useful in controlling AD induced cerebral amyloid deposits and behavioral deterioration (Pinnen et al., 2011).

4.2 Parkinson's disease (PD)

Systemic inflammation has been shown to promote microglial activation in PD, on the other hand genes implicated in PD may also influence inflammatory mediators. Over expression of wild-type α-synuclein in neurons is associated with the activation of microglia, and the release of TNF, IL-1β, IL-6, COX-2, and iNOS (Tarawneh & Galvin, 2010). Minocycline, a tetracycline derivative, has been shown to possess anti-inflammatory and anti-apoptotic properties, which reduces microglial activation and inhibit the release of potentially toxic cytokines in the striatal region of MPTP mice. Pretreatment with minocycline improved survival of dopaminergic neurons in animal models of PD (Peng et al., 2006). Based on the efficacy, safety and tolerability of minocycline in a randomized, double-blind, Phase II clinical trial (The NINDS NET -PD 2006), it has been recommended for long-term treatment of PD.

NSAIDs have been associated with a 45% reduction in the risk of developing PD in one prospective study with 14 years of follow up (Wahner et al., 2007). On the other hand a case control study of 22,007 patients did not find evidence that NSAIDs use reduces PD (Driver et al., 2011). Triptolide, an active component of Tripterygium extracts, which possesses potent anti-inflammatory and immunosuppressive properties, exerts neuroprotective and neurotrophic activities in animal models of PD (Chen et al., 2010). Currently, the application of triptolide for PD is in preclinical stages. Similarly, the synthetic triterpenoid CDDO-Me, an inhibitor of NFκB attenuates production of TNF and other glial-derived inflammatory mediators has been shown to protect dopaminergic neurons (Trans et al., 2008). Glatiramer acetate (GA) is an artificial copolymer of a pool of peptides (45 ~ 100 amino acids, MW 4.7 ~ 11 kDa) (Kipnis and Schwartz, 2002) which exerts anti-inflammatory effects through adaptive immunomodulation. Tsai (2007) suggested that it enhances the production of brain derived neuroprotective factor (BDNF) and has therapeutic potential for the treatment of familial PD. On the other hand immunomodulatory drugs including pargyline, selegiline (Deprenyl) and pentoxifylline, have all shown neuroprotective activity in both MPTP- (Liu and Hong, 2007) and the 6-OHDA rodent models of PD (Sanchez-Pernaute et al., 2004). Similarly, the glucocorticoid dexamethasone was shown to be protective against MPTP (Kurkowska-Jastrzebska et al., 2004). Other anti-inflammatory regimens such as steroids, which have been shown to be effective at arresting DA neuron loss in rodents, need further studies. At this time use of anti inflammatory drugs as a potential preventive therapeutic measure in PD remains but a promising possibility.

4.3 Huntington's disease (HD)

Neuroinflammation is a prominent feature associated with HD and may constitute a novel target for neuroprotection. Increased expression of several key inflammatory mediators, including IL-6, IL-8, and MMP9, in the striatum, cortex and cerebellum in experimental and clinical HD has been reported (Silvestroni, 2009). Treatment of quinolic acid induced HD rats with minocyline resulted in the attenuation of inflammation, and reduction of striatal lesions (Ryu et al., 2006). In a first open-label safety and efficacy trial, 10 out of 14 HD patients treated with minocycline (100mgday−1) showed an improvement in their Unified HD Rating (Bonelli et al., 2004). In striking disagreement with this study, subsequent studies using higher doses of minocycline (200mgday−1) showed good tolerance and apparent safety, but failed to exhibit any improvement in HD features (Reynolds, 2007). Besides these conflicting results, the safety of minocycline has recently been questioned when two-thirds of subjects who were administered minocycline discontinued the drug after developing serious hyperpigmentation only 1 year into the 5-year treatment regime (Reynolds, 2007).

Treatment with acetylsalicylate or rofecoxib in transgenic mice model of HD failed to show any beneficial effects (Norfus et al., 2004). Dexamethasone treatment (4mg daily for 20 days followed by 8mg daily for an additional 20 days) in HD patients has demonstrated improvement of abnormal involuntary movements, and manual dexterity, with no observable side-effects (Bonnucelli et al., 1992). Accumulating evidence suggests that changes in the immune system may critically contribute to the pathology of HD. However, the nature of this contribution remains unclear, to the extent that it is not even known whether the immune activation has a beneficial or detrimental role in HD patients (Soulet and Cicchetti, 2011).

4.4 Amyotrophic lateral sclerosis (ALS)

Inflammation has been shown to play a critical role in the pathogenesis of ALS. Markers of inflammation, including microglial stimulating factors and pro-inflammatory cytokines, such as TNF alpha and FasL are increased in ALS (Kiaei et al., 2006).Several places in the inflammatory events that appear to accompany ALS might be amenable to drug action. Animal experiments have suggested that Cox 2 inhibitors might be of use in ALS, but a clinical trial of a direct inhibitor of Cox2 has failed to give a definite answer.

Lenalidomide a potent immunomodulatory agent with abiity to down regulate pro-inflammatory cytokines prolong survival in the transgenic mouse model of ALS (G93A mice) by destabilizing DNA coding for TNFα and other cytokines (Kiaei, 2006). Lenalidomide significantly attenuated neuronal loss, improved motor performance, and survival. These data encourage clinical evaluation of lenalidomide to slow or block progression of ALS (Neymotin et al 2009). Pioglitazone, a peroxisome proliferator-activated receptor-gamma (PPAR γ) agonist with anti-inflammatory properties, has been shown to improve motor performance, delay weight loss, attenuate motor neuron loss, and extend survival of transgenic mouse models of ALS (Kiaei, 2005). A clinical trial for safety and efficacy of pioglitazone in ALS patients - models is expected to be completed by the end of 2011. Although immune modulators/anti inflammatory drugs including minocycline, celecoxib, rofecoxib, and sulindac showed protection in mouse models of ALS, but these drugs failed in human ALS trials (Gordon et al., 2007).

4.5 Multiple sclerosis (MS)

Multiple Sclerosis is an idiopathic disease in which the body's immune response attacks the central nervous system resulting in demyelination. Although its exact etiology and pathogenesis are still unclear, there is much evidence to suggest the involvement of T cell triggered inflammation. In MS, peripheral T cells gain entry into the brain via the BBB, recognize myelin as foreign body and attack it as if it were an invading virus. This triggers inflammatory processes and stimulates other immune cells and soluble factors such as cytokines and antibodies (Leary and Thompson, 2005).

In a large clinical trial, immunomodulatory drug, glatiramer acetate was found to be efficient in the treatment of relapsing remitting multiple sclerosis, however the trial had to be terminated prematurely because the drug failed to stop disease progression after two years (Wolinsky et al., 2007). The results of trials with the immunomodulatory drug, interferon beta (IFN beta), in patients with MS were also disappointing (Montalban, 2004). Recently, a single-center, phase two pilot study with interferon beta-1b on primary progressive MS disease showed no effect on sustained disability assessed by expanded disability status scale (EDSS), but surprisingly revealed statistically significant differences for the multiple sclerosis functional composite score and for T1 and T2 lesion volume (Montalban et al., 2009). Studies on humanized monoclonal antibody, alemtuzumab (Campath-1H), which induces the cytolysis of CD52 positive cells leading to a T cell depletion is highly effective in reducing relapse rate, MRI lesion load and disease progression in relapsing remitting multiple sclerosis (The CAMMS223 Trial 2008), However, it does not seem to protect from disease progression once patients have progressed to secondary progressive stage (SPMS) (Coles et al., 2006). Laquinimod (ABR-215062) is another orally administered investigational agent that, in animal models of MS, has been shown to decrease leukocyte infiltration into the central nervous system and to induce a shift from T-helper type 1 (Th1; proinflammatory) cells to Th2/3 (anti-inflammatory) cells (Miron et al., 2008). Phase III clinical trials suggested a significant activity of laquinimod (as shown on MRI measures) against the relapsing form of MS (Miron et al., 2008). The agent also appears to exhibit synergistic immune modulating effects when given with interferon therapy (Miron et al., 2008).

5. Oxidative stress

Neuronal cells in the brain are highly sensitive to oxidative stress due to their large dependence on oxidative phosphorylation for energy, normal functioning and survival. In brain the demand for oxygen consumption is extremely high with 1-2% of the oxygen being converted into superoxide anion radicals ($O_2^{\bullet -}$) and hydrogen peroxide, leading to oxidative stress (Moura et al., 2010). Oxidative stress results when there is an imbalance of reactive oxygen species (ROS) production and availability of endogenous antioxidants to scavenge the ROS. Generation of high levels of ROS, and down regulation of anti-oxidant mechanisms, results in neuronal cell death in neurodegenerative diseases (Farooqui and Farooqui, 2009). The role of oxidative stress and use of antioxidants as neuroprotective agents in some of the common neurodegenerative disorders is discussed below:

5.1 Alzheimer's disease (AD)

Oxidative stress has been associated in beta amyloid (Aβ) toxicity; It is clearly evident from in vitro studies that oxidation of soluble Aβ promotes its transformation into the aggregated form creating a vicious cycle of aggregation and oxidative damage (Lee, 2010). There is ample evidence to suggest that amyloidal aggregation can be inhibited by antioxidants, and free radical scavengers, such as vitamin E and propyl gallate, have been shown to protect neuronal cells against Aβ toxicity (Behl, 1999).The most common antioxidant vitamin E has been found to delay clinical progression in AD patients from moderate to severe impairment, although no cognitive benefit was found (Wyttenbach et al., 2000). On the other hand Masaki et al. (2000), reported that vitamin E improves cognitive performance in AD. According to some recent reports antioxidant supplementation has not been effective for the treatment of AD (Mecocci and Polidori, 2011). In spite of these conflicting reports there remains considerable interest in vitamin E, and an important ongoing study (Dysken, 2010), is expected to clarify these doubts.

Recent studies have shown that melatonin levels are lower in AD patients compared to age-matched control subjects (Mahlberg et al., 2008). Treatment with melatonin provides protection against AD by inhibiting Aβ-induced toxicity (Zhou et al., 2008; Wang, 2009). However there is insufficient evidence to support the effectiveness of melatonin for managing cognitive impairment in AD (Jansen et al., 2006). Further clinical phase II trial to determine the effect of melatonin on cognitive function in mild cognitive impaired (MCI) patients is presently undergoing (ClinicalTrials.gov Identifier: NCT00544791).

Statins by virtue of their hypocholestremic, antioxidant and anti inflammatory properties have been shown to lower Aβ production and to reduce Aβ-mediated neurotoxicity. On the contrary no significant clinical benefit on cognition or global functioning was shown by atorvastatin in a phase 3 clinical trial in patients with mild-to-moderate AD already taking donepezil (Feldman et al., 2010). Another clinical trial, to test the effectiveness of statins in prevention and therapy of Alzheimer's disease, is ongoing (Mangialasche et al., 2010).

Recent experimental studies using a wide range of antioxidants including P- P methoxy – diphenyl diselenide (Pinton et al., 2011), S allyl cysteine (Javed et al., 2011), conjugates of ibuprofen and glutathione (Pinnen et al., 2011), tirilazad (Youdim et al., 2004), Ibuprofen and lipoic acid (Distefano et al., 2010), and chlorogenic acid (Kwon et al., 2010), have shown neuroprotective effects in animal models of AD. On the other hand mitochondria specific antioxidants such as acetyl-L-carnitine and R-alpha lipoic acid have been suggested to be beneficial for treatments for AD (Palacios et al., 2011). Further clinical studies are warranted to establish the therapeutic efficacy of these drugs in AD.

5.2 Parkinson's disease (PD)

Oxidative damage to proteins, lipids, and nucleic acids has been found in the substantia nigra of patients with PD (Fasano, 2006). The metabolism of dopamine (DA) itself creates a favorable environment for oxidative damage through intermediates such as DA-quinone and 3, 4- dihydroxy phenylacetaldehyde (Jackson and Smeyne , 2005). On the other hand reduced plasma levels of anti-oxidants such as glutathione and uric acid have been reported in PD patients (Elokda et al., 2010).

An open label study of Vitamin E and Vitamin C, suggested that these antioxidants delay the need to initiate levodopa therapy for the treatment of PD by 2.5 years (Fahn et al., 1992), while other randomized placebo controlled trials showed no disease-modifying effect for Vitamin E, (Shoulson, 1998), but a modest protective effect and slowing of disease progression was observed when vitamin E was given with with Deprenyl, (Olanow, 1995). The use of glutathione (600 mg twice daily) in patients with PD resulted in significant decrease in their disability scores (Sechi, 1996). Selegeline and rosagiline the inhibitors of monoamine oxidase B (MAOB) also significantly delayed the onset of L dopa in PD patients. Oral Coenzyme Q10 (CoQ10), a cofactor in electron transport chain in mitochondria, was shown to slow motor deterioration, and improve activities of daily living in patients with mild PD (Shults, 2002). Studies on beneficial effect of lycopene supplementation suggest its therapeutic potential in PD (Kaur et al., 2011). A small number of controlled trials indicate that melatonin is useful to treat disturbed sleep in PD (Medeiros et al., 2007), particularly rapid eye movement-associated sleep behavior disorder (Aurora et al., 2010). Melatonin and the recently introduced melatonergic agents (ramelteon, agomelatine) merit further investigations (Srinivasan et al., 2011).

5.3 Huntington's disease (HD)

Oxidative stress has been shown to play an important role in the pathogenesis of HD. Elevated levels of oxidative damage products such as malondialdehyde, 8 hydroxy-guanosine, 3 nitrotyrosine and heme oxygenase in the brain of HD patients and increased free radical production in animal models indicates the involvement of oxidative stress either as a causative event, or as a secondary constituent of the cell death cascade. Recently Lee et al (2011), observed an increase in the level of 4 hydroxynonenal (4 HNE) a useful marker for the oxidative stress in both human and animal models of HD, suggesting that the lipid peroxidation pathway may be a novel therapeutic target for preventing oxidative damage in HD.

Treatment with CoQ10 was associated with reduced levels of 8-hydroxyguanosine (a marker of oxidative damage) and improved survival in experimental model of HD mice. In a multicenter, blinded, randomized study on HD patients administered 300 mg CoQ10 slowed the decline of total functional capacity (Huntington Study Group 2001). A higher dose of coenzyme Q10 (2400 mg) for HD, is now in phase III of clinical trial (NCT00608881). Results of a recent study using antioxidant dimebon (the old Russian cold medicine), showed that 60 mg per day was safe and well tolerated and improved cognition in individuals with HD (Kieburtz, 2010). However in a clinical trial on late stage HD patients dimebon failed to show a significant improvement in cognition or global functioning.

The antioxidant response element (ARE) signaling pathway is an important pathway involved in antioxidant and anti-inflammatory responses (Johnson et al., 2008). The ARE is activated through the binding of its transcription factor, Nrf2 (NF-E2-related factor 2). In addition to the typical induction of detoxification enzymes, Nrf2-ARE activation results in increased cellular energy and redox potential, inhibitory neurotransmitter signaling, and metabolic processes (Nguyen et al., 2004). Synthetic triterpenoids, which are derived from 2-Cyano-3,12-Dioxooleana1,9-Dien-28-Oic acid (CDDO) have been shown to up-regulate Nrf2/ARE induced genes in the brain and peripheral tissues, reduce oxidative stress, improve motor impairment and increase longevity in HD mice (Stack 2010). This compound showed a great potential for treatment of HD. Eriodictyol, a flavonoid found in citrus fruits, induces the nuclear translocation of Nrf2, enhances the expression of heme-oxygenase-1 (HO-1) and quinone oxidoreductase 1 (NQO-1), and increases the levels of endogenous antioxidant glutathione (Johnson et al., 2009), these findings suggest its potential use for the treatment for HD and other neurodegenerative disorders.

5.4 Amyotrophic lateral sclerosis (ALS)

Oxidative damage mediated by toxic free radicals has been implicated in the pathogenesis of ALS (Graf et al 2005). Abundant evidence of oxidative stress has been found in autopsy specimens of ALS, including elevated protein carbonyl levels, increased 3-nitrotyrosine levels, 8-hydroxy-2-deoxyguanosine (a marker for oxidative DNA damage) and 4 HNE levels (an indicator of lipid peroxidation) (Barber et al., 2006).

About 20% of familial ALS is caused by a genetic defect in an antioxidant enzyme called super oxide dismutase -1 (SOD-1). A study on AEOL 10150, a manganoporphyrin antioxidant that catalytically neutralizes superoxide, hydrogen peroxide, and peroxynitrite, and inhibits lipid peroxidation showed that administration of this drug to SOD1G93A transgenic mice at symptom onset improved the survival period by 196% (Crow et al., 2005). In 2005 a phase I single dose escalating study of AEOL 10150 showed that the drug was well tolerated with no serious adverse events [www.rideforlife.com]. Clinical trials with promising second-generation antioxidant, edavarone which was shown to slow motor decline and neuron degeneration in a - a mice model of ALS are underway (Kuzma-Kozakiewicz and Kwiecinski, 2011). A recent study utilizing dietary supplementation with S adenosyl methionine (SAM) altered the course of motor neuron pathology in G93A mutant SOD1 mice by preventing loss of motor neurons and reducing gliosis, SOD-1 aggregation, protein carbonylation, and induction of antioxidant activity (Suchy et al., 2010).

5.5 Multiple sclerosis (MS)

It has been suggested that mitochondrial injury and subsequent energy failure is a major factor driving axonal injury in MS patients (Witte et al., 2010). As the mitochondrial proteins and DNA are highly vulnerable to oxidative damage (Higgins et al., 2010), it has been proposed that free radical-mediated mechanisms may lead to mitochondrial injury in MS (van Horssen et al., 2011). Oxidized lipids and oxidized DNA have been detected in the brain tissues from patients with MS (Quin et al., 2007). Results from a recent study (Haider et al., 2011), on autopsy material from HD patients provide extensive evidence for an important role of oxidative damage in the pathogenesis of demyelination and neurodegeneration in MS.

Treatment with lipoic acid and anti-acrolein compound hydrazine both potent antioxidants, were observed to reduce axonal injury in experimental models of MS (Chaudhary et al., 2011). Recently C-Phycocyanin and saffron naturally occurring antioxidants improved experimental Autoimmune Encephalitis (EAE) and peripheral blood mononuclear cells from MS patients (Penton -Rol et al., 2011; Ghazavi et al., 2009). Viral mediated delivery of antioxidant genes of superoxide dismutase and catalase in EAE mice has also been observed to suppress neuronal and axonal loss (Qi et al., 2007). Inosine is a widely distributed nucleoside in the body and is a potent scavenger of free radicals. Administration of inosine in MS patients resulted in a significant decrease in the number of lesions and improved disability status (Markowitz et al., 2009). Erythropoietin (Epo), a hematopoietic growth factor and an antioxidant, showed clinical and electrophysiological improvement of motor function as well as improved cognitive performance in MS patients (Ehrenreich et al., 2007).

6. Targeting glutamate excitotoxicity

Excessive activation of glutamate receptors by excitatory amino acids leads to a number of deleterious consequences, including impairment of calcium buffering, generation of free radicals, activation of the mitochondrial permeability transition and secondary excitotoxicity (Berliocchi et al., 2005). A pivotal role for excitotoxicity in neurodegenerative diseases is gaining increasingly more acceptance (Kim et al., 2011). Progress in the use of anti-excitotoxic drugs for the treatment of neurodegenerative disorders is discussed below.

6.1 Alzheimer's disease (AD)

Several studies have linked tau and amyloid aggregation to glutamate mediated toxicity and clearly suggest the involvement of N-methyl-D-Aspartate (NMDA) receptor subunits (NR1 and NR2) in the pathogenesis of AD (Koutsilieri and Riederer, 2007). Alzheimer's disease is associated with reduced levels of two mRNA isoform subsets of the NR1 receptor and changes in the expression of NR2A and NR2B in the superior temporal cortex, cingulate cortex and hippocampus (Hynd et al., 2004). The presence of presenilin-1 in a macromolecular complex with NR1 and NR2A further supports a role for excitotoxicity in AD (Saura et al., 2004).

Memantine is an uncompetitive NMDA receptor antagonist that can decrease pathological activation of NMDA receptors without affecting physiological NMDA receptor activity (Farlow, 2008). Memantine is associated with functional improvement in AD patients and has been approved by FDA for the treatment of AD (Farlow, 2008). Latrepirdine (Dimebon), a nonselective antihistamine and weak NMDA receptor blocker was found to have beneficial effects in animal models of AD (Santamaría et al., 2001). It has also been shown to enhance mitochondrial function (Wyttenbach et al., 2002). In a clinical trial (Goswami et al., 2006), on 183 patients with mild to moderate AD, latrepirdine, improved performance on the primary cognitive outcome, behavioral activities of daily living, and global function. The most common side effects were dry mouth and depressed mood, in some patients. However, a recent phase III AD trial of Dimebon in 598 patients did not show any significant improvement in primary or secondary outcomes (Bezprozvanny, 2010).

6.2 Parkinson's disease (PD)

Brain glutamate over activity is well documented in Parkinson's disease (Morin et al., 2010). Studies on dopamine denervated rats and MPTP-treated Parkinsonian monkeys have clearly provided insight into the relative abundance of different NMDA subunits in the striatum. Dopamine depletion in the 6-OHDA rat models, and MPTP primate models results in relative decrease in the abundance of NMDA receptor subtype 1 (NR1) and subtype 2B (NR2B) subunits in the synaptosomal membranes, which is restored by chronic levodopa therapy (Dunah, 2000; Hallett et al., 2005). Since stimulation of NR2B-containing NMDA receptors contributes to the generation of Parkinsonian symptoms (Hallett and Standaert, 2004), NR2B-selective NMDA receptor antagonists may be therapeutically beneficial for Parkinsonian patients. Prior administration of NMDA receptor antagonist dizocilpine suppresses the dopa-induced increase in glutamate in 6-hydroxydopamine-lesioned rats and may therefore offer neuroprotection (Jonkers, 2002).

Several NMDA antagonists have been studied in PD (Tarawneh and Galvin, 2010). Both amantidine and dextromethorphan have antidyskinetic effects. Amantidine has been associated with increased lifespan (Uitti, 1996; Verhagen, 1998). Selective NMDA receptor antagonists, such as ifenprodil and CP-101,606, have been developed in an attempt to avoid the side effects of non-selective blockers. Ifenprodil, has anti-Parkinsonian actions in rat and, and nonhuman primates (Nash and Brotchie, 2002). CP-101,606 reduced Parkinsonian symptoms, in both haloperidol-treated rats, and MPTP-lesioned nonhuman primates (Steece, 2000). Pretreatment of 6-OHDA lesioned rats with 4-trifluoromethoxy-N-(2-trifluoromethyl-benzyl)-benzamidine (BZAD-01), a novel selective inhibitor of the NMDA NR1A/2B receptor, significantly reduced the amount of dopaminergic cell loss and significantly improved all behavioral measures (Leaver et al., 2008). When given in combination with levodopa-carbidopa, the NMDA-antagonist remacemide, has been shown to reduce parkinsonism in rodent and monkey models of Parkinson's disease (Greenamyre, 1994). A clinical study confirmed that remacemide is safe and well tolerated in PD patients who are treated with L-DOPA (Clarke, 2001).

The simultaneous blockade of AMPA (α-amino-3-hydroxy-5-methyl-4- isoxazolepropionic acid) and NMDA receptor offers substantially greater reduction in the response alterations induced by levodopa than inhibition of either of these receptors alone in both rat and primate models of PD. Simultaneous blockade of the AMPA receptors with GYKI-47261 and NMDA receptor with amantadine or MK-801 resulted in significant reductions in levodopa-induced dyskinesias in a primate model, while the wearing-off dyskinesias were completely ameliorated in rat models of PD (Bibbiani, 2005). Treatment with NMDA glutamate receptor antagonist memantine for 52 weeks resulted in the improvements in cognitive functions and stabilization of motor impairments in PD patients (Litivinenko et al., 2010).

6.3 Huntington's disease (HD)

The major hypothesis driving HD synaptic research is the excitability of medium spiny projection neurons (MSNs). Injections of excitatory amino acids into the striatum of rodents, and primates results in neuronal death and a neurologic phenotype similar to that of Huntington's disease. Intrastriatal injections of NMDA glutamate agonists, such as quinolinic acid, have been used to create animal models of HD. Animal models and human studies show evidence of decreased glutamate receptors, in particular the mGluR2 subtypes, down-regulation of the GLT-1 glial glutamate transporter, and increased sensitization of NMDA receptors (Leegwater and Cha, 2004). Since excitotoxicity is known to be involved in the development of HD, approaches to reduce extra synaptic glutamate signaling have been explored and include modulation of NR2 B signaling (Heng et al., 2009), lowering glutamate receptor activation with NMDA receptor antagonists (Ketamine and memantine), and modulating the interplay of glutamate and dopamine on MSNs (Andre et al., 2010). The efficacy of memantine in slowing down the rate of progression of HD was studied in a two year, open and multicenter trial with promising results (Beister et al., 2004).

Cannabinoid-derived drugs also hold great promise in protecting neurons from glutamate mediated toxicity. Activation of neuronal CB (1) or CB (2) cannabinoid receptors attenuates excitotoxic glutamatergic neurotransmission and triggers prosurvival signaling pathways. The administration of CB (2) receptor-selective agonists reduced neuroinflammation, brain edema, striatal neuronal loss and motor symptoms in wild-type mouse models subjected to excitotoxicity (Palazuelos, 2009). Treatment with the analogue of the antiglutamatergic agent and the tryptophan metabolite kynurenic acid (KYNA), in transgenic mouse model of HD resulted in prolonged survival, reduction in hypo-locomotion, and prevention of atrophy of the striatal neurons (Zadori et al., 2011).

6.4 Amyotrophic lateral sclerosis (ALS)

Glutamate-mediated excitotoxicity arising from repetitive firing or elevation of intracellular calcium by calcium permeable glutamate receptors has long been postulated to have an important role in motor neuron degeneration in ALS (Rowland and Schneider, 2001). Glutamate levels are increased in cerebrospinal fluid of patients with sporadic ALS (Rothstein et al 1990) and clearance of glutamate from neuromuscular synapses is diminished in patients with ALS due to loss of the astroglial glutamate transporter EAAT2 (excitatory amino acid transporter 2), that is of major importance for synaptic glutamate reuptake (Rothstein et al., 1995).

Cephalosporins increase EAAT2 promoter activity and protect motor neurons from glutamate toxicity in organotypic spinal cord slice cultures of rats (Rothstein et al., 1993). Controversial but mainly negative data on the efficacy of cephalosporins in ALS have been published (Norris, 1994). However, gabapentin, lamotrigine, and topiramate, and other agents known to alter glutamate synthesis and release, appeared promising in pre-clinical studies (Maragakis et al., 2003) but showed no benefit in ALS patients (Cudkowicz et al., 2003). Beta-lactam antibiotics exert neuroprotective effects by up-regulating GLT-1 receptors in vitro and in vivo in normal rats (Rothstein et al., 1995) and in transgenic ALS mice treated with ceftriaxone (Rothstein et al., 2005). Harvey and Martz (2007) have reported prolonged treatment with atovaquone, an antimalaric drug, showed a persistent disease remission. This observation confirms the previous reports of a possible therapeutic effect of beta-lactam antibiotics in ALS. A double blind placebo controlled clinical trial on about 600 patients using a β lactam antibiotic ceftriaxone which is a safe EAAT2 expression enhancer, is being carried out in the United States of America (NCT00349622) since July 2006. Final data collection for the primary outcome measure (survival and rate of change in ALSFRSr - stage 3) will be available in March 2012. Talampanel (8-methyl-7H-1,3-dioxolo(2,3)benzodiazepine), is a noncompetitive modulator of AMPA glutamate receptors which is under development as an antiepileptic agent, has been shown to prolong survival of SOD1G93A ALS mouse (Traynor et al., 2006). The ALS Functional Rating Scale-revised (ALSFRS-r) scores declined at a slower rate in a 9-month phase II study of talampanel in 60 patients (Traynor et al., 2006). The inhibitor of presynaptic glutamate release, riluzole, is currently the only drug that has shown efficacy in a phase 3 study in ALS patients (Zinman and Cudkowicz, 2011). On the other hand memantine was well tolerated in combination with riluzole in patients with ALS resulting in some improvement in function rating of disease (Levine et al., 2010).

6.5 Multiple sclerosis (MS)

Glutamate excitotoxicity mediated by the AMPA /kainate type of glutamate receptors not only damage neurons but also the myelin producing of oligodendrocytes of the CNS. In MS, oligodendrocytes and some axons are lost as a result of excessive relaease of glutamate by activated immune cells. It has been suggested that glutamate activates immune cells and inflammation and contributes to lesion formation in MS (Gonsette, 2008). The hypothesis that the excitatory neurotransmitter glutamate contributes to axonal damage has been strengthened by several studies demonstrating the neuroprotective effects of AMPA receptor antagonists such as NBQX (2,3-dihydroxy-6-nitro-7-sulfamoyl-benzo(F)quinoxaline) in animals (Pitt et al., 2003). In addition, memantine, a NMDA antagonist currently available for the management of Alzheimer's disease, ameliorates disability in experimental autoimmune encephalomyelitis-affected rats, raising the possibility of its neuroprotective effect in MS (Wallström et al., 1996). The protective effects of glutamate antagonists are important, especially as it has been hypothesized that AMPA/kainate receptors become the primary mediators of axonal injury during prolonged and intensified injury exposure in the chronic phase (Ouardouz et al., 2006) suggesting the possibility of a potential benefit in targeting these receptors. Riluzole inhibits the release of glutamate from nerve terminals and modulates the activities of both kainate and NMDA receptors is presently undergoing a clinical trial alone and in combination with interferon β (NCT 00501943) at University of California, USA.

Another promising compound for treating MS is minocycline, which has been found to be protective in many neurodegenerative diseases (Fong et al., 2008). Experimental studies using both invitro (Defaux et al., 2011) and invivo (Chen et al., 2010) models of MS showed protective effects of minocycline. Combination of minocycline with methylprednisolone and atorvastatin was observed to synergistically suppress EAE severity in mice (Chen et al 2010). At the same time results of a clinical trial, involving minocyline alone and in combination with glatiramer acetate in patients with MS, showed minocyline to be safe and well tolerated with a reduction in the relapse rate (Zhang et al., 2008). The encouraging results from the animal models and clinical experiments on minocycline make it a promising candidate for MS treatment whether used alone or combined with other drugs (Chen, 2011).

7. Apoptosis

Apoptosis is a form of cell death in which programmed sequence of events lead to elimination of cells without releasing harmful substances in surrounding area. It plays a crucial role in developing and maintaining health by eliminating old cells, unnecessary cells and unhealthy cells. However premature apoptosis and/or an aberration in apoptosis regulation may lead to degenerative disorders. Neuronal apoptosis can be induced both in vivo and in vitro by different stimuli including oxidative stress, calcium toxicity, excitotoxicity, inhibition of the mitochondrial respiratory chain, and deficiency of survival factors which may contribute to disorders including Alzheimer's disease, Huntington's disease, Parkinson's disease, amyotrophic lateral sclerosis and multiple sclerosis. Inhibition of apoptosis could constitute a suitable therapeutic strategy for delaying the progression of neurodegenerative disease (Sureda et al., 2011).

7.1 Alzheimer's disease (AD)

Extensive evidence showed that apoptosis is involved in neuronal loss in AD. Postmortem analysis of AD brain showed DNA fragmentation in neurons and glia of hippocampus and cortex as detected by TdT-mediated dUTP nick end labeling (TUNEL) (Vila and Przedborski, 2003). Rohn, et al. (2002) demonstrated the activation of mitochondrial and receptor-mediated apoptotic pathways in AD hippocampal brain sections wherein active caspase-9 was co-localized with active caspase-8. Recently, a marked co-localization of pathological hyperphosphorylated tau, cleaved caspase-3 and caspase-6 has been reported in TUNEL-positive neurons in the brain stem of AD patients (Wai et al., 2009). Furthermore, in vitro studies have shown that amyloid beta protein (Aβ) provokes a significant down regulation of antiapoptotic proteins such as Bcl-2, Bcl-xl and Bcl-w and a significant up-regulation of pro-apoptotic proteins such as bax (Yao et al., 2005).

The activation of Poly ADP-ribose polymerase (PARP) plays a critical role in caspase-independent apoptosis. Therefore, PARP inhibitors represent one possible therapeutic strategy in AD. Insulin like growth factor-binding protein-3 (IGFBP-3) modulates cell growth and survival. Humanin (HN) a peptide and IGFBP3 coactivator significantly inhibited neuronal cell death induced by familial Alzheimer's disease mutant gene and amyloid β (Aβ) (Ikonen et al., 2003). Thus HN acts as AD related survival factor by interacting with IGFBP-3. Recently, it has been suggested that a potent humanin derivative may be a promising alternative strategy for AD therapy (Matsuoka & Hashimoto, 2009). Pycnogenol (PYC), a potent antioxidant suppressed caspase-3 activation, DNA fragmentation, PARP cleavage, and eventually protected against Aβ-induced apoptosis in animal model of AD. PYC is a promising candidate for clinical trials in AD (Ishrat et al., 2009).

Invitro studies demonstrated antiapoptotic activity of the endogenous antioxidants geniposide and estrogen (Liu et al., 2009). Recently Puerarin, a phytoestrogen was observed to prevent Aβ-induced neurotoxicity through inhibiting neuronal apoptosis. Further studies are warranted to study these antiapoptotic drugs for their, preventive or therapeutic efficacy in AD (Xing et al., 2011).

Melatonin is a natural hormone secreted by the pineal gland. In vitro experiments showed that Aβ−treated cultures exhibited characteristic features of apoptosis, and melatonin attenuated Aβ-induced apoptosis and activated the survival signal pathways stabilizing mitochondrial function by acting as anti-apoptotic Bcl-2 family modulator (Jang et al., 2005). Melatonin significantly delays the development of the signs of AD, prevents cognitive impairment, and ameliorates sundowning in AD patients (Gehrman et al., 2009).

7.2 Parkinson's disease (PD)

Accumulating evidence suggests that the molecular and biochemical pathways of apoptosis are involved in dopaminergic cell death in PD. This evidence includes the activation of the mitogen activated protein (MAP) kinase pathway, the induction of Bax, prostate apoptosis response-4 (Pa 4) and glyceraldehyde 3 phosphate dehydrogenase, as well as the activation of caspases. In cell culture and animal models therapeutic interference with the signaling phase of apoptosis, e.g. inhibition of the MAP kinase pathway, provides morphological and function protection. In contrast, inhibition of the propagation and execution phase of apoptosis (e.g. by inhibition of the caspases), blocks cell death but may result in survival of dysfunctional neuron. For full functional recovery, the combination of an antiapoptotic together with a neuro-restorative therapy may be necessary (Tatton et al., 2003).

Dopaminergic cells from animal models of PD exhibit increased expression of the pro-apoptotic protein Bax effector protease caspase-3 and caspase-8 (Tatton et al., 2003). Treatment with L-Dopa and dopamine agonists is associated with lower levels of antiapoptotic Bcl-2 in the blood (Blandini, 2004).The peptidyl inhibitor carbobenzoxy-Val-Ala-Asp-fluoromethylketone (zVADfmk) can protect neurons from apoptosis induced by mitochondrial toxins. However, its therapeutic efficacy is limited by its poor penetrability into the brain (Yang et al., 2004). The more potent broad-spectrum caspase inhibitor, Q-VD-OPH, may be more promising. Specific caspase inhibitor such as acetyl-tyrosinyl-valyl-alanyl-aspartyl-chloro-methylketone (Ac-YVAD-cmk), has also demonstrated efficacy in several experimental paradigms of Parkinson's disease (Yang et al., 2004).

Propargylamines including selegeline and rasagiline besides their MAO -B activity have proven to be potent anti-apoptotic agents in both in vitro and in vivo studies (Olanow, 2006). These drugs inhibit apoptosis through caspase inhibition (Bonuccelli & Del Dotto, 2006). Moreover, rasagiline appears to induce anti-apoptotic pro-survival proteins, Bcl-2 and glial cell-line derived neurotrophic factor (Maruyama, 2004). Selegiline has also been shown to delay the need for symptomatic therapy in untreated Parkinson's disease patients (Shoulson, 1998). Further studies to determine utility of these propargylamines in the treatment of PD and their mechanism of neuroprotective activity are in progress.

In an experimental study, melatonin showed neuroprotective effects against MPP+- induced apoptosis by inhibiting the calpain/cdk5 signaling cascade in cerebellar granule neurons(CGNs) (Alvira et al., 2006). Mounting evidence indicates that melatonin blocks the MPT dependent apoptotic fragmentation of nuclear DNA in rat astrocytes (Jou et al., 2004). On the other hand, human trials of melatonin showed significantly improved effect on sleep disturbances in PD (Medeiros et al., 2007; Dowling et al., 2005), but there were undetected differences in motor dysfunction (Medeiros et al., 2007).

Oral administration of Co Q10 resulted in amelioration of mitochondria induced apoptosis by dose-dependent restoration of striatal complex I activity, increase in expression of Bcl-2 as well as decrease in catalepsy score in an animal model of PD (Abdin & Hamouda, 2008). Treatment with CoQ10 also resulted in restoration of striatal dopamine levels (Abdin & Hamouda, 2008). In a multicenter clinical trial Co Q10 appears to slow progressive deterioration of function in PD through increased expression of Bcl-2 (Shults et al., 2002). However these findings were questioned in a later trial (Storch et al., 2007).

7.3 Huntington's disease (HD)

Several lines of evidence point to a role for apoptosis in HD in animal models and in postmortem tissues. Caspase 3 has been shown to cleave mutant huntingtin and the activation of caspase 1 in HD brain. The expression of expanded polyglutamine residues has been associated with apoptotic mechanisms via caspase activation, cleavage of the death substrates lamin B and inhibition of caspase-activated DNAse. Bax expression in peripheral B and T lymphocytes and monocytes is increased in HD, and lymphoblasts derived from HD patients show increased stress-induced apoptotic cell death associated with caspase-3 activation (Vis, 2005).

Recent findings suggest a possible role for the hypoxia-inducible factor 1 (HIF-1) in HD. HIF-1 regulates the expression of several genes, including mediators of apoptosis, making it a potential target for future therapies (Correia and Moreira, 2010). Extracellular ATP stimulates apoptosis through stimulation of purinergic P2X7 receptors, and subsequent alterations in calcium permeability, both of which have been described in HD. The administration of the P2X7-antagonist Brilliant Blue-G (BBG) to HD mice prevented neuronal apoptosis, and attenuated motor-coordination deficits (Diaz-Hernandez et al., 2009), suggesting the role of P2X7 in pathogenesis of HD and highlighting the therapeutic potential of a PsX7 antagonist for its treatment.

Melatonin has been shown to defer the signs of HD in a 3-nitropropionic acid-induced rat animal model of HD (Tunez et al., 2004). In a human study administration of tryptophan, resulted in melatonin levels rising significantly in both of control and HD groups (Christofides et al., 2006). Moreover, the delayed onset of the diurnal melatonin rise in patients with HD has been currently reported (Aziz et al., 2009). Larger scale studies in detecting the level of melatonin in HD patients and further human trials on the impact of melatonin on HD are needed.

7.4 Amyotrophic lateral sclerosis (ALS)

Apoptosis is a potential mechanism of motor neuron death in ALS. Morphological studies are difficult as dying motor neurons may exhibit features of apoptotic as well as cytoplasmic and autophagic neuronal death and distinctly apoptotic cells are found only rarely in spinal cord specimens. Caspases, members of the cysteine protease family, are known effectors or executioners of apoptosis. The activity of caspase-1 (Li, et al., 2000) and caspase-9 were found higher in the spinal cords of patients with ALS (Inoue et al 2003). Activation of caspase 1 has been shown to be an early event in SOD1G37R and SOD1G85R transgenic ALS mice, occurring months before neuronal death, whereas activation of caspase 3 is coincident with the onset of motor axon loss in three different mSOD1 lines (G93A, G37R and G85R) (Pasinelli et al., 2000). Intraventricular injection of zVADfmk, a broad caspase inhibitor, suppresses caspase upregulation and delays disease onset and mortality in mouse models of ALS (Li et al., 2000).

Members of the Bcl-2 family of proteins are important regulators of apoptosis, including both suppressors (Bcl-2, Bcl-XL) and promoters (Bax, Bad, Bak and Bcl-xS) of programmed cell death. Decreased expression of the anti-apoptotic proteins and increased expression of the proapoptotic proteins has been found in human ALS as well as transgenic mouse models (Guegan and Przedborski, 2003). Over-expression of Bcl-2 (Kostic et al., 1997) and deletion of Bax (Gould et al., 2006) independently result in delayed onset of motor decline and prolonged survival without reducing disease duration.

Minocycline prolonged survival by 10-22% in transgenic mouse models of ALS (van den Bosch et al., 2002). In these SOD1 G37R mice, minocycline reduces the activity of caspase 1, caspase 3, inducible nitric oxide synthase, and p38 mitogen-activated protein kinase, and diminishes loss of motor neurons. Minocycline has been tested in two preliminary human trials and has been shown to be safe in patients with ALS (Pontieri et al., 2005). However, in a multicentre, phase III trial (NCT00047723) minocyline failed to show any protective effect.

Lithium is a neuroprotective and antiapoptotic agent that promotes autophagy. It prolonged survival in SOD1-transgenic mice and increased the number of autophagic vacuoles in motor neurons (Fornai et al., 2008). Preliminary results of a small open-label study suggested longer survival and slower disease progression in ALS patients treated with lithium (Fornai et al., 2008). At least two other Phase II trials with lithium carbonate are under way (Clinical Trials.gov NCT00790582, NCT00925847).

7.5 Multiple sclerosis (MS)

Apoptosis is important for the homeostasis of the immune system and presumably plays a two sided role in the pathogenesis of MS. On the other hand evidnce has been provided that impaired apoptosis might result in increased numbers or persistence of activated myelin - specific T cells, thus inducing the pathophysiologic processes in MS. On the other hand, local tissue damage might involve apoptosis of glial and neuronal cells and lead to the clinical symptoms (Todaro et al., 2004). It has been hypothesized that a failure of auto-reactive T- and B-lymphocytes, as well as activated macrophages, to undergo apoptosis contributes to the pathogenesis of MS (Pender and Rist, 2001). Inhibitor of apoptosis (IAP), a family of anti-apoptotic genes were shown to be elevated in peripheral blood immune cells (monocytes T cells), in MS patients (Hebb et al., 2008). Moreover antisense mediated knock down of inhibitor of apoptosis (IAP) family member known as X linked IAP (XIAP) reverses paralysis in an animal model of MS (Zehutner et al., 2007) suggesting that treatments targeting XIAP and perhaps other IAPs may have utility in the treatment of MS.

Histone deacetylase 3 (HDAC 3) belongs to a family of proteins which plays an important role in protein acetylation, chromatin remodeling and transcription of genes, including those that are involved in cell proliferation and cell death. An increased expression of HDAC3 and relative resistance to Trichostat A (TSA) induced apoptosis in T cells in MS patients has been reported (Zhang et al., 2011). A number of selective and non selective HDAC inhibitors have been developed that could also become part of the therapeutic strategy in the treatment of immune disorders including MS (Zhang et al., 2011).

8. Conclusion

Neuroprotection in neurodegenerative diseases remains an important but elusive goal. A successful neuroprotective treatment could transform neurodegenerative diseases from a relentless progressive and disabling disease to a problem that can be managed with only a modest effect on quality of life. Current barriers include a lack of knowledge of the basic mechanism of neurodegenerative diseases and deficiencies in the methodology used to study disease progression. Overall, however the activity aimed at understanding and treating neurodegenerative diseases has grown exponentially and should ultimately result in better therapy for these diseases.

The authors would like to make clear that this review cannot cover all drugs under investigation for the therapy of neurodegenerative diseases. For a more accurate list of these molecules the reader has to refer to reviews on each single neurodegenerative disorder.

9. References

Abdin, A. A.; & Hamouda, H. E. (2008). Mechanism of the Neuroprotective Role of Coenzyme Q10 With or Without L-Dopa in Rotenone-Induced Parkinsonism. *Neuropharmacology*, Vol.55, No.8, (December 2008), pp. 1340-346, ISSN 1873-7064

Aggarwal, S. P.; Zinman, L.; Simpson, E.; McKinley, J.; Jackson, K.E.; Pinto, H.; Kaufman, P.; Conwit, R. A.; Schoenfeld, D.; Shefner, J. & Cudkowicz, M. (2010). Northeast and Canadian Amyotrophic Lateral Sclerosis Consortia. *Lancet Neurol*, Vol.9, No.5, (April 2010), pp. 481-488, *ISSN:* 1474-4422

Ahtoniemi, T.; Jaronen, M.; Keksa-Goldsteine, V.; et al. (2008). Mutant SOD1 from Spinal Cord of G93A Rats is Destabilized and Binds to Inner Mitochondrial Membrane. *Neurobiol Dis*, Vol.32, No.3, (December 2008), pp. 479-85, *ISSN:* 0969-9961

Aliev, G.; Liu, J.; Shenk, J. C.; Fischbach, K.; Pacheco, G. J.; Chen, S. G.; Obrenovich, M. E.; Ward, W. F.; Richardson, A. G.; Smith, M. A.; Gasimov, E.; et al. (2009). Neuronal Mitochondrial Amelioration by Feeding Acetyl-1-Carnitine and Lipoic Acid to Aged Rats. *J Cell Mol Med*, Vol.13, No.2, (February 2009), pp. 320-333, ISSN: 1582-1838

Alvira, D.; Tajes, M.; Verdaguer, E.; Acuña-Castroviejo, D.; Folch, J.; Camins, A. & Pallas, M. (2006). Inhibition of the cdk5/p25 Fragment Formation may Explain the Antiapoptotic Effects of Melatonin in an Experimental Model of Parkinson's Disease. *J Pineal Res*, Vol.40, No.3, (April 2006), pp. 251-8, ISSN: 0742-3098

Andre, V. M.; Cepeda, C. & Levine, M. S. (2010). Dopamine and Glutamate in Huntington's Disease: A Balancing Act. *CNS Neurosci Ther*, Vol.16, No.3, (June 2010), pp. 163–178, ISSN: 1755-5930

Andreassen, O. A.; Dedeoglu, A.; Ferrante, R. J.; et al. (2001). Creatine Increase Survival and Delays Motor Symptoms in a Transgenic Animal Model of Huntington's Disease. *Neurobiol Dis*, Vol.8, No.3, (December 2001), pp. 479-491, ISSN: 0969-9961

Asuni, A. A.; Boutajangout, A.; Quartermain, D. & Sigurdsson, E. M. (2007). Immunotherapy Targeting Pathological Tau Conformers in a Tangle Mouse Model Reduces Brain Pathology with Associated Functional Improvements. *J Neurosci*, Vol.22, No.34, (August 2007), pp. 9115-9129, ISSN: 0270-6474

Atkin, J. D.; Farg, M. A.; Turner, B. J.; et al. (2006). Induction of the Unfolded Protein Response in Familial Amyotrophic Lateral Sclerosis and Association of Protein-Disulfide Isomerase with Superoxide Dismutase 1. *J Biol Chem*, Vol.281, No.40, (October 2006), pp. 30152-65, *ISSN:* 00219258

Aurora, R. N.; Zak, R. S.; Maganti, R. K.; Averbach, S. H.; Casey K. R.; Chowdhuri, S.; Karripot, S.; Ramar, K.; Kristo D. A.; Bista, S. R.; Lamm C. I.; Morgenthaler T.I.; et al. (2010). Best Practice Guide for the Treatment of REM Sleep Behavior Disorder (RBD). *Journal of Clinical Sleep Medicine*, Vol.15, No.1, (February 2010), pp. 85–95, ISSN: 15509389

Aziz, N. A.; Pijl, H.; Frölich, M.; Schröder-van der Elst, J. P.; van der Bent, C.; Roelfsema, F. & Roos, R. A. (2009). Delayed Onset of the Diurnal Melatonin Rise in Patients with Huntington's disease. *J Neurol*, Vol.256, No.12, (December 2009), pp. 1961-5, ISSN: 34055354

Barber, S. C.; Mead, R. J. & Shaw, P. J. (2006). Oxidative Stress in ALS: A Mechanism of Neurodegeneration and a Therapeutic Target. *Biochim Biophys Acta*, Vol.1762, No.11-12, (November-December 2006), pp. 1051-67, ISSN: 0006-3002

Bar-On, P.; Crews, L.; Koob, A. O.; Mizuno, H.; Adame, A.; Spencer, B. & Masliah, E. (2008). Statins Reduce Neuronal Alpha-Synuclein Aggregation in Vitro Models of Parkinson's Disease. *J Neurochem*, Vol.105, No.5, (June 2008), pp. 1656-67, ISSN: 00943509

Behl, C. (1999). Alzheimer's Disease and Oxidative Stress: Implications for Novel Therapeutic Approaches. *Prog Neurobiol*, Vol.57, Vol.3, (February 1999), pp. 301, ISSN: 0360-8972

Beister, A.; Kraus, P.; Kuhn, W.; et al. (2004). The N-methyl-D-Aspartate Antagonist Memantine Retards Progression of Huntington's disease. *J Neural Transm Suppl*, No.68, (2004), pp. 117-122, ISSN: 03036975

Berliocchi, L.; et al. (2005). Botulinum Neurotoxin C Initiates Two Different Programs for Neurite Degeneration and Neuronal Poptosis. *J Cell Biol*, Vol.168, No.4, (February 2005), pp. 607–618, ISSN: 1540-8140

Bezprozvanny, I. (2010). The Rise and Fall of Dimebon. *Drug News Perspect*, Vol.23, No.8, (October 2010), pp. 518-23, ISSN: 0214-0934

Bibbiani, F.; Oh, J. D.; Kielaite, A.; et al. (2005). Combined Blockade of AMPA and NMDA Glutamate Receptors Reduces Levodopa-Induced Motor Complications in Animal Models of PD. *Exp Neurol*, Vol.196, No.2, (December 2005), pp. 422-429, ISSN: 1351-5101

Bjørkøy, G.; Lamark, T.; Brech, A.; Outzen, H.; Perander, M.; Overvatn, A.; Stenmark, H. & Johansen, T. (2005). P62/SQSTM1 Forms Protein Aggregates Degraded by Autophagy and has a Protective Effect on Huntington-Induced Cell Death. *J Cell Biol*, Vol.21, No.4, (November 2005), pp. 603-14, ISSN: 0021-9525

Blandini, F.; Cosentino, M.; Mangiagalli, A.; Marino, F.; Samuele, A.; Rasini, E.; Fancellu, R.; Tassorelli, C.; Pacchetti, C., Martignoni, E., Riboldazzi, G., calandrella, D., Lecchini, S.; Frigo, G. & Nappi, G. (2004). Modifications of Apoptosis-Related Protein Levels in Lymphocytes of Patients with Parkinson's Disease. The Effect of Dopaminergic Treatment. *J Neural Transm*, Vol.111, No.8, (August 2004), pp. 1017-30, ISSN: 0300-9564

Blazquez, C.; Chiarlone, A.; Sagredo, O.; Aguado, T.; Pazos, M. R.; Resel, E.; Palazuelos, J.; Julien, B.; Salazar, M.; Borner, C.; Benito, C.; Carrasco, C.; Diez-Zaera, M.; Paoletti, P.; Diaz-Hernandez, M.; Ruiz, C.; Sendtner, M.; Lucas, J. J.; de Yebenes, J. G.; Marsicano, G.; Monory, K.; Lutz, B.; Romero, J.; Alberch, J.; Gines, S.; Kraus, J.; Fernandez-Ruiz, J.; Galve-Ropeh, I. & Guzman, M. (2011). Loss of Striatal Type 1 Cannabinoid Receptors is a Key Pathogenic Factor in Huntington's Disease. *Brain*, Vol.134, No.1, (January 2011), pp. 119-36, ISSN: 00068950

Blokhin, A.; Vyshkina, T.; Komoly, S. & Kalman, B. (2008). Variations in mitochondrial DNA copy numbers in MS brains. *J Mol Neurosci*, Vol.35, Issue No.3, (July 2008), pp. 283-7, ISSN: 1662-5099

Bonelli, R. M.; Hodl, A. K.; Hofmann, P. & Kapfhammer, H. P. (2004). Neuroprotection in Huntington's Disease: A 2-Year Study on Minocycline. *Int Clin Psychopharmacol*, Vol.19, No.6, (November 2004), pp. 337-342, ISSN: 26811315

Bonuccelli, U. & Del Dotto, P. (2006). New Pharmacologic Horizons in the Treatment of Parkinson's Disease. *Neurology*, Vol. 67, No.7, (October 2006), pp. S30-8, ISSN: 0028-3878

Bonuccelli, U.; Nuti, A.; Maremmani, C.; Ceravolo, R. & Muratorio, A. (1992). Steroid Therapy in Huntington's Disease. *Adv Biochem Psychopharmacol*, Vol.47, (1992), pp. 149-54, ISSN: 0065-2229

Bordet, T.; Buisson, B.; Michaud, M.; et al. (2007). Identification and Characterization of Cholest-4-en-3-one, Oxime (TRO19622), A Novel Drug Candidate for Amyotrophic Lateral Sclerosis. *J Pharmacol Exp Ther*, Vol.322, No.2, (August 2007), pp. 709–20, ISSN:00223565

Bosco, D. A.; Morfini, G.; Karabacak, N. M.; Song, Y.; Gros-Lows, F.; Pasinelli, P.; Goolaby H.; Fontaine B. A.; Lemay, N.; McKenna-Yasek, D.; Frosch, M. P.; Agar, J. N.; Julien, J. Pl; Brady, S. T.; Brown, R. H. Jr.; et al. (2010). Wild-Type and Mutant SOD1 Share an Aberrant Conformation and a Common Pathogenic Pathway in ALS. *Nat Neurosci*, Vol.13, No.11, (November 2010), pp. 1396–403, ISSN: 00223565

Breitner, J. C.; Baker, L. D.; Montine, T. J.; Meinert, C. L.; Lyketsos, C. G.; Ashe, K. H.; Brandt, J.; Craft, S.; Evans, E. D.; Green, R. C.; Ismail, M. S.; Martin, B. K.; Mullan, M. J.; Sabbagh, M. & Tariot, P. N. (2011). ADAPT Research Group, Extended Results of the Alzheimer's Disease Anti-inflammatory Prevention Trial. *Alzheimers Dement*, Vol.7, No.4, (July 2011), pp. 402-11, ISSN: 1552-5260

Brunden, K. R.; Trojanowski, J. Q. & Lee, V. M. (2009). Advances in Tau-Focused Drug Discovery for Alzheimer's Disease and Related Tauopathies. *Nat Rev Drug Discov*, Vol.8, No.10, (October 2009), pp. 783-93, ISSN: 1474-1776

Burchell, V. S.; Gandhi, S.; Deas, E.; Wood, N. W.; Abramov, A. Y. & Plun-Favreau, H. (2010). Targeting Mitochondrial Dysfunction in Neurodegenerative Disease: Part II, *Expert Opin Ther Targets*, Vol.14, No.5, (May 2010), pp. 497-511, ISSN: 1472-8222

Burchell, V. S.; Gandhi, S.; Deas, E.; Wood, N. W.; Abramov, A. Y. & Plun-Favreau, H. (2010). Targeting Mitochondrial Dysfunction in Neurodegenerative Disease: Part I, *Expert Opin Ther Targets*, Vol.14, No.4, (April 2010), pp. 369-85, ISSN: 1472-8222

CAMMS223 Trial Investigators. (2008). Alemtuzumab vs. Interferon Beta-1a in Early Multiple Sclerosis. *N Engl J Med*, Vol.23, No.359, (October 2008), pp. 1786-1801, ISSN: 284793

Chaturvedi, R. K. & Beal, M. F. (2008). Mitochondrial Approaches for Neuroprotection. *Ann N Y Acad Sci*, Vol.1147, (December 2008), pp. 395, ISSN: 00778923

Chaudhary, P.; Marracci, G. Y. X.; Galipeau, D.; Morris, B. & Bourdette, D. (2011). Lipoic Acid Decreases Inflammation and Confers Neuroprotection in Experimental Autoimmune Optic Neuritis. *J. Neuroimmunol*, Vol.233, No.1-2, (April 2011), pp. 90-6, ISSN: 01655728

Chen, C. (2011). Mitochondrial Dysfunction, Metabolic Deficits, and Increased Oxidative Stress in Huntington's Disease. *Chang Gung Med J*, Vol.34, No.2, (March-April 2011), pp. 135-52, ISSN: 20720939

Chen, X.; Pi, R.; Liu, M.; Ma, X.; Jiang, Y.; Liu, Y.; Mao, X. & Hu, X. (2010). Combination of Methylprednisolone and Minocycline Synergistically Improves Experimental Autoimmune Encephalomyelitis in C57 BL/6 Mice. *J Neuroimmunol*, Vol.14, No.1-2, (September 2010), pp. 104-9, ISSN: 0165-5728

Chiang, M. C.; Chen, C. M.; Lee, M. R.; Chen, H. W.; Chen, H. M.; Wu, Y. S.; Hung, C. H.; Kang, J. J.; Chang, C. P.; Chang, C.; Wu, Y. R.; Tsai, Y. S. & Chern, Y. (2010). Modulation of Energy Deficiency in Huntington's Disease Via Activation of the Peroxisome Proliferator-Activated Receptor Gamma. *Hum Mol Genet*, Vol.15;19, No.20, (October 2010) pp. 4043-58, ISSN: 9646906

Christofides, J.; Bridel, M.; Egerton, M.; Mackay, G. M.; Forrest, C. M.; Stoy, N.; Darlington, L. G. & Stone, T. W. (2006). Blood 5-Hydroxytryptamine, 5-Hydroxyindoleacetic Acid and Melatonin Levels in Patients With Either Huntington's Disease or Chronic Brain Injury. *J Neurochem*, Vol.97, No.4, (May 2006), pp.1078-88, ISSN: 00943509

Clarke, C. E.; Cooper, J. A. & Holdich, T. A.; TREMOR Study Group. (2001). A Randomized, Double-Blind, Placebo-Controlled, Ascending-Dose Tolerability and Safety Study of Remacemide as Adjuvant Therapy in Parkinson's Disease with Response Fluctuations, *Clin Neuropharmacol,* Vol.24, No.3, (May-June 2011), pp. 133-8, ISSN 3625664

Coles, A. J.; Cox, A.; Le Page, E.; Jones, J.; Trip, S. A.; Deans, J.; Seaman, S.; Miller, D. H.; Hale, G.; Waldmann, H. & Compston, D. A. (2006). The window of therapeutic opportunity in multiple sclerosis: evidence from monoclonal antibody therapy. *J Neurol*, Vol.253, Issue No.1, (January 2006), pp. 98-108, ISSN: 3405354

Corona, C.; Frazzini, V.; Silvestri, E.; Lattanzio, R.; La Sorda, R.; Piantelli, M.; Canzoniero, L. M.; Ciavardelli, D.; Rizzarelli, E. & Sensi, S. L. (2011). Effects of Dietary Supplementation of Carnosine on Mitochondrial Dysfunction, Amyloid Pathology, and Cognitive Deficits in 3xTg-AD Mice. *PLoS One*, Vol.15, No.3, (March 2011), pp. e17971, ISSN: 19326203

Correia, S. C. & Moreira, P. I. (2010). Hypoxia-inducible Factor 1: A New Hope to Counteract Neurodegeneration? *J Neurochem*, Vol.112, No.1, (January 2010), pp.1-12, ISSN: 00943509

Crow, J. P.; Calingasan, N. Y.; Chen, J.; Hill, J. L. & Beal, M. F. (2005). Manganese Porphyrin Given at Symptom Onset Markedly Extends Survival of ALS Mice. *Ann Neurol,* Vol.58, No.2, (August 2005), pp. 258-265, ISSN: 3645134

Cudkowicz, M. E.; Shefner, J. M.; Schoenfeld, D. A.; et al. (2003). A Randomized, Placebo-Controlled Trial of Topiramate in Amyotrophic Lateral Sclerosis. *Neurology,* Vol.26, No.61, (August 2003), pp. 456–64, ISSN: 283878

Cudkowicz, M. E.; Katz, J.; Moore, D. H.; et al. (2010). Toward More Efficient Clinical Trials for Amyotrophic Lateral Sclerosis. *Amyotroph Lateral Scler,* Vol.11, No. 3, (May 2010), pp. 259-65, ISSN: 17482968

Defaux, A.; Zurich, M. G.; Honegger, P. & Monnet-Tschudi, F. (2011). Minocycline Promotes Remyelination in Aggregating Rat Brain Cell Cultures After Interferon-y Plus Lipopolysaccharide-Induced Demyelination, *Neuroscience*, Vol.28, No.187 (July 2010), pp. 84-92, ISSN: 13196138

Di Stefano, A.; Sozio, P.; Cerasa, L. S.; Iannitelli, A.; Cataldi, A.; Zara, S.; Giorgioni, G. & Nasuti, C. (2010). Ibuprofen and Lipoic Acid Diamide as Co-Drug with Neuroprotective Activity: Pharmacological Properties and Effects in Beta-Amyloid (1-40) Infused Alzheimer's Disease Rat Model. *Int J Immunopathol Pharmacol,* Vol.23, No.2, (April-June 2010), pp. 589-99, ISSN: 3946320

Diaz-Hernandez, M.; Diez-Zaera, M.; Sanchez-Nogueiro, J.; et al. (2009). Altered P2X7-Receptor Level and Function in Mouse Models of Huntington's Disease and Therapeutic Efficacy of Antagonist Administration. *FASEB J,* Vol.23, No.6, (June 2009), pp. 1893- 1906, ISSN: 0892-6638

Dowling, G. A.; Mastick, J.; Colling, E.; Carter, J. H.; Singer, C. M. & Aminoff, M. J. (2005). Melatonin for Sleep disturbances in Parkinson's Disease. *Sleep Med,* Vol.6, No.5, (September 2005), pp. 459-66, ISSN: 1389-9457

Driver, J. A.; Logroscino, G.; Lu, L.; Gaziano, M. & Kurth, T. (2011). Use of Non-Steroidal Anti-Inflammatory Drugs and Risk of Parkinson's Disease: Nested Case-Control Study. *BMJ,* Vol.20, No.342, (January 2011), pp. 198, ISSN: 0959535

Dumont, M.; Kipiani, K.; Yu, F.; Wille, E.; Katz, M.; Calingasan, N. Y.; Gouras, G. K.; Lin, M. T. & Beal, M. F. (2011). Coenzyme Q10 Decreases Amyloid Pathology and Improves Behavior in a Transgenic Mouse Model of Alzheimer's Disease. *J Alzheimers Dis*, Volumes 1;27, No.1, (January 2011), pp. 211-23, ISSN: 13872877

Dunah, A. W.; Wang, Y.; Yasuda, R. P.; et al. (2000). Alterations in Subunit Expression, Composition, and Phosphorylation of Striatal N-Methyl-D-Aspartate Glutamate Receptors in a Rat 6-Hydroxydopamine Model of Parkinson's Disease. *Mol Pharmacol*, Vol.57, No.2, (February 2000), pp. 342-52, ISSN: 0026-895X

Dutta, R.; McDonough, J.; Yin, X.; Peterson, J.; Chang, A.; Torres, T.; Gudz, T.; Macklin, W. B.; Lewis, D. A.; Fox, R. J.; Rudick, R.; Mirnics, K.; & Trapp B. D. (2006). Mitochondrial Dysfunction as a Cause of Axonal Degeneration in Multiple Sclerosis Patients. *Ann Neurol*, Vol.59, No.3, (March 2006), pp. 478–89, ISSN: 3645134

Dysken, M. W. (2010). A Randomized Clinical Trial of Vitamin E and Memantine in Alzheimer's Disease, VA Coop Study (CSP #546)

Ehrenreich, H.; Fischer, B.; Norra, C.; Schellenberger, F.; Stender, N.; Stiefel, M.; et al (2007). Exploring Recombinant Human Erythropoietin in Chronic Progressive Multiple Sclerosis. *Brain*, Vol.130, No.10, pp. 2577–2588, ISSN: 00068950

Ehrnhoefer, D. E.; Duennwald, M.; Markovic, P.; Wacker, J. L.; Engenmann, S.; Roark, M.; Legleiter, J.; Marsh, J. L.; Thompson, L. M.; Lindquist, S.; Muchowski, P. J. & Wanker, E. E. (2006). Green Tea (-)-epigallocatechin-Gallate Modulates Early Events in Huntingtin Misfolding and Reduces Toxicity in Huntington's Disease Models. *Hum Mol Genet*, Vol.15, No.18, (September 2006), pp. 2743-51, ISSN: 0964-6906

Elokda, A.; DiFrancisco-Donoghue, J.; Lamberg, E. M. & Werner, W. G. (2010). Effects of Exercise Induced Oxidative Stress on Glutathione Levels in Parkinson's Disease On and Off Medication. *Neurology* Vol. 257, No.10, (October 2010), pp. 1648-53, ISSN: 283878

Ereshefsky, L.; Jhee, S.; Yen, M.; Moran, S.; Pretorius, S. & Adams, J. (2009). Cerebrospinal Fluid Beta-Amyloid and Dynabridging in Alzheimer's Disease Drug Development. *Biomark Med*, Vol.3, No.6, (December 2009), pp. 711-21, ISSN: 17520363

Fahn, S. & Cohen, G. (1992). The Oxidant Stress Hypothesis in Parkinson's Disease: Evidence Supporting It. *Annals of Neurology*, Vol.32, No.6, (December 1992), pp. 804–812, ISSN: 3645134

Farlow, M. R.; Graham, S. M. & Alva, G. (2008). Memantine for the Treatment of Alzheimer's Disease: Tolerability and Safety Data from Clinical Trials. *Drug Saf*, Vol.31, No.7, (2008), pp. 577-585, ISSN: 0114-5916

Farooqui, T. & Farooqui, A. A. (2009). Aging: An Important Factor for the Pathogenesis of Neurodegenerative Diseases. *Mech Ageing Dev*, Vol.130, No.4, (April 2009), pp. 203–15, ISSN: 0047-6314

Fasano, M.; Bergamasco, B. & Lopiano, L. (2006). Modifications of the Iron-Neuromelanin System in Parkinson's Disease. *J Neurochem*, Vol.96, No. 4, (February 2006), pp. 909, ISSN: 00943509

Faust, K.; Gehrke, S.; Yang, Y.; et al. (2009). Neuroprotective Effects of Compounds with Antioxidant and Anti-inflammatory Properties in a Drosophila Model of Parkinson's Disease. *BMC Neurosci*, Vol.1, No.10, (September 2009), pp. 109, ISSN: 1471-2202

Feldman, H. H.; Doody, R. S.; Kivipelto, M.; Sparks, D. L.; Waters, D. D.; Jones, R. W.; Schwam, E.; Schindler, R.; Hey-Hadavi, J.; DeMicco, D. A. & Breazna, A. (2010). Randomized Controlled Trial of Atorvastatin in Mild to Moderate Alzheimer Disease. *Neurology*, Vol.23, No.12, (March 2010), pp. 956-64, ISSN: 283878

Ferrante, R. J.; Andreassen, O. A.; Dedeoglu, A.; et al. (2002). Therapeutic Effects of Coenzyme Q10 and Remacemide in Transgenic Mouse Models of Huntington's Disease. *J Neurosci*, Vol.1, No.22, (March 2002), pp. 1592, ISSN: 13196138

Fong, J. S.; Rae-Grant, A. & Huang, D. (2008). Neurodegeneration and Neuroprotective Agents in Multiple Sclerosis. *Recent Pat CNS Drug Discov*, Vol.3, No.3, (November 2008), pp. 153-165, ISSN: 15748898

Fornai, F.; Longone, P.; Ferrucci, M.; et al. (2008). Autophagy and Amyotrophic Lateral Sclerosis: The Multiple Roles of Lithium. *Autophagy*, Vol.4, No.4, (May 2008), pp. 527-530, ISSN: 1554-8627

Forte, M.; Gold, B. G.; Marraci, G.; Chaudhary, P.; Basso, E.; Johnsen, D.; Yu, X.; Fowlkes, J.; Rahder, M.; Stern, K.; Bernardi, P. & Bourdette, D. (2007). Cyclophilin D Inactivation Protects Axons in Experimental Autoimmune Encephalomyelitis an Anmal Model of Multiple Sclerosis. *Proc Natl Acad Sci USA*, Vol.1;104, No.18, (May 2007), pp. 7558-7563, ISSN: 10916490

Gehrman, P. R.; Connor, D. J.; Martin, J. L.; Shochat, T.; Corey-Bloom, J. & Ancoli-Israel, S. (2009). Melatonin Fails to Improve Sleep or Agitation in Double-Blind Randomized Placebo-Controlled Trial of Institutionalized Patients with Alzheimer Disease. *Am J Geriatr Psychiatry*, Vol.17, No.2, (February 2009), pp. 166-9, ISSN: 10647481

Ghaznavi, A.; Mosayebi, G.; Salehi, H. & Abtahi, H. (2009). Effect of Ethanol Extract of Saffron (Crocus Sativus L.) on the Inhibition of Experimental Autoimmune Encephalomyelitis in C57bl/6 Mice. *Pak J Biol Sci*, Vol.12, No.9, (May 2009), pp. 690-5, ISSN: 1028-8880

Glass, M.; Dragunow, M. & Faull, R. L. (2000). The Pattern of Neurodegeneration in Huntington's Disease: A Comparative Study of Cannabinoid, Dopamine, Adenosine and GABA(A) Receptor Alterations in the Human Basal Ganglia in Huntington's Disease. *Neuroscience*, Vol.97, No.3, (2000), pp. 505-519, ISSN: 13196138

Gordon, P. H.; Moore, D. H.; Miller, R. G.; et al. (2007). Efficacy of Minocycline in Patients with Amyotrophic Lateral Sclerosis: A Phase III Randomized Trial. *Lancet Neurol*, Vol.6, No.12, (December 2007), pp. 1045-53, ISSN: 14744422

Gonsette, R. E. (2008). Neurodegeneration in Multiple Sclerosis: the Role of Oxidative Stress and Excitotoxicity. *J Neurol Sci*, Vol.15, No.274(1-2), (November 2008), pp. 48-53, ISSN: 13001817

Goswami, A.; Dikshit, P.; Mishra, A.; Mulherkar, S.; Nukina, N. & Jana, N. R. (2006). Oxidative Stress Promotes Mutant Huntington Aggregation and Mutant Huntington-Dependent Cell Death by Mimicking Proteasomal Malfunction. *Biochem Biophys Res Commun*, Vol.342, No.1, (March 2006), pp. 184-90, ISSN: 0006-291X

Gould, T. W.; Buss, R. R.; Vinsant, S.; Prevette, D.; Sun, W.; Knudson, C. M.; Milligan, C. E.; Oppenheim, R. W. (2006). Complete Dissociation of Motor Neuron Death from Motor Dysfunction by Bax Deletion in a Mouse Model of ALS. *J Neurosci*, Vol.26, No.34, (August 2006), pp. 8774-86, ISSN: 02706474

Graf, M.; Ecker, D.; Horowski, R.; et al. (2005). High Dose Vitamin E Therapy in Amyotrophic Lateral Sclerosis as Add-On Therapy to Riluzole: Results of a Placebo-Controlled Double-Blind Study. *J Neural Transm,* Vol.112, No.5, (May 2005), pp. 649-60, ISSN: 0300-9564

Greenamyre, J. T.; Eller, R. V.; Zhang, Z.; et al. (1994). Antiparkinsonian Effects of Remacemide Hydrochloride, a Glutamate Antagonist, in Rodent and Primate Models of Parkinson's Disease. *Ann Neurol,* Vol.35, No.6, (June 1994), pp. 655-661, ISSN: 3645134

Guegan, C. & Przedborski, S. (2003). Programmed Cell Death in Amyotrophic Lateral Sclerosis. *J Clin Invest,* Vol.111, No.2, (January 2003), pp. 153-61, ISSN: 219738

Haider, L.; Fischer, M.; Frischer, J.; Bauer, J.; Hoftberger, R.; Botond, G.; Esterbauer, H.; Binder, C.; Witztum, J. and Lassmann, H. (2011). Oxidative Damage in Multiple Sclerosis Lesions. *Brain,* Vol.134, No.7, (July 2011), pp. 1914-24, ISSN: 68950

Hallett, P. J.; Dunah, A. W.; Ravenscroft, P.; et al. (2005). Alterations of Striatal NMDA Receptor Subunits Associated with the Development of Dyskinesia in the MPTP-Lesioned Primate Model of Parkinson's Disease. *Neuropharmacology,* Vol.48, No.4, (March 2005), pp. 503, ISSN: 18737064

Hallett, P. J. & Standaert, D. G. (2004). Rationale For and Use of NMDA Receptor Antagonists in Parkinson's Disease. *Pharmacol Ther,* Vol.102, No.2, (May 2004), pp. 155, ISSN: 1637258

Hanger, D.; Anderton, B. & Noble, W. (2009). Tau Phosphorylation: The Therapeutic Challenge for Neurodegenerative Disease. *Trends in Molecular Medicine,* Vol.15, No.3, (March 2009), pp. 112-119, ISSN: 1471-4914

Harvey, W. T. & Martz, D. (2007). Motor Neuron Disease Recovery Associated with IV Ceftriaxone and Anti-Babesia Therapy. *Acta Neurol Scand,* Vol.115, No.2, (February 2007), pp. 129-131, ISSN: 16314

Hebb, A. L.; Moore, C. S.; Bhan, W. & Robertson, G. S. (2008). Targeting Apoptosis to Treat Multiple Sclerosis. *Current Drug Discovery Technologies,* Vol.5, No.1, (March 2008), pp. 75-77, ISSN: 1570-1638

Heller, K. (2010). Targeting Misfolded Proteins to Fight Neurodegenerative Diseases. *PLoS Biol,* Vol.8, No.1, (January 2010), pp. e1000290, ISSN: 1544-9173

Heng, M. Y.; Detloff, P. J.; Wang, P. L.; Tsien, J. Z. & Albin, R.L. (2007). In Vivo Evidence for NMDA Receptor-Mediated Excitotoxicity in a Murine Genetic Model of Huntington Disease. *J Neurosci,* Vol.29, No.10, (September 2009), pp. 3200-3205, ISSN: 02706474

Heng, M. Y.; Tallaksen-Greene, S. J.; Detloff, P. J. & Albin, R. L. (2007). Longitudinal Evaluation of the Hdh(CAG)150 Knock-in Murine Model of Huntington's Disease. *J Neurosci,* Vol.27, No.34, (August 2007), pp. 8989-98, ISSN: 0270-6474

Higgins, G. C.; Beart, P. M.; Shin, Y. S.; Chen, M. J.; Cheung, N. S. & Nagley, P. (2010). Oxidative Stress: Emerging Mitochondrial and Cellular Themes and Variations in Neuronal Injury. *J Alzheimer's Dis,* Vol.20, No.2, (2010), pp. S453-73, ISSN: 13872877

Holmes, C.; Cunningham, C.; Zotova, E.; et al. (2009). Systemic Inflammation and Disease Progression in Alzheimer Disease. *Neurology,* Vol.74, No.14, (April 2010), pp. 768, ISSN: 283878

Huntington Study Group. (2001). A Randomized, Placebo-Controlled Trial of Coenzyme Q10 and Remacemide in Huntington's Disease. *Neurology,* Vol.57, No.3, (2001), pp. 397-404, ISSN: 283878

Hynd, M. R.; Scott, H. L. & Dodd, P. R. (2004). Differential Expression of N-Methyl-D-Aspartate Receptor NR2 Isoforms in Alzheimer's Disease. *J Neurochem* Vol.90, No.4, (August 2004), pp. 913, ISSN: 00943509

Ikonen, M.; Liu, B.; Hashimoto, Y.; Ma, L.; Lee, K. W.; Niikura, T.; Nishimoto, I. & Cohen, P. (2003). Interaction Between the Alzheimer's Survival Peptide Humanin and Insulin-Like Growth Factor-Binding Protein 3 Regulates Cell Survival and Apoptosis. *Proc Natl Acad Sci USA,* Vol.100, No.22, (October 2003), pp. 13042-7, ISSN: 10916490

Illieva, E. V.; Ayala, V.; Jove, M.; Dalfo, E.; Cacabelos, D.; Povedano, M.; Bellmunt, M. J.; Ferrer, I.; Pamplona, R. & Portero-Otin, M. (2007). Oxidative and Endoplasmic Reticulum Stress Interplay in Sporadic Amyotrophic Lateral Sclerosis. *Brain,* Vol.130, No.12, (December 2007), pp. 3111-23, ISSN: 0006-8950

Inoue, H.; Tsukita, K.; Iwasato, T.; Suzuki, Y.; Tomioka, M.; Tateno, M.; Nagao, M.; Kawata, A.; Saido, T.C.; Miura, M.; Misawa, H.; Itohara, S. & Takahashi, R. (2003). The Crucial Role of Caspase-9 in the Disease Progression of a Transgenic ALS Mouse Model. *EMBO J,* Vol.22, No.24, (December 2003), pp. 6665-6674, ISSN: 0261-4189

Ishrat, T.; Parveen, K.; Hoda, M. N.; Khan, M. B.; Yousuf, S.; Ansari, M. A.; Saleem, S. & Islam, F. (2009). Effects of Pycnogenol and Vitamin E on Cognitive Deficits and Oxidative Damage Induced by Intracerebroventricular Streptozotocin in Rats. *Behav Pharmacol,* Vol.20, No.7, (October 2009), pp. 567-75, ISSN: 9558810

Jackson-Lewis, V. & Smeyne, R. J. (2005). MPTP and SNpc DA Neuronal Vulnerability: Role of Dopamine, Superoxide and Nitric Oxide in Neurotoxicity. *Minireview Neurotox Res,* Vol.7, No.3, (2005), pp. 193, ISSN: 1029-8429

Jacobsen, S.; Comery, T.; Kreft, A.; et al. (2009). GSI-953 is a Potent APP-Selective Gamma-Secretase Inhibitor for the Treatment of Alzheimer's Disease. *Alzheimer Dement,* Vol.5, No.4, (2009), pp. 139-P139, ISSN: 15525260

Jang, M. H.; Jung, S. B.; Lee, M. H.; Kim, C. J.; Oh, Y. T.; Kang, I.; Kim, J. & Kim, E. H. (2005). Melatonin Attenuates Amyloid Beta25-35-Induced Apoptosis in Mouse Microglial BV2 Cells. *Neurosci Lett,* Vol.380, No.1-2, (May 2005), pp. 26-31, ISSN: 0304-3940

Jansen, S. L.; Forbes, D. A.; Duncan, V. & Morgan, D. G. (2006). Melatonin for Cognitive Impairment. *Cochrane Database Syst Rev,* Vol.25, No.1, (January 2006), CD003802, ISSN: 1469493X

Javed, H.; Khan, M. M.; Khan, A.; Vaibhav, K.; Ahmad, A.; Khuwaja, G.; Ahmed, M. E.; Raza, S. S.; Ashafaq, M.; Tabassum, R.; Siddiqui, M. S.; El-Agnaf, O. M.; Safhi, M. M. & Islam, F. (2011). S-Allyl Cysteine Attenuates Oxidative Stress Associated Cognitive Impairment and Neurodegeneration in Mouse Model of Streptozotocin-Induced Experimental Dementia of Alzheimer's Type. *Brain Res,* Vol.1389, (May 2011), pp. 133-42, ISSN: 68993

Jeong, H.; Then, F.; Melia, T. J. Jr.; Mazzukki, J. R.; Cui, L.; Savas, J. N.; Voisine, C.; Paganetti, P.; Tanese, N.; Hart, A. C.; Yamamoto, A.; Kraine, D.; et al. (2009). Acetylation Targets Mutant Huntington to Auto phagosomes for Degradation. *Cell,* Vol.137, No.1, (May 2009), pp. 60-72, ISSN: 0092-8674

Johnson, J. A.; Johnson, D. A.; Kraft, A. D.; Calkins, M. J.; Jakel, R. J.; Vargas, M. R. & Chen, P. C. (2008). The Nrf2-ARE Pathway: An Indicator and Modulator of Oxidative Stress in Neurodegeneration. *Ann N Y Acad Sci,* Vol.1147, (December 2008), pp. 61-9, ISSN: 1460404

Johnson, J.; Maher, P. & Hanneken, A. (2009). The Flavonoid, Eriodictyol, Induces Long-Term Protection in ARPE-19 Cells Through its Effects on Nrf2 Activation and Phase 2 Gene Expression. *Invest Ophthalmol Vis Sci,* Vol.50, No.5, (May 2009), pp. 2398-406, ISSN: 1460404

Jonkers, N.; Sarre, S.; Ebinger, G.; et al. (2002). MK801 Suppresses the L-DOPA-Induced Increase of Glutamate in Striatum of Hemi-Parkinson Rats. *Brain Res,* Vol.926, No.1-2, (February 2002), pp. 149, ISSN: 68993

Jou, M. J.; Peng, T. I.; Reiter, R. J.; Jou, s. B.; Wu, H. Y. & Wen, S. T. (2004). Visualization of the Antioxidative Effects of Melatonin at the Mitochondrial Level During Oxidative Stress-Induced Apoptosis of Rat Brain Astrocytes. *J Pineal Res,* Vol.37, No.1, (August 2004), pp. 55-70, ISSN: 0742-3098

Kaur, H.; Chauhan, S. & Sandhir, R. (2011). Protective Effect of Lycopene on Oxidative Stress and Cognitive Decline in Rotenone Induced Model of Parkinson's Disease. *Neurochem Res,* Vol.36, No.8 (August 2011), pp. 1435-43, ISSN: 0364-3190

Kerchner, G. A. & Boxer, A. L. (2010). Bapineuzumab. *Expert Opin Biol Ther,* Vol.10, No.7, (July 2010), pp. 1121-1130, ISSN: 1471-2598

Kerman, A.; Liu, H. N.; Croul, S.; et al. (2010). Amyotrophic Lateral Sclerosis is a Non-Amyloid Disease in Which Extensive Misfolding of SOD1 is Unique to the Familial Form. *Acta Neuropathol,* Vol.119, No.3, pp. 335–44, ISSN: 0001-6322

Khare, S. D.; Ding, F.; Gwanmesia, K. N. & Dokholyan, N. V. (2005). Molecular Origin of Polyglutamine Aggregation in Neurodegenerative Diseases. *PLoS Comp Biol,* Vol.1, No.3, pp. e30, ISSN: 15537358

Kiaei, M.; Kipiani, K.; Petri, S.; Choi, M. K.; Chen, J. & Beal, M. F. (2005). Integrative Role of Cpla WITH cox-2 and the Effect of Non-Steriodal Anti-Inflammatory Drugs in a Transgenic Mouse Model of Amyotrophic Lateral Sclerosis. *J Neurochem,* Vol.93, No.2, pp. 403-11, ISSN: 0022-3042

Kiaei, M.; Petri, S.; Kipiani, K.; et al. (2006). Thalidomide and Lenalidomide Extend Survival in a Transgenic Mouse Model of Amyotrophic Lateral Sclerosis. *J Neurosci* Vol.26, No.9, (March 2006), pp. 2467-73, ISSN: 0270-6474

Kieburtz, K.; McDermott, M. P.; Voss, T. S.; Corey-Bloom, J.; Deuel, L. M.; Dorsey, E. R.; Factor, S.; Geschwind, M. D.; Hodgeman, K.; Kayson, E.; Noonberg, S.; Pourfar, M.; Rabinowitz, K.; Ravina, B.; Sanchez-Ramos, J.; Seely, L.; Walker, F.; Feigin, A.; Huntington Disease Study Group DIMOND Investigators. (2010). A Randomized, Placebo-Controlled Trial of Latrepirdine in Huntington's Disease. *Arch Neurol,* Vol.67, No.2, (February 2010), pp. 154-60, ISSN: 39942

Kim, S. H.; Lu, H. F. & Alano, C. C. (2011). Neuronal Sirt3 Protects Against Excitotoxic Injury in Mouse Cortical Neuron Culture. *PLoS ONE,* Vol.6, No.3, (March 2011), pp. e14731, ISSN: 19326203

Kipnis, J. & Schwartz, M. (2002). Dual Action of Glatiramer Acetate (Cop-1) in the Treatment of CNS Autoimmune and Neurodegenerative Disorders. *Trends Mol Med,* Vol.8, No.7, (August 2002), pp. 319-323, ISSN: 1471-4914

Kirkinezos, I. G.; Hernandez, D.; Bradley, W. G. & Moraes, C. T. (2004). An ALS Mouse Model with a Permeable Blood-Brain Barrier Benefits from Systemic Cyclosporine A Treatment. *J Neurochem,* Vol.88, No.4, (February 2004), pp. 821-6, ISSN: 0022-3042

Komatsu, M.; Waguri, S. & Koike, M. (2007). Homeostatic Levels of p62 Control Cytoplasmic Inclusion Body Formation in Autophagy-Deficient Mice. *Cell,* Vol.131, No.6, (December 2007), pp. 1149-1163, ISSN: 0092-8674

Kostic, V.;Jackson-Lewis, V.; de Bilbao, F.; Dubois-Dauphin, M. & Przedborski, S. (1997). Bcl-2: Prolonging Life in a Transgenic Mouse Model of Familial Amyotrophic Lateral Sclerosis. *Science,* Vol.277, No.5325, (July 1997), pp. 559-563, ISSN: 0036-8075

Koutsilieri, E. & Riederer, P. (2007). Excitotoxicity and New Antiglutamatergic Strategies in Parkinson's Disease and Alzheimer's Disease. *Parkinsonism Relat Disord,* Vol.12, No.3, (2007), pp. S329-31, ISSN: 13538020

Krainc, D. (2010). Clearance of Mutant Proteins as a Therapeutic Target in Neurodegenerative Diseases. *Arch Neurol,* Vol.67, No.4, (April 2010), pp. 388-92, ISSN: 39942

Kramer, M. L. & Schulz-Schaeffer, W. J. (2007). Presynaptic Alpha-Synuclein Aggregates, Not Lewy Bodies, Cause Neurodegeneration in Dementia with Lewy Bodies. *J Neurosci,* Vol.27, (February 2007), pp. 1405, ISSN: 0003-9942

Kuzma-Kozakiewicz, M. & Kwiecinski, H. (2011). New Therapeutic Targets for Amyotrophic Lateral Sclerosis. *Expert Opin Ther Targets,* Vol.15, No.2, (February 2011), pp. 127-43, ISSN: 15675769

Kurkowska-Jastrzebska, I.; Litwin, T.; Joniec, I.; Ciesielska, A.; Przybyłkowski, A.; Członkowski, A.; Członkowska, A. (2004). Dexamethasone Protects Against Dopaminergic Neurons Damage in a Mouse Model of Parkinson's Disease. *Int Immunopharmacol,* Vol.4, No.10-11, (October 2004), pp. 1307-18, ISSN: 15675769

Kwon, S. H.; Lee, H. K.; Kim, J. A.; Hong, S. I.; Kim, H. C.; Jo, T. H.; Park, Y. I.; Lee, C. K.; Kim, Y. B.; Lee, S. Y. & Jang, C. G. (2010). Neuroprotective Effects of Chlorogenic Acid on Scopolamine-Induced Amnesia Via Anti-Acetylcholinesterase and Anti-Oxidative Activities in Mice. *Eur J Pharmacol,* Vol.649, No.1-3, (15 December 2010), pp. 210-7, ISSN: 0014-2999

Lanka, V.; Wieland, S.; Barber, J. & Cudkowicz, M. (2009). Arimoclomol: A Potential Therapy Under Development for ALS. *Expert Opin Investig Drugs* Vol.8, No.12, (December 2009), pp. 1907-18, ISSN: 13543784

Leary, S. M. & Thompson, A. J. (2005). Primary progressive multiple sclerosis : current and future treatment options. *CNS Drugs,* Vol. 19, No.5, (2005), pp. 369-376, ISSN: 1172-7047

Leaver, K. R.; Allbutt, H. N.; Creber, N. J.; et al. (2008). Neuroprotective effects of a selective N-methyl-D-aspartate NR2B receptor antagonist in the 6-hydroxydopamine rat model of Parkinson's disease. *Clin Exp Pharmacol Physiol,* Vol. 35, No.11, (November 2008), pp. 1388, ISSN: 0305-1870

Lee, H. P.; Zhu, X.; Casadesus, G.; Castellani, R. J.; Nunomura, A.; Smith, M. A.; Lee, H. G. & Perry, G. (2010). Antioxidant Approaches for the Treatment of Alzheimer's Disease. *Expert Rev Neurother,* Vol.10, No.7, (July 2010), pp. 1201-8, ISSN: 13543784

Lee, J.; Kosaras, B.; Del Signore, S. J.; Cormier, K.; McKee, A.; Ratan, R. R.; Kowall, N. W. & Ryu, H. (2011). Modulation of Lipid Peroxidation and Mitochondrial Function Improves Neuropathology in Huntington's Disease Mice. *Acta Neuropathol,* Vol.121, No.4, (April 2011), pp. 487-98, ISSN: 0001-6322

Leegwater-Kim, J. & Cha, J. H. (2004). The Paradigm of Huntington's Disease: Therapeutic Opportunities in Neurodegeneration. *NeuroRx,* Vol.1, No.1, (January 2004), pp. 28-38, ISSN: 1545-5343

Leoutsakos, J. M.; Muthen, B. O.; Breitner, J. C. & Lyketsos, C. G. (2011). For the ADAPT Research Team. Effects of Non-Steroidal Anti-Inflammatory Drug Treatments on Cognitive Decline Vary by Phase of Pre-Clinical Alzheimer Disease: Findings from the Randomized Controlled Alzheimer's Disease Anti-Inflammatory Prevention Trial. *Int J Geriatr Psychiatry,* doi:10.1002/gps.2723. [Epub ahead of print], (10 May 2011), ISSN: 8856230

Levine, M. S.; Cepeda, C.; Cummings, D. M.; Hickey, M. A.; Kleiman-Weiner, M.; Chen, J. Y. & Watson, J. B. (2010). Rescuing the Corticostriatal Synaptic Disconnection in the R6/2 Mouse Model of Huntington's Disease: Exercise, Adenosine Receptors and Ampakines. *PLoS Curr,* Vol.2, (September 2010), pii: RRN1182, ISSN: 2157-3999

Li, M.; Ona, V. O.; Guégan, C.; Chen, M.; Jackson-Lewis, V.; Andrews, L. J.; Olszewski, A. J.; Stieg, P. E.; Lee, J. P.; Przedborski, S.; Friedlander, R. M. (2000). Functional Role of Caspase-1 and Caspase-3 in an ALS Transgenic Mouse Model. *Science,* Vol.288, No.5464, (14 April 2000), pp. 335-339, ISSN: 00308075

Litvinenko, I. V.; Odinak, M. M.; Moqil'naya, V. I. & Perstney, S. V. (2010). Use of Memantine (Akatinol) for the Correction of Cognitive Impairments in Parkinson's Disease Complicated by Dementia. *Neurosci Behav Physiol,* Vol.40, No.2, (February 2010), pp. 149-55, ISSN: 0097-0549

Liu, B. & Hong, J. S. (2003). Role of Microglia in Inflammation-Mediated Neurodegenerative Diseases: Mechanisms and Strategies for Therapeutic Intervention. *J Pharmacol Exp Ther, Vol.*304, No.1, (January 2003), pp. 1-7, ISSN: 0022-3565

Liu, J. H.; Yin, F.; Guo, L. X.; Deng, X. H. & Hu, Y. H. (2009). Neuroprotection of Geniposide Against Hydrogen Peroxide Induced PC12 Cells Injury: Involvement of PI3 Kinase Signal Pathway. *Acta Pharmacol Sin,* Vol.30, No.2, (February 2009), pp. 159-65, ISSN: 16714083

Lu, Y.; Ansar, S.; Michaelis, M. L. & Blagg, B. S. (2009). Neuroprotective Activity and Evaluation of Hsp90 Inhibitors in an Immortalized Neuronal Cell Line. *Bioorg Med Chem,* Vol.17, No.4, (February 2009), pp. 1709-15, ISSN: 9680896

Luo, W.; Sun, W.; Taldone, T.; Rodina, A. & Chiosis, G. (2010). Heat Shock Protein 90 in Neurodegenerative Diseases. *Molecular Neurodegeneration,* Vol.5, No.3, (June 2010), pp.24, ISSN: 17501326

Mahlberg, R.; Walther, S.; Kalus, P.; Bohner, G.; Haedel, S.; Reischies, F. M.; Kuhl, K. P.; Hellweg, R. & Kunz, D. (2008). Pineal Calcification in Alzheimer's Disease: an in Vivo Study Using Computed Tomography. *Neurobiol Aging,* Vol.29, No.2, (February 2008), pp. 203-209, ISSN: 1974580

Manczak, M.; Mao, P.; Calkins, M. J.; Cornea, A.; Reddy, A. P.; Murphy, M. P.; Szeto, H. H.; Park, B. & Reddy, P. H. (2010). Mitochondria-Targeted Antioxidants Protect Against Amyloid-Beta Toxicity in Alzheimer's Disease Neurons. *J Alzheimers Dis,* Vol.20, No.2, pp. (2010), S609-31, ISSN: 13872877

Mangialasche, F.; Solomon, A.; Winblad, B.; Mecocci, P. & Kivipelto M. (2010). Aging Research Center, Karolinska Institutet, Stockholm, Sweden, Alzheimer's disease: Clinical Trials and Drug Development. *Lancet Neurol,* Vol.9, No.7, (July 2010), pp. 702-16, ISSN: 14744422

Mangialasche, F.; Polidori, M. C.; Monastero, R.; Ercolani, S.; Camarda, C.; Cecchetti, R. & Mecocci, P. (2009). Biomarkers of Oxidative and Nitrosative Damage in Alzheimer's Disease and Mild Cognitive Impairment. *Ageing Res Rev,* Vol.8, No.4, (October 2009), pp. 285-305, ISSN: 1568-1637

Maragakis, N. J.; Jackson, M.; Ganel, R. & Rothstein, J. D. (2003). Topiramate Protects Against Motor Neuron Degeneration in Organotypic Spinal Cord Cultures but not in G93A SOD1 Transgenic Mice. *Neurosci Lett,* Vol.338, No.2, (February 2003), pp. 107-10, ISSN: 0304-3940

Markowitz, C. E.; Spitsin, S.; Zimmerman, V.; Jacobs, D.; Udupa, J. K.; Hooper, D. C. & Koprowski, H. (2009). The Treatment of Multiple Sclerosis with Inosine. *J Altern Complement Med,* Vol.15, No.6, (June 2009), pp. 619-25, ISSN: 10755535

Martin, I.; Dawson, V. L. & Dawson, T. M. (2011). Recent Advances in the Genetics of Parkinson's Disease. *Annu Rev Genomics Hum Genet,* Vol.22, No.12, (September 2011), pp. 301-25, ISSN: 15278204

Martone, R. L.; Zhou, H.; Atchison, K.; et al. (2009). Alzheimer Disease Amide Inhibitor of Amyloid Precursor Protein Gamma-Secretase for the Treatment of Alzheimer's Disease. *J Pharmacol Exp Ther,* Vol.331, No.2, (2009), pp. 598-608, ISSN: 0022-3565

Maruyama, W.; Nitta, A.; Shamoto-Nagai, M.; Hirata, Y.; Akao, Y.; Youdim, M.; Furukawa, S.; Nabeshima, T. & Naoi, M. (2004). N-Propargyl-1 R-Aminoindan, Rasagiline, Increases Glial Cell Line-Derived Neurotrophic Factor (GDNF) in Neuroblastoma SH-SY5Y Cells Through Activation of NF-KappaB Transcription Factor. *Neurochem Int,* Vol.44, No.6, (May 2004), pp. 393-400, ISSN: 0197-0186

Masaki, K. H.; Losonczy, K. G.; Izmirlian, G.; et al. (2000). Association of Vitamin E and C Supplement Use with Cognitive Function and Dementia in Elderly Men. *Neurology,*Vol.54, No.6, pp. 1265, ISSN: 283878

Matsuoka, M. & Hashimoto, Y. (2010). Humanin and the Receptors for Humanin. *Mol Neurobiol,* Vol.41, No.1, (February 2010), pp. 22-8, ISSN: 0893-7648

Matsuoka, Y.; Jouroukhin, Y.; Gray, A. J.; et al. (2008). A Neuronal Microtubule-Interacting Agent, NAPVSIPQ, Reduces Tau Pathology and Enhances Cognitive Function in a Mouse Model of Alzheimer's Disease. *J Pharmacol Exp Ther,* Vol.325, No.1, (April 2008), pp. 146-153, ISSN: 0022-3565

Mecocci, P. & Polidori, M. C. (2011). Antioxidant Clinical Trials in Mild Cognitive Impairment and Alzheimer's Disease. *Biochim Biophys Acta,* October 2011, [Epub ahead of print], ISSN: 0006-3002

Medeiros, C. A. M.; De Bruin, P. F.; Lopes, L. A.; Magalhaes, M. C.; Seabra, M. & De Bruin, V. M. (2007). Effect of Exogenous Melatonin on Sleep and Motor Dysfunction in Parkinson's Disease: A Randomized, Double Blind, Placebo-Controlled Study. *Journal of Neurology,* Vol.254, No.4, (April 2007), pp. 459–464, ISSN: 3405354

Medina, D.; Caccamo, A. & Oddo, S. (2011). Methylene Blue Reduces Aβ Levels and Rescues Early Cognitive Deficit by Increasing Proteasome Activity. *Brain Pathol,* Vol.21, No.2, (March 2011), pp. 140-49, ISSN: 10156305

Miron, V. E.; Schubart, A. & Antel, J. P. (2008). Central Nervous Systemdirected Effects of FTY720 (Fingolimod). *J Neurol Sci,* Vol.274, No. 1-2, (November 2008), pp. 13-17, ISSN: 13001817

Montalban, X.; Sastre-Garriga, J.; Tintore, M.; Brieva, L.; Aymerich, F. X.; Rio, J.; Porcel, J.; Borras, C.; Nos, C. & Rovira, A. (2009). A Single-Center, Randomized, Double-Blind, Placebo-Controlled Study of Interferon Beta-1b on Primary Progressive and Transitional Multiple Sclerosis. *Mult Scler* Vol.15, No.10, (October 2009), pp. 1195-1205, ISSN: 13524585

Montgomery, S. A.; Thal, L. J. & Amrein, R. (2003). Meta-Analysis of Double Blind Randomized Controlled Clinical Trials of Acetyl-L-Carnitine Versus Placebo in the Treatment of Mild Cognitive Impairment and Mild Alzheimer's Disease. *Int Clin Psychopharmacol*, Vol.18, No.2, (March 2003), pp. 61-71, ISSN: 2681315

Morin, N.; Grégoire, L.; Gomez-Mancilla, B.; Gasparini, F. & Di Paolo, T. (2010). Effect of the Metabotropic Glutamate Receptor Type 5 Antagonists MPEP and MTEP in Parkinsonian Monkeys. *Neuropharmacology*, Vol.8, No.7, (June 2010), pp. 981-986, ISSN: 0028-3908

Moura, M. B.; Dos Santos, L. S. & Van Houten, B. (2010). Mitochondrial Dysfunction in Neurodegenerative Diseases and Cancer. *Environmental and Molecular Mutagenesis*, Vol.51, No.5, (June 2010), pp. 391–405, ISSN: 8936692

Nagai, Y. & Popiel, H. A. (2008). Conformational Changes and Aggregation of Expanded Polyglutamine Proteins as Therapeutic Targets of the Polyglutamine Diseases: Exposed Beta-Sheet Hypothesis. *Curr Pharm Des*, Vol.14, No.30, pp. 3267, ISSN: 1381-6128

Nash, J. E. & Brotchie, J. M. (2002). Characterisation of Striatal NMDA Receptors Involved in the Generation of Parkinsonian Symptoms: Intrastriatal Microinjection Studies in the 6-OHDA-Lesioned Rat. *Mov Disord*, Vol.17, No.3, (May 2002), pp. 455, ISSN: 8853185

Neef, D. W.; Tursk, M. L. & Thiele, D. J. (2010). Modulation of Heat Shock Transcription Factor 1 as a Therapeutic Target for Small Molecular Intervention in Neurodegenerative Disease. *PLoS Biol*, Vol.8, No.1, (January 2010), pp. e1000291, ISSN: 1544-9173

Neymotin, A.; Petri, S.; Calingasan, N. Y.; et al. (2009). Lenalidomide (Revlimid) Administration at Symptom Onset is Neuroprotective in a Mouse Model of Amyotrophic Lateral Sclerosis. *Exp Neurol*, Vol.220, No.1, (November 2009), pp. 191-7, ISSN: 0014-4886

Nguyen, T.; Yang, C. S. & Pickett, C. B. (2004). The Pathways and Molecular Mechanisms Regulating Nrf2 Activation in Response to Chemical Stress. *Free Radic Biol Med*, Vol.37, No.4, (August 2004), pp. 433-41, ISSN: 8915849

Noble, W.; Planel, E.; Zehr, C.; et al. (2005). Inhibition of Glycogen Synthase Kinase-3 by Lithium Correlates with Reduced Tauopathy and Degeneration in Vivo. *Proc Natl Acad Sci USA*, Vol.102, No.19, (May 2005), pp. 6990-6995, ISSN: 10916490

Norfus, F.; Nanje, A.; Gutekunst, C. A.; Shi, G.; Chen, J.; Bejarano, M.; Fox, J.; Ferrrante, R. J. & Hersch, S. M. (2004). Anti Inflammatory Treatment with Acetylsalicylate or Rofecoxib is not Neuroprotective in Huntington's Disease Transgenic Mice. *Neurobiol Dis*, Vol.17, No.2, (November 2004), pp. 319-325, ISSN: 0969-9961

Norris, F. H. (1994). Ceftriaxone in amyotrophic lateral sclerosis. *Arch Neurol*, Vol.51, No.5, (May 1994), pp. 447, ISSN: 0003-9942

Olanow, C. W. (2006). Rationale for Considering that Propargylamines might be Neuroprotective in Parkinson's Disease. *Neurology*, Vol.66, No.10, (May 2006), pp. S69-79, ISSN: 0028-3878

Olanow, C. W.; Hauser, R. A.; Gauger, L.; et al. (1995). The Effect of Deprenyl and Levodopa on the Progression of Parkinson's Disease. *Ann Neurol*, Vol.38, No.5, (November 1995), pp. 771-777, ISSN: 3645134

Olcese, J. M.; Cao, C.; Mori, T.; Mamcarz, M. B., Maxwell, A.; Runfeldt, M. J.; Wang, L.; Zhang, C.; Lin, X.; Zhang, G. & Arendash, G. W. (2009). Protection Against Cognitive Deficits and Markers of Neurodegeneratin by Long-Term Oral Administration of Melatonin in a Transgenic Model of Alzheimer's Disease. *J Pineal Res,* Vol.47, No.1, (August 2009), pp. 82-96, ISSN: 15677249

Ono, K.; Hasegawa, K.; Naiki, H. & Yamada, M. (2005). Preformed Beta Amyloid Fibrils are Destabilized by Coenzyme Q10 in Vitro. *Biochem Biophys Res Commun,* Vol.330, No.1, (April 2005), pp. 111-116, ISSN: 0006-291x

Ouardouz, M.; Malek, S.; Coderre, E. & Stys, P. K. (2006). Complex Interplay Between Glutamate Receptors and Intracellular Ca2+ Stores During Ischaemia in Rat Spinal Cord White Matter. *J Physiol,* Vol.577, No.1, (November 2006), pp. 191-204, ISSN: 9284257

Oyanagi, K.; Yamazaki, M.; Takahashi, H.; et al. (2008). Spinal Anterior Horn Cells in Sporadic Amyotrophic Lateral Sclerosis Show Ribosomal Detachment from, and Cisternal Distention of the Rough Endoplasmic Reticulum. *Neuropathol Appl Neurobiol,* Vol.34, No.6, (December 2008) pp. 650-8, ISSN: 0305-1846

Palacino, J. J.; Sagi, D.; Goldberg, M. S.; et al. (2004). Mitochondrial Dysfunction and Oxidative Damage in Parkin Deficient Mice. *J Biol Chem,* Vol.279, No.18, (April 2004), pp. 18614, ISSN: 0021-9258

Palacios, H. H.; Yendluri, B. B.; Parvathaneni, K.; Shadlinski, V. B.; Obrenovich, M. E.; Leszek, J.; Gokhman, D., Gasiorowski, K.; Braqi, V. & Aliev, G. (2011). Mitochondrion-Specific Antioxidants as Drug Treatments for Alzheimer Disease. *CNS Neurol Disord Drug Targets,* Vol.10, No.2, (March 2011), pp. 149-62, ISSN: 1871-5273

Palazuelos, J.; Aguado, T.; Pazos, M. R.; et al. (2009). Microglial CB2 Cannabinoid Receptors are Neuroprotective in Huntington's Disease Excitotoxicity. *Brain,* Vol.132, No.11, (November 2009), pp. 3152-64, ISSN: 0068950

Paleologou, K. E.; Irvine, G. B. & El-Agnaf, O. M. (2005). Alpha-Synuclein Aggregation in Neurodegenerative Diseases and its Inhibition as a Potential Therapeutic Strategy. *Biochem Soc Trans,* Vol.33, No.5, (November 2005), pp. 1106-1110, ISSN: 0300-5127

Pallos, J.; Bodai, L.; Lukacsovich, T.; et al. (2008). Inhibition of Specific HDACs and Sirtuins Suppresses Pathogenesis in a Drosophila Model of Huntington's Disease. *Hum Mol Genet,* Vol.17, No.23, (December 2008), pp. 3767, ISSN: 9646906

Pandey, M.; Varghese, M.; Sindhu, K.M.; Sreetama, S.; Navneet, A. K.; Mohanakumar, K. P. & Usha, R. (2008). Mitochondrial NAD+-Linked State 3 Respiration and Complex-I Activity are Compromised in the Cerebral Cortex of 3-Nitropropionic Acid-Induced Rat Model of Huntington's Disease. *J Neurochem,* Vol.104, No.2, (January 2008), pp. 420-34, ISSN: 0022-3042

Pasinelli, P.; Houseweart, M. K.; Brown, R. H. Jr. & Cleveland, D. W. (2000). Caspase-1 and -3 are Sequentially Activated in Motor Neuron Death in Cu, Zn Superoxide Dismutase-Mediated Familial Amyotrophic Lateral Sclerosis. *Proc Natl Acad Sci USA,* Vol.97, No.25, (December 2000), pp. 13901-6, ISSN: 10916490

Pender, M. P. & Rist, M. J. (2001). Apoptosis of Inflammatory Cells in Immune Control of the Nervous System: Role of Glia. *Glia,* Vol.36, No.2, (November 2001), pp. 137-44, ISSN: 0894-1491

Peng, J.; Xie, L.; Stevenson, F.F.; Melov, S.; Di Monte, D.A. & Andersen, J.K. (2006). Nigrostriatal Dopaminergic Neurodegeneration in the Weaver Mouse is Mediated via Neuroinflammation and Alleviated by Minocycline Administration. *J Neurosci,* Vol.26, No.45, (November 2006), pp. 11644-11651, ISSN: 0270-6474

Penton-Rol, G.; Martinez-Sanchez, G.; Cervantes-Llanos, M.; Lagumersindez-Denis, N.; Acosta-Medina, E. F.; Falcon-Cama, V.; Alonso-Ramirez, R.; Valenzuela-Silva, C.; Rodriguez-Jimenez, E.; Llopiz-Arzuaga, A.; Marin-Prida, J.; Lopez-Saura, P. A.; Guillen-Nieto, G. E. & Penton-Arias, E. C. (2011). Phycocyanin Ameliorates Experimental Autoimmune Encephalomyelitis and Indices Regulator T Cells. *Int Immunopharmacol,* Vol.11, No.1, (January 2011), pp. 29-38, ISSN: 15675769

Phiel, C. J.; Wilson, C. A.; Lee, V. M. & Klein, P. S. (2003). GSK-3Alpha Regulates Production of Alzheimer's Disease Amyloid-Beta Peptides. *Nature,* Vol.423, No.6938, (May 2003), pp. 435-439, ISSN: 0028-0836

Pinnen, F.; Sozio, P.; Cacciatore, I.; Comacchia, C.; Mollica, A.; Iannitelli, A.; D'Aurizio, E.; Cataldi, A.; Zara, S.; Nasuti, Q. & Di Stefano, A. (2011). Ibuprofen and Glutathione Conjugate as a Potential Therapeutic Agent for Treating Alzheimer's Disease. *Arch Pharm (Weinheim),* Vol.344, No.3, (March 2011), pp. 139-48, ISSN: 1521-4184

Pinton S, da Rocha JT, Gai BM, Prigol M, da Rosa LV, Nogueira CW (2011). Neuroprotector Effect of p,p'-Methoxvl-Diphenyl Diselenide in a Model of Sporadic Dementia of Alzheimer's Type in Mice: Contribution of Antioxidant Mechanism. *Cell Biochem Funct,* Vol.29, No.3, (April 2011), pp. 235-45, ISSN: 0263-6484

Pitt, D.; Nagelmeier, I. E.; Wilson, H. C. & Raine, C. S. (2003). Glutamate Uptake by Oligodendrocytes: Implications for Excitotoxicity in Multiple Sclerosis. *Neurology,* Vol.61, No.8, (October 2003), pp. 1113-1120, ISSN: 283878

Pontieri, F.E.; Ricci, A.; Pellicano, C.; Benincase, D. & Buttarelli, F.R. (2005). Minocycline in Amyotrophic Lateral Sclerosis: A Pilot Study. *Neurol. Sci.,* Vol.26, No.4, (October 2005), pp. 285-287, ISSN: 15901874

Potter, P. (2010). Investigational Medications for Treatment of Patients With Alzheimer Disease, *J Am Osteopath Assoc.* Vol.110, No.9, (September 2010), pp. S27-S36, ISSN: 0098-6151

Qi, X.; Lewin, A. S.; Sun, L.; Hauswirth, W. W. & Guy, J. (2007). Suppression of Mitochondrial Oxidative Stress Provides Long Term Neuroprotection in Experimental Optic Neuritis. *Invest Opthalmol Vis Sci,* Vol.48, No.2, (February 2007), pp. 681-691, ISSN: 1460404

Qi, X.; Sun, L.; Lewin, A. S.; Hauswirth, W. W. & Guy, J. (2007). Long-Term Suppression of Neurodegeneration in Chronic Experimental Optic Neuritis: Antioxidant Gene Therapy, *Invest Ophthalmol Vis Sci,* Vol.48, No.12, (December 2007), pp. 5360-70, ISSN: 1552-5783

Quin, J.; Goswami, R.; Balabanov, R. & Dawson, G. (2007). Oxidised Phosphatidylcholine is a Marker for Neuroinflammation in Multiple Sclerosis Brain. *J Neurosci Res,* Vol85, No.5, (April 2007), pp. 977–84, ISSN 03604012

Quintanilla, R. A.; Jin, Y. N.; Fuenzalida, K.; Bronfman, M. & Johnson, G. V. (2008). Rosiglitazone Treatment Prevents Mitochondrial Dysfunction in Mutant Huntington-Expressing Cells: Possible Role of Peroxisome Proliferator-Activated Receptor-Gamma (PPARgamma) in the Pathogenesis of Huntington's Disease. *J Biol Chem,* Vol.283, No.37, (September 2008), pp. 25628-37, ISSN: 0021-9258

Ravikumar, B.; Vacher, C. & Berger, Z. (2004). Inhibition of mTOR Induces Autophagy and Reduces Toxicity of Polyglutamine Expansions in Fly and Mouse Models of Huntington Disease. *Nat Genet*, Vol.36, No.6, (June 2004), pp. 585-595, ISSN: 1061-4036

Reynolds, N. (2007). Revisiting Safety of Minocycline as Neuroprotection in Huntington's Disease. *Mov Disord*, Vol.22, No.2, (January 2007), pp. 292, ISSN: 8853185

Rinne, J. O.; Brooks, D. J.; Rossor, M. N.; et al. (2010). 11C-PiB PET Assessment of Change in Fibrillar Amyloid-Beta Load in Patients with Alzheimer's Disease Treated with Bapineuzumab: A Phase 2, Double-Blind, Placebo-Controlled, Ascending-Dose Study. *Lancet Neurol*, Vol.9, No.4, (April 2010), pp. 363-372, ISSN: 14744422

Rohn, T. T.; Rissman, R. A.; Davis, M. C.; Kim, Y. E.; Cotman, C. W. & Head, E. (2002). Caspase-9 Activation and Caspase Cleavage of Tau in the Alzheimer's Disease Brain. *Neurobiol Dis*, Vol.11, No.2, (November 2002), pp. 341-354, ISSN: 0969-9961

Rothstein, J. D.; Jin, L.; Dykes-Hoberg, M.; Kuncl, R.W. (1993). Chronic Inhibition of Glutamate Uptake Produces a Model of Slow Neurotoxicity. *Proc. Natl. Acad. Sci. USA*, Vol.90, No.14, (15 July 1993), pp. 6591- 6595, ISSN:10916490

Rothstein, J. D.; Patel, S.; Regan, M.R.; Haenggeli, C.; Huang, Y.H.; Bergles, D.E.; Jin, L.; Dykes Hoberg, M.; Vidensky, S.; Chung, D.S.; Toan, S.V.; Bruijn, L.I.; Su, Z.Z.; Gupta, P.; Fisher, P.B. (2005). Beta-Lactam Antibiotics Offer Neuroprotection by Increasing Glutamate Transporter Expression. *Nature*, Vol.433, No. 7021, (January 2005), pp. 73-77, ISSN: 0028-0836

Rothstein, J.D.; Tsai, G.; Kuncl, R.W.; Clawson, L.; Cornblath, D.R.; Drachman, D.B.; Pestronk, A.; Stauch, B.L.; Coyle, J.T. (1990). Abnormal Excitatory Amino Acid Metabolism in Amyotrophic Lateral Sclerosis. *Ann. Neurol.*, Vol.28, No.1, (July 1990), pp. 18-25, ISSN: 3645134

Rothstein, J.D.; Van Kammen, M.; Levey, A.I.; Martin, L.J.; Kuncl, R.W. (1995). Selective Loss of Glial Glutamate Transporter GLT-1 in Amyotrophic Lateral Sclerosis. *Ann. Neurol.*, Vol.38, No.1, (July 1995), pp. 73-84, ISSN: 3645134

Rowland, L.P.; Shneider, N.A. (2001). Amyotrophic Lateral Sclerosis. *N. Engl. J. Med.*, Vol.344, No.22, (May 2001), pp. 1688-700, ISSN: 284793

Rubinsztein, D. C.; DiFiglia, M. & Heintz, N. (2005). Autophagy and its Possible Roles in Nervous System Diseases, Damage and Repair. *Autophagy.*; Vol.1, No.1, (April 2005), pp. 11-22, ISSN: 15548627

Ryu, J. K.; Choi, H. B. & McLarnon, J. G. (2006). Combined Minocycline Plus Pyruvate Treatment Enhances Effects of Each Agent to Inhibit Inflammation, Oxidative Damage, and Neuronal Loss in an Excitotoxic Animal Model of Huntington's Disease. *Neuroscience*, Vol.141, No.4, (September 2006), pp. 1835-48, ISSN: 03064522

Sae-Ung, K.; Ueda, K.; Govitrapong, P. & Phansuwan-Pujito, P. (2011). Melatonin Reduces the Expression of Alpha-Synuclein in the Dopamine Containing Neuronal Regions of Amphetamine-Treated Postnatal Rats. *J Pineal Res*, doi: 10.1111/j.1600-079X.2011.00927.x. Abstract (26 July 2011), ISSN: 0742-3098

Salloway, S.; Sperling, R.; Gilman, S.; et al. (2009). A Phase 2 Multiple Ascending Dose Trial of Bapineuzumab in Mild to Moderate Alzheimer Disease. *Neurology*, Vol.73, No.24, (15 December 2009), pp. 2061-2070, ISSN: 0028-3878

Sánchez-Pernaute, R.; Cooper, A. F.; Meixiang, Yu; Brownell, A. N. & Ole, Isacson. (2004). Selective COX-2 Inhibition Prevents Progressive Dopamine Neuron Degeneration in a Rat Model of Parkinson's Disease *Journal of Neuroinflammation*, Vol.1, No.1, (17 May 2004), pp. 6-13, ISSN: 17422094

Santamaría, A.; Pérez-Severiano, F.; Rodríguez-Martínez, E.; Maldonado, P. D.; Pedraza-Chaverri, J.; Ríos, C. & Segovia, J. (2001). Comparative Analysis of Superoxide Dismutase Activity Between Acute Pharmacological Models and a Transgenic Mouse Model of Huntington's Disease. *Neurochem Respondents*, Vol.26, No.4, (April 2001), pp. 419-24, ISSN: 0364-3190

Sasaki, S.; Warita, H.; Abe, K. & Iwata, M. (2005). Impairment of Axonal Transport in the Axon Hillock and the Initial Segment of Anterior Horn Neurons in Transgenic Mice with a G93A Mutant SOD1 Gene. *Acta europathol,* Vol.110, No.1, (July 2005), pp. 48-56, ISSN: 21527806

Sastre, M. & Gentleman, S. M. (2010). NSAIDs: How They Work and Their Prospects as Therapeutics in Alzheimer's Disease. *Front Aging Neurosci*, Vol.2, No.20, (May 2010), ISSN: 00986151

Saura, C. A.; Choi, S. Y.; Beglopoulos, V.; et al. (2004). Loss of Presenilin Function Causes Impairments of Memory and Synaptic Plasticity Followed by Age-Dependent Neurodegeneration. *Neuron*, Vol.42, No.1, (8 April 2004), pp. 23-36, ISSN: 0896-6273

Scotter, E. L.; Goodfellow, C. E.; Graham, E. S.; Dragunow, M. & Glass, M. (2010). Neuroprotective Potential of CB_1 Receptor Agonists in an in Vitro Model of Huntington's Disease, *British Journal of Pharmacology,*Vol.160, No.3, (June 2010), pp. 747-761, ISSN: 14765381

Sechi, G.; Deledda, M. G.; Bua, G.; et al. (1996). Reduced Intravenous Glutathione in the Treatment of Early Parkinson's Disease. *Prog Neuropsychopharmacol Biol Psychiatry;* Vol.20, No.7, (October 1996), pp. 1159, ISSN: 02785846

Shim, J. H.; Yoon, S. H.; Kim, K. H.; Han, J. Y.; Ha, J. Y.; Hyun, D. H.; Paek, S. H.; Kang, U. J.; Zhuang, X. & Son, J. H. (2011). The Antioxidant Trolox Helps Recovery From the Familial Parkinson's Disease-Specific Mitochondrial Deficits Caused by PINK1- and DJ-1-Deficiency in Dopaminergic Neuronal Cells. *Mitochondrion*, Vol.11, No.5, (September 2011), pp. 707-15, ISSN: 0017-3495

Shoulson, I. (1998). DATATOP: A Decade of Neuroprotective Inquiry. Parkinson Study Group. Deprenyl And Tocopherol Antioxidative Therapy Of Parkinsonism. *Ann Neurol*, Vol.44, No.3, (September 1998), S160-6, ISSN: 1938-3207

Shults, C. W.; Oakes, D.; Kieburtz, K.; et al. (2002). Effects of Coenzyme Q10 in Early Parkinson Disease: Evidence of Slowing of the Functional Decline. *Arch Neurol*, Vol.59, No.10, (October 2002), pp. 1541-50, ISSN: 0003-9942

Shults, C. W.; Flint Beal, M.; Song, D. & Fontaine, D. (2004). Pilot Trial of High Dosages of Coenzyme Q10 in Patients with Parkinson's Disease. *Exp Neurol*, Vol.188, No.2, (August 2004), pp. 491-4, ISSN: 0014-4886

Singh, O. ((2010). Protein-Misfolding Diseases and the Paradigm of Proteomics-Based Therapeutic Targets, *Expert Rev. Proteomics,* Vol.7, No.4, (August 2010), pp. 463-464, ISSN: 14789450

Soares, H.; Raha, N.; Sikpi, M.; et al. (2009). Abeta Variability and Effect of Gamma Secretase Inhibition on Cerebrospinal Fluid Levels of Abeta in Healthy Volunteers. *Alzheimer Dement*. Vol.5, No.4, (September 2010), pp. 252-P253, ISSN: 1945-1997

Soto, C. (2003). Unfolding the Role of Protein Misfolding in Neurodegenerative Diseases. *Nat. Rev. Neurosci*, Vol.4, No.1, (January 2003), pp. 49–60, ISSN: 1471003X

Soulet, D & Cicchetti, F. (2011). The Role of Immunity in Huntington's Disease. *Mol Psychiatry*, Vol.16, No.9, (September 2011), pp. 889-902, ISSN: 1359-4184

Srinivasan, V.; Cardinali, D. P.; Srinivasan, U. S.; Kaur, C.; Brown, G. M.; Spence, D. W.; Hardeland, R. & Pandi-Perumal, S. R. (2011). Therapeutic Potential of Melatonin and its Analogs in Parkinson's Disease: Focus on Sleep and Neuroprotection. *Ther Adv Neurol Disord*, Vol.4, No.5, (September 2011), pp. 297-317, ISSN: 1756-2864

St-Pierre, J.; Drori, S.; Uldry, M.; Silvaggi, J. M.; Rhee, J.; Jäger, S.; Handschin, C.; Zheng, K.; Lin, J.; Yang, W.; Simon, D. K.; Bachoo, R. & Spiegelman, B. M. (2006). Suppression of Reactive Oxygen Species and Neurodegeneration by the PGC-1 Transcriptional Coactivators. *Cell*, Vol.127, No.2, (October 2006), pp. 397-408, ISSN: 0092-8674

Stack, C.; Ho, D.; Wille, E.; Calingasan, N. Y.; Williams, C.; Liby, K.; Sporn, M.; Dumont, M. & Beal, M. F. (2010). Triterpenoids CDDO-ethyl Amide and CDDO-Trifluoroethyl Amide Improve the Behavioral Phenotype and Brain Pathology in a Transgenic Mouse Model of Huntington's Disease. Free Radic Biol Med, Vol.49, No.2, (July 2010), 147-58, ISSN: 0891-5849

Staff, R. T.; Ahearn, T. S.; Murray, A. D.; Bentham, P.; Seng, K. M. & Wischik, C. (2008). Tau Aggregation Inhibitor (TAI) Therapy with Rember(TM) Arrests the Trajectory of rCBF Decline in Brain Regions Affected by Tau Pathology in Mild and Moderate Alzheimer's Disease (AD). *Alzheimer Dement*, Vol.4, No.4, (September 2010), T775-T775, ISSN: 1945-1997

Steece-Collier, K.; Chambers, L. K.; Jaw-Tsai, S. S.; et al. (2000). Antiparkinsonian Actions of CP-101,606, An Antagonist of NR2B Subunit-Containing N-Methyl-d-Aspartate Receptors. *Exp Neurol*, Vol.163, No.1, (May 2000), pp. 239, ISSN: 0036-8075

Steffan, J. S.; Bodai, L.; Pallos, J.; et al. (2001). Histone Deacetylase Inhibitors Arrest Polyglutamine-Dependent Neurodegeneration in Drosophila. *Nature*, Vol.413, No.6857, (October 2001), pp. 739-743, ISSN: 00280836

Storch, A.; Jost, W. H.; Vieregge, P.; Spiegel, J.; Greulich, W.; Durner, J.; Müller, T.; Kupsch, A.; Henningsen, H.; Oertel, WH.; Fuchs, G.; Kuhn, W.; Niklowitz, P.; Koch, R.; Herting, B.; Reichmann, H.; German. (2007). Coenzyme Q(10) Study Group. Randomized, Double-Blind, Placebo-Controlled Trial on Symptomatic Effects of Coenzyme Q(10) in Parkinson Disease. *Arch Neurol*, Vol.64, No.7, (July 2007), pp. 938-44, ISSN: 1176-5178

Su, B.; Wang, X.; Zheng, L.; et al (2009). Abnormal Mitochondrial Dynamics and Neurodegenerative Diseases. *Biochim Biophys Acta*, Vol.1802, No.1, (January 2010), pp. 135-41, ISSN: 09254439

Suchy, J.; Lee, S.; Ahmed, A. & Shea, T. B. (2010). Dietary Supplementation with S-Adenosyl Methionine Delays the Onset of Motor Neuron Pathology in a Murine Model of Amyotrophic Lateral Sclerosis. *Neuromolecular Med*, Vol.12, No.1, (March 2010), pp. 86-97, ISSN: 1535-1084

Sureda, F. X.; Junyent, F.; Verdaguer, E.; Auladell, C.; Pelegri, C.; Vilaplana, J.; Folch, J.; Canudas, A. M.; Zarate, C. B.; Pallès, M. & Camins, A. (2011). Antiapoptotic Drugs: A Therapautic Strategy for the Prevention of Neurodegenerative Diseases. *Curr Pharm. Des*, Vol.17, No.3, (2011), pp. 230-45, ISSN: 1381-6128

Suwa, M.; Egashira, T.; Nakano, H.; Sasaki, H. & Kumagai, S. (2006). Metformin Increases the PGC-1alpha Protein and Oxidative Enzyme Activities Possibly Via AMPK Phosphorylation in Skeletal Muscle in Vivo. *J Appl Physiol*, Vol.101, No.6, (December 2006), pp. 1685-92, ISSN: 87507587

Takeuchi, S.; Fujiwara, N.; Ido, A.; et al (2010). Induction of Protective Immunity by Vaccination with Wild-Type Apo Superoxide Dismutase 1 in Mutant SOD1 Transgenic Mice. *J Neuropathol Exp Neurol*, Vol.69, No.10, (October 2010), pp. 1044-56, ISSN: 00223069

Tansey, M. G. & Goldberg, M. S. (2010). Neuroinflammation in Parkinson's Disease: Its Role in Neuronal Death and Implications for Therapeutic Intervention. *Neurobiol Dis*, Vol.37, No.3, (March 2010), pp. 510–518, ISSN: 0969-9961

Tarawneh, R. & Galvin, J. (2010). Potential Future Neuroprotective Therapies for Neurodegenerative Disorders and Strokes. *Clin Geriatr Med*. 2010 February, Vol.26, No.1, (February 2010) pp. 125–147, ISSN: 0749-0690

Tatton, W. G.; Chalmers-Redman, R.; Brown, D. & Tatton, N. (2003). Apoptosis in Parkinson's Disease: Signals for Neuronal Degradation. *Ann Neurol*, Vol.53, Suppl.3, pp. S61-70, ISSN: 0364-5134

Todaro, M.; Zeuner, A. & Stassi, G. (2004). Role of Apoptosis in Autoimmunity. *J Clin Immunol*, Vol.24, No.1, (January 2004), pp. 1-11, ISSN: 02719142

Tomita, T. (2009). Secretase Inhibitors and Modulators for Alzheimer's Disease Treatment. *Expert Rev Neurother*, Vol.9, No.5, (May 2009), pp. 661 -679, ISSN: 1473-7175

Trans, T. A.; McCoy, M. K.; Sporn, M. B. & Tansey, M. G. (2008). The Synthetic Triterpenoid CDDO-Methyl Ester Modulates Microglial Activities, Inhibits TNF Production, and Provides Dopaminergic Neuroprotection. *J Neuroinflammation*, Vol.12, No.5, (May 2008), pp. 14, ISSN: 1742-2094

Traynor, B. J.; Bruijn. L.; Conwit, R.; Beal, F.; O'Neill, G.; Fagan, S. C. & Cudkowicz, M. E. (2006). Neuroprotective Agents for Clinical Trials in ALS: A Systematic Assessment. *Neurology*, Vol.67, No.1, (11 July 2006), pp. 20-27. ISSN:0028 3878

Tsai, S. J. (2005). Glatiramer Acetate Could Be a Potential Antidepressant Through its Neuroprotective and Anti-Inflammatory Effects. *Med. Hypotheses*, Vol.69, No.6, (2007), pp. 145-148, ISSN: 0306-9877

Túnez, I.; Montilla, P.; Del Carmen Muñoz, M.; Feijóo, M. & Salcedo, M. (2004). Protective Effect of Melatonin on 3-Nitropropionic Acid-Induced Oxidative Stress in Synaptosomes in an Animal Model of Huntington's Disease. *J Pineal Res*, Vol.37, No.4, (November 2004), pp. 252-256, ISSN: 07423098

Turturici, G.; Sconzo, G. & Geraci, F. (2011). Hsp70 and Its Molecular Role in Nervous System Diseases. *Biochem Res Int*, 2011;2011:618127, (24 February 2011), ISSN: 20902255

Uitti, R. J.; Rajput, A. H.; Ahlskog, J. E.; et al. (1996). Amantadine Treatment is an Independent Predictor of Improved Survival in Parkinson's Disease. *Neurology*, Vol.46, No.6, (June 1996), pp. 1551, ISSN: 00283878

Van Den Bosch, L.; Tillkin, P.; Lemmens, G.; & Robberecht, W. (2002). Minocycline Delays Disease Onset and Mortality in a Transgenic Model of ALS. *Neuroreport*, Vol.13, No.8, (July 2002), pp. 1067-1070, ISSN: 00283878

Van Horssen, J.; Witte, M. E.; Schreibelt, G. & de Vries, H. E. (2011). Radical Changes in Multiple Sclerosis Pathogenesis, *Biochim Biophys Acta*. Vol.1812, No.2, (February 2011), pp. 141-50, ISSN: 0006-3002

van Meeteren, M. E.; Teunissen, C. E.; Dijkstra, C. D. & van Tol, E. A. (2005). Antioxidants and Polyunsaturated Fatty Acids in Multiple Sclerosis. *European Journal of Clinical Nutrition*, Vol.59, No.12, (August 2005), pp. 1347–1361, ISSN: 0954-3007

Verhagen, L.; Blanchet, P. J.; van den Munckhof, P.; Del Dotto, P.; Natte, R. & Chase, T. N. (1998). A Trial of Dextromethorphan in Parkinsonian Patients with Motor Response Complications. *Mov Disord*, Vol.13, No.3, (May 1998), pp. 414-417, ISSN: 0146-0404

Vila, M.; Przedborski, S. (2003). Targeting Programmed Cell Death in Neurodegenerative Diseases. *Nat. Rev. Neurosci*, Vol.4, No.5, (May 2003), pp. 365-375, ISSN: 1471-003X

Vis, J. C.; Schipper, E.; de Boer-van Huizen, R. T.; Verbeek, M. M.; de Waal, R. M.; Wesseling, P.; ten Donkelaar, H. J. & Kremer, B. (2005). Expression Pattern of Apoptosis-Related Markers in Huntington's Disease. *Acta Neuropathol,* Vol.109, No.3, (March 2005), pp. 321-8, ISSN: 0001-6322

Wahner, A. D.; Bronstein, J. M.; Bordelon, Y. M. & Ritz, B. (2007). Nonsteroidal Anti-Inflammatory Drugs May Protect Against Parkinson Disease. *Neurology,* Vol.69, No.19, (November 2007), pp. 1836–1842, ISSN: 0028-3878

Wai, M.S.; Liang, Y.; Shi, C.; Cho, E.Y.; Kung, H.F.; Yew, D. T. (2009). Co-Localization of Hyperphosphorylated Tau and Caspases in the Brainstem of Alzheimer's Disease Patients. *Biogerontology*, Vol.10, No.4, (August 2009), pp. 457-469, ISSN: 1389-5729

Wallström, E.; Diener, P.; Ljungdahl, A.; Khademi, M.; Nilsson, C. G.; & Olsson, T. (1996). Memantine Abrogates Neurological Deficits, But Not CNS Inflammation, in Lewis Rat Experimental Autoimmune Encephalomyelitis *J Neurol Sci*, Vol.137, No.2, (May 1996) pp. 89-96, ISSN: 0317-1671

Wang, X. (2009). The Anti-Apoptotic Activity of Melatonin in Neurodegenerative Diseases, Published in final edited for as: *CNS Neurosci Ther*, Vol.15, No.4, (2009), pp. 345-357, ISSN: 1755-5930

Wang, H.; Larriviere, K. S. & Keller, K. E. (2008). R+ Pramipexole as a Mitochondrially Focused Neuroprotectant: Initial Early Phase Studies in ALS. *Amyotroph Lateral Scler*, Vol.9, No.1, (February 2008), pp. 50–58, ISSN: 1466-0822

Weinstock- Guttman, B. B.; Baier, M.; Park, Y.; Feichter, J.; Lee-Kwen, P.; Gallagher, E.; Venkatraman, J.; Meksawan, K.; Deinehert, S.; Witte, M. E.; Geurts, J. J.; deVires, H. E.; van der Valk, P.; van Horssen, J. (2010). Mitochondrial Dysfunction: A Potential Link Between Neuroinflammation and Neurodegeneration. *Mitochondrion,* Vol.10, No.5, (August 2010), pp. 411–8, ISSN: 1567-7269

Witte, M. E.; Geurts, J. J.; de Vries, H. E.; van der Valk, P. & van Horssen, J. (2010). Mitochondrial Dysfunction: a Potential Link Between Neuroinflammation and Neurodegeneration? *Mitochondrion,* Vol.10, No.15, (August 2010), pp. 411-8, ISSN: 15677249

Wolinsky, J. S.; Narayana, P.A.; O'Connor, P.; Coyle, P. K.; Ford, C.; Johnson, K.; Miller, A.; Pardo, L.; Kadosh, S. & Ladkani, D. (2007). Glatiramer Acetate in Primary Progressive Multiple Sclerosis: Results of a Multinational, Multicenter, Double-Blind, Placebo-Controlled Trial. *Ann .Neurol*, Vol.61, No.6, (January 2007), pp. 14-24, ISSN: 0028-3878

Wyttenbach, A.; Carmichael, J.; Swartz, J.; Furlong, R. A.; Narain, Y.; Rankin, J. & Rubinsztein, D. C. (2000). Effects of Heat Shock, Heat Shock Protein 40 (HDJ-2), and Proteasome Inhibition on Protein Aggregation in Cellular Models of Huntington's Disease. *Proc Natl Acad Sci U S A*, Vol.97, No.6, (March 2000), pp. 2898-903, ISSN: 00278424

Wyttenbach, A.; et al. (2002). Heat Shock Protein 27 Prevents Cellular Polyglutamine Toxicity and Suppresses the Increase of Reactive Oxygen Species Caused by Huntington. *Hum Mol Genet*, Vol.11, No.9, (May 2002), pp. 1137-1151, ISSN: 1460-2083

Xing, G.; Dong, M.; Li, X.; Zou, Y.; Fan, L.; Wang, X.; Cai, D.; Li, C.; Zhou, L.; Liu, J. & Niu, Y. (2011). Neuroprotective Effects of Puerarin Against Beta-Amyloid-Induced Neurotoxicity in PC12 Cells via a PI3K-Dependent Signaling Pathway. *Brain Res Bull*, Vol.85, No.3-4, (May 2011), pp. 212-8, ISSN: 0361-9230

Yang, L.; Sugama, S.; Mischak, R. P.; Kiaei, M.; Bizat, N.; Brouillet, E.; Joh, T. H. & Beal, M. F. (2004). A Novel Systemically Active Caspase Inhibitor Attenuates the Toxicities of MPTP, Malonate, and 3NP in vivo. *Neurobiol Dis*, Vol.17, No.2, (November 2004), pp. 250-9, ISSN: 0969-9961

Yao, M.; Nguyen, T.V. & Pike, C. J. (2005). Beta-Amyloid-Induced Neuronal Apoptosis Involves c-Jun N-Terminal Kinase-Dependent Downregulation of Bcl-w. *J. Neurosci*, Vol.25, No.5, (February 2005), pp. 1149-1158, ISSN: 1525-8882

Yoshiyama, Y.; Higuchi, M.; Zhang, B.; et al. (2007). Synapse Loss and Microglial Activation Precede Tangles in a P301S Tauopathy Mouse Model. *Neuron*, Vol.115, No.6, (June 2008), pp. 337 -351, ISSN: 1422-0067

Youdim, M. B.; Fridkin, M. & Zheng, H. (2004). Novel Bifunctional Drugs Targeting Monoamine Oxidase Inhibition and Iron Chelation as an Approach to Neuroprotection in Parkinson's Disease and Other Neurodegenerative Diseases. *Neural Transm*, Vol.111, No.10-11, (October 2004), pp. 1455-71, ISSN: 0014-2999

Zádori, D.; Nyiri, G.; Szonyi, A.; Szatmári, I.; Fülöp, F.; Toldi, J.; Freund, T. F.; Vécsei, L. & Klivényi, P. (2011). Neuroprotective Effects of a Novel Kynurenic Acid Analogue in a Transgenic Mouse Model of Huntington's Disease. *J Neural Transm*, Vol.118, No.6, (June 2011), pp. 865-75, ISSN: 1540-8140

Zehutner, S. P.; Bourbonniere, I.; Moore, C. S.; Morris, S.; Meltrol, D.; St. Jean, M.; Lacasse, E. & Hebb, A. L. (2007). Linked Inhibitor of Apoptosis (IAP), Regulates T Cell Effector Function, *J Immunol*, Vol.179, No.11, (December 2007), pp. 7553-60, ISSN: 1938-3207

Zhang, Y.; Metz, L. M.; Yong, V. W.; Bell, R. B.; Yeung, M.; Patry, D. G. & Mitchell, J. R. (2008). Pilot Study of Minocycline in Relapsing-Remitting Multiple Sclerosis. *Can J Neurol Sci*, Vol.35, No.2, (May 2008), pp. 185-91, ISSN: 0317-1671

Zhao, Q.; Landen, J.; Burstein, A. H.; et al. (2010). Pharmacokinetics and Pharmacodynamics of Ponezumab (PF-04360365) Following a Single-Dose Intravenous Infusion in Patients with Mild to Moderate Alzheimer's Disease. *Alzheimer Dement*, Vol.6, No.4, pp. S143-S143, ISSN: 1552-5260

Zhou, J.; Zhang, S.; Zhao, X. & Wei, T. (2008). Melatonin Impairs NADPH Oxidase Assembly and Decreases Superoxide Anion Production in Microglia Exposed to Amyloid-Beta1-42. *J Pineal Res*, Vol.45, No.2, (September 2008), pp. 157–165, ISSN: 0185-3325

Zinman, L. & Cudkowicz, M. (2011). Emerging Targets and Treatments in Amyotrophic Lateral Sclerosis. *Lancet Neurol*, Vol.10, No.5, (May 2011), pp. 481-90, ISSN: 1474-4465

6

Emerging Concepts Linking Mitochondrial Stress Signalling and Parkinson's Disease

Ana C. Costa, L. Miguel Martins and Samantha H. Y. Loh
Cell Death Regulation Laboratory, MRC Toxicology Unit, Leicester, UK

1. Introduction

Neurodegenerative diseases comprise of a large group of pathologies that affect a considerable number of individuals among the world's population with a higher incidence in elderly people. The most common neurodegenerative diseases, such as Alzheimer's disease (AD) and Parkinson's disease (PD), are characterised by the presence of protein aggregates in different regions of the brain. The causes of these diseases remain undetermined. Nevertheless, new information on this topic is continuously being brought to light.

Mitochondrial dysfunction has been implicated in the pathogenesis of PD. The first evidence for this came from studies using the neurotoxin MPTP (1-methyl-4-phenyl-1,2,3,6-tetrahydropyridine) and the complex I inhibitor rotenone, which cause parkinsonism in animal models, making them a useful system for investigating the mechanisms underlying PD. The subsequent discovery of several gene mutations responsible for causing heritable forms of PD that are directly linked to mitochondria (either genes encoding proteins that are localised to mitochondria (PINK1) or have some role in mitochondrial function (parkin, DJ-1)) provided further insights into the importance of mitochondria in the pathogenesis of PD. More recently, some of the gene products of PARK loci have been found to participate in mitochondrial quality control systems. In this review, we describe, in detail the molecular mechanism of mitochondrial quality control as well as the importance of a mitochondrial unfolded protein response and its possible relevance to the symptoms of PD.

2. Mitochondria: Essential organelles of eukaryotic cells

Mitochondria are cellular organelles with a multitude of functions, ranging from the production of the majority of ATP in the cell, storage of calcium and buffering of its cytosolic concentration to participation in different pathways that influence cellular homeostasis and fate, including cell death cascades.

Mitochondria are two-membrane organelles with an outer membrane facing the cytosol and an inner membrane facing the mitochondrial matrix; the space between the membranes is referred to as the inter-membrane space (IMS). Both the outer and inner membranes are composed of phospholipids and proteins; however, they have different properties. The outer membrane is highly permeable to small molecules due to the presence of porins within its structure, which allows the IMS to maintain approximately the same concentrations of ions and sugars as the cytosol. However, the inner membrane does not exhibit such permeability, thus the passage of molecules to the matrix is highly selective. Most IMS proteins have well-characterised roles in apoptosis following release from the mitochondria into the cytosol, such as cytochrome c, Smac/DIABLO, HtrA2/Omi, and endonuclease G (Endo G) (Radke *et al.*, 2008).

The inner mitochondrial membrane exhibits a particular organisation including several invaginations that form the mitochondrial cristae. This organisation makes the length of the membrane much greater and enables a higher efficiency of energy production. It is in the inner membrane of the mitochondria where the electron transport chain (ETC) is located. The ETC is comprised of five protein complexes and is responsible for the oxidative phosphorylation (OXPHOS) that results in the production of energy in the form of adenosine triphosphate (ATP), which is accompanied by consumption of oxygen and production of water. Complexes I, III and IV pump protons (H^+) into the IMS and create a gradient essential for the generation of ATP by complex V (ATP synthase). This proton gradient is crucial for the normal functioning of mitochondria and is known as the mitochondrial membrane potential ($\Delta\Psi m$). Reactive oxygen species (ROS) are also generated as a by-product of OXPHOS. ROS production can be partially modulated by two cofactors, coenzyme Q_{10} at complex III and cytochrome c at complex IV (Mattson *et al.*, 2008).

The mitochondrial matrix is a sub-compartment with a high protein content. It contains all of the enzymes required for the Krebs cycle, fatty acid oxidation and haeme synthesis and also incorporates several chaperones and proteases involved in the folding and degradation of proteins. In addition, the matrix contains mitochondrial DNA (mtDNA), together with the proteins required for its transcription and translation. Although most mitochondrial proteins (~1500) are encoded by nuclear DNA, thirteen proteins involved in the ETC are mitochondrially encoded (Ryan and Hoogenraad, 2007). This constitutes a challenge for the cell as both nuclear and mitochondrial transcription must be tightly coordinated. Due to its localisation near the ETC, mtDNA is susceptible to oxidative damage, which may result in mutations.

The number of mitochondria is variable according to the tissue and cell type, and it reflects the energetic needs of the cell. For example, neurons and muscle cells have a high mitochondrial content compared to other cell types. The number of mitochondria can be modulated, but these organelles cannot be generated de novo. Mitochondrial biogenesis consists of an increase in the translation of mitochondrial proteins (both nuclearly and mitochondrially encoded); recruitment of these proteins to the mitochondria, which results in mitochondrial enlargement; and finally, division and generation of additional mitochondrion units (Ryan and Hoogenraad, 2007). Within a cell, a mitochondrion cannot be considered as an individual and independent organelle. Mitochondria behave as a network exhibiting successive cycles of fusion (mitochondrion units combining with each other) and fission (separation of mitochondrion units). Mitochondrial dynamics make these organelles more capable of responding to different cellular demands. The proteins responsible for mitochondrial dynamics are relatively well characterised, although new proteins are constantly being identified that play roles in this active process.

Due to the importance of mitochondria for cellular homeostasis, it is obvious that the dysfunction of this organelle may result in severe consequences. Depending on the extent of damage, different signalling pathways will be activated. If the extent of damage is too severe, it might cause dissipation of the mitochondrial membrane potential and release of pro-apoptotic proteins (such as cytochrome c and HtrA2), resulting in cell death.

Mitochondrial dysfunction has long been associated with the natural chronic process of ageing as well as with neurodegenerative diseases, such as AD and PD, and metabolic diseases, such as diabetes. Neurons are particularly sensitive to mitochondrial dysfunction, which probably reflects their high energetic needs and their absolute dependence on mitochondria to obtain most of the ATP required for neuronal function (de Castro *et al.*, 2010). The presence of protein aggregates is also a characteristic of the neurodegenerative diseases PD and AD. The importance of proper protein folding has long been recognised, and the effects of un-/misfolding and aggregation have been linked to many pathological conditions. These aggregates may be cytosolic, such as Lewy bodies in PD and fibrillary tangles in AD, or extracellular, such as amyloid plaques in AD. However, little is known about the effects of unfolded proteins in the mitochondria.

Protein homeostasis is important to maintain cells in a healthy state; therefore, it is essential to prevent the accumulation of proteins in non-native forms. A recent study in the nematode *C. elegans* has shown that in this multicellular animal, a considerable number of proteins aggregate with age (David *et al.*, 2010). These aggregation-prone proteins may also be related to the deregulation of proteostasis in some neurodegenerative diseases. A better understanding of the mechanisms involved in protein misfolding and aggregation will certainly help to explain the causes and/or progression of certain diseases.

3. Concepts of mitochondrial quality control

As mentioned above, oxidative damage is likely to occur in mitochondria (the main ROS source), possibly affecting proteins, lipids and mtDNA. Multiple quality control systems exist to protect mitochondria and ultimately, the cell against damage (Figure 1). Primarily, as part of a molecular quality control system within the organelle, mitochondrial chaperones and proteases play roles in the processes of protein folding, the assembly of protein complexes and the degradation of misfolded or damaged proteins. Second, at the organellar level, there is another mechanism of quality control that depends on the dynamic nature of mitochondrial fusion and fission events (Tatsuta and Langer, 2008). When fusing with healthy mitochondria, damaged mitochondria can recover by sharing essential solutes, metabolites and other components from the healthy partner. However, if the damage is too severe, mitochondria will not undergo fusion but instead will lose their mitochondrial membrane potential and be eliminated by autophagy, a process also known as mitophagy. Finally, under sufficiently severe damage, cellular quality control mechanisms can be activated. In this case, upon the opening of the mitochondrial permeability transition pore (mPTP) and release of pro-apoptotic proteins from the IMS, the cell may undergo apoptosis.

The focus of this review will be on the molecular quality control of mitochondria because both the organellar and cellular aspects of mitochondrial quality control have been extensively reviewed (de Castro *et al.*, 2010, Knott and Bossy-Wetzel, 2008, Tatton *et al.*, 2003).

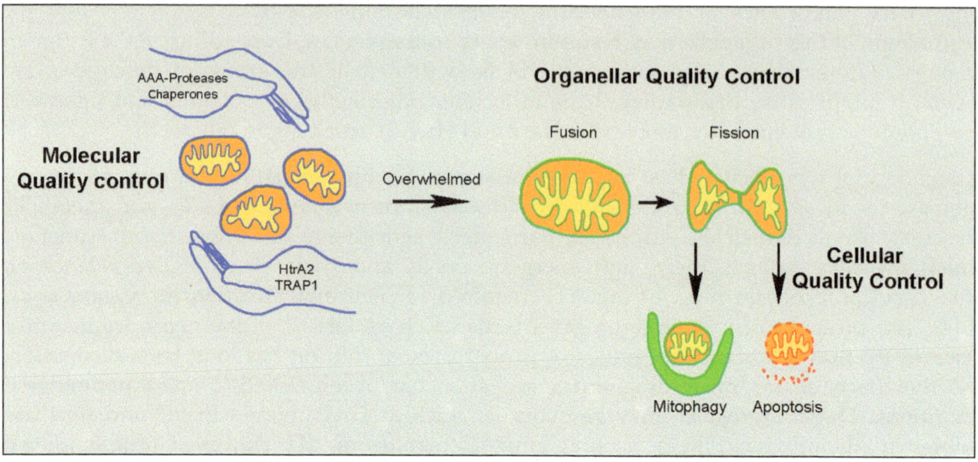

Fig. 1. Mitochondrial Quality Control is assured by different mechanisms and effectors; at the molecular level, it is assured through the protective action of chaperones and proteases, such as molecular chaperones in the mitochondrial matrix, AAA-proteases in the inner membrane, and HtrA2 and TRAP1 in the IMS (drawing highlighted in blue). When this mechanism of defence is not sufficient to maintain fully functional mitochondria, a second level of quality control exists at the organellar level. Fusion with healthy mitochondria might be sufficient to restore the functionality of a mitochondrion. Otherwise, fission might occur, producing small mitochondria that will not fuse again but will be degraded by autophagy (mitophagy) (highlighted in green). If the damage to the mitochondria is too severe, it might lead to the opening of the mitochondrial permeability transition pore (mPTP), releasing pro-apoptotic proteins into the cytosol, such as cytochrome c and HtrA2, resulting in the activation of apoptosis (drawing highlighted in red).

3.1 Effectors of molecular quality control: Chaperones and proteases

Molecular chaperones play critical roles in the maintenance of protein homeostasis by aiding in the folding of newly synthesised and/or imported proteins, the assembly of multimeric protein complexes, protein translocation across membranes and protein degradation. In addition, molecular chaperones are essential for cellular signalling. In eukaryotes, chaperones are segregated to specific places, such as the cytosol, endoplasmic reticulum (ER) and mitochondria. The mechanisms through which the levels of chaperones are modulated have not been well studied. Nevertheless, it is known that signalling pathways activating chaperone-encoding genes are repressed by free chaperones that are not engaged by client proteins (Yoneda *et al.*, 2004). In contrast, if the levels of client proteins are too high, the availability of free chaperones can be dramatically decreased, and the repressor effect will not occur, possibly resulting in increased transcription of chaperones.

The mitochondrial chaperones and proteases are essential components of the mitochondrial quality control mechanism because they selectively remove unfolded or misfolded proteins, avoiding their deleterious accumulation. A failure in molecular quality control is emerging as a feature of neurodegenerative diseases, such as PD.

3.1.1 AAA protease chaperones

ATP-dependent proteases are present in the mitochondrial matrix as well as in the inner membrane. The AAA+ (ATPases associated with various cellular activities) superfamily of peptidases is able to eliminate misfolded proteins from the mitochondria and plays a regulatory role during mitochondrial biogenesis by processing proteins. Mammalian inner mitochondrial membranes possess hetero- and homo-oligomeric *m*-AAA and homo-oligomeric *i*-AAA protease complexes. The *m*-AAA protease presents its catalytic site on the mitochondrial matrix, while the *i*-AAA protease catalytic site is directed to the IMS. The homo-oligomeric complexes are composed of AFG3L2 subunits, while the hetero-oligomeric are composed of paraplegin and AFG3L2 subunits. Mutations in these proteases have been implicated in neurodegenerative conditions; mutations in the paraplegin subunit cause hereditary spastic paraplegia which is characterised by cell-specific axonal degeneration, and mutations in *AFG3L2* lead to a dominant heritable form of spinocerebellar ataxia (Lee *et al.*, 2011). Furthermore, a mutation in the mitochondrial chaperone Hsp60 has also been identified in hereditary spastic paraplegia. The mitochondrial matrix chaperone Hsp60 mediates ATP-dependent folding of a wide variety of proteins, making it an important player in the molecular mitochondrial quality control system.

3.1.2 PINK1, HtrA2 and TRAP1

The mitochondrial protein PTEN-induced putative kinase 1 (PINK1) plays important roles in mitochondrial quality control. It participates in molecular quality control through interactions with high-temperature-requirement protein A2 (HtrA2) and possibly TNF receptor–associated protein 1 (TRAP1) and at the organellar level via its activity in a signalling pathway involving parkin and mitophagy. The *PINK1* and *PARK13* (HtrA2) genes have been found to be associated with PD. Mutations in *PINK1* cause an autosomal recessive form of the disease, which can be characterised by early onset (Valente *et al.*, 2004). Additionally, mutations in the HtrA2 gene have been found in sporadic PD patients, and HtrA2 protein has been detected in Lewy bodies (Strauss *et al.*, 2005). Furthermore, an increase in phosphorylated HtrA2 in brain tissues of sporadic PD patients and, conversely, reduced phosphorylation in PD patients with *PINK1* mutations have also been reported (Plun-Favreau *et al.*, 2007).

3.1.2.1 HtrA2

HtrA2 (also known as Omi) was first identified as a mammalian homologue of the bacterial endoprotease HtrA (high temperature requirement A). In bacteria, HtrA acts as a chaperone at normal temperatures and as a protease at high temperatures and removes damaged or denatured proteins from the periplasm (Faccio *et al.*, 2000). HtrA2 is a serine protease with an amino-terminal inhibitor of apoptosis (IAP) domain identical to those in the *Drosophila* protein Reaper. It is localised in the IMS, and following certain stimuli, it is released into the cytosol, where it binds to IAPs, inhibiting their effects and promoting apoptosis. In addition to its caspase-dependent action, HtrA2 promotes cell death in a caspase-independent manner through increased proteolytic activity (Martins *et al.*, 2003). HtrA2 was initially thought to be a pro-apoptotic protein homologous to Reaper. However, the observation that HtrA2-mutant mice present an extremely shortened lifespan (~30 days) and a neurological phenotype with parkinsonian features has promoted a different view of the role of this protein (Martins *et al.*, 2004).

The phosphorylation state of HtrA2 influences its proteolytic activity and is dependent on PINK1 (Plun-Favreau *et al.*, 2007). PINK1 and HtrA2 interact with each other, although it is not clear whether PINK1 phosphorylates HtrA2. Nevertheless, phosphorylation of HtrA2 occurs upon p38 MAPK activation and requires PINK1. It appears that p38, PINK1 and HtrA2 are components of a stress-sensing pathway and that phosphorylation of HtrA2 increases its proteolytic activity and enhances its cell-protective effects. The observation that higher levels of phosphorylated HtrA2 are present in the brains of sporadic PD patients has led to the hypothesis that this stress-sensing pathway is activated in PD. However, the precise stimulus that originates the stress is not known. Interestingly, in brains from PD patients with *PINK1* mutations, the levels of phosphorylated HtrA2 are reduced, emphasising the importance of PINK1 for HtrA2 phosphorylation. This reduced HtrA2 phosphorylation might account for the pathogenic effects of PD-linked *PINK1* mutations. Thus, HtrA2 appears to be part of a quality control pathway, acting downstream of PINK1.

HtrA2 knockout (KO) mice show accumulation of unfolded proteins in the mitochondria as well as a defect in respiration. Loss of HtrA2 augments ROS levels, and treatment with anti-oxidants is neuroprotective in this condition. The up-regulation of the transcription factor C/EBP homology protein (CHOP) specifically in the brain of the HtrA2 KO mice indicates activation of the integrated stress response. Enhanced levels of CHOP have also been detected in brain tissue of idiopathic PD patients (Moisoi *et al.*, 2009). This increased level of CHOP specifically in the brain may account for the neuronal loss observed in this mouse model. However, the observation that CHOP is also up-regulated in regions of the brain that do not undergo neuronal death indicates that CHOP up-regulation is an early event that precedes neuronal loss.

HtrA2 also interacts with both intracellular amyloid β (Aβ) and the C-terminal tail of presenilins, although the functional significance of these interactions is obscure (Gupta *et al.*, 2004, Park *et al.*, 2004). More recently, HtrA2 has been linked to amyloid precursor protein (APP) metabolism (Huttunen *et al.*, 2007). A small percentage of HtrA2 localises alongside ER membranes and binds to immature APP *in vitro*. Finally, in HtrA2$^{-/-}$ cells, APP is stabilised, and Aβ production is increased. These observations further suggest that HtrA2 has a protective effect and functions in protein homeostasis.

3.1.2.2 TRAP1

Another piece of evidence relating PINK1 to mitochondrial molecular quality control comes from an *in vitro* study that revealed a physical interaction between PINK1 and the mitochondrial chaperone TRAP1 (Hsp75) (Pridgeon *et al.*, 2007). PINK1 phosphorylates TRAP1 (also located in the IMS), and this protects the cell against apoptosis induced by H_2O_2 treatment. Notably, the PINK1-dependent phosphorylation of TRAP1 inhibits the release of cytochrome c from mitochondria and thereby increases cell survival under certain stress conditions (Pridgeon *et al.*, 2007). TRAP1 may therefore be another downstream effector of PINK1 involved in the molecular mitochondrial quality control pathway. TRAP1 is structurally related to the HSP90 family, possesses an ATP-binding domain and shows ATPase activity *in vitro*. TRAP1 activity can be inhibited by the Hsp90 inhibitors radicicol and geldanamycin. Nevertheless, TRAP1 does not form complexes with the classic co-chaperones of Hsp90 and might have distinct functions from the other members of the HSP90 family (Felts *et al.*, 2000). In addition, TRAP1 exerts a protective effect against apoptosis when cells are subjected to various apoptotic stimuli (Hua *et al.*, 2007, Masuda *et al.*, 2004). Moreover, high levels of TRAP1 protein may be involved in drug resistance in certain cancer treatments (Costantino *et al.*, 2009, Landriscina *et al.*, 2010). More detailed studies are necessary to better understand the roles of TRAP1 in mitochondrial quality control and possibly in other signalling pathways.

It is clear that maintenance of proteostasis is crucial for the health of the cell, and it is logical to hypothesise that regulation of quality control mechanisms must be of great importance when an insult occurs. As mentioned above, the various sub-compartments of the cell exhibit different subsets of chaperones and proteases that have location-specific functions. Accordingly, depending on the insult and the organelles affected, different stress responses might be activated.

3.2 A mitochondrial unfolded protein response (UPR^{mt}) with its origin in the mitochondrial matrix

The concept of anterograde communication between the nucleus and mitochondria is well established; however, the communication process from the mitochondria to the cytosol and nucleus, so-called retrograde signalling, remains unclear. The main problem in understanding this process lies in identification of the molecules responsible for the initiation of the signal in the mitochondria and determination of how this signal is transmitted to the nucleus to alter nuclear gene expression. The mitochondrial retrograde signalling pathway is associated with both normal and pathophysiological conditions. This retrograde signalling pathway exists in simple organisms, such as yeast, where it has primarily been studied, and in multicellular organisms. Despite the fact that this signalling pathway is conserved, the proteins and molecular mechanisms involved do not seem to be.

Compartment specificity in signalling by chaperones has been demonstrated for the ER, the cytoplasm and the mitochondrial matrix. These compartment-specific signals are responses to the presence of unfolded proteins in each of these compartments. Following the accumulation of unfolded proteins in the cytosol, heat shock–sensitive transcription factors (HSFs) are activated and increase the transcription of proteins involved in adaptation to this stress, a process known as the heat-shock response (HSR). The signal derived from an excess of unfolded proteins in the ER, on the other hand, is sensed by the lumenal domains of transmembrane proteins and is propagated through their cytoplasmic domains, ultimately leading to the transcription of nuclear genes encoding proteins that alleviate the stress in the ER (e.g., the ER chaperone BiP). This process is known as the unfolded protein response of the ER (UPR^{ER}) (Benedetti *et al.*, 2006).

The stress responses can also be induced by drug treatments. For example, treatment of cells with arsenite, which results in the accumulation of unfolded proteins in the cytoplasm, selectively activates cytoplasmic chaperone gene expression. On the other hand, treatment of cells with tunicamycin, which blocks ER-specific N-linked glycosylation, activates the UPR^{ER}, resulting in increased expression of ER-localised chaperones (Yoneda *et al.*, 2004).

Remarkably, little is known about the specific stress response resulting from the accumulation of unfolded proteins in the mitochondria, despite the fact that many different model systems have been used to study it. Here, we describe recent findings achieved in *C. elegans* and, to a lesser extent, mammalian model systems in detail.

3.2.1 *C. elegans*

The nematode *C. elegans* has been extensively used to study the UPR^{mt}. The ability to use sensitive reporter genes as well as the ease of genetically manipulating these worms makes them convenient models to address this issue. The existence of a UPR^{mt} in *C. elegans* became evident after it was observed that provoking stress in the mitochondrial matrix, either by reduction of mtDNA through treatment with ethidium bromide or down-regulation of mitochondrial chaperones or proteases (*spg-7*), resulted in transcriptional up-regulation of the mitochondrial chaperones *hsp-6* (the *C. elegans* orthologue of human mtHsp70) and *hsp-60* (Yoneda *et al.*, 2004). Up-regulation is a specific response for these stress modulator molecules, as the cytosolic or ER chaperones are not up-regulated nor are other mitochondrial enzymes. Further studies using RNAi library screening led to the discovery of several genes required for UPR^{mt} signalling (Figure 2).

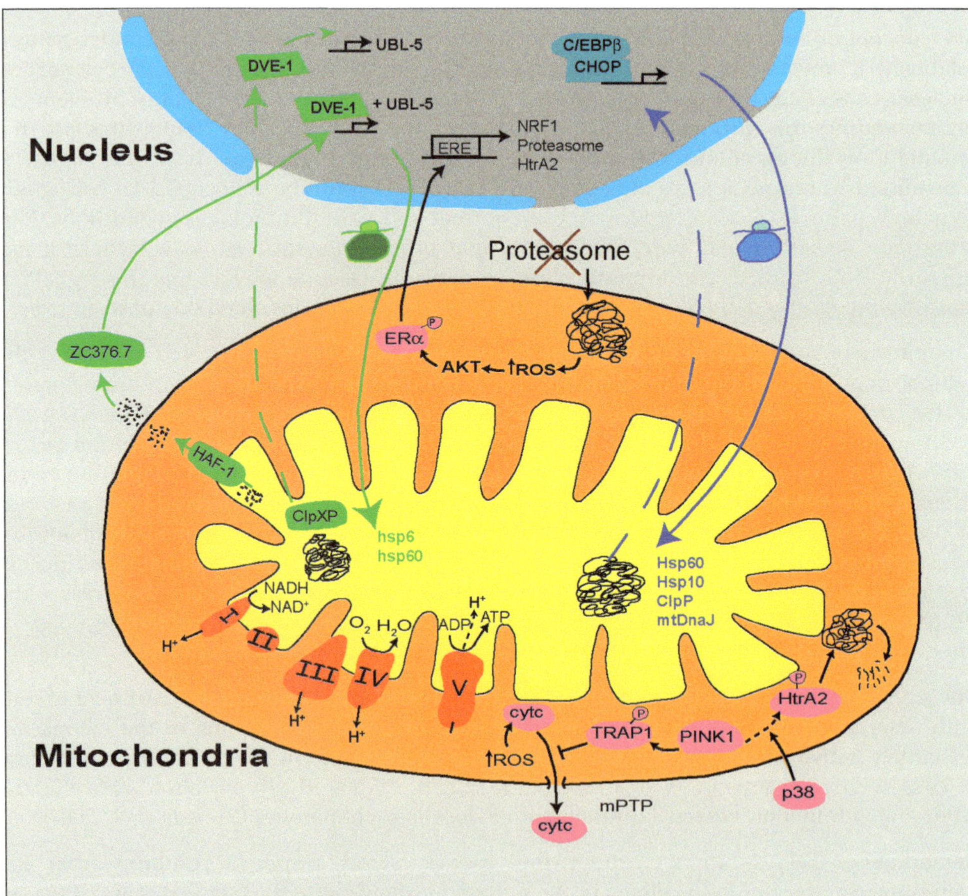

Fig. 2. Mitochondrial stress signalling

Key components of the molecular quality control machinery and mitochondrial unfolded protein response (UPR^{mt}) are represented here. Communication between mitochondria and the nucleus is tightly regulated. Retrograde signalling transmits information from the mitochondria to the nucleus (dashed lines), whereas anterograde signalling transmits information in the opposite direction (solid lines). The mechanism of UPR^{mt} activation in the nematode *C. elegans* is highlighted in green on the left. In *C. elegans*, the accumulation of unfolded proteins in the mitochondrial matrix may be sensed by the ClpXP complex, which might generate a signal leading to certain nuclear events. The nature of this signal remains elusive, although ClpXP activity is known to result in the formation of small peptides that are actively extruded to the IMS through the peptide transporter HAF-1. Once in the IMS, the peptides can be released to the cytosol and activate a receptor or other effector molecules. The bZIP transcription factor ZC3376.7 is activated by this peptide efflux from mitochondria and translocates to the nucleus, where it up-regulates UPR^{mt}-responsive genes. Nuclear events occur on UPR^{mt} include the transcriptional up-regulation of ubl-5 and redistribution of DVE-1 in the nucleus. While both events are downstream of ClpXP, only *ubl-5* transcription activation is downstream of HAF-1. This UPR^{mt} activation results in increased levels of both hsp60 and hsp6 mitochondrial chaperones. The mechanism of UPR^{mt} activation in mammalian cells is highlighted in blue on the right. The presence of excess unfolded proteins in the mitochondrial matrix promotes transcriptional up-regulation of Chop and formation of a complex between the transcription factor CHOP and C/EBPβ in the nucleus, resulting in transcriptional activation of mitochondrial stress responsive genes, such as Hsp60, Hsp10, ClpP and mtDnaJ and increased levels of their encoded proteins in the mitochondria. HtrA2 is located in the IMS and is part of the protein quality control machinery. The proteolytic activity of HtrA2 is phosphorylation-dependent, requires the presence of PINK1 and is mediated through p38 pathway activation. The molecular chaperone TRAP1 is also located in the IMS and might be responsible for the proper folding and assembly of other proteins or complexes. TRAP1 also has a cytoprotective effect in inhibiting the release of cytochrome c when there is an increase level of ROS in mitochondrial. The unfolded protein response of the IMS is represented in the upper middle part of the mitochondria in the figure. This stress response can be activated on accumulation of aggregates of misfolded proteins in the IMS, which can be a result of failure of the proteasome, or due to failure of the molecular quality control in this compartment. The presence of protein aggregates leads to overproduction of ROS, activation of AKT and phosphorylation of the Estrogen Receptor α (ERα). Activation of ERα receptor results in transcription of genes, such as transcription factor NRF1, proteasome and HtrA2.

Ubiquitin-like protein 5 (UBL-5) is essential for UPR^{mt} activation, although its down-regulation does not result in the accumulation of misfolded proteins in the mitochondria, suggesting that it must act downstream of this event. Moreover, upon mitochondrial stress, *ubl-5* is transcriptionally up-regulated, and its protein levels are increased in the nucleus (Benedetti *et al.*, 2006). This might be a feed-forward mechanism to amplify the stress response. It is of note that UBL-5 mRNA levels are reasonably high in mitochondrion-rich human tissues, such as heart, skeletal muscle, liver, and kidney, and that polymorphisms in UBL-5 have been linked to obesity and diabetes (Benedetti *et al.*, 2006).

dve-1 is another gene involved in the UPR^{mt} (Haynes *et al.*, 2007). The DVE-1 protein is a putative transcription factor that is localised to the nucleus and possesses a predicted homeobox-related DNA-binding domain. Under mitochondrial stress, DVE-1 exhibits an altered nuclear distribution (punctate) and binds to the promoters of the mitochondrial chaperone genes *hsp-6* and *hsp-60*. Furthermore, in stressed worms, DVE-1 forms a complex with UBL-5. Interestingly, UBL-5 is also able to form a complex with the mammalian orthologue of DVE-1, SATB2, but the relevance of the formation of this complex in the UPR^{mt} in mammalian cells is unknown (Haynes *et al.*, 2007).

CLPP-1 is also essential for UPR^{mt} signalling. CLPP-1, the *C. elegans* orthologue of the bacterial ClpP protease, is localised to the mitochondrial matrix. ClpP is the ATP-dependent proteolytic subunit (with a cylindrical shape) of a heteromeric complex formed with a partner AAA+ ATPase (Ortega *et al.*, 2004). Bacterial ClpP functions in conjunction with two partner chaperones, ClpX and ClpA, associated with a wide range of substrates. Moreover, an increase in the levels of misfolded proteins enhances the degradation of these substrates. ClpX is the only ClpP partner known in eukaryotes, and to date, the substrates of mitochondrial ClpP remain unknown. In *C. elegans*, CLPP-1 is necessary for DVE-1 activation. Silencing of CLPP-1 by RNAi prevents the redistribution of DVE-1 in the nucleus and the transcriptional up-regulation of UBL-5, suggesting an upstream action of CLPP-1 in the activation of the UPR^{mt}. Once CLPP-1 is localised to the mitochondria, it is likely that it senses the mitochondrial perturbation and mediates the proteolysis signal that is sent to the nucleus. Interestingly, CLPP-1-dependent proteolysis is required for the UPR^{mt} as an inhibitor of CLPP-1 proteolytic activity abolishes its effect in activating the stress response (Haynes *et al.*, 2007). ClpX is also relevant for UPR^{mt} signalling in *C. elegans*. There are two isoforms of *ClpX* genes in *C. elegans*, both of which encode proteins homologous to bacterial ClpX, and when both genes are silenced, the UPR^{mt} is attenuated. It appears that the function of ClpX in the worm is comparable to that in bacteria and mammals (Haynes *et al.*, 2010). In bacteria, ClpP breaks down proteins into small peptides. Furthermore, studies in yeast have shown that mitochondrial peptides can be extruded to the IMS and subsequently to the cytosol.

The mitochondrial transporter responsible for the extrusion of peptides from the mitochondrial matrix in yeast is Mdl1p. Interestingly, there are multiple orthologues of Mdl1p in *C. elegans*, and the most evolutionarily conserved of these, HAF-1, plays a role in UPR^{mt} signalling as deletion mutations in the *haf-1* gene cause an impairment of this response. Additionally, HAF-1 seems to be located in the inner mitochondrial membrane, which is consistent with its function in transporting cargo from the matrix to the IMS (Haynes *et al.*, 2010). Epistasis analysis has placed HAF-1 upstream of *ubl-5* transcriptional induction, but not of DVE-1 redistribution in the nucleus, which suggests the existence of other transcription factors involved in the UPR^{mt}.

Subsequently, the protein ZC376.7, which includes a C-terminal leucine zipper domain, a predicted nuclear localisation sequence, and a nuclear export sequence, was identified. In unstressed worms, ZC376.7 is localised diffusely in the cytosol, but following mitochondrial stress, it is translocated to the nucleus. ZC376.7 appears to act downstream of HAF-1 and CLPP-1 because the nuclear localisation of this transcription factor in stressed worms is attenuated by down-regulation of both HAF-1 and CLPP-1 (Haynes *et al.*, 2010). Further studies will be required to better understand this signalling mechanism. It is still unclear how small peptides can activate UPR^{mt} signalling and influence the subcellular distribution of ZC376.7. Is there a cytoplasmic receptor for these small peptides? Is the nature of the peptides important, or rather, is the rate of efflux the most important feature? It is also of particular interest to determine the downstream effectors that influence DVE-1 function. Many questions remain unanswered, although knowledge on this topic is progressively increasing.

Interestingly, a recent study using *C. elegans* as a model system demonstrated that the UPR^{mt} can be activated in a cell-non-autonomous manner (Durieux *et al.*, 2011). Mitochondrial stress caused by down-regulation of a component of the ETC in the nervous system results in activation of the UPR^{mt} in the intestine of the animal. However, it appears that UBL-5 is not required for UPR^{mt} activation in this cell-non-autonomous manner. It is still not known which signal is transmitted from the nervous system to the periphery, and additional research will be required to address these questions further (Figure 3).

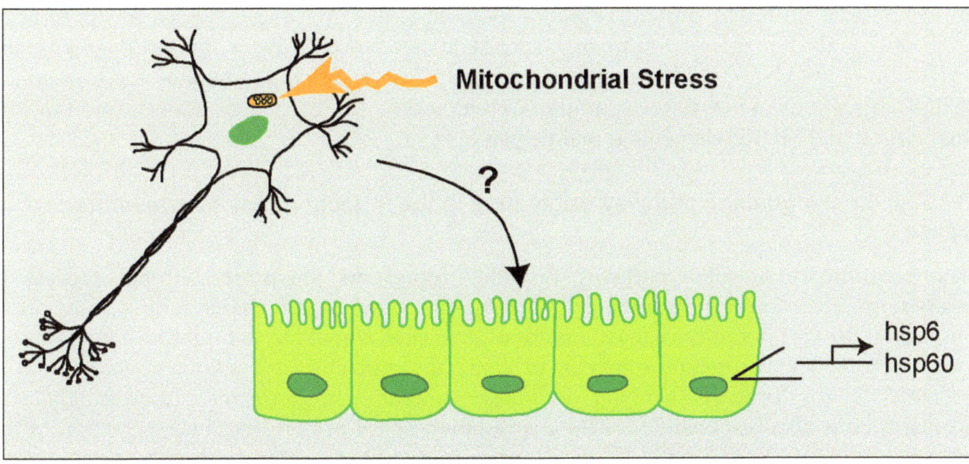

Fig. 3. Cell-non-autonomous activation of the UPR^{mt} in *C. elegans*.

Generation of mitochondrial stress in the central nervous system by depletion of an ETC protein subunit results in the activation of the UPR^{mt} in distant tissues, such as the worm intestine (transcriptional up-regulation of *hsp6* and *hsp60* in intestinal cells). The nature of the signal transmitted from the brain to the intestine is presently unknown.

3.2.2 Mammalian cells

Work by Zhao and colleagues brought to light the existence of an UPR^{mt} (Zhao *et al.*, 2002). The expression of a truncated form of the mitochondrial matrix protein ornithine transcarbamylase (ΔOTC), which accumulates in an insoluble state in the matrix, results in the activation of nuclear genes encoding mitochondrial stress proteins. Upon accumulation of ΔOTC in mitochondria, the mitochondrial chaperones Hsp60, Hsp10, and mtDnaJ as well as the protease ClpP are up-regulated. In mammalian cells, mtHsp70 is not up-regulated by ΔOTC accumulation, which is consistent with its function as a protein transporter across membranes, rather than a stress-sensing molecule. The transcription factors CHOP and CCAAT/enhancer-binding protein β (C/EBPβ) form a hetero-dimer and participate in this mitochondrial stress response by binding to the promoters of UPR^{mt}-responsive genes.

Furthermore, CHOP protein levels are increased by ΔOTC accumulation, indicating that *Chop* itself is a UPR^{mt}-responsive gene.

Subsequently, an AP-1 element, which is essential for CHOP function in the UPR^{mt}, was identified within the *Chop* promoter. Interestingly, C/EBPβ (but not C/EBPα) also contains an AP-1 site. Because c-Jun binds to AP-1 sites, the effect of a MEK inhibitor on the phosphorylation state of JNK upon UPR^{mt} induction was tested, and the results suggest that the MEK/JNK2 pathway could play a role in UPR^{mt} signalling (Horibe and Hoogenraad, 2007).

Six novel UPR^{mt}-responsive genes, encoding the mitochondrial proteases YME1L1 and MPPβ, the import component Tim17A, and the enzymes NDUFB2, Endo G and thioredoxin 2, have recently been identified (Aldridge *et al.*, 2007). In addition to the CHOP recognition element, these genes contain two other conserved elements in their promoters: mitochondrial unfolded protein response element (MURE) 1 and 2, which are present in nine out of the ten genes found to be up-regulated specifically in the UPR^{mt}, with the exception of the Hsp60/10 bidirectional promoter. The transcription factors that bind to the CHOP element are known (for example, CHOP and C/EBPβ), but the transcription factors that bind to the MURE elements remain elusive.

3.3 A distinct signalling pathway originating in the mitochondrial inter-membrane space

The ubiquitin-proteasome pathway probably represents the most common process of protein quality control within the cell. Conjugation of ubiquitin chains with a substrate is important for various physiological functions, from cell signalling to targeting substrates for degradation. The proteasome exists in both the nucleus and the cytoplasm and is responsible for protein turnover in these cellular compartments. Interestingly, the proteasome is also responsible for the degradation of ER proteins because a fraction of the proteasome is associated with ER membranes (Kalies *et al.*, 2005). In the ER, misfolded or damaged proteins are recognised by chaperones, such as BiP, and transported to the cytosol, where the proteasome degrades them. Inhibition of proteasome activity results in accumulation of misfolded proteins in the ER.

Similarly, inhibition of the proteasome also results in accumulation of unfolded proteins in the IMS (Radke *et al.*, 2008). Inhibition of either Hsp90 or the proteasome causes proteins to accumulate in the mitochondria (Margineantu *et al.*, 2007).

Endo G is an IMS protein that accumulates in the IMS following proteasome inhibition (Radke *et al.*, 2008). Overexpression experiments using either wild-type or a mutant form of Endo G have shown that both forms are substrates for ubiquitination, although the mutant form is ubiquitinated at a much higher level. The mitochondrial targeting signal is not required for conjugation with ubiquitin. These observations are consistent with the existence of a protein quality control system in the cytoplasm prior to the import of proteins to the mitochondria. Further analyses have shown that upon proteasome inhibition, wild-type Endo G is cleaved by HtrA2, while the mutant forms of the protein are not. Elimination of mutant Endo G appears to depend on the proteasome pathway.

A defect in proteasome activity may cause the accumulation of mitochondrial proteins and deregulate their activity. HtrA2 seems to be part of a second checkpoint following the action of the proteasome in the cytosol (Radke *et al.*, 2008). Consistent with this, mutations in HtrA2 may impair its function and lead to unwanted accumulation of its putative substrates. Furthermore, mutant forms of IMS proteins are resistant to HtrA2 degradation, and this could augment their deleterious effect and result in mitochondrial collapse.

The consequences of unfolded protein accumulation in the IMS have not been explored, although a recent study by Papa and Germain showed that upon IMS stress, a distinct protective pathway is activated (Papa and Germain, 2011). Overexpression of a mutant form of the protein Endo G results in the formation of aggregates in the IMS and mitochondrial stress. Under these conditions, HtrA2 and proteasome components increase in an oestrogen receptor α (ERα)-dependent manner. Accumulation of mutant Endo G does not result in the up-regulation of CHOP or Endo G, in contrast to what is observed during the UPR^{mt}. Endo G accumulation also does not cause increased expression of BiP or BIM, which is a characteristic feature of the UPR^{ER}. Using a luciferase reporter with oestrogen-responsive elements (EREs), it has been observed that the accumulation of various IMS proteins activates ERE-containing genes. Additionally, the activation of EREs depends on ERα phosphorylation and not ERβ. ERα appears to be phosphorylated by AKT, which in turn is activated by ROS. ROS overproduction has been reported following mutant Endo G overexpression and is inhibited by the anti-oxidant *N*-acetylcysteine (NAC), suppressing the activation of the ERE reporter. Nuclear respiratory factor 1 (NRF1) is a transcription factor that activates the expression of genes involved in mitochondrial respiration and can be induced by ER activation. IMS stress results in enhanced *NRF1* transcription. Furthermore, increased levels of HtrA2 have been detected following IMS stress induction, as have increases in proteasome activity.

4. Conclusions

Neurodegenerative diseases include a vast number of pathologies, all of which involve the progressive degeneration of neurons. Many of these diseases are directly linked to the ageing process, such as AD and PD (meaning that age is the main, but not the sole, risk factor). The underlying mechanisms associated with the neurodegeneration remain undetermined. A better understanding of the causes and mechanisms involved in these diseases is essential to develop efficient treatments that not only attenuate their symptoms but also alter and possibly reverse disease progression.

Both mitochondrial dysfunction and protein aggregation have been implicated in PD. However, little is known about protein aggregation in the mitochondria and its possible links to PD. Mitochondria are essential organelles in the eukaryotic cell with a variety of functions, including energy production in the form of ATP. Maintenance of a functional ETC in the inner mitochondrial membrane is of extreme importance because dysfunction could considerably increase the generation of ROS, causing damage to different components of the organelle and subsequently the cell.

The majority of mitochondrial proteins are produced in the cytosol and imported to the organelle as precursors. To cross the mitochondrial membranes, these precursors need to be in an unfolded state and need to bind to membrane transporters to reach the mitochondrial matrix. Mitochondrial chaperones are therefore extremely important in assisting in the folding of the newly imported proteins as well as that of newly synthesised proteins in the matrix.

Through evolution, mitochondria have gained defence mechanisms against damage. Different lines of defence, termed molecular, organellar and cellular quality control, can be successively activated to respond to such damage. In this review, we focused on the molecular mechanisms of mitochondrial quality control, which rely on the actions of chaperones and proteases to maintain a healthy pool of mitochondria. Failure of this molecular quality control has been linked to neurodegeneration; it appears that many of the proteins involved in this aspect of mitochondrial quality control are associated with PD. For example, both PINK1 and HtrA2 have been linked to PD. PINK1 and HtrA2 are part of a stress-sensing pathway in which PINK1 facilitates HtrA2 phosphorylation, increasing its proteolytic activity and subsequently its protective effect (through a mechanism that is not clearly understood). Additionally, PINK1 acts upstream of the chaperone TRAP1, which might also be involved in mitochondrial quality control as its protective effect against various apoptotic stimuli has been well documented.

The discovery of an UPR^{mt} is also extremely interesting, and revealing the components and mechanisms involved in this stress response may shed light on new strategies for disease treatments.

Up-regulation of chaperones has been proposed for the treatment of a number of pathologies, but the results have not always been satisfactory. For example, up-regulation of Hsp70 can ameliorate some conditions and increase lifespan in animal models, but it also increases tumour development. Understanding the roles of mitochondrial stress modulators is therefore essential for the identification of putative targets for drug treatments.

5. References

Aldridge JE, *et al.* (2007) Discovery of genes activated by the mitochondrial unfolded protein response (mtUPR) and cognate promoter elements. *PLoS One*, Vol. 2, No. 9; (9): pp. e874.

Benedetti C, *et al.* (2006) Ubiquitin-like protein 5 positively regulates chaperone gene expression in the mitochondrial unfolded protein response. *Genetics*, Vol. 174, No. 1 Sep; (1): pp. 229-239.

Costantino E, *et al.* (2009) TRAP1, a novel mitochondrial chaperone responsible for multi-drug resistance and protection from apoptotis in human colorectal carcinoma cells. *Cancer Lett*, Vol. 279, No. 1, Jun 28; (1): pp. 39-46.

David DC, *et al.* (2010) Widespread protein aggregation as an inherent part of aging in C. elegans. *PLoS Biol*, Vol. 8, No. 8; (8): pp. e1000450.

de Castro IP, *et al.* (2010) Mitochondrial quality control and neurological disease: an emerging connection. *Expert Rev Mol Med*, Vol. 12: pp. e12.

Durieux J, *et al.* (2011) The cell-non-autonomous nature of electron transport chain-mediated longevity. *Cell*, Vol. 144, No. 1, Jan 7; (1): pp. 79-91.

Faccio L, *et al.* (2000) Characterization of a novel human serine protease that has extensive homology to bacterial heat shock endoprotease HtrA and is regulated by kidney ischemia. *J Biol Chem*, Vol. 275, No. 4, Jan 28; (4): pp. 2581-2588.

Felts SJ, *et al.* (2000) The hsp90-related protein TRAP1 is a mitochondrial protein with distinct functional properties. *J Biol Chem*, Vol. 275, No. 5, Feb 4; (5): pp. 3305-3312.

Gupta S, *et al.* (2004) The C-terminal tail of presenilin regulates Omi/HtrA2 protease activity. *J Biol Chem*, Vol. 279, No. 44, Oct 29; (44): pp. 45844-45854.

Haynes CM, *et al.* (2007) ClpP mediates activation of a mitochondrial unfolded protein response in C. elegans. *Dev Cell*, Vol. 13, No. 4, Oct; (4): pp. 467-480.

Haynes CM, *et al.* (2010) The matrix peptide exporter HAF-1 signals a mitochondrial UPR by activating the transcription factor ZC376.7 in C. elegans. *Mol Cell*, Vol. 37, No. 4, Feb 26; (4): pp. 529-540.

Horibe T, Hoogenraad NJ. (2007) The chop gene contains an element for the positive regulation of the mitochondrial unfolded protein response. *PLoS One*, Vol. 2, No. 9; (9): pp. e835.

Hua G, *et al.* (2007) Heat shock protein 75 (TRAP1) antagonizes reactive oxygen species generation and protects cells from granzyme M-mediated apoptosis. *J Biol Chem*, Vol. 282, No. 28, Jul 13; (28): pp. 20553-20560.

Huttunen HJ, *et al.* (2007) HtrA2 regulates beta-amyloid precursor protein (APP) metabolism through endoplasmic reticulum-associated degradation. *J Biol Chem*, Vol. 282, No. 38, Sep 21; (38): pp. 28285-28295.

Kalies KU, *et al.* (2005) The protein translocation channel binds proteasomes to the endoplasmic reticulum membrane. *EMBO J*, Vol. 24, No. 13, Jul 6; (13): pp. 2284-2293.

Knott AB, Bossy-Wetzel E. (2008) Impairing the mitochondrial fission and fusion balance: a new mechanism of neurodegeneration. *Ann N Y Acad Sci*, Vol. 1147, Dec: pp. 283-292.

Landriscina M, *et al.* (2010) Mitochondrial chaperone Trap1 and the calcium binding protein Sorcin interact and protect cells against apoptosis induced by antiblastic agents. *Cancer Res*, Vol. 70, No. 16, Aug 15; (16): pp. 6577-6586.

Lee S, *et al.* (2011) Electron cryomicroscopy structure of a membrane-anchored mitochondrial AAA protease. *J Biol Chem*, Vol. 286, No. 6, Feb 11; (6): pp. 4404-4411.

Margineantu DH, *et al.* (2007) Hsp90 inhibition decreases mitochondrial protein turnover. *PLoS One*, Vol. 2, No. 10; (10): pp. e1066.

Martins LM, *et al.* (2003) Binding specificity and regulation of the serine protease and PDZ domains of HtrA2/Omi. *J Biol Chem*, Vol. 278, No. 49, Dec 5; (49): pp. 49417-49427.

Martins LM, *et al.* (2004) Neuroprotective role of the Reaper-related serine protease HtrA2/Omi revealed by targeted deletion in mice. *Mol Cell Biol*, Vol. 24, No. 22, Nov; (22): pp. 9848-9862.

Masuda Y, *et al.* (2004) Involvement of tumor necrosis factor receptor-associated protein 1 (TRAP1) in apoptosis induced by beta-hydroxyisovalerylshikonin. *J Biol Chem*, Vol. 279, No. 41, Oct 8; (41): pp. 42503-42515.

Mattson MP, *et al.* (2008) Mitochondria in neuroplasticity and neurological disorders. *Neuron*, Vol. 60, No. 5, Dec 10; (5): pp. 748-766.

Moisoi N, *et al.* (2009) Mitochondrial dysfunction triggered by loss of HtrA2 results in the activation of a brain-specific transcriptional stress response. *Cell Death Differ*, Vol. 16, No. 3, Mar; (3): pp. 449-464.

Ortega J, *et al.* (2004) ClpA and ClpX ATPases bind simultaneously to opposite ends of ClpP peptidase to form active hybrid complexes. *J Struct Biol*, Vol. 146, No. 1-2, Apr-May; (1-2): pp. 217-226.

Papa L, Germain D. (2011) Estrogen receptor mediates a distinct mitochondrial unfolded protein response. *J Cell Sci*, Vol. 124, No. 9, May 1; (9):pp.1396-1402.

Park HJ, *et al.* (2004) Alzheimer's disease-associated amyloid beta interacts with the human serine protease HtrA2/Omi. *Neurosci Lett*, Vol. 357, No. 1, Feb 26; (1): pp. 63-67.

Plun-Favreau H, *et al.* (2007) The mitochondrial protease HtrA2 is regulated by Parkinson's disease-associated kinase PINK1. *Nat Cell Biol*, Vol. 9, No. 11, Nov; (11): pp. 1243-1252.

Pridgeon JW, *et al.* (2007) PINK1 protects against oxidative stress by phosphorylating mitochondrial chaperone TRAP1. *PLoS Biol*, Vol. 5, No. 7, Jul; (7): pp. e172.

Radke S, *et al.* (2008) Mitochondrial protein quality control by the proteasome involves ubiquitination and the protease Omi. *J Biol Chem*, Vol. 283, No. 19, May 9; (19): pp. 12681-12685.

Ryan MT, Hoogenraad NJ. (2007) Mitochondrial-nuclear communications. *Annu Rev Biochem*, Vol. 76: pp. 701-722.

Strauss KM, *et al.* (2005) Loss of function mutations in the gene encoding Omi/HtrA2 in Parkinson's disease. *Hum Mol Genet*, Vol. 14, No. 15, Aug 1; (15): pp. 2099-2111.

Tatsuta T, Langer T. (2008) Quality control of mitochondria: protection against neurodegeneration and ageing. *EMBO J*, Vol. 27, No. 2, Jan 23; (2): pp. 306-314.

Tatton WG, *et al.* (2003) Apoptosis in Parkinson's disease: signals for neuronal degradation. *Ann Neurol* Vol. 53, Suppl 3: pp. S61-70; discussion S70-62.

Valente EM, *et al.* (2004) Hereditary early-onset Parkinson's disease caused by mutations in PINK1. *Science*, Vol. 304, No. 5674, May 21; (5674): pp. 1158-1160.

Yoneda T, *et al.* (2004) Compartment-specific perturbation of protein handling activates genes encoding mitochondrial chaperones. *J Cell Sci*, Vol. 117, No. Pt 18, Aug 15; (Pt 18): pp. 4055-4066.

Zhao Q, *et al.* (2002) A mitochondrial specific stress response in mammalian cells. *EMBO J*, Vol. 21, No. 17 Sep 2; (17): pp. 4411-4419.

7

Melanocortins: Anti-Inflammatory and Neuroprotective Peptides

Carla Caruso, Lila Carniglia, Daniela Durand,
Teresa N. Scimonelli and Mercedes Lasaga
*Research Institute for Reproduction, School of Medicine, University of Buenos Aires,
IFEC-CONICET Department of Pharmacology, School of Chemistry,
National University of Córdoba, Córdoba,
Argentina*

1. Introduction

The melanocortin system includes the melanocortins, their receptors and two endogenous antagonists. This system is involved in several physiological processes in the brain. Melanocortins have potent anti-inflammatory and neuroprotective effects in the central nervous system (CNS). Therefore, they are suitable candidates for the treatment of inflammatory and neurodegenerative disorders within the brain.

2. Melanocortins

Melanocortins include α, β, and γ-melanocyte stimulating homones (MSH), and adrenocorticotropin (ACTH). These neuropeptides derive from pro-opiomelanocortin (POMC) proteolytic cleavage (Fig. 1). POMC is a 31 KDa pro-hormone that is processed by pro-hormone convertases (PCs) in secretory vesicles of the cell. PCs belong to the family of serine proteases and recognize pairs of basic amino acid residues. PC expression is tissue specific and their presence induces secretion of different products generated from POMC, thereby determining melanocortins' selective expression (Bicknell, 2008). Intact POMC was also shown to be released into the circulation (Gibson et al., 1994). α-MSH is produced in the presence of PC1 and PC2 (Benjannet et al., 1991) and additional modifications such as glycosylation, phosphorylation, amidation, and acetylation may occur. For example, acetylation gives α-MSH increased resistance to degradation, this modification resulting in increased biological activity (Wilkinson, 2006).

Although α-MSH is synthesized in several tissues such as skin, placenta, testis, ovary, kidney, and adrenal gland, the main source of α-MSH is the pars intermedia of the pituitary gland (Usategui et al., 1976). In the CNS, α-MSH is produced in the arcuate nucleus of the hypothalamus (O'Donohue & Dorsa, 1982) and in the nucleus of the solitary tract in the brain stem (Bronstein et al., 1992). Melanocortin fibers project from these sites to the paraventricular nucleus, the lateral hypothalamus, and throughout the brain, e.g., amygdala, hippocampus, nucleus accumbes, and spinal cord (Bagnol et al., 1999). ACTH is produced mainly in the anterior pituitary gland and released into circulation, although it is also expressed in the skin (Wakamatsu et al., 1997). γ-MSH was detected in adrenal medulla (Bjartell et al., 1987), intestine neurons (Wolter, 1985), and the brain (Kawai et al., 1984) whereas β-MSH was found in human hypothalamus (Bertagna et al., 1986), but not in rodent brain. All melanocortins share a conserved sequence of aminoacids: Met-Glu(Gly)-His-Phe-Arg-Trp necessary for their biological activity. Rare mutations in POMC gene have been found in humans, and are associated with severe early-onset obesity, adrenal insufficiency and red hair pigmentation (Krude et al., 1998).

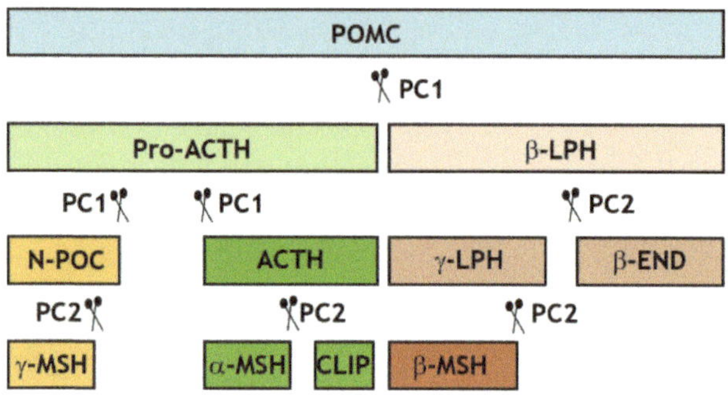

Fig. 1. Hypothalamic post-translational processing of POMC. PC1 (also known as PC3) cleaves POMC protein to generate pro-ACTH and β-lipotropin (β-LPH). Pro-ACTH is further cleaved by PC1 to generate ACTH and N-terminal peptide (N-POC). In the brain and in the intermediate lobe of pituitary, PC2 cleaves ACTH to generate corticotropin-like intermediate peptide (CLIP) and α-MSH. Then, two more peptidases, carboxipeptidase E and peptidyl α-amidating monooxygenase, are needed to produce mature α-MSH. PC2 also generates γ-lipotropin (γ-LPH) and β-endorphin (β-END) from β-LPH cleavage, β-MSH from γ-LPH, and γ-MSH from N-POC cleavage.

2.1 Melanocortin receptors

Cloning of melanocortin receptors (MCRs) led to the characterization of five distinct MCRs which help to explain the wide range of physiological functions of melanocortins. Each receptor is the product of a small, intronless separate gene. MCRs belong to class A of seven transmembrane G protein-coupled receptors (GPCRs) and are positively coupled to adenylate cyclase. MCRs exhibit sequence homology from 40% to 60%. All MCRs have several potential N-glycosylation sites in their N-terminal domains, conserved cysteine residues in their carboxyl termini for potential acetylation with fatty acids, and consensus recognition sites for protein kinase A (PKA) and C. ACTH, α-MSH, and β-MSH are agonists of all MCRs except MC2R which only recognizes ACTH (Schiöth et al., 1996), whereas γ-MSH is a selective MC3R agonist (Roselli-Rehfuss et al., 1993) (Table 1).

MC1R was the first receptor cloned from a melanoma cell line (Chhajlani & Wikberg, 1992) and from normal melanocytes (Mountjoy et al., 1992), and is expressed predominantly in the skin where it mediates α-MSH induction of melanogenesis. MC1R mutations are associated with increased risk of developing melanoma (Kennedy et al., 2001). MC1R is also found in immune cells such as macrophages (Lam et al., 2005), monocytes (Bhardwaj et al., 1997), neutrophils (Catania et al., 1996), and B lymphocytes (Cooper et al., 2005). It is also expressed in endothelial cells (Hartmeyer et al., 1997) and fibroblasts (Böhm et al., 1999).

MC1R is involved in the anti-inflammatory action of α-MSH in leukocytes (Taherzadeh et al., 1999). Indeed, MC1R involvement in the anti-inflammatory effects of melanocortins has been widely studied in peripheral cells (Catania et al., 2004). Recently, MC1R expression was also found in rat heart (Catania et al., 2010). In the CNS, MC1R was detected only in neurons of periaqueductal grey matter (Xia et al., 1995) and in mouse brain (Rajora et al., 1997a). However, nothing is known about the role of MC1R in central effects of melanocortins.

MC2R is present in the adrenal gland and is selectively activated by ACTH leading to production and release of steroids (Mountjoy et al., 1992). Mutations in MC2R gene that produce a non functional receptor are associated with familial glucocorticoid deficiency (Elias et al., 1999), a rare autosomal recessive disorder. MC2R is also present in rodent adipocytes (Boston & Cone, 1996), suggesting a role for melanocortins in lipolysis, although it was not found in human adipocytes (Chhajlani, 1996). MC2R was found in human keratinocytes where its activation by ACTH induced cortisol synthesis (Slominski et al., 1996), and it was recently shown to be present in bone cells as well (Isales et al., 2010).

MC3R is widely distributed in the CNS, highly expressed in the hypothalamus and the limbic system (Roselli-Rehfuss et al., 1993). It has been proposed to function as an auto-receptor since it is expressed in POMC neurons where it might regulate melanocortin release (Jégou et al., 2000). However, MC3R knock-out mice are obese and hyperphagic and have increased fat mass (Chen et al., 2000), indicating that MC3R may have other actions in the brain. MC3R is present in the digestive tract in stomach, duodenum and pancreas and in human placenta (Gantz et al., 1993), as well as in human heart, kidney, testis, ovary, mammary gland, and skeletal muscle (Chhajlani, 1996). Immune cells such as macrophages (Lam et al., 2005) and B lymphocytes (Cooper et al., 2005) express this receptor which is involved in anti-inflammatory effects of melanocortins in macrophages (Getting et al., 2006). MC3R plays a role in sodium homeostasis having natriuretic actions (Lin et al., 1987) and has protective effects in heart ischemia in rats (Guarini et al., 2002).

MC4R is expressed throughout the brain including the cortex, thalamus, hypothalamus, and the spinal cord (Gantz et al., 1994; Mountjoy et al., 1994), and it was shown to be more widely distributed than MC3R in the brain. Outside the CNS, it has been detected in human adipose tissue (Chhajlani, 1996), and it was recently detected in human epidermal melanocytes where it regulates pigmentation (Spencer & Schallreuter, 2009). MC4R is involved in neuroendocrine and autonomic functions, being a key factor in the regulation of food intake and metabolism (Huszar et al., 1997). The anorexigenic effect of α-MSH involves this receptor (Marsh et al., 1999). In this regard, mutations in MC4R gene in humans are associated with obesity (Yeo et al., 1998) and are now considered the most common monogenic cause of obesity. In contrast, no MC3R variants are associated with obesity in humans. MC4R is also involved in the antipyretic actions of α-MSH (Sinha et al., 2004), and it also mediates the neurotrophic effect of α-MSH on cultured neurons (Adan et al., 1996) and on neurite elongation of dorsal root ganglia neurons (Tanabe et al., 2007). MC4R is involved in melanocortins anti-inflammatory action in the brain (Lasaga et al., 2008). MC4R is the only MCR expressed in astrocytes (Selkirk et al., 2007; Caruso et al., 2007) where it exerts anti-inflammatory effects (Caruso et al., 2007). We recently showed that hypothalamic cultured neurons express MC4R and MC3R, and α-MSH also exerts an anti-inflammatory action on these cells (Caruso et al., 2010). Activation of MC4R in astrocytes also induces the expression of brain-derived neurotrophic factor (BDNF) (Caruso et al., 2011), which suggests that BDNF could mediate melanocortins effects.

MC5R is found in adipocytes, kidney, liver, lung, bone marrow, thymus, mammary gland, testis, ovary, uterus, pituitary, stomach and skin (Chhajlani, 1996; Gantz et al., 1994; Labbé et al., 1994; van der Kraan et al., 1998). Observation of MC5R knock-out mice indicates that its main functions involve regulation of lacrimal glands and of secretion of sebaceous glands (Chen et al., 1997). These mice showed no changes in anti-inflammatory, neuroprotective or analgesic actions induced by administration of α-MSH. MC5R was also found in the adrenal gland (Liakos et al., 1998) where α-MSH induces aldosterone production *in vitro*, although to a lesser extent. MC5R is expressed in B and T lymphocytes, indicating that it could be involved in immune regulation. This receptor has also been detected in some areas of the CNS but its physiological functions are unknown (Griffon et al., 1994).

Receptor subtype	Ligand affinity	Physiological functions	Tissue distribution
MC1	α-MSH= β-MSH ≥ACTH >>γ-MSH	Melanocyte differentiation Synthesis of melanin Pigmentation Anti-inflammatory	Melanocytes, keratinocytes, macrophages,monocytes, neutrophils, endothelial cells
MC2	ACTH	Steroidogenesis	Adrenal cortex, keratinocytes, adipocytes
MC3	γ-MSH = ACTH >α-MSH = β-MSH	Anti-inflammatory Energy homeostasis Natriuretic activity	Hypothalamus and limbic system, digestive tract, heart, kidney, immune cells and placenta
MC4	α-MSH= β-MSH= ACTH >>γ-MSH	Energy homeostasis Sexual behavior Anti-inflammatory Neuroprotection Antipyretic	Widely distributed in the brain
MC5	α-MSH ≥ β-MSH= ACTH >>γ-MSH	Exocrine gland secretion	Widely distributed in peripheral tissues, specially in glands

Table 1. Ligand, function and distribution of MCRs

The melanocortin system is unique in that it is the only system with endogenous antagonists. The Agouti protein (Miller et al., 1993) produced in the skin of rodents is a competitive antagonist of MC1R and also of MC4R albeit with lower affinity (Blanchard et al., 1995). In humans, Agouti is expressed in the skin, adipose tissue, testis, ovary, liver, heart and kidney (Wikberg et al., 2000) and regulates skin pigmentation. The Agouti-related protein (AGRP) was cloned based on its homology with Agouti (Shutter et al., 1997). It is present in the brain only in neurons of the arcuate nucleus (Dinulescu & Cone, 2000) where it promotes increased feeding and decreased energy expenditure by binding MC4R (Cone, 2005). Ubiquitous expression of AGRP causes obesity in mice (Ollman et al., 1997). AGRP is a competitive antagonist of MC3R and MC4R and it was shown to inhibit constitutive MC4R activity (Haskell-Luevano & Monek, 2001).

2.2 MCR signaling pathways

The classical signaling pathway for MCRs couples to stimulatory G protein that activates adenylate cyclase and increases intracellular cyclic AMP (cAMP) production. In turn, cAMP can activate PKA. This kinase was reported to be involved in melanocortins effects in melanoma cells (Ao et al., 1998) and in adrenal cells (Roy et al., 2011). In Agouti mice PKA constitutive activity even rescued mice from obesity syndrome (Czyzyk et al., 2008). As a result of its activation, PKA can phosphorylate and activate the cAMP responsive element binding protein (CREB), which then acts within the nucleus as a transcription factor. CREB is activated by α-MSH in neurons of the hypothalamic paraventricular nucleus (Sarkar et al., 2002), in neurons of the solitary nucleus (Sutton et al., 2005), in hypothalamic cultured neurons (Caruso et al., 2010), and also in cultured rat astrocytes (Caruso et al., 2011). Apart from the cAMP-PKA-CREB pathway MCRs also activate other signaling pathways. MC3R has been shown to induce inositol phosphate signaling (Konda et al., 1994) and MC5R was reported to activate the Janus kinase/signal transducer and activator of transcription (Jak/STAT) pathway in B cells (Buggy, 1998). Stimulation of all MCRs leads to activation of mitogen-activated protein kinases (MAPK) ERK-1/2 (Chai et al., 2006; Chai et al., 2007; Herraiz et al., 2011; Patten et al., 2007, Rodrigues et al., 2009; Roy et al., 2011). Depending on the cell type this effect may involve phosphoinositol 3 kinase activation (Rodrigues et al., 2009; Vongs et al., 2004). Some reports also show that ERK activation may be PKA-independent in MCR transfected cell lines (Chai et al., 2006; Vongs et al., 2004). Intracellular calcium is also elevated by MC1R, MC3R, and MC4R stimulation (Eves et al., 2003; Konda et al., 1994; Newman et al., 2006). Although these data show some insight into MCR signaling, much work is still needed to fully elucidate signaling pathways of MCRs and to evaluate their importance in *in vivo* models. Pathways may also interact with each other as cross-talk between receptors, adding complexity to the picture. For example, MC4R activation enhances insulin-stimulated mTOR signaling (Chai et al., 2010) and potentiates leptin signaling (Zhang et al., 2009).

In addition to G proteins, MCRs can interact with other proteins that regulate their function. Some accessory proteins help folding and trafficking GPCRs to the cell membrane whereas others are found associated with the receptor and are involved in ligand binding. It is now established that a functional MC2R requires the expression of melanocortin 2 receptor accessory protein (MRAP). MRAP interacts with MC2R and facilitates MC2R cell surface expression, thereby producing an ACTH-responsive receptor (Webb et al., 2009). MRAP has two isoforms, MRAPα and MRAPβ, both expressed in the human adrenal gland (Metherell et al., 2005). Both MRAP isoforms interact directly with MC2R enabling ligand binding and activation (Roy et al., 2007). Individuals lacking MRAP have familial glucocorticoid deficiency disease (Metherell et al., 2005), which highlights the role of MRAP in MC2R functionality. Another accessory protein, MRAP-2, is expressed in the brain and the adrenal gland (Chan et al., 2009). MRAP and MRAP-2 act as negative regulators of MCRs other than MC2R since they reduce cAMP production in response to receptor activation (Chan et al., 2009). In addition, mahoghany, mahoganoid (also called mahogunin ring finger-1), and syndecan-3 were identified as accessory proteins for MCRs. Mahoghany, a transmembrane protein present in the brain and skin, was shown to be a low-affinity receptor for Agouti but not for AGRP (He et al., 2001). Recently, mahoganoid was shown to reduce MC1R and MC4R coupling to cAMP (Perez-Oliva et al., 2009). Finally, syndecan-3 is a proteoglycan that enhances AGRP antagonism of α-MSH at MC4R (Reizes et al., 2003). In spite of all this evidence, interaction between MCRs and accessory proteins is still not fully understood.

2.3 Synthetic compounds acting on MCRs

Some synthetic compounds for MCRs have been developed. (Nle^4, D-Phe^7) α-MSH (NDP-MSH), also known as melanotan I (MTI), is the most potent linear analogue of α-MSH (Sawyer et al., 1980). It shows high affinity for all MCRs and has been widely used in radioligand binding studies. Other agonist peptides are melanotan II (MTII), a small cyclic peptide that is a non selective agonist of all MCRs except MC2R, and HP-228, a linear analogue that is also a non selective agonist for MCRs but shows greater affinity for MC1R (Abou-Mohamed et al., 1995). Several MC4R agonists have also been developed. Ro27-3225 is a full agonist in human cells that express MC4R (Benoit et al., 2000) and was shown to protect against haemorrhagic shock (Giuliani et al., 2007b). Also, THIQ is a MC4R agonist that reduced food intake less effectively than MTII (Muceniece et al., 2007). Antagonists have also been developed. SHU9119 is a potent non-selective antagonist of MC3R and MC4R (Schiöth et al., 1999). HS014 (Schiöth et al., 1999), is the first selective MC4R antagonist since it has 20-fold higher affinity for MC4R over MC3R. HS024 is a competitive analog of α-MSH (Kask et al., 1998) with 100 times more affinity for MC4R over MC3R, although it antagonizes cAMP accumulation induced by all MCRs except MC2R. All antagonists stimulate food intake when administered centrally.

3. Anti-inflammatory effects of melanocortins

Inflammation is a physiological response to infection or tissue damage which, if properly controlled, ultimately leads to the restoration of homeostasis. Cytokines, chemokines, nitric oxide (NO) and prostaglandins (PGs) are mediators of inflammatory processes that induce vasodilation and extravasation of immune cells into injured tissues, activation of pathogen clearance mechanisms and tissue regeneration. These factors have also been linked to the pathology of several CNS disorders with an exacerbated inflammatory component, such as Alzheimer´s disease (AD), Parkinson disease (PD), multiple sclerosis (MS), HIV infection, and brain ischemia/reperfusion. Among their many physiological functions, melanocortins play an important role in the regulation of immune and inflammatory reactions. These effects can be exerted through their binding to centrally expressed MCRs which in turn regulate descending neural anti-inflammatory pathways, or by acting directly on immune cells or non-immune cells present in peripheral tissues (Lasaga et al., 2008), where they modulate the production of inflammatory mediators and the migration of inflammatory cells. Different MCRs may be responsible for the anti-inflammatory properties of melanocortins depending on the tissue or cell type involved. MC1R, MC3R and MC5R are the subtypes most commonly associated with these peripheral effects, whereas MC3R and MC4R are more likely responsible for melanocortins anti-inflammatory action within the CNS. Some studies also indicate that alternative non-MCR-mediated pathways may be involved in the signaling of certain melanocortin peptides such as γ-MSH (Langouche et al., 2002) and α-MSH C-terminal tripeptide Lys-Pro-Val (KPV).

3.1 Peripheral effects

3.1.1 *In vitro* studies

Melanocortins effects on peripheral tissues have been studied in a broad range of *in vitro* systems, particularly in immune cells where they appear to act mainly by decreasing the production and release of inflammatory mediators and impairing leukocyte activation and infiltration into damaged tissues. For instance, it was shown that α-MSH inhibits synthesis and release of pro-inflammatory cytokines such as interleukin-1β (IL-1β), tumor necrosis factor-α (TNF-α), interferon-γ (IFN-γ), and IL-2 in cells of the immune system (Lipton et al., 1999; Luger et al., 2003; Manna et al., 2006; Star et al., 1995; Taherzadeh et al., 1999). It enhances the release of the anti-inflammatory cytokine IL-10 in monocytes (Bhardwaj et al., 1996) and keratinocytes (Redondo et al., 1998) as well. α-MSH can also inhibit chemokine production in a human retinal epithelial cell line that expresses MC1R (Cui et al., 2005), and IL-8 in fibroblasts and in human adipocytes, (Böhm et al., 1999, 2002). Melanocortins modulate the expression of adhesion molecules in response to inflammatory stimuli. For instance, α-MSH inhibits the expression of adhesion molecules induced by LPS or TNF-α in endothelial cells (Scholzen et al., 2003), leading to impaired lymphocyte adhesion. Another target of melanocortins is the inducible NO synthase (iNOS). This enzyme is induced by inflammatory stimuli and produces a high output of NO, a short-lived molecule which plays a major role in the regulation of immune, nervous and cardiovascular systems. Beyond its many physiological roles, excessive NO production may be harmful and mediate tissue damage and cell death. Several studies indicate that melanocortin peptides exert a protective role by inhibiting iNOS expression in stimulated macrophages, thus leading to decreased NO production (Mandrika et al., 2001; Star et al., 1995; Taylor, 2005). PGs are a family of lipid molecules derived enzymatically from fatty acids with a broad spectrum of physiological functions. They participate in multiple homeostatic effects and play a dual role in immunomodulation, different members of the family being involved in both the onset and resolution of the inflammatory response. Their production is catalyzed by cyclooxygenase (COX) 1 and 2, COX-2 being the isoform specifically activated by inflammation. α-MSH inhibits pro-inflammatory PG synthesis from fibroblasts induced by IL-1β (Cannon et al., 1986). Furthermore, in melanocyte and keratinocyte cell lines α-MSH was shown to reduce the release of PGE_2 induced by TNF-α (Nicolaou et al., 2004).

3.1.2 *In vivo* studies

Some of the *in vivo* anti-inflammatory actions of melanocortins in the periphery are due to ACTH binding to its receptor MC2R in the adrenal cortex which promotes the production of glucocorticoids with a consequent systemic anti-inflammatory response. Melanocortin peptides can have anti-inflammatory effects acting via central MCRs through descending neurogenic pathways or directly on peripheral tissues through other MCR subtypes. Both α-MSH and γ-MSH are capable of inhibiting the effects of IL-1β on the activation of the hypothalamic-pituitary-adrenal axis by acting on central melanocortin receptors (Cragnolini et al., 2004). Several studies show that systemic and/or central administration of α-MSH exerts protective effects in diverse models of peripheral inflammation. Circulating levels of α-MSH have also been shown to be increased in inflammatory diseases such as rheumatoid arthritis, MS, PD, and HIV infection (Catania et al., 2000). Anti-inflammatory actions of melanocortins have been widely studied in animal models of systemic inflammation such as septic shock where α-MSH has been shown to reduce circulating levels of pro-inflammatory cytokines TNF-α and IL-1α (Gonindard et al., 1996) and to improve animals' survival rate from 10% to 50% by 24 h (Lipton et al., 1994). Treatment with ACTH and POMC-derived peptides was also shown to inhibit cytokine release and neutrophil migration in a mouse model of acute experimental inflammation (Getting et al., 1999). In a model of acute hepatitis induced by LPS, Chiao et al. (1996) showed that α-MSH was able to prevent liver inflammation by inhibiting NO production, TNF-α and IL-8 mRNA increase, and neutrophil infiltration. α-MSH was also shown to reduce chemokine synthesis and prevent damage to lungs and kidneys under hypoxic conditions in a model of renal ischemia (Chiao et al., 1997; Deng et al., 2004). It also reduced heart injury and size of the ischemic area in a rat model of myocardial ischemia, through activation of MC3R (Bazzani et al., 2001; Guarini et al., 2002). Research on experimental inflammatory bowel disease showed that treatment with α-MSH effectively reduces inflammatory mediators in experimental colitis (Rajora et al., 1997b). As for skin inflammation, both centrally and locally administered α-MSH has been shown to modulate the cutaneous immune response in several mouse models of contact dermatitis or cutaneous vasculitis (Brzoska et al., 2008). Furthermore, this peptide was proved to induce hapten-specific tolerance *in vivo* by a mechanism involving IL-10 as a crucial mediator (Grabbe et al., 1996). Since α-MSH and MC1R protein levels are up-regulated in human burns and scars a role in cutaneos injury is also suggested (Muffley et al., 2011). A gene therapy approach based on an α-MSH expression vector has been tested in a model of experimental autoimmune uveitis, in which the treatment was successful in suppressing this condition by a mechanism dependent on MC5R expression, suggesting that this approach might provide effective therapy for uveitis (Lee et al., 2009).

MC1R involvement in the anti-inflammatory effects of melanocortins has been widely observed in peripheral cells (Catania et al., 2004). Recently, it was shown that the selective MC1R agonist BMS-470539 was succesful in inhibiting leukocyte trafficking in the vasculature of mice subjected to mesenteric ischemia-reperfusion. This anti-inflammatory effect was lost when examining the vasculature of mice with mutant inactive MC1Rs (Leoni et al., 2010), indicating that MC1R plays a prominent role in melanocortins effects. In models of allergic and nonallergic lung inflammation, melanocortins inhibited leukocyte accumulation, a protective effect that was associated with MC3R activation (Getting et al., 2008). On the other hand, Ro27-3225, a selective MC4R agonist, reduced the expression of TNF-α and IL-6, and reduced pancreatitis severity, effects that were blocked by HS024, a selective MC4R antagonist (Minutoli et al., 2011). On the other hand, several MCR-independent effects of melanocortin C terminal sequence-derived peptides were described. The melanocortin-derived tripeptide KPV was shown to reduce the inflammatory infiltrate in a model of inflammatory bowel disease, leading to recovery (Kannengiesser et al., 2008). Another synthetic peptide $(CPVK)_2$ also showed anti-inflammatory activity similar to NDP-MSH against endotoxin treatment *in vitro* and *in vivo* by reducing TNF-α and NO production (Gatti et al., 2006). The mechanism of action of these peptides seems to involve interaction with the IL-1 receptor I, thereby preventing IL-1β binding (Mastrofrancesco et al., 2010).

3.2 Central effects

3.2.1 *In vitro* studies

Inflammatory reactions within the CNS constitute a physiological host-defense mechanism by which damaging agents are cleared and tissue homeostasis is restored. As part of this response, glial cells become reactive and release a wide variety of inflammatory mediators such as cytokines, chemokines, complement factors and acute phase reactants. These factors are necessary for an adequate immune or inflammatory response, but if the response is not properly controlled, they may also lead to tissue damage and cytotoxicity. Therefore, the discovery of compounds with the ability to modulate inflammatory responses in the brain is of paramount importance.

Activation of MCRs in the brain is known to be essential to the anti-inflammatory circuit of melanocortins. Expression of MC1R (Xia et al., 1995; Rajora et al., 1997a) and MC5R (Griffon et al., 1994) has been described but their physiological functions in the CNS are unknown. Considering that α-MSH has anti-inflammatory action in brain of mice with non-functional MC1R (Ichiyama et al., 1999), this receptor may not be an important mediator of anti-inflammatory effects of melanocortins in the CNS. Therefore, the main candidates to mediate central effects of melanocortins are MC3R and MC4R since these are the subtypes expressed in the brain. Astrocytes are the most abundant glial cell population in the brain. The only MCR subtype found in these cells is MC4R (Caruso et al., 2007; Selkirk et al., 2007). On the other hand, subtypes 1, 3, 4 and 5 were detected in a human microglial cell line (Lindberg et al., 2005). Melanocortins were shown to inhibit production of IL-6, TNF-α and NO in a murine microglial cell line, where endogenous α-MSH released from microglial cells was proposed to act as an autocrine immunomodulatory factor (Delgado et al., 1998). They also inhibited the release of both NO and TNF-α from microglia stimulated with β-amyloid peptides and IFN-γ (Galimberti et al., 1999), suggesting that these peptides might modulate the local response to β-amyloid deposition. In human astrocytoma cells, α-MSH inhibits LPS-induced TNF-α release (Wong et al., 1997). We showed that α-MSH attenuates LPS+IFN-γ-induced inflammation in rat astrocytes by decreasing iNOS and COX-2 expression and NO and PGE_2 release (Caruso et al., 2007). These effects were prevented by HS024, strongly suggesting a role for MC4R in brain anti-inflammatory melanocortin effects. However, α-MSH had no effect on basal or IL-1β-induced PGE_2 levels in astrocytes (Katsuura et al., 1989), although it inhibited LPS- or IL-1β-induced PGE_2 production from hippocampus fragments (Weidenfeld et al., 1995), but not IL-1β-induced PGE_2 release from hypothalamic fragments (Mirtella et al., 1995). We recently showed that hypothalamic neurons express MC3R and MC4R and that α-MSH reduces TNF-α expression in these cells where it induces CREB activation (Caruso et al., 2010).

3.2.2 *In vivo* studies

A typical reaction to inflammatory processes in the CNS is the induction of fever as a host-defense response. Melanocortin anti-pyretic action has been known for some time (Tatro, 2000) and is considered adrenal-independent (Murphy et al., 1983). α-MSH central administration reduces fever caused by LPS (Huang et al., 1997), IL-1β (Daynes et al., 1987) and TNF-α (Martin et al., 1991). Also, during fever episodes, levels of α-MSH increase in the brain (Bell & Lipton, 1987) suggesting a physiological role for melanocortins in fever control. α-MSH circulating levels increase in response to endotoxin administration in humans (Catania et al., 1995). Intraperitoneal (i.p.) administration of α-MSH was shown to inhibit fever by activating central MCRs, since their blockade prevented an α-MSH anti-pyretic effect (Huang et al., 1998). This effect was also blocked by HS014, a selective MC4R antagonist, thereby highlighting MC4R involvement in α-MSH effect over LPS-induced fever (Sinha et al., 2004). Central administration of α-MSH in mice reduces the expression of iNOS in lungs and liver and serum TNF-α levels induced by endotoxemia (Delgado

Hernandez et al., 1999). Conversely, i.p. injection of α-MSH has no effect over endotoxemia-induced iNOS expression in lung and liver, supporting the notion that activation of central MCRs is responsible for the peripheral anti-inflammatory effect of α-MSH. Moreover, treatment with α-MSH reduces expression of TNF-α and IL-1β after cerebral ischemia (Huang & Tatro, 2002), lowers TNF-α and NO production induced by LPS+IFN-γ in the CNS (Delgado et al., 1998), and also reduces TNF-α production in brain inflammation (Rajora et al., 1997a). Furthermore, melanocortins inhibit the IL-1β-induced production of NO and PGs in rat hypothalamus (Cragnolini et al., 2006). We demonstrated that α-MSH reduces induction of iNOS and COX-2 gene expression at hypothalamic level in rats during endotoxemia, and that this effect is mediated by MC4R activation (Caruso et al., 2004). Together with α-MSH, γ-MSH and β-MSH were found to exert anti-inflammatory action in a model of neuroinflammation in mice by reducing LPS-induced NO production (Muceniece et al., 2004).

3.3 Mechanisms of anti-inflammatory actions of melanocortins

The nuclear factor-κB (NF-κB) is an essential regulator of the immune response since it drives the expression of several pro-inflammatory genes such as cytokines, chemokines, iNOS and COX-2 induced by diverse inflammatory stimuli (Li & Verma 2002). Under resting conditions it is held within the cytoplasm in an inactive state by its inhibitor (IκB). Upon proper stimulation, IκB is phosphorylated and dissociates from the complex, allowing NF-κB to translocate to the nucleus where it acts as a transcription factor. The most attractive feature of melanocortins is that they reduce production of a variety of inflammatory mediators but do not enterily suppress the inflammatory response. α-MSH is able to inhibit the activation of NF-κB induced by a great diversity of inflammatory stimuli in different cell lines (Manna & Aggarwal, 1998), and in brain inflammation (Ichiyama et al., 1999). This inhibitory action, thought to be the main mechanism responsible for the anti-inflammatory effects of melanocortins, appears to be mediated by cAMP production and PKA activation (Manna & Aggarwal, 1998). α-MSH regulates NF-κB and also p38-MAPK pathways probably through a common upstream element by inducing the binding of the IL-1R-associated kinase 1 (IRAK 1) to its inhibitor IRAK-M in activated macrophages (Taylor, 2005). However, NF-κB inhibition might not be the mechanism of action of melanocortins in all cell types studied. Apart from NF-κB, melanocortins activate CREB, a transcription factor acting on cell proliferation, differentiation and survival. It also regulates the expression of genes involved in immune responses and long term memory. In rat astrocytes, MC4R activation by α-MSH stimulates the cAMP-PKA-CREB pathway without involving inhibition of NF-κB (Caruso et al., 2011). CREB activation by α-MSH occurs in hypothalamic neurons as well, and also without modifying NF-κB activation (Caruso et al., 2010). Similarly, α-MSH failure to modify NF-κB activation was reported in H4 glioma cells (Sarkar et al., 2003).

Another important mediator in α-MSH effects is IL-10, an anti-inflammatory cytokine capable of inhibiting NF-κB activity and the release of many pro-inflammatory mediators such as IL-1, IL-6, TNF-α, and IL-8 (Sabat et al., 2010). This cytokine is induced by α-MSH in monocytes and keratinocytes, and knock-out mice for IL-10 were found to be resistant to α-MSH treatment in a model of allergic inflammation (Raap et al., 2003), strongly supporting a role for IL-10 as a mediator in melanocortin effect. Furthermore, a MC3R/4R antagonist, SHU9119, reduces LPS-induced IL-10 release in monkeys (Vulliémoz et al., 2006), thereby establishing a physiological role for endogenous melanocortins as modulators of this cytokine's release.

4. Neuroprotective effects of melanocortins

Melanocortins neuroregenerative actions were described long ago. The first reports showed that melanocortin peptides improve nerve regeneration following peripheral nerve injury. ACTH administration improved recovery of adrenalectomized rats subjected to sciatic nerve denervation (Strand & Kung, 1980). α-MSH and ACTH also induced recovery after crushing the sciatic nerve (Bijlsma et al., 1983). α-MSH-like peptides stimulate neurite outgrowth in peripheral nerve injury *in vivo* (Plantinga et al., 1995), and axonal outgrowth from fetal spinal cord slices (van der Neut et al., 1988), and regrowth of injured axons in rat adult spinal cord (Joosten et al., 1999). Endogenous α-MSH also improved recovery of rats with destruction of dopamine neurons of the nucleus accumbens (Wolterink et al., 1990). Its analog MTII also induced nerve regeneration and neuroprotection by preventing toxic neuropathy induced by cisplatin (Ter Laak et al., 2003). Several studies suggested that MC4R is the receptor involved in the neuroregenerative properties of melancortins. α-MSH-induced neurite-like outgrowth in the neuroblastoma cell line 2A was shown to be blocked with a specific MC4R antagonist (Adan et al., 1996). The MC4R agonist ME10501 is neuroprotective in spinal cord injury (Sharma et al., 2006). In mouse dorsal root ganglia neuron cultures, α-MSH promoted neurite outgrowth, an effect entirely inhibited by a selective MC4R blocker, JKC-363 (Tanabe et al., 2007). This study also showed that only MC4R mRNA expression was induced after sciatic nerve injury, suggesting that MC4R could play a central role in nerve regeneration. The mechanism of neurotrophic effects of melanocortins remains largely unknown although it is suggested to be a consequence of the anti-inflammatory effects of these peptides.

Several models of brain injury were shown to improve after melanocortin treatment. In rats subjected to four-vessel occlusion global cerebral ischemia, i.p. administration of α-MSH prevented CA1 pyramidal cell death and reduced glial activation (Forslin Aronsson et al., 2006). NDP-MSH protects hippocampal neurons from dying after cerebral ischemia in gerbils (Giuliani et al., 2006), and after excitotoxicity (Forslin Aronsson et al., 2007). Also, delayed treatment with α-MSH diminished stratial damage and neuronal death after focal cerebral ischemia (Giuliani et al., 2007a). Melanocortins reduced hippocampal damage and improve learning and memory as long as 50 days after ischemia (Giuliani et al., 2009). These studies showed that neuroprotection by melancortins involved MC4R whereas the selective MC3R agonist γ-MSH had no protective effect on cerebral ischemia (Giuliani et al., 2006). In addition, melanocortins through MC4R blocked memory impairment (Gonzalez et al., 2009) as well as memory reconsolidation impairment (Machado et al., 2010) induced by IL-1β administration in the hippocampus. We showed that MC4R activation protects astrocytes from apoptosis induced by LPS+IFN-γ (Caruso et al., 2007), and other authors showed that it also protects hypothalamic neurons from serum deprived-induced apoptosis (Chai et al., 2006). Protection of astrocytes by melanocortins involved decreasing caspase 3 activity induced by LPS+IFN-γ and inducing expression of the anti-apoptotic protein Bcl-2 as well as decreasing expression of the apoptotic protein Bax induced by LPS+IFN-γ (Caruso et al.,

2007). This protective effect was also shown to involve ERK activation in a cell line of hypothalamic neurons (Chai et al., 2006). These data strongly suggest that melanocortins are neuroprotective through MC4R.

A common feature of neurodegenerative diseases is chronic immune activation in the brain. Cytokines have a dual role in inflammation and disease. They contribute to the acute phase of inflammation but also play protective roles in later stages of injury. This is also the case in neurodegeneration: given that IL-1β and TNF-α are increased in neurodegenerative diseases such as AD, PD, and MS, they are believed to be involved in the etiology of these pathologies. However, the role of inflammation in the development of neurodegenerative disorders is not clear. A general understanding indicates that inflammatory processes contribute to the onset of neurodegenerative diseases. Although there is no evidence of melanocortin effects on models of PD or AD, anti-inflammatory therapies such as nonsteroidal anti-inflammatory drugs (NSAIDs) were neuroprotective (Asanuma & Miyazaki, 2008; McGeer & McGeer, 2007). However, the use of NSAIDs for long periods of time can have undesired side effects. Melanocortins could be a better approach for treating these disorders since they could preserve the benefits of the inflammatory response and at the same time prevent its harmful effects. In fact, α-MSH was suggested to be useful in the treatment of inflammatory experimental autoimmune encephalomyelitis (EAE), a T-cell mediated inflammatory autoimmune process that resembles the human demyelinating disease MS. Alterations in plasma concentrations of α-MSH were shown to occur during exacerbation of MS (Sandyk & Awerbuch, 1992). However, in cerebrospinal fluid of MS patients concentrations of α-MSH-like peptides were normal (Pinessi et al., 1992). Orally administered α-MSH can reduce signs of EAE and inhibit CNS inflammation by reducing Th1-cytokines released by CNS lymphocytes (Brod & Hood, 2011). Injection of α-MSH at the onset of EAE also profoundly diminished the severity of EAE in mice (Taylor & Kitaichi, 2008). Furthermore, it was shown that modified T- cells that express and release α-MSH reduce the signs of this disease when they are transferred into mice with EAE, suggesting the possibility of their use in future therapeutic applications (Han et al., 2007).

Astrocytes actions help neurons to perform their physiological functions and contribute to maintain brain homeostasis. They have both beneficial and damaging responses in the CNS. Astrocytes proliferate in response to trauma and provide an environment that can help neurons to survive injury. They are activated by pro-inflammatory agents or by injury and contribute to brain-repair processes, but when inflammation is chronic their sustained activation can have harmful effects. Astrogliosis was found to be present in neurodegenerative diseases (Maragakis & Rothstein, 2006). However, mice deficient in glial fibrillary acidic protein having consequently impaired astrocyte functions develop more severe EAE disease compared to wild type mice (Liedtke et al., 1998). Astrocytes are able to produce neurotrophic factors that can promote neuron survival. We recently showed that MC4R activation induces expression of BDNF in rat astrocytes (Caruso et al., 2011). BDNF has proved to be neuroprotective in AD, MS and PD (Nagahara & Tuszynski, 2011). Indeed, MS patients have decreased levels of BDNF compared to healthy controls (Frota et al., 2009). Therefore, BDNF is a possible mediator of melanocortin action in the brain. It is likely that melanocortins may induce neuroprotective genes such as Bcl-2 and BDNF, thereby contributing to ameliorate neurodegenerative diseases. However, much study is needed to prove this hypothesis.

5. Conclusions

Acute inflammatory response usually ends once the insult is eliminated and tissue is repaired. If this does not occur, inflammation becomes chronic, leading to harmful effects. Since local inflammation is necessary for pathogen clearance, tissue recovery and regeneration, ideal anti-inflammatory agents should prevent exacerbated immune reaction without completely eliminating inflammatory response. Thus, modulation rather than abolishment of inflammation seems to be the best option, and provides an opening to new treatment approaches in acute and chronic diseases of the CNS. Melanocortins are suitable candidates for this task. Their anti-inflammatory properties are well known and they also have neuroregenerative and neuroprotective properties that can help preserve neuron function. However, in view of the variety of effects produced by these peptides, we need to develop more selective and potent agonists for each receptor in order to avoid undesired side effects. Neurodegenerative diseases are tightly linked to chronic inflammation. The extent to which inflammatory mediators functionally impair cognition and memory is largely unknown. Astrocytes in particular might be especially attractive and underappreciated targets for neurodegenerative disease therapeutics. Finally, future studies need to determine the underlying mechanisms of inflammation that lead to neurodegeneration in order to advance towards the development of effective treatments for neurodegenerative diseases.

6. References

Abou-Mohamed, G.; Papapetropoulos, A.; Ulrich, D.; Catravas, J.D.; Tuttle, R.R. & Caldwell, R.W. (1995). HP-228, a novel synthetic peptide, inhibits the induction of nitric oxide synthase in vivo but not in vitro. J Pharmacol Exp Ther, Vol.275, No.2, (November 1995), pp. 584-591, ISSN 0022-3565.

Adan, R.A.; van der Kraan, M.; Doornbos, R.P.; Bar, P.R.; Burbach, J.P. & Gispen, W.H. (1996). Melanocortin receptors mediate α-MSH-induced stimulation of neurite outgrowth in neuro 2A cells. *Brain Res Mol Brain Res*, Vol.36, No.1, (February 1996), pp. 37-44, ISSN 0169-328X.

Ao, Y.; Park, H.Y.; Olaizola-Horn, S. & Gilchrest, B.A. (1998). Activation of cAMP-dependent protein kinase is required for optimal alpha-melanocyte-stimulating hormone-induced pigmentation. *Exp Cell Res*, Vol.244, No.1, (October 1998), pp. 117-124, ISSN 0014-4827.

Asanuma, M. & Miyazaki, I. (2008). Nonsteroidal anti-inflammatory drugs in experimental parkinsonian models and Parkinson's disease. *Curr Pharm Des*, Vol.14, No.14, pp. 1428-1434, ISSN 1381-6128.

Bagnol, D.; Lu, X.Y.; Kaelin, C.B.; Day, H.E.; Ollmann, M.; Gantz, I.; Akil, H.; Barsh, G.S. & Watson, S.J. (1999). Anatomy of an endogenous antagonist: relationship between Agouti-related protein and proopiomelanocortin in brain. *J Neurosci*, Vol.15, No.19, (September 1999), pp. RC26, ISSN 0270-6474.

Bazzani, C.; Guarini, S.; Botticelli, A.R.; Zaffe, D.; Tomasi, A.; Bini, A.; Cainazzo, M.M.; Ferrazza, G.; Mioni, C. & Bertolini, A. (2001). Protective effect of melanocortin peptides in rat myocardial ischemia. *J Pharmacol Exp Ther, Vol.*297, No.3, (June 2001), pp. 1082-1087, ISSN 0022-3565.

Bell, R.C. & Lipton, J.M. (1987). Pulsatile release of antipyretic neuropeptide alpha-MSH from septum of rabbit during fever. *Am J Physiol*, Vol.252, (June 1987), pp. R1152-R1157, ISSN 0002-9513.

Benjannet, S.; Rondeau, N.; Day, R.; Chrétien, M. & Sedah, N.G. (1991). PC1 and PC2 are protein convertases capable of cleaving proopiomelanocortin at distinct pairs of basic residues. *Proc Natl Acad Sci USA*, Vol.88, No.9, (May 1991), pp. 3564-3568, ISSN 0027-8424.

Benoit, S.C.; Schwartz, M.W.; Lachey, J.L.; Hagan, M.M.; Rushing, P.A.; Blake, K.A.; Yagaloff, K.A.; Kurylko, G.; Franco, L.; Danhoo, W. & Seeley, R.J. (2000). A novel selective melanocortin-4 receptor agonist reduces food intake in rats and mice without producing aversive consequences. *J Neurosci*, Vol.20, No.9, (May 2000), pp. 3442-3448, ISSN 0270-6474.

Bertagna, X.; Lenne, F.; Comar, D.; Massias, J.F.; Wajcman, H.; Baudin, V.; Luton, J.P. & Girard, F. (1986). Human beta-melanocyte-stimulating hormone revisited. *Proc Natl Acad Sci USA*, Vol.83, No.24, (December 1986), pp. 9719-9723, ISSN 0027-8424.

Bhardwaj, R.S., Schwarz, A., Becher, E., Mahnke, K., Aragane, Y., Schwarz, T. & Luger, T.A. (1996). Pro-opiomelanocortin-derived peptides induce IL-10 production in human monocytes. *J Immunol*, Vol.156, No.7, (April 1996), pp. 2517-2521, ISSN 0022-1767.

Bhardwaj, R.S.; Becher, E.; Mahnke, K.; Hartmayer, M.; Schwarz, T.; Scholzen, T. & Luger, T.A. (1997). Evidence for the differential expression of the functional alpha-melanocyte-stimulating hormone receptor MC-1 on human monocytes. *J Immunol*, Vol.158, No.7, (April 1997), pp. 3378-33884, ISSN 0022-1767.

Bicknell, A.B. (2008). The tissue-specific processing of pro-opiomelanocortin. *J Neuroendocrinol*, Vol.20, No.6, (June 2008), pp. 692-699, ISSN 0953-8194.

Bijlsma, W.A.; Schotman, P.; Jennekens, F.G.; Gispen, W.H. & De Wied, D. (1983). The enhanced recovery of sensorimotor function in rats is related to the melanotropic moiety of ACTH/MSH neuropeptides. *Eur J Pharmacol*, Vol.92, No.3-4, (September 1983), pp. 231-236, ISSN 0014-2999.

Bjartell, A.; Ekman, R. & Sundler, F. (1987). Gamma 2-[corrected]-MSH-like immunoreactivity in porcine pituitary and adrenal medulla. An immunochemical and immunocytochemical study. *Regul Pept*, Vol.19, No.5-6, (December 1987), pp. 291-306, ISSN 0167-0115.

Blanchard, S.G.; Harris, C.O.; Ittoop, O.R.; Nichols, J.S.; Parks, D.J.; Truesdale, A.T. & Wilkinson W.O. (1995). Agouti antagonism of melanocortin binding and action in the B16F10 murine melanoma cell line. *Biochemistry*, Vol.34, No.33, (August 1995), pp. 10406-10411, ISSN 0006-2960.

Böhm, M.; Schulte, U.; Kalden, H. & Luger, T.A. (1999). Alpha-melanocyte-stimulating hormone modulates activation of NF-kappa B and AP-1 and secretion of interleukin-8 in human dermal fibroblasts. *Ann NY Acad Sci*, Vol.885, (October 1999), pp. 277-286, ISSN 0077-8923.

Böhm, M.; Schiller, M.; Ständer, S.; Seltmann, H.; Li, Z.; Brzoska, T.; Metze, D.; Schiöth, H.B.; Skottner, A.; Seiffert, K.; Zouboulis, C.C. & Luger, T.A. (2002). Evidence for expression of melanocortin-1 receptor in human sebocytes in vitro and in situ. *J Invest Dermatol*, Vol.118, No.3, (March 2002), pp. 533-539, ISSN 0022-202X.

Boston, B.A. & Cone, R.D. (1996). Characterization of melanocortin receptor subtype expression in murine adipose tissues and in the 3T3-L1 cell line. *Endocrinology*, Vol.137, No.5, (May 1996), pp. 2043-2050, ISSN 0013-7227.

Brod, S.A. & Hood, Z.M. (2011). Ingested (oral) ACTH inhibits EAE. *J Neuroimmunol*, Vol.232, No.1-2, (March 2011), pp. 131-135, ISSN 0165-5728.

Bronstein, D.M.; Schafer, M.K.H.; Watson, S.J. & Akil H. (1992). Evidence that β-endorphin is synthesized in cells in the nucleus tractus solitarius: detection of POMC mRNA. *Brain Res*, Vol.587, No.2, (August 1992), pp. 269-275, ISSN 0006-8993.

Brzoska, T.; Luger, T.A.; Maaser, C.; Abels, C. & Böhm, M. (2008). α-Melanocyte-stimulating hormone and related tripeptides: biochemistry, anti-inflammatory and protective effects in vitro and in vivo, and future perspectives for the treatment of immune-mediated inflammatory diseases. *Endocrine Reviews*, Vol.29, No.5, (August 2008), pp. 581-602, ISSN 0163-769X.

Buggy, J. (1998). Binding of alpha-melanocyte-stimulating hormone to its G-protein-coupled receptor on B-lymphocytes activates the Jak/STAT pathway. *Biochemical J*, Vol.331, No.1, (April 1998), pp. 211-216, ISSN 0264-6021.

Cannon, J.G.; Tatro, J.B.; Reichlin, S. & Dinarello, C.A. (1986). α-Melanocyte stimulating hormone inhibits immunostimulatory and inflammatory actions of interleukin 1. *J Immunol*, Vol.137, No.7, (October 1986), pp. 2232-2236, ISSN 0022-1767.

Caruso, C.; Mohn, C.; Karara, A.L.; Rettori, V.; Watanobe, H.; Schiöth, H.B.; Seilicovich, A. &, Lasaga, M. (2004). Alpha-melanocyte-stimulating hormone through melanocortin-4 receptor inhibits nitric oxide synthase and cyclooxygenase expression in the hypothalamus of male rats. *Neuroendocrinology*, Vol.79, No.5, pp. 278-286, ISSN 0028-3835.

Caruso, C.; Durand, D.; Schiöth H.B.; Rey, R.; Seilicovich, A. & Lasaga, M. (2007). Activation of melanocortin 4 receptors reduces the inflammatory response and prevents apoptosis induced by lipopolysaccharide and interferon-gamma in astrocytes. *Endocrinology*, Vol.148, No.10, (October 2007), pp. 4918-4926, ISSN 0013-7227.

Caruso, C.; Sánchez, M.; Durand, D.; Pérez, M.C.; Lasaga, M. & Scimonelli, T. (2010). α-Melanocyte-stimulating hormone modulates lipopolysaccharide plus interferon-γ-induced tumor necrosis factor-α expression but not tumor necrosis factor-α receptor expression in cultured hypothalamic neurons. *J Neuroimmunol*, Vol.227, No.1-2, (October 2010), pp. 52-59, ISSN 0165-5728.

Caruso, C.; Carniglia, L.; Durand, D.; Gonzalez, P.V.; Scimonelli, T. & Lasaga, M. (2011). Melanocortin 4 receptor activation induces brain-derived neurotrophic factor expression in rat astrocytes through cyclic AMP - Protein kinase A pathway. *Mol Cell Endocrinol*, doi:10.1016/j.mce.2011.07.036, in press, ISSN 0303-7207.

Catania, A.; Suffredini, A.F. & Lipton, J.M. (1995). Endotoxin causes release of alpha-melanocyte-stimulating hormone in normal human subjects. *Neuroimmunomodulation*, Vol.2, No.5, (September-October 1995), pp. 258-262, ISSN 1021-7401.

Catania, A.; Rajora, N.; Capsoni, F.; Minonzio, F.; Star, R.A. & Lipton, J.M. (1996). The neuropeptide alpha-MSH has specific receptors on neutrophils and reduces chemotaxis in vitro. *Peptides*, Vol.17, No.4, pp. 675-679, ISSN 0196-9781.

Catania, A.; Airaghi, L.; Colombo, G. & Lipton, J.M. (2000). α-melanocyte-stimulating hormone in normal human physiology and disease states. *Trends Endocrinol Metab*, Vol.11, No.8, (October 2000), pp. 304-308, ISSN 1043-2760.

Catania, A.; Gatti, S.; Colombo, G. & Lipton, J.M. (2004). Targeting melanocortin receptors as a novel strategy to control inflammation. *Pharmacol Rev*, Vol.56, No.1, (March 2004), pp. 1-29, ISSN 0031-6997.

Catania, A.; Lonati, C.; Sordi, A.; Leonardi, P.; Carlin, A. & Gatti, S. (2010). The peptide NDP-MSH induces phenotype changes in the heart that resemble ischemic preconditioning. *Peptides*, Vol.31, No.1, (January 2010), pp. 116-122, ISSN 0196-9781.

Chai, B.; Li, J.Y.; Zhang, W.; Newman, E.; Ammori, J. & Mulholland, M.W. (2006). Melanocortin-4 receptor-mediated inhibition of apoptosis in immortalized hypothalamic neurons via mitogen-activated protein kinase. *Peptides*, Vol.27, No.11, (November 2006), pp. 2846-2857, ISSN 0196-9781.

Chai, B.; Li, J.Y.; Zhang, W., Ammori, J.B. & Mulholland, M.W. (2007). Melanocortin-3 receptor activates MAP kinase via PI3 kinase. *Regul Pept*, Vol.139, No.1-3, (March 2007), pp. 115-121, ISSN 0167-0115.

Chai, B.; Li, J.Y.; Zhang, W., Wu, X.; Zhang, C. & Mulholland, M.W. (2010). Melanocortin-4 receptor activation promotes insulin-stimulated mTOR signaling. *Peptides*, Vol.31, No.10, (October 2010), pp. 1888-1893, ISSN 0196-9781.

Chan, L.F.; Webb, T.R.; Chung, T.T.; Meimaridou, E.; Cooray, S.N.; Guasti, L.; Chapple, J.P.; Egertová, M.; Elphick, M.R.; Cheetham, M.E.; Metherell, L.A. & Clark, A.J. (2009). MRAP and MRAP2 are bidirectional regulators of the melanocortin receptor family. *Proc Natl Acad Sci U S A*, Vol.106, No.15, (April 2009), pp. 6146-6151, ISSN 0027-8424.

Chen, A.S.; Marsh, D.J.; Trumbauer, M.E.; Frazier, E.G.; Guan, X.M.; Yu, H.; Rosenblum, C.I.; Vongs, A.; Feng, Y.; Cao, L.; Metzger, J.M.; Strack, A.M.; Camacho, R.E.; Mellin, T.N.; Nunes, C.N.; Min, W.; Fisher, J.; Gopal-Truter, S.; MacIntyre, D.E.; Chen, H.Y. & Van der Ploeq, L.H. (2000). Inactivation of melanocortin type 3 receptor results in increased fat mass and reduced lean body mass. *Nat Genet*, Vol.26, No.1, (September 2000), pp. 97-102, ISSN 1061-4036.

Chen, W.; Kelly, M.A.; Opitz-Araya, X.; Thomas, R.E.; Low, M.J. & Cone R.D. (1997). Exocrine gland dysfunction in MC5-R-deficient mice: evidence for coordinated regulation of exocrine gland function by melanocortin peptides. *Cell*, Vol.91, No.6, (December 1997), pp. 789-798, ISSN 0092-8674.

Chhajlani, V. & Wikberg, J.E. (1992). Molecular cloning and expression of the human melanocyte stimulating hormone receptor cDNA. *FEBS Lett*, Vol.309, No.3, (September 1992), pp. 417-420, ISSN 0014-5793.

Chhajlani, V. (1996). Distribution of cDNA for melanocortin receptor subtypes in human tissues. *Biochem Mol Biol Int*, Vol.38, No.1, (February 1996), pp. 73-80, ISSN 1039-9712.

Chiao, H.; Foster, S.; Thomas, R.; Lipton, J. & Star, R.A. (1996). Alpha-melanocyte-stimulating hormone reduces endotoxin-induced liver inflammation. *J Clin Invest*, Vol.97, No.9, (May 1996), pp. 2038-2044, ISSN 0021-9738.

Chiao, H.; Kohda, Y.; McLeroy, P.; Craig, L.; Housini, I. & Star, R.A. (1997). Alpha-melanocyte-stimulating hormone protects against renal injury after ischemia in mice and rats. *J Clin Invest*,Vol.99, No.6, (March 1997), pp. 1165-1172, ISSN 0021-9738.

Cone, RD. (2005). Anatomy and regulation of the central melanocortin system. *Nat Neurosci*, Vol.8, No.5, (May 2005), pp. 571-578, ISSN 1097-6256.

Cooper, A.; Robinson, S.J.; Pickard C.; Jackson C.L.; Friedman P.S. & Healy E. (2005). Alpha-melanocyte-stimulating hormone suppresses antigen-induced lymphocyte proliferation in humans independently of melanocortin 1 receptor gene status. *J Immunol*, Vol.175, No.7, (October 2005), pp. 4806-4813, ISSN 0022-1767.

Cragnolini, A.B.; Perelló, M.; Schiöth, H.B. & Scimonelli, T.N. (2004). Alpha-MSH and gamma-MSH inhibit IL-1beta induced activation of the hypothalamic-pituitary-adrenal axis through central melanocortin receptors. *Regul Pept*, Vol.122, No.3, (November 2004), pp. 185-190, ISSN 0167-0115.

Cragnolini, A.; Caruso, C.; Lasaga, M. & Scimonelli, T.N. (2006). alpha-MSH and gamma-MSH modulate early release of hypothalamic PGE2 and NO induced by IL-1beta differently. *Neurosci Lett*, Vol.409, No.3, (December 2006), pp. 168-172, ISSN 0304-3940.

Cui, H.S.; Hayasaka, S.; Zhang, X.Y.; Chi, Z.L. & Hayasaka, Y. (2005). Effect of alpha-melanocyte-stimulating hormone on interleukin 8 and monocyte chemotactic protein 1 expression in a human epithelial cell line. *Ophthalmic Res*, Vol.37, No.5, (September-October 2005), pp. 279-288, ISSN 0030-3747.

Czyzyk, T.A.; Sikorski, M.A.; Yang, L. & McKnight, S. (2008). Disruption of the RIIβ subunit of PKA reverses the obesity syndrome of agouti lethal yellow mice. *Proc Natl Acad Sci U S A*, Vol.105, No.1, (January 2008), pp. 276-281, ISSN 0027-8424.

Daynes, R.A.; Robertson, B.A.; Cho, B.H.; Burnham, D.K. & Newton, R. (1987). Alpha-melanocyte-stimulating hormone exhibits target cell selectivity in its capacity to affect interleukin 1-inducible responses in vivo and in vitro. *J Immunol*, Vol.139, No.1, (July 1987), pp. 103-109, ISSN 0022-1767.

Delgado Hernandez, R.; Demitri, M.T.; Carlin, A.; Meazza, C.; Villa, P.; Ghezzi, P.; Lipton, J.M. & Catania, A. (1999). Inhibition of systemic inflammation by central action of the neuropeptide α-melanocyte-stimulating hormone. *Neuroimmunomodulation*, Vol.6, No.3, (May-June 1999), pp. 187-192, ISSN 1021-7401.

Delgado, R.; Carlin, A.; Airaghi, L.; Demitri, M.T.; Meda, L.; Galimberti, D.; Baron, P.; Lipton, J.M. & Catania, A. (1998). Melanocortin peptides inhibit production of proinflammatory cytokines and nitric oxide by activated microglia. *J Leukoc Biol*, Vol.63, No.6, (June 1998), pp. 740-745, ISSN 0741-5400.

Deng, J.; Xuzhen, H.; Yuen, P. & Star, R. (2004). α-Melanocyte-stimulating hormone inhibits lung injury after renal ischemia/reperfusion. *Am J Respir Crit Care Med*, Vol.169, No.6, (March 2004), pp. 749-756, ISSN 1073-449X.

Dinulescu, D.M. & Cone, R.D. (2000). Agouti and agouti-related protein: Analogies and contrasts. *J Biol Chem*, Vol.275, Nro.10, (March 2000), pp. 6695-6698, ISSN 0021-9258.

Elias, L.L., Huebner, A.; Pullinger, G.S.; Mirtella, A. & Clark, A.J. (1999). Functional characterization of naturally occurring mutations of the human adrenocorticotropin receptor: poor correlation of phenotype and genotype. *J Clin Endocrinol Metab*, Vol.84, No.8, (August 1999), pp. 2766-2770, ISSN 0021-972X.

Eves, P.; Haycock, J.; Layton, C.; Wagner, M.; Kemp, H.; Szabo, M.; Morandini, R.; Ghanem, G.; García-Borrón, J.C.; Jiménez-Cervantes, C. & Mac Neil, S. (2003). Anti-inflammatory and anti-invasive effects of alpha-melanocyte-stimulating hormone in human melanoma cells. *Br J Cancer*, Vol.89, No.10, (November 2003), pp. 2004-2015, ISSN 0007-0920.

Forslin Aronsson, A.; Spulber, S.; Popescu, L.M.; Winblad, B.; Post, C.; Oprica, M. & Schultzberg M. (2006). α-Melanocyte-stimulating hormone is neuroprotective in rat global cerebral ischemia. *Neuropeptides*, Vol.40, No.1, (February 2006), pp. 65-75, ISSN0143-4179.

Forslin Aronsson, A.; Spulber, S.; Oprica, M.; Winblad, B.; Post, C. & Schultzberg, M. (2007). α-MSH rescues neurons from excitotoxic cell death. *J Mol Neurosci*, Vol.33, No.3, pp. 239-251, ISSN 0895-8696.

Frota, E.R.; Rodrigues, D.H.; Donadi, E.A.; Brum, D.G.; Maciel, D.R. & Teixeira AL. (2009). Increased plasma levels of brain derived neurotrophic factor (BDNF) after multiple sclerosis relapse. *Neurosci Lett*, Vol.460, No.2, (August 2009), pp. 130-132, ISSN 0304-3940.

Galimberti, D.; Baron, P.; Meda, L.; Prat, E.; Scarpini, E.; Delgado, R.; Catania, A. & Lipton, J.M. (1999). α-MSH peptides inhibit production of nitric oxide and TNF-α by activated microglial cells activated with β-amyloid and interferon-γ. *Biochem Biophys Res Commun*, Vol.263, No.1, (September 1999), pp. 251-256, ISSN 0006-291X.

Gantz, I.; Konda, Y.; Tashiro, T.; Shimoto, Y.; Miwa, H.; Munzert, G.; Watson, S.J.; DelValle, J. & Yamada T. (1993). Molecular cloning of a novel melanocortin receptor. *J Biol Chem*, Vol.268, No.11, (April 1993), pp. 8246-8250, ISSN 0021-9258.

Gantz, I.; Shimoto, Y.; Konda, Y.; Miwa, H.; Dickinson, C.J. & Yamada, T. (1994). Molecular cloning, expression, and characterization of a fifth melanocortin receptor. *Biochem Biophys Res Commun*, Vol.200, No.3, (May 1994), pp. 1214-1220, ISSN 0006-291X.

Gatti, S.; Carlin, A.; Sordi, A.; Leonardi, P.; Colombo, G.; Fassati, L.R.; Lipton, J.M. & Catania, A. (2006). Inhibitory effects of the peptide (CKPV)2 on endotoxin-induced host reactions. *J Surg Res*, Vol.131, No.2, (April 2006), pp. 209-214, ISSN 0022-4804.

Getting, S.J; Gibbs, L.; Clark, A.J.; Flower, R.J. & Perretti, M. (1999). POMC Gene-Derived Peptides Activate Melanocortin Type 3 Receptor on Murine Macrophages, Suppress Cytokine Release, and Inhibit Neutrophil Migration in Acute Experimental Inflammation. *J Immunol*, Vol.162, No.12, (June 1999), pp. 7446-7453, ISSN 0022-1767.

Getting, S.J.; Lam, C.W.; Leoni, G.; Gavins, F.N.; Grieco, P. & Perretti, M. (2006). [D-Trp8]-gamma-melanocyte-stimulating hormone exhibits anti-inflammatory efficacy in mice bearing a nonfunctional MC1R (recessive yellow e/e mouse). *Mol Pharmacol*, Vol.70, No.6, (December 2006), pp. 1850-1855, ISSN 0026-895X.

Getting, S.J.; Riffo-Vasquez, Y.; Pitchford, S.; Kaneva, M.; Grieco, P.; Page, C.P.; Perretti, M. & Spina, D. (2008). A role for MC3R in modulating lung inflammation. *Pulm Pharmacol Ther*, Vol.21, Nro.6, (December 2008), pp. 866-873, ISSN 1094-5539.

Gibson, S.; Crosby, S.R.; Stewart, M.F.; Jennings, A.M.; McCall, E. & White, A. (1994). Differential release of proopiomelanocortin-derived peptides from the human pituitary: evidence from a panel of two-site immunoradiometric assays. *J Clin Endocrinol Metab*, Vol.78, No.4, (April 1994), pp. 835-841, ISSN 0021-972X.

Giuliani, D.; Mioni, C.; Altavilla, D.; Leone, S.; Bazzani, C.; Minutoli, L.; Bitto, A.; Cainazzo, M.; Marini, H.; Zaffe, D.; Botticelli, A.; Pizzala, R.; Savio, M.; Necchi, D.; Schioth, H.B.; Bertolini, A.; Squadrito, F. & Guarini, S. (2006). Both early and delayed treatment with melanocortin 4 receptor-stimulating melanocortins produces neuroprotection in cerebral ischemia. *Endocrinology*, Vol.147, No.3, (March 2006), pp. 1126-1135, ISSN 0013-7227.

Giuliani, D.;Ottani, A.; Mioni, C.; Bazzani, C.;Galantucci, M.; Minutoli, L.; Bitto, A.; Zaffe, D.; Botticelli, A.R.; Squadrito, F. & Guarini, S. (2007a). Neuroprotection in focal cerebral ischemia owing to delayed treatment with melanocortins. *Eur J Pharmacol*, Vol.570, No.1-3, (September 2007), pp. 57-65, ISSN 0014-2999.

Giuliani, D.; Mioni, C.; Bazzani, C.; Zaffe, D.; Botticelli, A.R.; Capolongo, S.; Sabba, A. Galantucci, M.; Iannone, A.; Grieco, P.; Novellino, E.; Colombo, G.; Tomasi, A.; Catania, A. & Guarini, S. (2007b). Selective melanocortin MC4 receptor agonists reverse haemorrhagic shock and prevent multiple organ damage. *Br J Pharmacol*, Vol.150, No.5, (March 2007), pp. 595-603, ISSN 0007-1188.

Giuliani, D.; Ottani, A.; Minutoli, L.; Stefano, V.D.; Galantucci, M.; Bitto, A.; Zaffe, D.; Altavilla, D.; Botticelli, A.R.; Squadrito, F. & Guarini, S. (2009). Functional recovery after delayed treatment of ischemic stroke with melanocortins is associated with overexpression of the activity-dependent gene Zif268. *Brain Behav Immun*, Vol.23, No.6, (August 2009), pp. 844-850, ISSN 0889-1591.

Gonindard, C.; Goigoux, C.; Hollande, E. & D'Hinterland, L.D. (1996). The Administration of an α-MSH Analogue Reduces the Serum Release of IL-1α and TNFα Induced by the Injection of a Sublethal Dose of Lipopolysaccharides in the BALB/c Mouse. *Pigment Cell Res*, Vol.9, No.3, (June 1996), pp. 148-153, ISSN 0893-5785.

Gonzalez, P.V.; Schiöth, H.B.; Lasaga, M. & Scimonelli, T.N. (2009). Memory impairment induced by IL-1beta is reversed by alpha-MSH through central melanocortin-4 receptors. *Brain Behav Immun*, Vol.23, No.6, (Aug 2009), pp. 817-822, ISSN 0889-1591.

Grabbe, S.; Bhardwaj, R.S.; Mahnke, K.; Simon, M.M.; Schwarz, T. & Luger, T.A. (1996). Alpha-melanocyte-stimulating hormone induces hapten-specific tolerance in mice. *J Immunol*, Vol.156, No.2, (January 1996), pp. 473-478, ISSN 0022-1767.

Griffon, N.; Mignon, V.; Facchinetti, P.; Diaz, J.; Schwartz, J.C. & Sokoloff, P. (1994). Molecular cloning and characterization of the rat fifth melanocortin receptor. *Biochem Biophys Res Commun*, Vol.200, No.2, (April 1994), pp. 1007-1014, ISSN 0006-291X.

Guarini, S.; Schiöth, H.B.; Mioni, C.; Cainazzo, M.; Ferraza, G.; Giuliani, D.; Wikberg, J.E.; Bertoni, A. & Bazzani, C. (2002). MC(3) receptors are involved in the protective effect of melanocortins in myocardial ischemia/reperfusion-induced arrhythmias. *Naunyn Schmiedeberg's Arch Pharmacol*, Vol.366, No.2, (August 2002), pp. 177-182, ISSN 0028-1298.

Han, D.; Tian, Y.; Zhang, M.; Zhou, Z. & Lu, J. (2007). Prevention and treatment of experimental autoimmune encephalomyelitis with recombinant adeno-associated virus-mediated alpha-melanocyte-stimulating hormone-transduced PLP139-151-specific T cells. *Gene Ther, Vol.*14, No.5, (March 2007), pp. 383-395, ISSN 0969-7128.

Hartmeyer, M.; Scholzen, T.; Becher, E.; Bhardwaj, R.S.; Schwarz, T. & Luger, T.A. (1997). Human dermal microvascular endothelial cells express the melanocortin receptor type 1 and produce increased levels IL-8 upon stimulation with α-melanocyte-stimulating hormone. *J Immunol*, Vol.159, No.4, (August 1997), pp. 1930-1937, ISSN 0022-1767.

Haskell-Luevano, C. & Monek, E.K. (2001). Agouti-related protein functions as an inverse agonist at a constitutively active brain melanocortin-4 receptor. *Regul Pept*, Vol.99, No.1, (May 2001), pp. 1-7, ISSN 0167-0115.

He, L.; Gunn, T.M.; Bouley, D.M.; Lu, X.Y.; Watson, S.J.; Schlossman, S.F.; Duke-Cohan, J.S. & Barsh, G.S. (2001). A biochemical function for attractin in agouti-induced pigmentation and obesity. *Nat Genet*, Vol.27, No.1, (January 2001), pp. 40-47, ISSN 1061-4036.

Herraiz, C.; Journé, F.; Abdel-Malek, Z.; Ghanem, G.; Jiménez-Cervantes, C. & García-Borrón, J.C. (2011). Signaling from the human melanocortin 1 receptor to ERK1 and ERK2 mitogen-activated protein kinases involves transactivation of cKIT. *Mol Endocrinol*, Vol.25, No.1, (January 2011), pp. 138-156, ISSN 0888-8809.

Huang, Q.H.; Entwistle, M.L.; Alvaro, J.D.; Duman, R.S.; Hruby, V.J. & Tatro, J.B. (1997). Antipyretic role of endogenous melanocortins mediated by central melanocortin receptors during endotoxin-induced fever. *J Neurosci*, Vol.17, No.9, (May 1997), pp. 3343-3351, ISSN 0270-6474.

Huang, Q.H.; Hruby, V.J. & Tatro, J.B. (1998). Systemic α-MSH suppresses LPS fever via central melanocortin receptors independently of its suppression of corticosterone and IL-6 release. *Am J Physiol*, Vol.275, No.2Pt2, (August 1998), pp. R524-R530, ISSN 0002-9513.

Huang, Q. & Tatro, J.B. (2002). Alpha-MSH suppress intracerebral tumor necrosis factor-α and interleukin-1β gene expression following transient cerebral ischemia in mice. *Neurosci Lett*, Vol.334, No.3, (December 2002), pp. 186-190, ISSN 0304-3940.

Huszar, D.; Lynch, C.A.; Fairchild-Huntress, V.; Dunmore, J.H.; Fang, Q.; Berkemeier, L.R.; Gu, W.; Kesterson, R.A.; Boston, B.A. & Cone, R.D. (1997). Targeted disruption of the melanocortin-4 receptor results in obesity in mice. *Cell*, Vol.88, No.1, (January 1997), pp. 131-141, ISSN 0092-8674.

Ichiyama, T.; Sakai, T.; Catania, A.; Barsh, G.S.; Furukawa, S. & Lipton, J.M. (1999). Systemically administered α-melanocyte-stimulating peptides inhibit NF-kappaB activation in experimental brain inflammation. *Brain Res*, Vol.836, No.1-2, (July 1999), pp. 31-37, ISSN 0006-8993.

Isales, C.M.; Zaidi. M. & Blair, H.C. (2010). ACTH is a novel regulator of bone mass. *Ann N Y Acad Sci*, Vol.1192, (March 2010), pp. 110-116, ISSN 0077-8923.

Jégou, S.; Boutelet, I. & Vaudry, H. (2000). Melanocortin-3 receptor mRNA expression in pro-opiomelanocortin neurones of the rat arcuate nucleus. *J Neuroendocrinol*, Vol.12, Nro.6, (June 2000), pp. 501-505, ISSN 0953-8194.

Joosten, E.A.; Majewska, B.; Houweling, D.A.; Bar, P.R. & Gispen W.H. (1999). Alpha-melanocyte stimulating hormone promotes regrowth of injured axons in the adult rat spinal cord. *J Neurotrauma*, Vol.16, No.6, (June 1999), pp. 543-553, ISSN 0897-7151.

Kask, A.; Mutulis, F.; Muceniece, R.; Pähkla, R.; Mutule, I.; Wikberg, J.S.; Rägo, L. & Schiöth H.B. (1998). Discovery of a novel superpotent and selective melanocortin 4 receptor antagonist (HS024): Evaluation in vitro and in vivo. *Endocrinology*, Vol.139, No.12, (December 1998), pp. 5006-5014, ISSN 0013-7227.

Katsuura, G.; Gottschall, P.E.; Dahl, R.R. & Arimura, A. (1989). Interleukin-1 beta increases prostaglandin E2 in rat astrocyte cultures: modulatory effect of neuropeptides. *Endocrinology*, Vol.124, No.6, (June 1989), pp. 3125-3127, ISSN0013-7227.

Kawai, Y.; Inagaki, S.; Shiosaka, S.; Shibasaki, T.; Ling, N.; Tohyama, M. & Shiotani, Y. (1984). The distribution and projection of gamma-melanocyte stimulating hormone in the rat brain: an immunohistochemical analysis. *Brain Res*, Vol.29, No.1, (April 1984), pp. 21-32, ISSN 0006-8993.

Kennedy, C.; ter Huurne, J.; Berkhout, M.; Gruis, N.; Bastiaens, M.; Bergman, W.; Willemze, R. & Bavinck, J.N. (2001). Melanocortin 1 receptor (MC1R) gene variants are associated with an increased risk for cutaneous melanoma which is largely independent of skin type and hair color. *J Invest Dermatol*, Vol.117, No.2, (August 2001), pp. 294-300, ISSN 0022-202X.

Kannengiesser, K.; Maaser, C.; Heidemann, J.; Luegering, A.; Ross, M.; Brzoska, T.; Böhm, M.; Luger, T.A.; Domschke, W. & Kucharzik, T. (2008). Melanocortin-derived tripeptide KPV has anti-inflammatory potential in murine models of inflammatory bowel disease. *Inflamm Bowel Dis*, Vol.14, No.3, (March 2008), pp. 324-331, ISSN 1078-0998.

Konda, Y.; Gantz, I.; Del Valle, J.; Shimoto, Y.; Miwa, H. & Yamada, T. (1994). Interaction of dual intracellular signaling pathways activated by the melanocortin-3 receptor. *J Biol Chem*, Vol. 269, No.18, (May 1994), pp. 13162-13166, ISSN 0021-9258.

Krude, H.; Biebermann, H.; Luck, W.; Horn, R.; Brabant, G. & Grüters, A. (1998). Severe early-onset obesity, adrenal insufficiency and red hair pigmentation caused by POMC mutations in humans. *Nat Genet*, Vol.19, No.2, (June 1998), pp. 155-157, ISSN 1061-4036.

Labbé, O.; Desarnaud, F.; Eggerickx, D.; Vassart, G. & Parmentier, M. (1994). Molecular cloning of a mouse melanocortin 5 receptor gene widely expressed in peripheral tissues. *Biochemistry*, Vol.33, No.15, (April 1994), pp. 4543-4549, ISSN 0006-2960.

Lam, C.W.; Getting, S.J. & Perretti, M. (2005). In vitro and in vivo induction of heme oxygenase 1 in mouse macrophages following melanocortin receptor activation. *J Immunol*, Vol.174, No.4, (February 2005), pp. 2297-2304, ISSN 0022-1767.

Langouche, L.; Pals, K. & Denef, C. (2002). Structure–activity relationship and signal transduction of γ-MSH peptides in GH3 cells: further evidence for a new melanocortin receptor. *Peptides*, Vol.23, No.6, (June 2002), pp. 1077-1086, ISSN 0196-9781.

Lasaga, M.; Debeljuk, L.; Durand, D.; Scimonelli, T.N. & Caruso, C. (2008). Role of alpha-melanocyte stimulating hormone and melanocortin 4 receptor in brain inflammation. *Peptides*, Vol.29, No.10, (October 2008), pp. 1825-1835, ISSN 0196-9781.

Lee, D.J.; Biros, D.J. & Taylor, A.W. (2009). Injection of an alpha-melanocyte stimulating hormone expression plasmid is effective in suppressing experimental autoimmune uveitis. *Int Immunopharmacol*, Vol.9, No.9, (August 2009), pp. 1079-1086, ISSN 1567-5769.

Leoni, G.; Voisin, M.B.; Carlson, K.; Getting, S.; Nourshargh, S. & Perretti, M. (2010). The melanocortin MC(1) receptor agonist BMS-470539 inhibits leucocyte trafficking in the inflamed vasculature. *Br J Pharmacol*, Vol.160, No.1, (May 2010), pp. 171-180, ISSN 0007-1188.

Li, Q. & Verma, I.M. (2002). NF-kappaB regulation in the immune system. *Nat Rev Immunol*, Vol.2, No.10, (October 2002), pp. 725-734, ISSN 1474-1733.

Liakos, P.; Chambaz, E.M.; Feige, J.J. & Defaye, G. (1998). Expression of ACTH receptors (MC2-R and MC5-R) in the glomerulosa and the fasciculata-reticularis zones of bovine adrenal cortex. *Endocr Res*, Vol.24, No.3-4, (Aug-Nov 1998), pp. 427-432, ISSN 0743-5800.

Liedtke, W.; Edelman, W.; Chiu, F-C.; Kucherlapati, R. & Raine, C. (1998). Experimental autoinmune encephalomyelitis in mice lacking glial fibrillary acidic protein is characterized by a more severe clinical course and an infiltrative central nervous system lesion. *Am J Pathol*, Vol.152, No.1, (January 1998), pp. 251-259, ISSN 0002-9440.

Lin, S.Y.; Chaves, C.; Wiedemann, E. & Humphreys, M.H. (1987). A γ-melanocyte stimulating hormone-like peptide causes reflex natriuresis after acute unilateral nephrectomy. *Hypertension*, Vol.10, No.6, (December 1987), pp. 619-627, ISSN 0194-911X.

Lindberg, C.; Hjorth, E.; Post, C.; Winblad, B. & Schultzberg, M. (2005). Cytokine production by a human microglial cell line: effects of β-amyloid and α-melanocyte-stimulating hormone. *Neurotox Res*, Vol.8, No.3-4, (November 2005), pp. 267-276, ISSN 1029-8428.

Lipton, J.M.; Ceriani, G.; Macaluso, A.; McCoy, D.; Carnes, K.; Biltz, J. & Catania, A. (1994). Anti-inflammatory effects of the neuropeptide α-MSH in acute, chronic and systemic inflammation. *Ann NY Acad Sci*, Vol.741, (November 1994), pp. 137-148, ISSN 0077-8923.

Lipton, J.M.; Zhao, H.; Ichiyama, T.; Barsh, G.S. & Catania, A. (1999). Mechanism of antiinflammatory action of α-MSH peptides: in vivo and in vitro evidence. *Ann NY Acad Sci*, Vol.885, (October 1999), pp. 173-182, ISSN 0077-8923.

Luger, T.A.; Scholzen, T.E.; Brzoska, T. & Böhm, M. (2003). New insights into the functions of alpha-MSH and related peptides in the immune system. *Ann NY Acad Sci*, Vol.994, (June 2003), pp. 133-140, ISSN 0077-8923.

Machado, I.; González, P.; Schiöth, H.B.; Lasaga, M. & Scimonelli, T.N. (2010). α-Melanocyte-stimulating hormone (α-MSH) reverses impairment of memory reconsolidation induced by interleukin-1 beta (IL-1 beta) hippocampal infusions. *Peptides*, Vol.31, No.11, (November 2010), pp. 2141-2144, ISSN 0196-9781.

Manna, S.K. & Aggarwal, B.B. (1998). Alpha-melanocyte-stimulating hormone inhibits the nuclear transcription factor NF-kappa B activation induced by various inflammatory agents. *J Immunol*, Vol.161, No.6, (September 1998), pp. 2873-2880, ISSN 0022-1767.

Manna, S.K.; Sarkar, A. & Sreenivasan, Y. (2006). Alpha-melanocyte-stimulating hormone down-regulates CXC receptors through activation of neutrophil elastase. *Eur J Immunol*, Vol.36, No.3, (March 2006), pp. 754-769, ISSN 0014-2980.

Mandrika, I.; Muceniece, R. & Wikberg, J.E. (2001). Effects of melanocortin peptides on lipopolysaccharide/interferon-gamma-induced NF-kappaB DNA binding and nitric oxide production in macrophage-like RAW 264.7 cells: evidence for dual mechanisms of action. *Biochem Pharmacol*, Vol.61, No.5, (March 2001), pp. 613-621, ISSN 0006-2952.

Maragakis, N.J. & Rothstein, J.D. (2006). Mechanism of disease: astrocytes in neurodegenerative disease. *Nat Clin Pract Neurol*, Vol.2, No.12, (December 2006), pp. 679-689, ISSN 1745-834X.

Marsh, D.J.; Hollopeter, G.; Huszar, D.; Laufer, R.; Yagaloff, K.A.; Fisher, S.L.; Burn, P. & Palmiter, R.D. (1999). Response of melanocortin-4 receptor-deficient mice to anorectic and orexigenic peptides. *Nat Genet*, Vol.21, No.1, (January 1999), pp. 119-122, ISSN 1061-4036.

Martin, L.W.; Catania, A.; Hiltz, M.E. & Lipton, J.M. (1991). Neuropeptide α-MSH antagonizes IL-6 and TNF-induced fever. *Peptides,* Vol.12, No.2, (March-April 1991), pp. 119-122, ISSN 0196-9781.

Mastrofrancesco, A.; Kokot, A.; Eberle, A.; Gibbons, N.C.; Schallreuter, K.U.; Strozyk, E.; Picardo, M.; Zouboulis, C.C.; Luger, T.A. & Böhm, M. (2010). KdPT, a tripeptide derivative of alpha-melanocyte-stimulating hormone, suppresses IL-1 beta-mediated cytokine expression and signaling in human sebocytes. *J Immunol,* Vol.185, No.3, (August 2010), pp. 1903-1911, ISSN 0022-1767.

McGeer, P.L. & McGeer, E.G. (2007). NSAIDs and Alzheimer disease: epidemiological, animal model and clinical studies. *Neurobiol Aging,* Vol.28, No.5, (May 2007), pp. 639-647, ISSN 0197-4580.

Metherell, L.A.; Chapple, J.P.; Cooray, S.;David, A.; Becker, C.; Rüschendorf, F.; Naville, D.; Begeot, M.; Khoo, B.; Nürnberg, P.; Huebner, A.; Cheetham, M.E. & Clark, A.J. (2005). Mutations in MRAP, encoding a new interacting partner of the ACTH receptor, cause familial glucocorticoid deficiency type 2. *Nat Genet,* Vol.37, No.2, (February 2005), pp. 166-170, ISSN 1061-4036.

Miller, M.W.; Duhl, D.M.; Vrieling, H.; Cordes, S.P.; Ollman, M.M.; Winkes, B.M. & Barsh G.S. (1993). Cloning of the mouse agouti gene predicts a secreted protein ubiquitously expressed in mice carrying the lethal yellow mutation. *Genes Dev,* Vol.7, No.3, (March 1993), pp. 454-467, ISSN 0890-9369.

Minutoli, L. ; Squadrito, F. ; Nicotina, P.A. ; Giuliani, D. ; Ottani, A. ; Polito, F. ; Bitto, A. ; Irrera, N. ; Guzzo, G. ; Spaccapelo, L. ; Fazzari, C. ; Macrì, A. ; Marini, H. ; Guarini, S. & Altavilla, D. (2011). Melanocortin 4 receptor stimulation decreases pancreatitis severity in rats by activation of the cholinergic anti-inflammatory pathway. *Crit Care Med,* Vol.162, No.4, (February 2011), pp. 917-928, ISSN 0090-3493.

Mirtella, A.; Tringali, G.; Guerriero, G.; Ghiara, P.; Parente, L.; Preziosi, P. & Navarra, P. (1995). Evidence that the interleukin-1 beta-induced prostaglandin E2 release from rat hypothalamus is mediated by type I and type II interleukin-1 receptors. *J Neuroimmunol,* Vol.61, No.2, (September 1995), pp. 171-177, ISSN 0165-5728.

Mountjoy, K.; Robbins, L.; Mortrud, L. & Cone, R.D. (1992). The cloning of a family of genes that encode the melanocortin receptors. *Science,* Vol.257, No.5074, (August 1992), pp. 1248-1251, ISSN 0036-8075.

Mountjoy, K.; Mortrud, L.; Low, M.J.; Simerkly, R.B. & Cone, R.D. (1994). Localization of the melanocortin-4 receptor (MC4-R) in neuroendocrine and autonomic control circuits in the brain. *Mol Endocrinol,* Vol.8, No.10, (October 1994), pp. 1298-1308, ISSN 0888-8809.

Muceniece, R.; Zvejniece, L.; Kirjanova, O.; Liepinsh, E.; Krigere, L.; Baumane, L.; Kalvinsh, I.; Wikberg, J.E. & Dambrova, M. (2004). Beta- and gamma-melanocortins inhibit lipopolysaccharide induced nitric oxide production in mice brain. *Brain Res,* Vol.995, No.1, (January 2004), pp. 7-13, ISSN 0006-8993.

Muceniece, R.; Zvejniece, L.; Vilskersts, R.; Liepinsh, E.; Baumane, L.; Kalvinsh, I.; Wikberg, J.E. & Dambrova, M. (2007). Functional evaluation of THIQ, a melanocortin 4 receptor agonist, in models of food intake and inflammation. *Basic Clin Pharmacol Toxicol,* Vol.101, No.6, (December 2007), pp. 416-420, ISSN 1742-7835.

Muffley, L.A.; Zhu, Q.K.; Engray, L.H.; Gibran, N.S. & Hocking, A.M. (2011). Spatial and temporal localization of the melanocortin 1 receptor and its ligand α-melanocyte-stimulating hormone during cutaneous wound repair. *J Histochem Cytochem*, Vol.59., No.3, (March 2011), pp. 278-288, ISSN 0022-1554.

Murphy, M.T.; Richards, D.B. & Lipton, J.M. (1983). Antipyretic potency of centrally administered alpha-melanocyte stimulating hormone. *Science*, Vol.221, No.4606, (July 1983), pp. 192-193, ISSN 0036-8075.

Nagahara, A.H. & Tuszynski, M.H. (2011). Potential therapeutic uses of BDNF in neurological and psychiatric disorders. *Nat Rev Drug Discov*, Vol.10, No.3, (March 2011), pp. 209-219, ISSN 1474-1776.

Newman, E.A.; Chai, B.X.; Zhang, W.; Li, J.Y.; Ammori, J.B. & Mulholland, M.W. (2006). Activation of the melanocortin-4 receptor mobilizes intracellular free calcium in immortalized hypothalamic neuron. *J Surg Res*, Vol.132, No.2, (May 2006), pp. 201-2077, ISSN 0022-4804.

Nicolaou, A.; Estdale, S.E.; Tsatmali, M.; Herrero, D.P. & Thody, A.J. (2004). Prostaglandin production by melanocytic cells and the effect of alpha-melanocyte stimulating hormone. *FEBS Lett*, Vol.570, No.1-3, (July 2004), pp. 223-226, ISSN 0014-5793.

O´Donohue, T.L. & Dorsa, D.M. (1982). The opiomelanotropinergic neuronal and endocrine systems. *Peptides*, Vol. 3, Nro.3, (May-June 1982), pp. 353-395, ISSN 0196-9781.

Ollman, M.M.; Wilson, B.D.; Yang, Y.K.; Kerns, J.A.; Chen, Y.; Gantz, I. & Barsh, G.S. (1997). Antagonism of central melanocortin receptors in vitro and in vivo by agouti-related protein. *Science*, Vol.278, No.5335, (October 1997), pp. 135-138, ISSN 0036-8075.

Patten, C.S.; Daniels, D.; Suzuki, A.; Fluharty, S.J. & Yee, D.K. (2007). Structural and signaling requirements of the human melanocortin 4 receptor for MAP kinase activation. *Regul Pept*, Vol.142, No.3, (August 2007), pp. 111-122, ISSN 0167-0115.

Pérez-Oliva, A.B.; Olivares, C.; Jiménez-Cervantes, C. & García-Borrón, J.C. (2009). Mahogunin ring finger-1 (MGRN1) E3 ubiquitin ligase inhibits signaling from melanocortin receptor by competition with Galphas. *J Biol Chem*, Vol.284, No.46, (November 2009), pp. 31714-31725, ISSN 0021-9258.

Pinessi, L.; Rainero, I.; de Gennaro, T.; Violante, A.; Cassano, D.; Matera, L. & Cesano, A. (1992). Cerebrospinal fluid and plasma concentrations of POMC-related peptides in multiple sclerosis. *Ann N Y Acad Sci*, Vol.650, (April 1992), pp. 351-354, ISSN 0077-8923.

Plantinga, L.C.; Verhaagen, J.; Edwards, P.M.; Hali, M.; Brakkee, J.H. & Gispen, W.H. (1995). Pharmacological evidence for the involvement of endogenous alpha-MSH-like peptides in peripheral nerve regeneration. *Peptides*, Vol.16, pp. 319-324, ISSN 0196-9781.

Raap, U.; Brzoska, T.; Sohl, S.; Päth, G.; Emmel, J.; Herz, U.; Braun, A.; Luger, T. & Renz, H. (2003). Alpha-melanocyte-stimulating hormone inhibits allergic airway inflammation. *J Immunol*, Vol.171, No.1, (July 2003), pp. 353-359, ISSN 0022-1767.

Rajora, N.; Boccoli, G.; Burns, D.; Sharma, S.; Catania, A. & Lipton, J.M. (1997a). α-MSH modulates local and circulating tumor necrosis factor-α in experimental brain inflammation. *J Neurosci*, Vol.17, No.6, (March 1997), pp. 2181-2186, ISSN 0270-6474.

Rajora, N.; Boccoli, G.; Catania, A. & Lipton, J.M. (1997b). α-MSH modulates experimental inflammatory bowel disease. *Peptides*, Vol.18, No.3, pp. 381-385, ISSN 0196-9781.

Redondo, P.; Garcia-Foncillas, J.; Okroujnov, I. & Bandrés, E. (1998). α-MSH regulates interleukin-10 expression by human keratinocytes. *Arch Dermatol Res*, Vol.290, No.8, (August 1998), pp. 425-428, ISSN 0340-3696.

Reizes, O.; Benoit, S.C.; Strader, A.D.; Clegg, D.J.; Akunuru, S. & Seeley, R.J. (2003). Syndecan-3 modulates food intake by interacting with the melanocortin/AgRP pathway. *Ann N Y Acad Sci*, Vol.994, (June 2003), pp. 66-73, ISSN 0077-8923.

Rodrigues, A.R.; Pignatelli, D.; Almeida, H. & Gouveia, A.M. (2009). Melanocortin 5 receptor activates ERK1/2 through a PI3K-regulated signalling mechanism. *Mol Cell Endocrinol*, Vol.303, No.1-2, (May 2009), pp. 74-81, ISSN 0303-7207.

Roselli-Rehfuss, L.; Mountjoy, K.; Robbins, L.; Mortrud, L.; Low, M.; Tatro, J.; Entwistle M.; Simerly, R. & Cone, R. D. (1993). Identification of a receptor for γ melanotropin and other proopiomelanocortin peptides in the hypothalamus and limbic system. *Proc Natl Acad Sci USA*, Vol.90, No.19, (October 1993), pp. 8856-8860, ISSN 0027-8424.

Roy, S.; Rached, M. & Gallo-Payet, N. (2007). Differential regulation of the human adrenocorticotropin receptor [melanocortin-2 receptor (MC2R)] by human MC2R accessory protein isoforms alpha and beta in isogenic human embryonic kidney 293 cells. *Mol Endocrinology*, Vol.21, No.7, (July 2007), pp. 1656-1669, ISSN 0888-8809.

Roy, S.; Pinard, S.; Chouinard, L. & Gallo-Payet, N. (2011). Adrenocorticotropin hormone (ACTH) effects on MAPK phosphorylation in human fasciculata cells and in embryonic kidney 293 cells expressing human melanocortin 2 receptor (MC2R) and MC2R accessory protein (MRAP)β. *Mol Cell Endocrinol*, Vol.336, No.1-2, (April 2011), pp 31-40, ISSN 0303-7207.

Sabat, R.; Grütz, G.; Warszawska, K.; Kirsch, S.; Witte, E.; Wolk, K. & Geginat, J. (2010). Biology of interleukin-10. *Cytokine Growth Factor Rev*, Vol.21, No.5, (October 2010), pp. 331-344, ISSN 1359-6101.

Sandyk, R. & Awerbuch, G.I. (1992). Nocturnal plasma melatonin and alpha-melanocyte stimulating hormone levels during exacerbation of multiple sclerosis. *Int J Neurosci*, Vol.67, No.1-4, (November-December 1992), pp. 173-186, ISSN 0020-7454.

Sarkar, A.; Sreenivasan, Y. & Manna, S.K. (2003). Alpha-melanocyte-stimulating hormone induces cell death in mast cells: involvement of NF-kappa B. *FEBS Lett*, Vol.549, No.1-3, (August 2003), pp. 87-93, ISSN 0014-5793.

Sarkar, S.; Légradi, G. & Lechan, R.M. (2002). Intracerebroventricular of alpha-melanocyte stimulating hormone increases phosphorylation of CREB in TRH- and CRH-neurons of the hypothalamic paraventricular nucleus. *Brain Res*, Vol.945, No.1, (July 2002), pp. 50-59, ISSN 0006-8993.

Sawyer, T.K.; Sanfilippo, P.J.; Hruby, V.J.; Engel, M.H.; Heward, C.B.; Burnett, J.B. & Hadley, M.E. (1980). 4-Norleucine, 7-D-phenylalanine-alpha-melanocyte-stimulating hormone: a highly potent alpha-melanotropin with ultralong biological activity. *Proc Natl Acad Sci USA*, Vol.77, No.10, (October 1980), pp. 5754-5758, ISSN 0027-8424.

Schiöth, H.B.; Chhajlani, V.; Muceniece, R.; Klusa, V. & Wikberg, J.E. (1996). Major pharmacological distinction of the ACTH receptor from other melanocortin receptors. *Life Sci*, Vol.59, No.10, pp. 797-801, ISSN 0024-3205.

Schiöth, H.B.; Muceniece, R.; Mutulis, F.; Bouifrouri, A.A.; Mutule, I. & Wikberg, J.E. (1999). Further pharmacological characterization of the selective melanocortin 4 receptor antagonist HS014: comparison with SHU9119. *Neuropeptides*, Vol.33, No.3, (June 1999), pp. 191-196, ISSN 0143-4179.

Scholzen, T.E.; Sunderkötter, C.; Kalden, D.H.; Brzoska, T.; Fastrich, M.; Fisbeck, T.; Armstrong, C.A.; Ansel, J.C. & Luger, T.A. (2003). Alpha-melanocyte stimulating hormone prevents lipopolysaccharide-induced vasculitis by down-regulating endothelial cell adhesion molecule expression. *Endocrinology*, Vol.144, No.1, (January 2003), pp. 360-370, ISSN 0013-7227.

Selkirk, J.V.; Nottebaum, L.M.; Lee, J.; Yang, W.; Foster, A.C. & Lechner S.M. (2007). Identification of differential melanocortin 4 receptor agonist profiles at natively expressed receptors in rat cortical astrocytes and recombinantly expressed receptors in human embryonic kidney cells. *Neuropharmacology*, Vol.52, No.2, (February 2007), pp. 459-466, ISSN 0028-3908.

Sharma, H.S.; Skottner, A.; Lundstedt, T.; Flärdh, M. & Wiklund, L. (2006). Neuroprotective effects of melanocortins in experimental spinal cord injury. An experimental study in the rat using topical application of compounds with varying affinity to melanocortin receptors. *J Neural Transm*, Vol.113, No.4, (April 2006), pp. 463-476, ISSN 0300-9564.

Shutter, J.R.; Graham, M.; Kinsey, A.C.; Scully, S.; Luthy, R. & Stark, K.L. (1997). Hypothalamic expression of ART, a novel gene related to agouti, is up-regulated in obese and diabetic mice. *Genes Dev*, Vol.11, No.5, (March 1997), pp. 593-602, ISSN 0890-9369.

Sinha, P.; Schiöth, H. & Tatro J. (2004). Roles of the melanocortin-4 receptor in antipyretic and hyperthermic actions of centrally administered alpha-MSH. *Brain Res*, Vol.1001, No. 1-2, (March 2004), pp. 150-158, ISSN 0006-8993.

Slominski, A.; Ermak, G. & Mihm, M. (1996). ACTH receptor, CYP11A1, CYP17 and CYP21A2 genes are expressed in skin. *J Clin Endocrinol Metab*, Vol.81, No.7, (July 1996), pp. 2746-2749, ISSN 0021-972X.

Spencer, J.D. & Schallreuter, K.U. (2009). Regulation of pigmentation in human epidermal melanocytes by functional high-affinity beta-melanocyte-stimulating hormone/melanocortin-4 receptor signaling. *Endocrinology*, Vol.150, No.3, (March 2009), pp. 1250-1258, ISSN 0013-7227.

Star, R.A.; Rajora, N.; Huang, J.; Stock, R.C.; Catania, A. & Lipton, J.M. (1995). Evidence of autocrine modulation of macrophage nitric oxide synthase by alpha-melanocyte-stimulating hormone. Proc *Natl Acad Sci U S A*, Vol.92, No.17, (August 1995), pp. 8016-8020, ISSN 0027-8424.

Strand, F.L. & Kung, T.T. (1980). ACTH accelerates recovery of neuromuscular function following crushing of peripheral nerve. *Peptides*, Vol.1, No.2, pp. 135-138, ISSN 0196-9781.

Sutton, G.M.; Duos, B.; Patterson, L.M. & Berthoud, H-R. (2005). Melanocortinergic modulation of cholecystokinin-induced suppression of feeding through extracellular signal-regulated kinase signalling in rat solitary nucleus. *Endocrinology*, Vol.146, No.9, (September 2005), pp. 3739-3747, ISSN 0013-7227.

Taherzadeh, S.; Sharma, S.; Chhajlani, V.; Gantz, I.; Rajora, N.; Demitri, M.T.; Kelly, L.; Zhao, H.; Ichiyama, T.; Catania, A. & Lipton, J.M. (1999). α-MSH and its receptors in regulation of tumor necrosis factor-α production by human monocyte/macrophages. *Am J Physiol*, Vol.276, No.5Pt2, pp. R1289-R1294, ISSN 0002-9513.

Tanabe, K.; Gamo, K.; Aoki, S.; Wada, K. & Kiyama, H. (2007). Melanocortin receptor 4 is induced in nerve-injured motor and sensory neurons of mouse. *J Neurochem*, Vol.101, No.4, (May 2007), pp. 1145-1152, ISSN 0022-3042.

Tatro, J.B. (2000). Endogenous antipyretics. *Clin Infect Dis*, Vol.31, No.5, (October 2000), pp. S190-S201, ISSN 1058-4838.

Taylor, A.W. & Kitaichi, N. (2008). The diminishment of experimental autoimmune encephalomyelitis (EAE) by neuropeptide alpha-melanocyte stimulating hormone (alpha-MSH) therapy. *Brain Behav Immun*, Vol.22, No.5, (July 2008), pp. 639-646, ISSN 0889-1591.

Taylor, A.W. (2005). The immunomodulating neuropeptide alpha-melanocyte-stimulating hormone (alpha-MSH) suppresses LPS-stimulated TLR4 with IRAK-M in macrophages. *J Neuroimmunol*, Vol.162, No.1-2, (May 2005), pp. 43-50, ISSN 0165-5728.

Ter Laak, M.P.; Brakkee, J.H.; Adan, R.A.; Hamers, F.P. & Gispen, W.H. (2003). The potent melanocortin receptor agonist melanotan-II promotes peripheral nerve regeneration and has neuroprotective properties in the rat. Eur J Pharmacol, Vol.462, No.1-3, (February 2003), pp. 179-183, ISSN 0014-2999.

Usategui, R.; Oliver, C.; Vaudry, H.; Lombardi, G.; Rozenberg, I. & Mourre, A.M. (1976). Immunoreactive alpha-MSH and ACTH levels in rat plasma and pituitary. *Endocrinology*, Vol.98, No.1, (January 1976), pp. 189-196, ISSN 0013-7227.

Van der Kraan, M.; Adan, R.A.; Entwistle, M.L.; Gispen, W.H.; Burbach, J.P. & Tatro, J.B. (1998). Expression of melanocortin-5 receptor in secretory epithelia supports a functional role in exocrine and endocrine glands. *Endocrinology*, Vol.139, No.5, (May 1998), pp. 2348-2355, ISSN 0013-7227.

Van der Neut, R.; Bär, P.R.; Sodaar, P. & Gispen, W.H. (1988). Trophic influences of alpha-MSH and ACTH4-10 on neuronal outgrowth in vitro. *Peptides*, Vol.9, No.5, (September-October 1988), pp. 1015-1020, ISSN 0196-9781.

Vongs, A.; Lynn, N.M. & Rosenblum, C.I. (2004). Activation of MAP kinase by MC4-R through PI3 kinase. *Regul Pept*, Vol.120, No.1-3, (August 2004), pp. 113-118, ISSN 0167-0115.

Vulliémoz, N.R.; Xiao, E.; Xia-Zhang, L.; Ferin, M. & Wardlaw, S.L. (2006). Melanocortin Modulation of Inflammatory Cytokine and Neuroendocrine Responses to Endotoxin in the Monkey. *Endocrinology*, Vol.147, No.4, (April 2006), pp. 1878-1883, ISSN 0013-7227.

Wakamatsu, K.; Graham, A.; Cook, D. & Thody, A.J. (1997). Characterisation of ACTH peptides in human skin and their activation of the melanocortin-1 receptor. *Pigment Cell Res*, Vol.10, No.5, (October 1997), pp. 288-297, ISSN 0893-5785.

Webb, T.R.; Chan, L.; Cooray, S.N.; Cheetham, M.E.; Chapple, J.P. & Clark, A.J. (2009). Distinct Melanocortin 2 Receptor Accessory Protein Domains Are Required for Melanocortin 2 Receptor Interaction and Promotion of Receptor Trafficking. *Endocrinology*, Vol.150, No.2, (February 2009), pp. 720-726, ISSN 0013-7227.

Weidenfeld, J.; Crumeyrolle-Arias, M. & Haour, F. (1995). Effect of bacterial endotoxin and interleukin-1 on prostaglandin biosynthesis by the hippocampus of mouse brain: role of interleukin-1 receptors and glucocorticoids. *Neuroendocrinology*, Vol.62, No.1, (July 1995), pp. 39-46, ISSN 0028-3835.

Wikberg, J.; Muceniece, R.; Mandrika, I.; Prusis, P.; Lindblom, J.; Post, C. & Skottner, A. (2000). New aspects on the melanocortins and their receptors. *Pharmacol Res*, Vol.42, No.5, (November 2000), pp. 393-420, ISSN 1043-6618.

Wilkinson, C.W. (2006). Roles of acetylation and other post-translational modifications in melanocortin function and interactions with endorphins. *Peptides*, Vol.27, No.2, (February 2006), pp. 453-471, ISSN 0196-9781.

Wolter, H.J. (1985). Dynorphin-A (1-8) and gamma-melanotropin exist within different myenteric plexus neurons of rat duodenum. *Biochem Biophys Res Commun*, Vol.131, No.2, (September 1985), pp. 821-826, ISSN 0006-291X.

Wolterink, G.; Van Zanten, E. & Van Ree, J.M. (1990). Functional recovery after destruction of dopamine systems in the nucleus accumbens of rats. IV. Delay by intra-accumbal treatment with ORG2766- or α-MSH antiserum. *Brain Res*, Vol.507, No.1, (January 1990), pp. 115-120, ISSN 0006-8993.

Wong, K.Y.; Rajora, N.; Boccoli, G.; Catania, A. & Lipton, J.M. (1997). A potencial mechanism of local anti-inflammatory action of alpha-melanocyte-stimulating hormone within the brain: modulation of tumor necrosis factor-alpha production by human astrocytic cells. *Neuroimmunomodulation*, Vol.4, No.1, (January-February 1997), pp. 37-41, ISSN 1021-7401.

Xia, Y.; Wikberg, J.E.S. & Chhajlani, V. (1995). Expression of melanocortin 1 receptor in periaqueductal gray matter. *Neuroreport*, Vol.6, No.16, (November 1995), pp. 2193-2196, ISSN 0959-4965.

Yeo, G.S.; Farooqi, I.S.; Aminiam, S.; Halsall, D.J.; Stanhope, R.G. & O'Rahilly, S. (1998). A frameshift mutation in MC4R associated with dominantly inherited human obesity. *Nat Genet*, Vol.20, No.2, (October 1998), pp. 111-112, ISSN 1061-4036.

Zhang, Y.; Wu, X.; He, Y.; Kastin, A.J.; Hsuchou, H.; Rosenblum, C.I. & Pan, W. (2009). Melanocortin potentiates leptin-induced STAT3 signaling via MAPK pathway. *J Neurochem*, Vol.110, No.1, (July 2009), pp. 390-399, ISSN 0022-3042.

8

Mechanisms and Patterns of Axonal Loss in Multiple Sclerosis

Zachary M. Harris and Jacob A. Sloane
Beth Israel Deaconess Medical Center, Harvard Medical School
USA

1. Introduction

After a variable or silent initial course, MS patients often enter a progressive neurological decline leading to permanent clinical disability. Axonal loss is considered the major factor behind this process. Elucidating the etiology and pathogenesis of this phenomenon is critical to developing treatments for progressive MS. Here we discuss pathologic presentation of axonal loss in MS, patterns of axonal loss at certain disease stages, and evidence that axonal loss in MS progresses independently of clinical relapses but coincides strongly with inflammation. Mechanisms behind axonal loss in MS include T cell attack, reactive nitrogen species-induced damage, loss of myelin (demyelination), and loss of trophic support from oligodendrocytes. Also, we will review animal models of neurodegeneration that share similar disease features with MS axonopathy. Finally, we will consider the progress of therapeutic strategies aimed at axonal preservation in MS including remyelination enhancement, blockage of Na+ channels and prevention of free radical formation.

2. Clinical overview of MS

In about 85% of patients, MS follows a biphasic course. In the first phase or relapsing-remitting multiple sclerosis (RRMS), patients suffer transient bouts of neurological deficit caused by neuroinflammation followed by rapid recovery (Noseworthy *et al.*, 2000). The pathologic hallmark of RRMS attacks is inflammatory demyelinated foci or lesions in the white and gray matter of the central nervous system visible on MRI. The clinical manifestations of RRMS attacks are variable from patient to patient, and may include paraesthesia (numbness), diplopia (double vision), scotoma (visual anomalies), sensory and motor disorders of limbs and cerebellar incoordination (lack of balance). In many cases, after a variable amount of time (approximately 10-20 years) patients will enter a progressive phase of the disease This more severe second stage is characterized by an irreversible neurological decline culminating in severe disability. Once this second phase is identified, patients exhibiting this biphasic couse are diagnosed with secondary progressive multiple sclerosis (SPMS). In some cases, patients will exhibit only a progressive phase of disease, which represents primary progressive multiple sclerosis (PPMS). These patients have symptomatic onset of the progressive form of the disease with no prior history of neuroinflammatory attacks.

3. History of axonal pathology in MS, 1868-1990s

Axonal pathology in multiple sclerosis was described by Charcot in 1868 (Charcot, 1868). From Charcot's identification of axonal damage up to the 1990s, two general observations on axonal pathology in multiple sclerosis come up frequently in the literature (Charcot, 1877; Dawson, 1916; Buzzard and Greenfield, 1921; Greenfield and King, 1936; Putnam, 1936; Adams and Kubik, 1952; Peters, 1968; Shintaku, *et al.*, 1988). First, MS lesions exhibit abnormal axonal anatomy. Second, Wallerian degeneration, the process of cellular degradation and necrosis far from zones of demyelination, is prevalent in long-standing MS cases. As more precise histological techniques have arisen, these broad features have been elaborated at the molecular level.

4. Histology of axonal pathology

4.1 Axonal injury

Axonal injury is defined as pathological changes in the cytoarchitecture of an axon happening within a short time window before axonal death (Gentleman *et al.*, 1993). Because debris of degenerating axons is rapidly cleared by CNS scavenger cells, quantification of axonal injury can often underestimate axonal loss accrued over long stretches of time (Trapp and Nave, 2008). Disturbance of fast axonal transport is the most accurate and sensitive method of determining axonal injury (Cochran *et al.*, 1991; Gentleman *et al.*, 1993; Ohgami *et al.*, 1992, Sherriff *et al.*, 1994a). Due to dystrophic changes, fast axonal transport mechanisms are unable to efficiently move cellular substances along the length of the axon. These substances accumulate as focal concentrations (spheroids), continuously and discontinuously, at certain points along the length of the axon (Figure 1). Axonal injury ranges from minor changes in the axoplasmic membrane to severe distentions as a result of disrupted fast axonal transport (Ferguson et al., 1997).

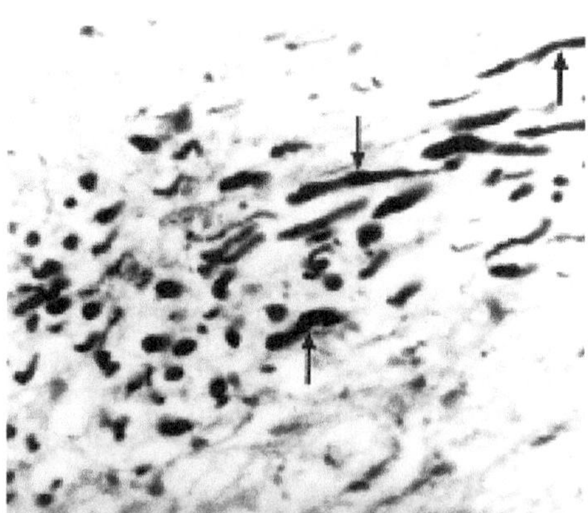

Fig. 1. Axonal injury in an active multiple sclerosis lesion. Immunocytochemistry staining with an anti-amyloid precursor protein (APP) antibody reveals stained spheroid elements 40-80 μm in diameter or in a beaded string-like appearance along the length of axons. Axonal dystrophy has caused these accumulations by interfering with fast axonal transport (from Ferguson *et al.*, 1997).

4.2 Axonal transection

Axonal transection in MS has been a main research focus since its discovery in the late 1990s (Trapp *et al.*, 1998; Lovas *et al.*, 2000; Peterson *et al.*, 2001). If axonal dystrophy exceeds a certain threshold, the axon cytoskeleton may dissolve resulting in a characteristic bulblike formation known as a transection (Figure 2). Axonal transections are also referred to as axonal end-bulbs, terminal ovoids or spheroids, or terminal swellings. Axonal end-bulbs are morphologically ovoid in shape. In acute MS white matter lesions, swellings average 40-80 µm in diameter (Trapp *et al.*, 1998). They are typically smaller in chronic lesions. Transections are positively identified by confirming the presence of only a single axonal connection to the swelling. Swellings that have two axonal connections represent intracellular protein accumulations that are pathological but not indicative of breakage (Ferguson *etl al.* 1997). Immunohistochemistry using anti-amyloid precursor protein (APP) antibodies is a useful method for identifying axonal transections (Sherriff *et al.*, 1994). APP and other fast axonal transport proteins accumulate in the end-bulb. Staining for non-phosphorylated neurofilament also detects ovoid formation (Sternberger *et al.*, 1983). Although demyelination is a key etiological factor in transection, end-bulbs may or may not be encircled with myelin (Trapp *et al.*, 1998; Bjartmar *et al.*, 2001; Aboul-Enein et al., 2006).

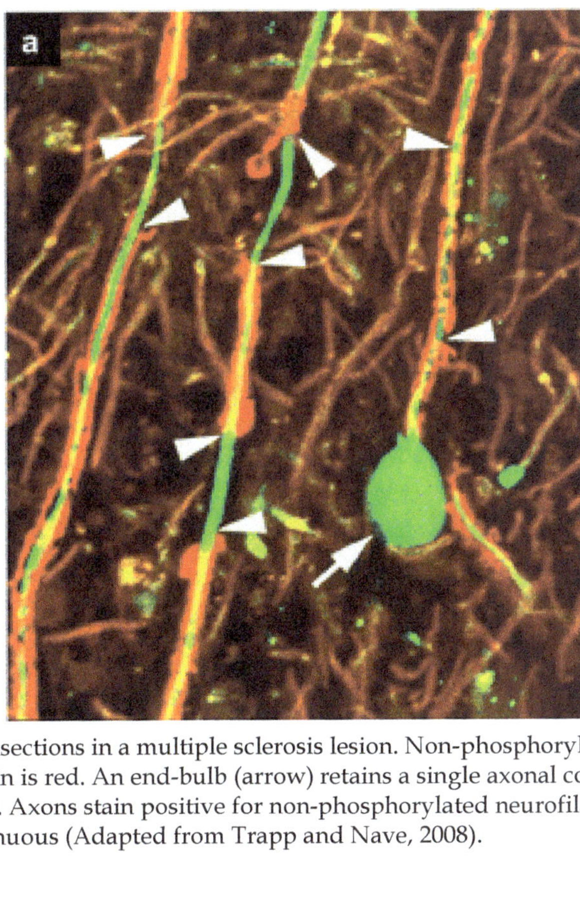

Fig. 2. Axonal transections in a multiple sclerosis lesion. Non-phosphorylated neurofilament is green and myelin is red. An end-bulb (arrow) retains a single axonal connection and is therefore terminal. Axons stain positive for non-phosphorylated neurofilament where myelin is discontinuous (Adapted from Trapp and Nave, 2008).

5. Molecular markers of axonal pathology

Immunocytochemistry staining of amyloid precursor protein (APP) or non-phosphorylated neurofilament is commonly used to identify axonal injury and axonal transection. Staining of these factors is often used in conjunction with antibodies to myelin antigens (i.e. myelin basic protein) in order to qualitatively determine the degree of demyelination coincident with axonal damage. Although less sensitive and accurate than immunocytological methods, Bielchowsky silver stain is a classic method still used to identify the general character of nerve fibers.

5.1 Bielchowsky silver stain

Before the era of immunocytochemistry, neurological studies relied on silver stains to visualize axonal pathology. Developed by Max Bielchowsky, the technique is a modified version of Santiago Ramón y Cajal's method of impregnating nerve fibers with silver. The method became known as the Bielchowsky silver stain. The classic technique is still used today to describe nerve fibers. Bielchowsky staining is particularly useful in identifying general axon morphology, such as axonal caliber and Wallerian degeneration (Galeano and Vav Ferriera, 1957; Wakita *et al.*, 2002). However, more sensitive laboratory techniques are needed in order to detect axonal injury and transection.

5.2 Nuclear magnetic resonance (NMR) spectroscopy

NMR spectroscopy is used to non-invasively measure chemical-pathologic changes in distinct brain slices of MS patients. Most notably, NMR studies have demonstrated whole brain reductions in the neuro-axonal marker N-acetylaspartate (NAA) in MS patients compared with normal controls (Gonen *et al.*, 2000). Because differences in NAA levels compared to controls are greater amongst older than younger MS patients, this neuronal marker is useful in charting the course of neurodegeneration in the disease (Gonen *et al.*, 2000). Reduced levels of NAA are detectable in inflammatory foci early on in the relapsing/remitting stage of the disease (Matthews *et al.*, 1996). Moreover, decreased NAA in the normal-appearing white matter (NAWM) of relapsing/remitting and progressive patients suggests that the neurodegenerative process is not confined to inflammatory lesions (Tourbah *et al.*, 1996). The ability to precisely localize changes in compounds such as NAA has made serial NMR of distinct brain slices a useful tool in human clinical trials looking at drug efficacy (Destefano *et al.*, 2007). Serial NMR has also been effective in tracking pathologic changes in animal models of MS, such as experimental autoimmune encephalomyelitis (EAE) (Stewart *et al.*, 1991).

5.3 Amyloid precursor protein (APP)

Detection of amyloid precursor protein (APP) positive foci within axons indicates axonal injury in MS lesions (Gehrmann *et al.*, 1995; Ferguson *et al.* 1997). This method derives from studies on axonal damage resulting from traumatic head injury (Gentleman *et al.*). APP is an integral membrane protein expressed primarily in neuronal synapses. Although its function is unknown, APP is thought to be associated with the endosomal/lysosomal system, synapse formation, neural plasticity, and iron transport (Haass *et al.*, 1992; Ferreira *et al.*, 1993). Normally, APP is transported by fast axonal transport along the axon (Koo *et al.*, 1990) and is undetectable by immunocytochemical methods. However, disruptions in the integrity of axonal structure inhibit the smooth transport of APP. Subsequently, APP builds up at certain points along the axon. Axonal damage appears microscopically as distinct, elongated APP+ blots following the course of the axon, or a succession of discontinuous APP+ punctate dots that look as if they are lodged within the axon (Figure 1). Immunocytochemistry for APP is a useful method of detecting axonal injury in human and animal nerve tissue preparations (Sherriff *et al.*, 1994b; Herrero-Herranz *et al*, 2008). Staining of other fast axonal transport substances is often used to determine or verify axonal injury, including synaptic vesicle terminal or synaptophisin protein (SPY) (Frischer *et al.* 2009).

5.4 Non-phosphorylated neurofilament

Detection of non-phosphorylated neurofilaments along axons or collected at the site of axonal transections is another efficient method of identifying axonal damage in MS (Sternberger *et al.*, 1983; Trapp *et al*; 1998). Neurofilament is the principal structural constituent of the axon, accounting for its shape and integrity. Phosphorylation of neurofilament ensures proper extension of neurofilament side arms (Dutta *et al.*, 2006). This process enhances axon diameter, neurofilament spacing, and conduction velocity of the axon. Normally, axons are insulated by myelin, a multilayered lipid sheath which enhances the conduction velocity of nerve impulses and protects the axonal cell membrane from the extracellular environment. Demyelination exposes the axolemma to phosphatases which dephosphorylate neurofilament fibers and subsequently induce structural damage. Dephosphorylated neurofilament fibers show fragmentation and decreased spacing between fibers due to reduced side-arm extensions (Dutta *et al.*, 2006). Demyelination/dysmyelination has also been shown to reduce axonal caliber and number of phosphorylated neurofilaments in animal models, as well as increase the number of non-phosphorylated neurofilament epitopes (deWaegh *et al.*, 1992, Hsieh S-T *et al.* 1993). Double-label immunohistochemistry for non-phosphorylated neurofilament and myelin antigens is an effective method for identifying axonal pathology concomitant with demyelination (Trapp *et al.*, 1998). In addition, axonal spheroids have been shown to contain many other substances (Table 1). Moreover, axonal spheroids are detectable in a number of other neurological conditions using immunocytochemistry for specific substances (Table 1).

6. Patterns of axonal pathology in MS

Although clinically axonal loss is being revealed as a pathological process independent of acute relapses (Kremenchutzky *et al.*, 1996), inflammation and neurodegenerative processes interface to accelerate neuronal death in MS (Frischer *et al.*, 2009). A comprehensive picture of the pathological changes taking place in axons in MS considers CNS lesions and normal brain and spinal cord tissue. Pathology in MS axons include dystrophic changes (i.e. thinning), non-terminal swellings (intracellular accumulations), intracellular vacuolization (Kornek *et al.*, 2001; Evangelou *et al.*, 2005; Miller and Leary, 2007) and end-bulb formation (transection). Distinct patterns of axonal pathology are present in different histopathogenetic stages of MS lesions (Table 2, Han *et al.*, 2008; Frischer *et al.*, 2009). Active and chronic MS white matter lesions exhibit axonal injury profiles corresponding with the degree of inflammation (Bitsch *et al.*, 2000; Herrero-Herranz, 2008; Frischer *et al.*, 2009).

Aging	MAP1A, tau, phosphorylated tau, synaptophysin, Hsp40, Hsp60, Hsp90, Hsp27, Hsp70, Hsp32, alpha ß-crystallin, ubiquitin, APP	(Fukuda et al., 2005; Dickson et al., 1990)
Alzheimer's disease	NF-M, ChAT, phosphorylated tau	(Nakazato et al., 1984; Stokin et al., 2005)
Amyotrophic lateral sclerosis	Kinesin, peripherin, neurofilament-M and -H, ßIII-tubulin, STOP proteins, galectin-1, superoxide dismutase-1, APP, 1-hexitol-lysine (AGE); chromogranin A	(Kato et al., 2001; Kikuchi et al., 2002; Letournel et al., 2003; Nakazato et al., 1984; Sasaki and Iwata, 1999; Shibata et al., 1996; Toyoshima et al., 1998; Yasuhara et al., 1994)
Brain abscess	APP	(Ohgami et al., 1992)
Central pontine Myelinolysis	APP	(Medana and Esiri, 2003)
CNS HIV infection	APP, ubiquitin	(Gray et al., 1998; Izycka-Swieszewska et al., 2000; Medana and Esiri, 2003; Raja et al., 1997; Smith et al., 1990)
CNS Malaria	APP	(Medana and Esiri, 2003)
Creutzfeldt-Jakob disease	NF-H, APP	(Guiroy et al., 1989; Kobayashi et al., 2008; Liberski and Budka, 1999)
Frontotemporal dementia	NF-H, tubulin	(Zhou et al., 1998)
Hallervorden-Spatz syndrome	APP, iron II, synuclein (alpha, beta, and gamma)	(Galvin et al., 2000; Neumann et al., 2000; Newell et al., 1999; Ohgami et al., 1992)
Infantile Neuroaxonal Dystrophy	Neurofilament	(Nakazato et al., 1984)
Multiple Sclerosis	Neurofilament, APP, N type calcium channel subunit alpha 1B (Cacna1b), oxidized phospholipids, synaptophysin	(Ferguson et al., 1997; Ghosh et al., 2004; Haider et al., 2011; Kornek et al., 2001; Raine and Cross, 1989; Trapp et al., 1998)
Multiple System Atrophy	Chromogranin A, NF-H	(Nakazato et al., 1984; Yasuhara et al., 1994)
Parkinson's disease	alpha-synuclein, phosphorylated tau, alphaß-crystallin, Bcl-x, parkin, chromogranin A, ubiquitin	(Choi et al., 2001; Choi et al., 2000; Jellinger, 2000; Yasuhara et al., 1994)
Parkinsonism-dementia of Guam	tau, ubiquitin, phosphorylated tau	(Schwab et al., 1997)
Periventricular leukomalacia	APP, fractin	(Arai et al., 1995; Haynes et al., 2008)
Stroke	APP, chromogranin A	(Ohgami et al., 1992; Yasuhara et al., 1994)
Traumatic brain injury	APP, synuclein	(Gentleman et al., 1993; Medana and Esiri, 2003; Newell et al., 1999; Raisanen et al., 1999)

Table 1. Neurological conditions presenting with axonal spheroid formation.

Lesion Subtype	Active Lesions	Chronic Active Lesions	Chronic Inactive Lesions
Myelin in lesion core	Present	Absent	Absent
Active demyelination	Present	Margins: Present Cores: Absent	Absent
Inflammation	Extensive throughout	Concentrated at margins	Comparable to aged-matched normal appearing white matter controls from non-MS brains
Axonal transections	Extensive throughout, arge in diameter	Margins: diffuse, small in diameter Core: few	- Few - similar to aged-matched controls
Axonal character	Continuous non-phosphorylated neurofilament along axons (intact demyelinated axons), axonal thinning	Same as active lesions but less prevalent and restricted mainly to lesion margins	- Unusually thick, demyelinated, axons - Occasional synaptophisin build up, - Occasional axonal tract degeneration
Axonal cell associations	- Cytotoxic T cells - Microglia and macrophages around degenerating axons	Same as active lesion but cell associations found mostly in lesion margins	Comparable to aged-matched normal appearing white matter controls from non-MS brains

Table 2. Axonal pathology within different MS white matter lesion subtypes.

6.1 Active lesions

Active white matter MS lesions are lesions undergoing demyelination with heavy infiltration of HLA-II reactive macrophages, microglia and leukocytes. In short, these lesions are white matter areas undergoing a hostile immune reaction. In active lesions, reactive CD8+ cytotoxic T cells and macrophages attack the myelin sheath of axons. Microglia and macrophages are commonly found surrounding degenerating axons (Trapp *et al.*, 1998; Barnett and Prineas, 2004). Macrophages phagocytose and clear myelin debris resultant from the destruction of myelin (Prineas and Wright, 1978; Ferguson *et al.*, 1997; Barnett and Prineas, 2004).

Active lesions display numerous small-caliber axons and relatively large transections throughout their entirety (Frischer *et al.*, 2009). The neurofilament fibers of dystrophic axons and swellings are commonly non-phosphorylated. Axonal spheroids or ovoids are usually positive for both non-phosphorylated neurofilament and amyloid precursor protein (APP), although ovoids positive for non-phosphorylated neurofilament positive and negative for APP have been reported (Ferguson *et al.*, 1997). Thin axons and transections may or may not be ensheathed with myelin (Trapp *et al.*, 1998; Bjartmar *et al.*, 2001), although contiguous demyelination is a common feature. Lengths of non-phosphorylated axons with intact myelin occasionally extend outside of the lesion zone (also observed in chronic lesions) (Trapp *et al.*, 1998). The degree of axonal pathology (i.e. number of ovoids, concentration of APP) correlates with the amount of inflammatory infiltrates within the lesion (Frischer *et al.*, 2009).

6.2 Chronic active lesions

Chronic active lesions are punched-out, demyelinated lesions with inflammation and active demyelination occurring mainly at their margins. Inflammation concentrated in the margins of chronic lesions is comparable to that in the cores of active lesions. For this reason they have been called "expanding lesions" (Frischer *et al.*, 2009). In their cores, chronic lesions contain fewer macrophages and T cells than active lesions. Inflammation in the cores of chronic active lesions is reduced compared to active lesions, and often non-existent. HLA-II reactive microglia and astrocytes are numerous in the borders of chronic lesions where inflammation and demyelination are prevalent.

Chronic lesions display fewer and smaller-diameter axonal swellings in their cores and margins than active lesions (Ferguson *et al.*, 1997). In chronic lesions, axonal ovoids are most numerous in the margins where inflammation is concentrated, further emphasizing the relationship between axonal injury and the inflammatory reaction. Likewise, the actively demyelinating margins of chronic lesions display far more axonal ovoids than their cores (Trapp *et al.*, 1998). However, since it is estimated that chronically demyelinated lesions show 60-70% loss of axons (Mews *et al.*, 1998), the lack of core axonal injury may reflect axonal destruction and loss. Axonal associations with leukocytes and monocytes are similar to those seen in active lesions, although these cell-to-cell interactions are concentrated at the margins where inflammation is most active.

6.3 Chronic inactive lesions

Chronic inactive lesions are punched-out, demyelinated lesions with no detectable inflammatory or actively demyelinating processes. Chronic inactive lesions display severe tissue vacuolization and diffuse astrocytosis. They contain few HLA-II reactive cells and are generally hypocellular (Frischer *et al.*, 2009).

Chronic inactive lesions contain few axonal spheroids in their cores and margins. Axons within chronic inactive lesions appear abnormally thicker than those within chronic active lesions, possibly due to axonal swelling associated with chronic disease processes (Shintaku *et al.*, 1988). The degree of axonal injury and inflammation in chronic inactive lesions is equal to that seen in normal appearing white matter from aged-matched, non-MS controls (Frischer *et al.*, 2009). This suggests that in these embattled lesions the disease process has died out.

6.4 Normal appearing white matter (NAWM): Relapsing/remitting and progressive patients

Axonal injury in the NAWM of progressive patients is more substantive compared to relapsing/remitting patients (Frischer *et al.*, 2009). NAWM of progressive patients is characterized by diffuse inflammation, axonal injury and microglia activation. Diffuse white matter injury can be profound in these patients even with a relatively minor focal lesion load (Kutzeinigg *et al.*, 2005). Similarly, focal demyelinating lesions show only a marginal correlation with inflammation in NAWM and cortical regions (Kutzeinigg *et al.*, 2005). This supports the idea that the formation of demyelinated foci occurs independently of inflammatory damage taking place in normal brain regions. However, pathologic changes occurring in the NAWM do so against a background of diffuse inflammation (Kutzeinigg *et al.*, 2005). This suggests that with disease chronicity inflammatory cells escape the control of the peripheral immune system and slowly accumulate in the whole brain. Over time, these infiltrates may inflict massive, cumulative white matter damage on a global scale, which manifests clinically as the progressive phase of the disease (Kutzeinigg *et al.*, 2005).

6.5 Axonal pathology in relapsing/remitting and progressive MS

Up until now, we have considered axonal pathology in lesions at different pathogenic stages of MS. Here, we will discuss axonal pathology as it occurs in patients with relapsing/remitting, primary progressive, and secondary progressive forms of MS.

In all MS subtypes (relapsing/remitting, primary and secondary progressive), the amount of axonal injury in any demyelinated lesion is tightly correlated with the degree of inflammation present in the lesion (Frischer *et al.*, 2009). This supports the idea that an inflammatory reaction is chiefly responsible for axonal injury in demyelinated zones. In line with this idea, active lesions show the highest density of axonal injury (Trapp *et al.*, 1998). Relapsing/remitting MS patient possess a higher number of active lesions than patients of any other disease phase. Because of this, relapsing/remitting patients have a higher degree of axonal injury than patients with progressive forms of the disease (Frischer *et al.*, 2009).

In spite of this, lesions at the same level of activity exhibit no significant differences in axonal injury between relapsing/remitting, primary progressive, and secondary progressive MS patients. That is, an active lesion from a relapsing/remitting patient contains the same extent of axonal injury as an active lesion from a progressive patient. The one important exception is with normal appearing white matter (NAWM) which shows a greater extent of axonal injury in progressive patients than in relapsing/remitting patients (Frischer *et al.*, 2009). As discussed above, one explanation for this is that in progressive patients inflammatory cells accumulate in the whole brain and inflict massive white matter damage, whereas in relapsing/remitting patients axonal injury is limited to inflammatory demyelinating foci (Kutzeinigg *et al.*, 2005). In summary, relapsing/remitting patients tend to exhibit high axonal injury associated with inflammatory demyelinating foci, whereas progressive patients tend to exhibit diffuse white matter damage that may be secondary to global inflammation.

Lesions from patients with progressive forms of MS (primary or secondary progressive) exhibit highly variable levels of axonal injury. However, the presence or absence of ongoing inflammation in progressive MS brains correlates with the extent of axonal damage. In order to demonstrate this, Frischer *et al.* classified progressive patients in a large post-mortem histological study as either pathologically active or pathologically inactive. Brains of pathologically active patients revealed the persistence of active or chronic active lesion activity (lesions with inflammatory activity). Brains of pathologically inactive patients contained inactive lesions only. Frischer *et al.* found that pathologically inactive patients lived significantly longer than pathologically active patients (mean 76 yrs., range 64-84 vs. mean 53 yrs., range 28-82). Chronic inactive lesions in the pathologically inactive group contained axonal injury equal to that of aged-match controls. Conversely, chronic inactive lesions in pathologically active patients exhibited significantly more axonal injury than those of the pathologically inactive group. This data suggests that in progressive MS axonal injury is intrinsically tied to an ongoing inflammatory reaction. In a subset of MS patients with significantly reduced axonal injury, the inflammatory reaction appears to die down to the level of aged-matched controls (Frischer *et al.*, 2009).

6.6 Axonal loss as a distant pathological process

Axonal loss is considered the primary cause of permanent clinical disability in patients with MS. The fact that axonal loss may approach 30-40% (Ganter *et al.*, 1999) in the spinal cord and possibly as high as 60-70% in lesioned white matter tissue (Mews *et al.*, 1998) demonstrates the severity of neurodegeneration in chronic disease pathogenesis. Evidence that the neurodegenerative component ensues independently of inflammatory disease derives from clinical data. These data include irresponsiveness of progressive MS to immunomodulatory therapies and inconclusive reports that pharmacological treatment of inflammatory bouts lessens morbidity and delays time of onset of progressive forms of the disease (Fisher *et al.*, 2008; Fisniku *et al.*, 2009).

Striking evidence that uncouples acute relapses and neurodegeneration comes from case-control studies examining the time of onset of progressive disability across different types of MS. In a poignant retrospective study using large cohorts of over 1000 patients per arm, Kremechutzky *et al.* showed that relapsing/remitting, primary progressive, and secondary progressive patients began irreversible neurological decline at about the same time (~2.6 years mean difference between time of onset). The clinical disability measured by the Expanded Disability Status Scale was similar across these patient groups and irrespective of preceding or subsequent relapse events.

Studies of the histopathogenesis of MS also indicate axonal loss as a distinct disease mechanism. Identification of degenerating nerve fibers outside inflammatory foci in the normal appearing white matter (NAWM) of post-mortem MS brains shows that the neurodegenerative process can occur independently - at least topgraphically- of inflammation and demyelination (Bjartmar *et al.*, 2001). However, there is a strong correlation between the degree of axonal injury and inflammation in all MS lesion stages and normal appearing white matter (Bitsch *et al.*, 2000; Herrero-Herranz, 2008; Frischer *et al.*, 2009). Moreover, progressive patients exhibit extensive neurodegeneration against a background of massive inflammation and glial activation (Kutzeinigg *et al.*, 2005). Although it is unclear precisely how the extent of inflammation definitely relates to axonal loss in MS. In the same way, the extent of axonal injury and the autoimmune inflammatory process concomitantly diminish to the level of aged-matched controls as the disease progresses (Frischer *et al.*, 2009).

7. Mechanisms of axonal injury

Extensive research has focused on determining the mechanisms responsible for axonal loss and findings have identified several pathogenic phenomena that might be responsible. Some mechanisms are thought to initiate other pathological events downstream, ultimately leading to the demise of the axon. Initiating factors include inflammatory and immunological attack of axons, exposure of demyelinated axons to the excitotoxic MS lesion environment, and loss of trophic support by oligodendrocytes and other resident CNS cells affected by the inflammatory milieu. These initiating factors are capable of setting up an energy imbalance in the axon, leading to a state of virtual hypoxia. The result is the eventual dissolution of the axonal cytoskeleton at the site of injury. Axonal damage can also cause a type of degradation distal to the site of injury referred to as Wallerian degeneration.

7.1 CD8+ cytotoxic T lymphocytes

Major histocompatibility complex (MHC) class I-restricted CD8+ cytotoxic T lymphocytes (CTLs) are thought to directly attack axons and dendrites (neurites) and neuronal soma in MS lesions. These cells outnumber class-I restricted CD4+ T cells approximately 10 fold in actively demyelinating MS white matter (Booss J *et al.*, 1983; Gay FW *et al.*, 1997). Interleukin-2 (IL-2), a cytokine released by CD4+ T helper cells, along with MHC class-I-antigen recognition, initiates differentiation of CD8+ T cells into effector CTLs. Because IL-2 concentrations are increased in the serum and CSF of MS patients (Gallo *et al.*, 1992), it is likely that in lesions CD8+ T cells differentiate into effector CTLs by recognizing MHC class I-peptide on CNS cells and receiving the IL-2 second signal. Because the CD8+ CTLs constitute a clonally expanded population, these effector cells are highly specified and reactive against a single antigen.

Activated CTLs are capable of causing detrimental damage to axons. CTLs have been shown to transect MHC class I-induced axons in culture (Medana I *et al.*, 2001). Axons and dendrites damaged by allogenic attack *in vitro* display degeneration characteristic of axonal injury (Manning *et al.*, 1987). In MS lesions, effector CTLs directly contact dystrophic axons and terminal ovoids (Neumann *et al.*, 2002). However, lesions at exceptionally early stages of demyelination contain few T or B cells (Henderson *et al.*, 2009). Once in contact with the axon, cytotoxic granules of CTLs polarize toward the surface (Figure 3). Perforin, an effector substance contained within these granules, polymerizes to form a pore that is inserted into the axonal membrane, allowing water and salt to flow into the axon. Na+ influx initiates reversal of the Na+/Ca++ exchanger, leading to a vicious cycle of increased Ca++ intracellular accumulation (Smith *et al.*, 2001). Granzyme, a second CTL effector substance, degrades axonal proteins, disrupting fast transport and potentially triggering apoptosis (Figure 4).

7.2 MHC induction

In the CNS, disparate cell lineages interact to ensure that the powerful immune defenses of the brain are not misguided. Autoimmune diseases such as MS must overcome these cell-to-cell interactions that hold the immune system at bay. For example, neurons are able to suppress MHC expression in surrounding cells, in particular microglia and astrocytes, through ligand-receptor interactions (Neumann H, 2001). However, disruption of Na+ membrane-dependent electrical activity has been shown to decrease the efficacy of these interactions and increase induction of MHC class-I by inflammatory cytokines such as interferon-γ. In the case of MS, demyelination and axonal injury are both capable of disrupting Na+ flow in axons. This helps explain the increased CTL differentiation and activation of microglia and astrocytes. Moreover, MHC class-I induction on neurons and axons makes these cells viable targets for immunological attack.

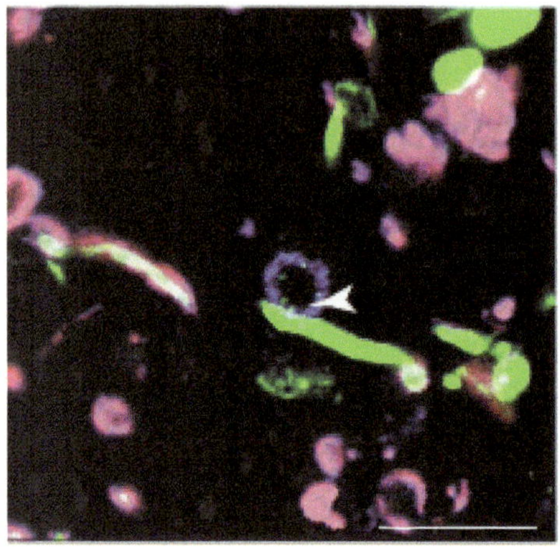

Fig. 3. A CD8+ cytotoxic T cell (blue) apposed to a demyelinated axon (green). The cytotoxic granules (light blue and arrowhead) are polarized toward the surface of the axon, indicating an "immunological synapse" (from Neumann *et al.*, 2002).

7.3 Nitric oxide intermediates

Activated microglia and macrophages are readily seen surrounding and engulfing degenerating axons and end-bulbs (Lassmann, 2003). These monocytes are thought to introduce toxic effector molecules capable of damaging axons. Two of these that have been identified are proteases and reactive nitrogen species. Proteases degrade intracellular structural elements, causing disturbances in fast axonal transport (Anthony *et al.*, 1998). High levels of nitric oxide (NO) radicals have been identified in MS lesions (Smith and Lassmann., 2002). NO radicals cause injury to mitochondria and disrupt axonal cytoarchitecture (Smith *et al.* 2001; Smith and Lassmann, 2002). NO radical-induced mitochondrial injury reduces generation of ATP and, if exceeding a certain threshold, triggers apoptotic mechanisms by cleavage and activation of caspases. Also, reactive nitrogen species disrupt the permeability of the axonal membrane, causing an influx of extracellular ions and axonal swelling. At low concentrations, NO species have been shown to block impulse conduction in axons even in the absence of structural damage (Redford *et al.*, 1997). This demonstrates how clinical deficit may manifest in MS patients before dramatic degenerative changes are detectable in axons (Lassmann *et al.*, 2003). Because reactive nitrogen species can also cause demyelination and oligodendrocyte damage, these substances fit well into the pathogenetic sequence of events in MS (Lassmann *et al.*, 2003). In line with this concept, early structural changes in mitochondria and oxidative DNA damage has recently been implicated in axonal injury preceding demyelination (Nikić *et al.*, 2011; Haider *et al.*, 2011).

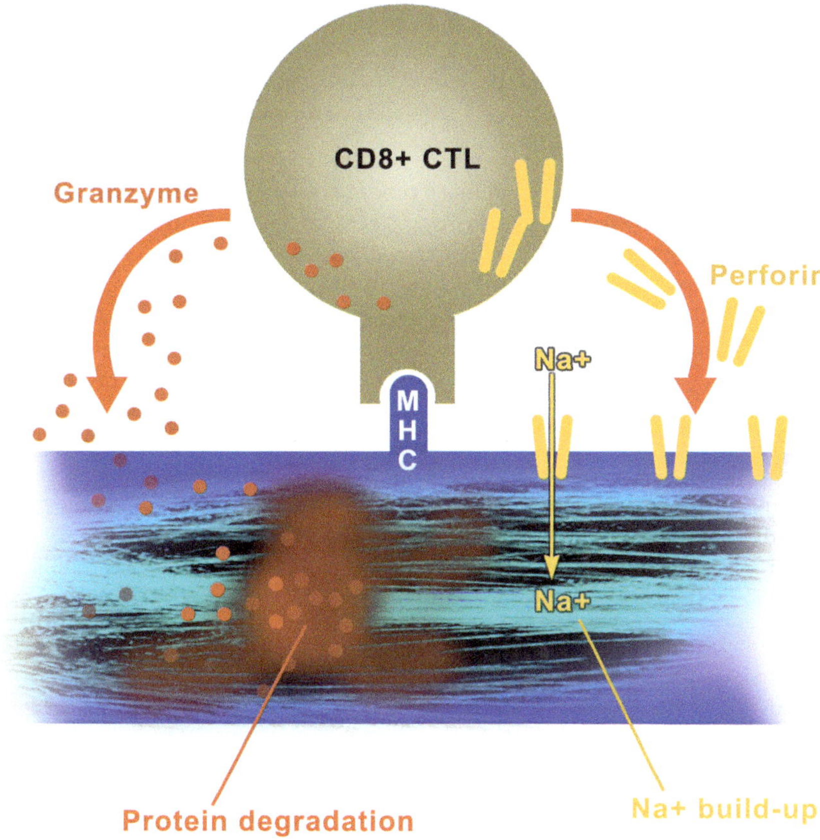

Fig. 4. A CD8+ CTL recognizes MHC-I on an MS axon and releases effector substances. Granzyme helps degrade the intracellular fast transport network. Perforin inserts into the axoplasmic membrane and allows Na+ to freely diffuse into the cell. Rising intracellular Na+ leads to detrimental effects in the axon.

7.4 Demyelination

The loss of myelin and glia causes severe dysregulation of physiologic and homeostatic mechanisms in axons ultimately ending in cell death. The duration from onset of injury to neuronal death depends on compensatory and reparative mechanisms of the cellular milieu of the CNS in addition to the extent further inflammatory reactions accelerate the process. The most striking evidence that loss of myelin is behind neurological progression in MS are post-mortem histological studies showing the tight correlation between inflammatory demyelination and axonal loss (Frischer *et al.*, 2009). Strong support also comes from experiments showing that myelin-protein deficient mice lose axons over time (Griffiths *et al.*, 1998). The relative slowness of axonal loss in these mice is comparable to the course of neurodegenerative progression in MS (Nave and Trapp, 2008). Further evidence includes histological data showing a 60-70% reduction in axonal density in chronically demyelinated lesions compared with normal tissue of the same area, and a 30% reduction in fresh lesions (Mews *et al.*, 1998). A similar percentage is seen in the spinal cord when the absolute number of nerve fibers are counted in a tract (Bjartmar *et al.*, 2000).

7.5 Energy imbalance in demyelinated axons

A state of energy imbalance is the hallmark predecessor to cell death. Because demyelinated axons are in a state of increased demand and decreased generation of energy in the form of ATP, chronic energy imbalance might significantly contribute to axonal loss in MS. In demyelinated axons, Na+ channels become diffusely arrayed along the cell surface in contrast to normal clustering around nodes of Ranvier (Figure 5, Craner *et al.*, 2004; Black *et al.*, 2007b). These axons have an increased energy requirement per action potential. Disruption of ion transport caused by cytoarchitectual disturbances further increases the metabolic load of the axon. Simultaneously, various pathologic mechanisms reduce generation of ATP. These mechanisms include disruption of the mitochondrial membrane by ambient nitric oxide and free radicals as well as down-regulation of mitochondrial protein transcripts (Mahad *et al.*, 2008). Using novel multiphoton imaging technology, a recent study identified mitochondrial pathology taking place within axonal swellings ensheathed with normal myelin in an animal model of multiple sclerosis (Nikić *et al.*, 2011). This data shows that energy imbalance in the axon can occur even in the absence of local demyelination.

Energy imbalance in the demyelinated axon leads to a reduction in protein synthesis and fast axonal transport. The cytoplasmic density of Na+/K+ATPase exchanger drops, and consequently the electrochemical gradient critical to the functionality and survival of the cell is compromised (Young *et al.*, 2008). The cell is overwhelmed with inrushing Na+ and is unable to compensate. Rising intracellular Na+ triggers a reversal of the Na+/Ca++ exchanger, leading to a Ca++mediated neurodegenerative cascade of events not unlike those seen in ischemia. This deleterious state has been called virtual hypoxia.

7.6 Oligodendrocyte decimation

The oligodendrocyte is an extraordinary glial cell derived from neuroepithelial stem cell progenitors. Its characteristic arbor projects numerous angular processes capable of myelinating up to 40 nerve axons (Weinshenker, 1994; Weiner, 1998; Compston and Coles, 2002). Classically oligodendrocyte processes wrap around the cell membrane of axons and produce concentric myelin layers. After myelination takes place, oligodendrocyte processes retain their physical connection with the myelin sheath of axons. *In vitro* studies using human oligodendrocytes and neurons cultured concomitantly show that molecular trophic factors released by oligodendrocytes significantly impact the survival and proliferation of axons (Wilkins *et al.*, 2003). Moreover, small molecule secretions by neurons and axons are thought to influence the structural viability and intracellular mechanisms of local oligodendrocytes well after the myelination phenomenon. Therefore, a bidirectional trophic interplay between neurons and oligodendrocytes supports the healthy maintenance of both these cell populations.

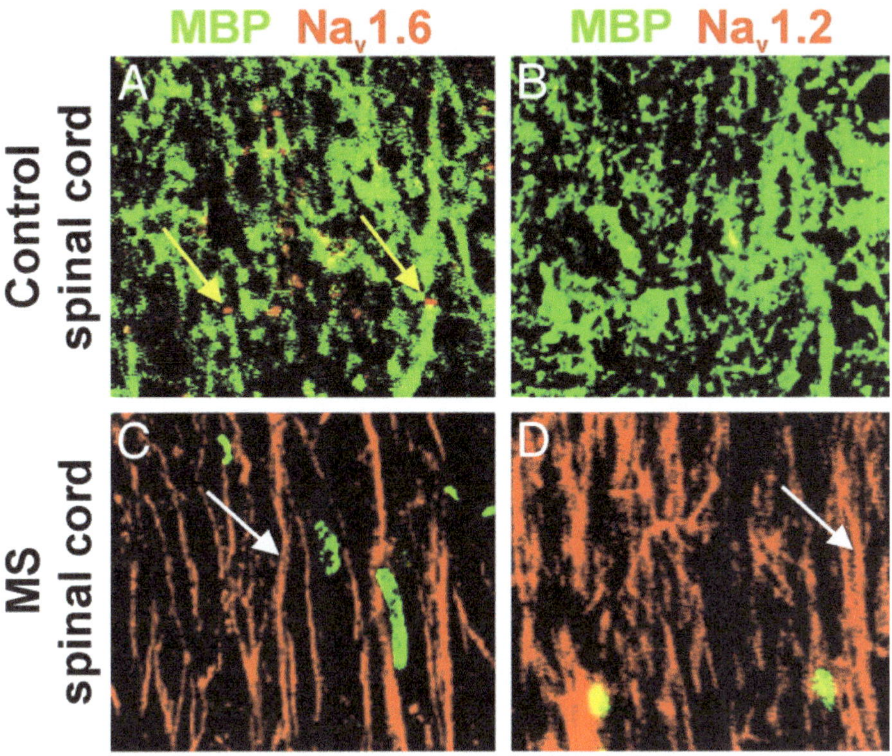

Fig. 5. MS spinal cord axons lacking myelin (green) exhibit increased expression of Na+ channels (red) along their surfaces. Panels A–B: Control spinal cord shows heavily myelinated fibers with (A) Nav1.6 channels concentrated at nodes of ranvier and (B) no detectable Nav1.2 sodium channel staining. Panels C–D: MS spinal cord shows severe demyelination with (A) Nav1.6 and (B) Nav1.2 sodium channels diffusely arrayed along naked axolemmas. Increased Na+ influx in MS axons leads to Na+/Ca++ exchanger reversal and subsequent degenerative changes (adapted from Craner *et al.*, 2004).

In MS, degenerating oligodendroyctes are numerous in white matter tissue adjacent to inflammatory foci and have been identified in NAWM regions distant from lesions (Henderson *et al.*, 2009). In both lesions and NAWM regions, oligodendrocyte processes "die back" from the axonal myelin sheath in some cases (Lucchinetti *et al.*, 2000). It is unclear whether the dying back phenomenon is resultant from contact with degenerating axons or dystrophy intrinsic to the oligodendrocyte. It is clear, however, that the environment of the MS lesion has a profound affect on oligodendrocyte survival. Compared to NAWM in both MS patients and controls, chronic lesions contained markedly decreased numbers of oligodendrocytes and oligodendrocyte progenitor cells (Kulmann *et al.*, 1999). Disruption in the secretion, integrity, and uptake of trophic factors released and/or delivered by neurons and glia might contribute to the oligodendrocyte demise in MS. Other possibilities include NO-mediated cytotoxicity, T cell-induced killing, or the presence of a currently unknown toxin or virus affecting oligodendrocyte health. Our group is currently studying molecular profiles of MS oligodendrocytes in order to find out what factors influence their survival.

7.7 Dissolution of the axonal cytoskeleton

As described above, various mechanisms interface to ultimately bring intracellular Ca++ concentrations to dangerous heights. These mechanisms include direct T cell-mediated axonal injury, diffusion of Na+ channels along demyelinated internodal regions of axons, and free radical-mediated increased membrane permeability and mitochondrial damage. Reduction in mitochondrial output establishes an energy imbalance within the cell, leading to stalled fast axonal transport and skewed ion channel densities in the axonplasmic membrane. Rising intracellular Ca++ activates Ca++ dependent proteases which degrade the axonal structural framework. The activity of ambient proteases and the loss of trophic factors from oligodendrocytes are thought to amplify this degenerative process in the MS lesion environment (Anthony *et al.*, 1998, Wilkins *et al.*, 2003). The active disintegration of the intra-axonal microtubule network and decreased ATP availability stall the machinery of fast axonal transport. Proteins like APP accumulate, causing swelling and increased tension in a manner not unlike that seen in acute traumatic head injury (Povlishock, 1992). Furthermore, disabled fast transport arrests movement of Ca++ channel proteins along axonal microtubules. Subsequent insertion of these channels into the membrane results in Ca++ channels discontinuously arrayed along the surface of MS lesion axons (Kornek *et al.* 2001). The result is a vicious cycle of Ca++ influx which eventually leads to the demise of the axon. The positive feedback loop of protease activation–cytoskeletal disruption–ion channel insertion continues as more Ca++ rushes into the cell (Smith *et al.*, 2001). Ultimately, swelling and structural damage reach a point where the axonal cytoskeleton dissolves (Lassmann *et al.*, 2003). The axon is transected, and conduction along the nerve fiber inhibited. Organelles and fast transport proteins such as APP remain and continue to accumulate in the terminus, causing axonal end-bulb formations with characteristic morphology (Povlishock, 1992).

7.8 Wallerian degeneration

Anterograde "Wallerian degeneration" or secondary degeneration has been proposed as a mechanism of axonal loss. In this process, acute ultrastructural changes at some point along the axon can cause degeneration in regions of the nerve fiber not immediately associated with the site of injury. Nerves passing through a focus of inflammatory demyelination might therefore manifest pathological changes distal to the injured or transected site (Shindler *et al.*, 2008). In this scope, degenerating nerves in the NAWM of MS patients might be spatially distinct from inflammatory foci but retain an intimate link to the cellular changes taking place at those sites of disease activity. That is, if axons and lesion are contained within the same tract, secondary degeneration helps explain the loss of axons in seemingly unaffected white matter areas contralateral to lesioned tissue (Evangelou *et al.*, 2000a; Lovas *et al.*, 2000; Evangelou *et al.*, 2000b; Evangelou *et al.*, 2004).

Demyelination however is not the only pathological phenomenon in MS capable of inducing Wallerian degeneration. Any subtle change in cytoarchitecture, due to its effects on fast axonal transport, will be felt downstream. Immunological attack of axons by CD8+ CTLs is capable of initiating secondary degeneration in the absence of demyelination (Manning *et al.*, 1987). In the same vein, NO-mediated axonal injury by monocytes could potentiate degenerative changes elsewhere in fiber tracts. Loss of important trophic factors can cause transynaptic secondary neuronal loss, which in turn leads to degeneration of the projecting axons (Wilkins *et al.*, 2003).

8. Animal models for MS axonopathy

8.1 Axonal injury in experimental autoimmune encephalomyelitis (EAE)

EAE is an inducible autoimmune condition in animals characterized by T cell mediated inflammatory demyelination and neurodegeneration (Gold *et al.*, 2006; Steinman and Zamvil, 2006). Animals are inoculated with CNS proteins often with complete Freund's adjuvant (CFA) to stimulate an inflammatory reaction to myelin antigens. Pertussis toxin is used in these models to break down the blood brain barrier and allow immune cell infiltration. Depending on the protocol and animal genotype, EAE can follow a monophasic, relapsing/remitting, or chronic course. In mice, symptoms usually become apparent within 2 weeks of inoculation. The classic first symptom is loss of tonus in the tail leading to paralysis, followed by loss of motor function in the hind and then forelimbs. Symptoms associated with MS also present in EAE, including ataxia, optic neuritis, emotional liability, and cognitive dysfunction.

Axonal pathology in EAE mice morphologically resembles changes seen in MS patients (Soulika *et al.*, 2009). EAE mice induced by immunization with myelin oligodendrocyte protein (MOG) peptide 35-55 show axonal vacuolization and fragmentation, as well as brain atrophy (Bannerman *et al.*, 2005; Wang *et al.*, 2005; Bannerman and Hahn, 2007; Herrero-Herranz *et al.*, 2008; Jones *et al.*, 2008). C57BL/6 mice immunized with MOG in CFA exhibit intra-axonal accumulations of APP and hyperphosphorylated heavy chains (NF-H). Neurological deficits manifest clinically in EAE mice at approximately the same time as characteristic SMI32+ spheroids are detectable in spinal cord axons (Figure 6, Soulika *et al.*, 2009). These spheroids contain high concentrations of Toll-like receptor 8 (TLR8) protein (Soulika *et al.*, 2009) shown to cause neuronal death via apoptosis and inhibit neurite formation (Ma *et al.*, 2006, 2007). In this same EAE model, innate immunity infiltrates are detectable early on in the disease course. Neutrophils in the early innate immunological wave permeabalize the blood brain barrier and perform neurotoxic effector functions via a contact-dependent, protease-mediated mechanism (Dinkel *et al.*, 2004). Moreover, a progressive, symmetric, severe loss of small diameter dorsal corticospinal axons is evident approximately 3 months post-innoculation (Soulika *et al.*, 2009). At this time, inflammation is diminished to the level of controls, while genes associated with the activation of innate immunity continue to be expressed (Soulika *et al. 2009)*. These data indicate that the innate arm of the immune system may play a key role in late-onset axonal loss in the MOG-induced EAE model (Weiner, 2009).

8.2 Neurodegeneration in mice lacking expression of 2'-3'-cyclic nuclotide 3'-phosphodiesterase (CNP)

CNP is an intrinsic protein of oligodendrocytes associated with cytoskeletal elements (Nishizawa *et al.*, 1985) and detectable in purified myelin (Kurihara *et al*, 1967). Engineered mice deficient in CNP (CNP-/-) display profound axonal loss, leading to a severe neurodegenerative disorder and premature death (Lapp-Siefke *et al.*, 2003). This animal model demonstrates that oligodendrocytes provide support for axons independent of the physical stability of myelin itself. Degenerating neurons of CNP-/- mice display pathologic changes characteristic of MS (Povlishock, 1992) including axonal swellings filled with microtubules, dense bodies, multivesicular bodies, and mitochondria. These cells were associated with phagocytic activity, reminiscent of macrophages and microglia often surrounding dystrophic axons in MS lesions. Moreover, the progressive neurological decline of CNP-/- mice is not unlike that seen in progressive MS patients. During the first 3 months, the knockout strain is indistinguishable from wildtype. This brings to mind the proposed clinical silence of the neurodegenerative component of MS preceding the progressive phase of the disease (Bjartmar and Trapp, 2003; Kremenchutsky *et al.*, 2006). At 4 months CNP-/- mice begin to show hindlimb impairments, convulsions, and ataxia. At 6 months, the mice are unable to grasp a round bar with their hindlimbs, and display a reduction in overall brain size. Less than 20% of CNP-/- mice reach 13 months. Those that do are unable to balance on a round bar for 1 second, and exhibit profound muscle weakness, weight loss, gait abnormalities, and kyphosis. The CNP-/- strain is of promising value to the MS research community. Not only does the model uncouple axonal loss from structurally intact myelin (demyelination), but it also demonstrates a relationship between intracellular processes of the oligodendrocyte and axonal survival.

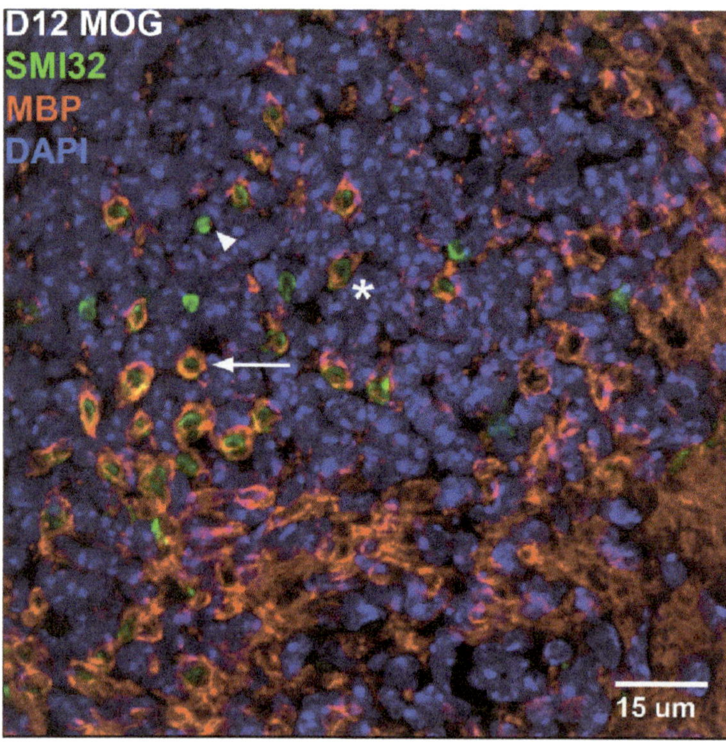

Fig. 6. Axonal spheroids (arrowhead) are evident in spinal cord axons in a mouse model of MOG-induced EAE. Although demyelination of the tract is evident, many of the spheroids are encircled with intact myelin (long arrow). This pathology is consistent with axonal changes in MS (adapted from Soulika *et al.*, 2009).

9. Overview of therapeutic strategies to counteract neuronal-axonal loss in MS

Developments in our understanding of axonal loss in MS have spearheaded the relatively recent realignment of our thinking about the disease as a neurodegenerative as well as immune-mediated disease process. The increased understanding of axonal loss in MS has opened exciting research avenues geared toward developing novel therapies. These therapies aim to increase neuroprotection, enhance the remyelinating capacity of the CNS, and address the incongruity of trophic support supposed in the multiple sclerosis CNS environment by replacing both important molecules and decimated cell populations. Elucidating the mechanisms of nerve degeneration and how they interface with inflammatory demyelination during the biphasic clinical course of MS remains a critical step toward therapeutic victory over the disease.

9.1 Remyelination

The brain has evolved mechanisms to counteract axonal degeneration. Most of the reparative focus is on rebuilding the myelin architecture devastated by the inflammatory milieu (Prineas *et al.*, 1993). Oligodendrocytes are responsible for repairing demyelinated axons through a process called remyelination. By repairing ultrastructural deficits accumulated through loss of myelin, remyelination not only partially restores saltatory conduction (Kriss *et al.*, 1988) but also ameliorates degenerative processes occurring elsewhere in the axon such as secondary Wallerian degeneration (Irvine *et al.*, 2008). In line with this, patients with robust remyelination live longer compared to patients showing few remyelinated brain regions (Patrikios *et al.*, 2006).

Chronic MS disease processes diminish the ability for specific brain regions to remyelinate (Hanafy and Sloane, 2011). For example, hyaluronic acid accumulates in chronic MS lesions and inhibits remyelination and oligodendrocyte progenitor maturation (Figure 7, Sloane *et al.*, 2010b). Activation of other molecular cascades such as the Notch1 pathway, Wnt pathway, and inflammation are thought to contribute to remyelination blockade (Hanafy and Sloane, 2011). The consequence of this is failure of the axon to successfully remediate injury and energy imbalance, further instigating dystrophic changes, transection, and secondary degeneration. A large sector of MS research is geared toward developing therapeutics that promote and amplify remyelination in MS. Strategies include enhancing oligodendrocyte proliferation and progenitor recruitment in chronic lesions (Patel *et al.*, 2010), grafting exogenous oligodendrocyte progenitor cells in proximity to affected tissue (Wang *et al.*, 2011), and blocking or genetically deleting receptors that inhibit remyelination (Mi *et al.*, 2007; Sloane *et al.*, 2010b). These efforts center around the idea that boosting remyelination capacity in MS patients would ameliorate long-term clinical outcomes and provide neuroprotection against progressive disease.

9.2 Na+ channel blockers

Increased Na+ influx into axons creates a state of virtual hypoxia in MS axons and contributes to axonal dissolution (Waxman, 2008). Irregular densities of Na+ channels detectable along demyelinated axons (Black *et al.*, 2007a) along with altered expression of Na+ channels in MS neurons provide strong support for this idea (Craner *et al.*, 2004).

Building on these observations, *in vitro* experiments show that selective Na+ channel blockers can prevent axonal injury from anoxia and ischemia (Stys *et al.*, 1992a, 1992b, 1996; Fern *et al.*, 1993;). Using a MOG-induced EAE mouse model, Lo *et al.* showed that administration of the Na+ channel blocker phenytoin ameliorates 28-30 day clinical outcomes in EAE and reduces loss of corticospinal axons from 63% to 28% (Lo *et al.*, 2002). Other studies have verified the neuroprotective effects of Na+ channel blockers in EAE (Bechtold *et al.* 2004). Moreover, phenytoin-treated mice in the Lo *et al.* study displayed 75% less inflammatory infiltration than normal EAE mice, possibly accounting for the dramatically improved clinical scores. This reduction has been attributed to hyperdensities of sodium channels on activated macrophages and microglia in the CNS of EAE mice (Craner *et al.*, 2005). Blockage of Na+ channels presumably curtails neurotoxic immune effector functions of these cells, including NO radical production and phagocytosis, and diminishes immune-mediated axonal destruction. Infiltrating monocytes in MS lesions also show increased sodium channel expression (Craner *et al.*, 2005). At present, three large scale phase-I human clinical trials have been launched to examine the efficacy of Na+ channel blockers in treating different stages of MS (Waxman, 2008). However, the progress of these trials has been disturbed by emerging evidence of acute disease exacerbation following withdrawl of Na+ channel blocker therapy. Black *et al.* found that EAE mice treated with phenytoin experienced marked inflammatory infiltration and increased vascular permeability once the drug was removed, with death occuring in approximately 50% of these mice (Black *et al.*, 2007).

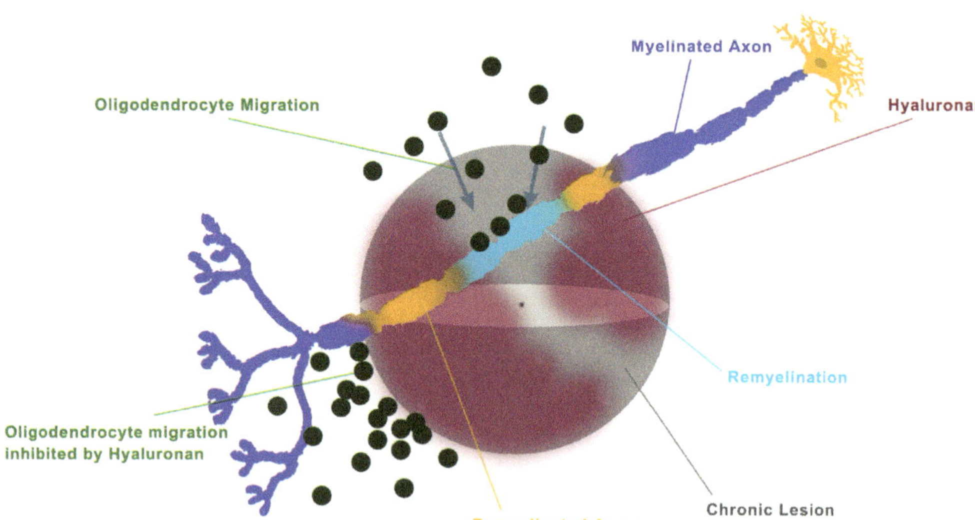

Fig. 7. MS axon passing through a chronic MS lesion. Oligodendrocytes migrate into the lesion environment to replace lost myelin on the axon (remyelination). Hyaluronan accumulates in the chronic MS lesion, preventing oligodendrocyte maturation and possibly influencing migration into the lesion.

9.3 Preventing free radical damage

NO is a double-edged sword in MS. On the one hand, NO is thought to modulate immunological functions. For example, prevention of NO production has been shown to exacerbate some forms of EAE (Giovanni *et al.*, 1998). On the other, NO-associated free radical damage has been implicated in the pathogenesis of axonal loss in MS and the clinical manifestations of the disease (Redford *et al.*, 1997; Smith *et al.*, 2001, 2002). NO can be converted into reactive nitrogen species, such as peroxynitrate (ONOO(-)), and inflict cellular damage (Jack *et al.*, 2007). In EAE, inducible nitric oxide synthase (iNOS) shows up in perivascular macrophages before demyelination, and is associated with transient functional disturbance in axons (Aboul-Enein *et al.*, 2006). This brings to mind early, reversible pathological changes seen in axons before inflammatory demyelination (About-Enein *et al.*, 2006; Nikić *et al.*, 2011). Furthermore, iNOS is highly expressed in actively demyelinating, remyelinating, and chronic MS lesions, and is extensive in normal brain matter regions (Hill *et al.*, 2004; Broholm *et al*, 2006). Because of these findings, blocking formation of reactive nitrogen species may be an attractive therapeutic target for the treatment of axonal loss in MS.

The neuroprotective ability of the drug glatiramer acetatate (GA, trade name Copaxone) is under active investigation. Subcutaneous injection of GA is currently used for the treatment of relapsing/remitting MS. GA is thought to work by inducing Th2/3 cells to cross the blood brain barrier, accumulate in the CNS, and express IL-10, TGF-β, and neurotrophic factors such as brain-derived neurotrophic factor (BDNF) (Aharoni *et al.*, 2003). GA has been reported to prevent free radical formation in peripheral blood adherent mononuclear cells *in vitro* (Iarlori *et al.*, 2008). One of these radicals, superoxide anion (O(2)(-)), reacts with NO to produce peroxynitrate. Peroxynitrate has been associated with extensive oligodendrocyte cell death in a subset of MS lesions (Jack *et al.*, 2007). Early animal studies on the neuroprotective effects of GA show promise. Spinal cords of glatiramer acetate-treated EAE mice show significantly reduced demyelination and enhanced remyelination compared to controls (Aharoni *et al.*, 2008). Moreover, when treatment was initiated at the time of manifestation of clinical symptoms, or even in the chronic disease phase when extensive demyelination had already accumulated, GA dramatically reduced pathological damage. Randomized human clinical trials measuring disease activity and burden using state-of-the-art imaging technology are currently investigating the neuroprotective effects of GA treatment in MS patients (García-Martín *et al.*, 2010). As more is discovered regarding the pathogenesis of axonal loss and mechanisms of substances such as GA, selectively shutting down the neurodegenerative machinery of MS will become more feasible.

10. Conclusion

Since Charcot's identification of axonal pathology in MS in 1869, two main attributes of the disease are clear. First, independent of the relapsing/remitting phase of MS, a pathologic process of accumulating axonal loss is chiefly responsible for the currently untreatable neurological decline in MS. Second, although it might not be the causative factor, inflammation definitely spatiotemporally coincides with the extent of axonal injury in affected tissue. The presence of cytotoxic CTLs targeted against axons, free radical-induced mitochondrial damage, and mislocalization of membrane ion channels point to an etiology that is immunological in nature. Loss of oligodendrocyte trophic support or other protective functions also cannot be disregarded as a cause of axonal dystrophy.

Brain cells are capable of releasing endogenous ligands in response to cellular damage which activate innate and cellular immune responses (Matzinger, 2002; Sloane *et al.*, 2010a). Recent evidence shows that, in an EAE mouse model, axonal dystrophy can occur in pre-lesion areas before hits of inflammatory demyelination (About-Enein et al., 2006; Nikić *et al.*, 2011). Moreover, axonal swellings in these areas often spontaneously resolve with no induced inflammation (Nikić *et al.*, 2011). It is possible that individual axons manifest dystrophic changes in the absence of inflammation and as a result release danger signals into the exocellular environment (Matzinger, 2002). Further axonal injury may amplify or modulate these chemical messengers until reaching a threshold that induces inflammation. Instigated innate and cellular immune effector cells target degenerating axons expressing MHC, resulting in active inflammation that amplifies structural damage to axons.

11. References

Aboul-Enein F, Weiser P, Höftberger R, Lassmann H, Bradl M. Transient axonal injury in the absence of demyelination: a correlate of clinical disease in acute experimental autoimmune encephalomyelitis. Acta Neuropathol 2006, 111:539–547.

Adams RD, Kubick CS. The morbid anatomy of the demyelinative disease. Am J Med. 1952 May;12(5):510-46.

Aharoni R, Herschkovitz A, Eilam R, Blumberg-Hazan M, Sela M, Bruck W, Arnon R. Demyelination arrest and remyelination induced by glatiramer acetate treatment of experimental autoimmune encephalomyelitis. Proc Natl Acad Sci U S A. 2008 Aug 12;105(32):11358-63.

Aharoni R, Kayhan B, Eilam R, Sela M, Arnon R. Glatiramer acetate-specific T cells in the brain express T helper 2/3 cytokines and brain-derived neurotrophic factor in situ. Proc Natl Acad Sci U S A. 2003 Nov 25;100(24):14157-62.

Anthony DC, Miller KM, Fearn S, et al. Matrix metalloproteinase expression in an experimentally-induced DTH model of multiple sclerosis in the rat CNS. J Neuroimmunol 1998;87:62–72.

Arai Y, Deguchi K, Mizuguchi M, and Takashima S. Expression of beta-amyloid precursor protein in axons of periventricular leukomalacia brains. Pediatr Neurol 1995 13:161-163.

Bannerman PG, Hahn A, Ramirez S, Morley M, Bönnemann C, Yu S, Zhang GX, Rostami A, Pleasure D. Motor neuron pathology in experimental autoimmune encephalomyelitis: studies in THY1-YFP transgenic mice. Brain. 2005 Aug;128(Pt 8):1877-86.

Bannerman PG, Hahn A. Enhanced visualization of axonopathy in EAE using thy1-YFP transgenic mice. J Neurol Sci. 2007 Sep 15;260(1-2):23-32.

Barnett MH, Prineas JW. Relapsing and remitting multiple sclerosis: pathology of the newly forming lesion. Ann Neurol. 2004 Apr;55(4):458-68.

Bechtold DA, Kapoor R, Smith KJ. Axonal protection using flecainide in experimental autoimmune encephalomyelitis. Ann Neurol. 2004 May;55(5):607-16.

Bitsch A, Schuchardt J, Bunkowski S, Kuhlmann T, Brück W. Acute axonal injury in multiple sclerosis. Correlation with demyelination and inflammation. Brain. 2000 Jun;123 (Pt 6):1174-83.

Bjartmar C, Kidd G, Mork S, et al. Neurological disability correlates with spinal cord axonal loss and reduced N-acetyl aspartate in chronic multiple sclerosis patients. Ann Neurol 2000;48:893–901.

Bjartmar C, Kinkel RP, Kidd G, Rudick RA, Trapp BD. Axonal loss in normal-appearing white matter in a patient with acute MS. Neurology. 2001 Oct 9;57(7):1248-52.

Bjartmar C, Trapp BD. Axonal degeneration and progressive neurologic disability in multiple sclerosis. Neurotox Res. 2003;5(1-2):157-64.

Black JA, Liu S, Carrithers M, Carrithers LM, Waxman SG. Exacerbation of experimental autoimmune encephalomyelitis after withdrawal of phenytoin and carbamazepine. Ann Neurol. 2007a Jul;62(1):21-33.

Black JA, Newcombe J, Trapp BD, Waxman SG. Sodium channel expression within chronic multiple sclerosis plaques. J Neuropathol Exp Neurol. 2007b Sep;66(9):828-37.

Booss J, Esiri MM, Tourtellotte WW, Mason DY. Immunohistological analysis of T lymphocyte subsets in the central nervous system in chronic progressive multiple sclerosis. J Neurol Sci. 1983 Dec;62(1-3):219-32.

Broholm H, Andersen B, Wanscher B, Frederiksen JL, Rubin I, Pakkenberg B, Larsson HB, Lauritzen M. Nitric oxide synthase expression and enzymatic activity in multiple sclerosis. Acta Neurol Scand. 2004 Apr;109(4):261-9.

Buzzard EF and Greenfield JG. Pathology of the nervous system. London: Constable, 1921: 288.

Charcot JM. Histologie de la sclerose en plaques. Gaz Hosp 1868;141:554-5, 557.

Charcot JM. Lectures on the diseases of the nervous system. Transl. by G. Sigerson. London: New Sydenham Society, 1877.

Choi P, Golts N, Snyder H, Chong M, Petrucelli L, Hardy J, Sparkman D, Cochran E, Lee JM, Wolozin B. Co-association of parkin and alpha-synuclein. Neuroreport 2001 12:2839-2843.

Choi P, Ostrerova-Golts N, Sparkman D, Cochran E, Lee JM, and Wolozin B. Parkin is metabolized by the ubiquitin/proteosome system. Neuroreport 2000 11:2635-2638.

Cochran E, Bacci B, Chen Y, Patton A, Gambetti P, Autilio-Gambetti L. Amyloid precursor protein and ubiquitin immunoreactivity in dystrophic axons is not unique to Alzheimer's disease. Am J Pathol. 1991 Sep;139(3):485-9.

Compston A, Coles A. Multiple sclerosis. Lancet. 2002 Apr 6;359(9313):1221-31. Review. Erratum in: Lancet 2002 Aug 24;360(9333):648.

Craner MJ, Damarjian TG, Liu S, Hains BC, Lo AC, Black JA, Newcombe J, Cuzner ML, Waxman SG. Sodium channels contribute to microglia/macrophage activation and function in EAE and MS. Glia. 2005 Jan 15;49(2):220-9.

Craner MJ, Newcombe J, Black JA, Hartle C, Cuzner ML, Waxman SG. Molecular changes in neurons in multiple sclerosis: altered axonal expression of Nav1.2 and Nav1.6 sodium channels and Na+/Ca2+ exchanger. Proc Natl Acad Sci U S A. 2004 May 25;101(21):8168-73.

Dawson JW. The histology of disseminated sclerosis. Part II Histological study. Edin Med J 1916; NS17: 311–344.

De Stefano N, Filippi M, Miller D, Pouwels PJ, Rovira A, Gass A, Enzinger C, Matthews PM, Arnold DL. Guidelines for using proton MR spectroscopy in multicenter clinical MS studies. Neurology. 2007 Nov 13;69(20):1942-52.

deWaegh SM, Lee VM, Brady ST. Local modulation of neurofilament phosphorylation, axonal caliber, and slow axonal transport by myelinating Schwann cells. Cell, 1992 Feb 7; 68(3): 451-63.

Dickson DW, Wertkin A, Kress Y, Ksiezak-Reding H, and Yen SH. Ubiquitin immunoreactive structures in normal human brains. Distribution and developmental aspects. Lab Invest 1990 63:87-99.

Dinkel K, Dhabhar FS, Sapolsky RM. Neurotoxic effects of polymorphonuclear granulocytes on hippocampal primary cultures. Proc Natl Acad Sci U S A. 2004 Jan 6;101(1):331-6.

Dutta R, McDonough J, Yin X, Peterson J, Chang A, Torres T, Gudz T, Macklin WB, Lewis DA, Fox RJ, Rudick R, Mirnics K, Trapp BD. Mitochondrial dysfunction as a cause of axonal degeneration in multiple sclerosis patients. Ann Neurol. 2006 Mar;59(3):478-89.

Evangelou N, DeLuca GC, Owens T, Esiri MM. Pathological study of spinal cord atrophy in multiple sclerosis suggests limited role of local lesions. Brain. 2005 Jan;128(Pt 1):29-34.

Evangelou N, Esiri MM, Smith S, et al. Quantitative pathological evidence for axonal loss in normal appearing white matter in multiple sclerosis. Ann Neurol 2000a;47:391–5.

Evangelou N, Konz D, Esiri MM, et al. Regional axonal loss in the corpus callosum correlates with cerebral white matter lesion volume and distribution in multiple sclerosis. Brain 2000b;123:1845–9.

Ferguson B, Matyszak MK, Esiri MM, and Perry VH. Axonal damage in acute multiple sclerosis lesions. Brain 1997 120 (Pt 3):393-399.

Fern R *et al.* (1993) Pharmacological protection of CNS white matter during anoxia: actions of phenytoin, carbamazepine and diazepam. J Pharmacol Exper Ther 266: 1549–1555

Ferreira A, Caceres A, Kosik KS. Intraneuronal compartments of the amyloid precursor protein. J Neurosci 1993; 13: 3112–23.

Fisher E, Lee JC, Nakamura K, Rudick RA. Gray matter atrophy in multiple sclerosis: a longitudinal study. Ann Neurol. 2008 Sep;64(3):255-65.

Fisniku LK, Chard DT, Jackson JS, Anderson VM, Altmann DR, Miszkiel KA, Thompson AJ, Miller DH. Gray matter atrophy is related to long-term disability in multiple sclerosis. Ann Neurol. 2008 Sep;64(3):247-54. Erratum in: Ann Neurol. 2009 Feb;65(2):232.

Frischer JM, Bramow S, Dal-Bianco A, Lucchinetti CF, Rauschka H, Schmidbauer M, Laursen H, Sorensen PS, Lassmann H. The relation between inflammation and neurodegeneration in multiple sclerosis brains. Brain. 2009 May;132(Pt 5):1175-89.

Fukuda, T., Shimizu, J., Furuhata, H., Abe, T., Shimizu, K., Oishi, T., Ogihara, M., Kubota, J., Sasaki, A., Sasaki, K., et al. Overexpression of heat shock proteins in pallido-nigral axonal spheroids of nonhuman aged primates. Acta Neuropathol 2005 110:145-150.

Galeano C, Vaz Ferriera A. A comparison of Cajal and Bielschowsky-Gros silver impregnations in Wallerian degeneration. Stain Technol. 1957 Jan;32(1):11-7.

Gallo P, Pagni S, Piccinno MG, Giometto B, Argentiero V, Chiusole M, Bozza F, Tavolato B. On the role of interleukin-2 (IL-2) in multiple sclerosis (MS). IL-2-mediated endothelial cell activation. Ital J Neurol Sci. 1992 Dec;13(9 Suppl 14):65-8.

Galvin JE, Giasson B, Hurtig HI, Lee VM, Trojanowski JQ. Neurodegeneration with brain iron accumulation, type 1 is characterized by alpha-, beta-, and gamma-synuclein neuropathology. Am J Pathol 2000 157:361-368.

Ganter P, Prince C, Esiri MM. Spinal cord axonal loss in multiple sclerosis: a post-mortem study. Neuropathol Appl Neurobiol. 1999 Dec;25(6):459-67.

García-Martín E, Pueyo V, Fernández J, Martín J, Ara JR, Almarcegui C, Dolz I. [Effect of treatment in loss of retinal nerve fibre layer in multiple sclerosis patients]. Arch Soc Esp Oftalmol. 2010 Jun;85(6):209-14.

Gay FW, Drye TJ, Dick GW, Esiri MM. The application of multifactorial cluster analysis in the staging of plaques in early multiple sclerosis. Identification and characterization of the primary demyelinating lesion. Brain. 1997 Aug;120 (Pt 8):1461-83.

Gehrmann J, Banati RB, Cuzner ML, Kreutzberg GW, Newcombe J. Amyloid precursor protein (APP) expression in multiple sclerosis lesions. Glia 1995; 15: 141–51.

Gentleman SM, Nash MJ, Sweeting CJ, Graham DI, Roberts GW. Beta-amyloid precursor protein (beta APP) as a marker for axonal injury after head injury. Neurosci Lett 1993; 160: 139–44.

Ghosh, N., DeLuca, G.C., and Esiri, M.M. Evidence of axonal damage in human acute demyelinating diseases. J Neurol Sci 2004 222:29-34.

Giovannoni G, Heales SJ, Land JM, Thompson EJ. The potential role of nitric oxide in multiple sclerosis. Mult Scler. 1998 Jun;4(3):212-6.

Gold R, Linington C, Lassmann H. Understanding pathogenesis and therapy of multiple sclerosis via animal models: 70 years of merits and culprits in experimental autoimmune encephalomyelitis research. Brain. 2006 Aug;129(Pt 8):1953-71.

Gonen O, Catalaa I, Babb JS, Ge Y, Mannon LJ, Kolson DL, Grossman RI. Total brain N-acetylaspartate: a new measure of disease load in MS. Neurology. 2000 Jan 11;54(1):15-9.

Gray F, Belec L, Chretien F, Dubreuil-Lemaire ML, Ricolfi F, Wingertsmann L, Poron F, Gherardi R. Acute, relapsing brain oedema with diffuse blood-brain barrier alteration and axonal damage in the acquired immunodeficiency syndrome. Neuropathol Appl Neurobiol 1998 24:209-216.

Greenfield JG, King LS. Observations on the histopathology of the cerebral lesions in disseminated sclerosis. Brain 1936; 59: 445–58.

Griffiths I, Klugmann M, Anderson T, Yool D, Thomson C, Schwab MH, Schneider A, Zimmermann F, McCulloch M, Nadon N, Nave KA. Axonal swellings and degeneration in mice lacking the major proteolipid of myelin. Science. 1998 Jun 5;280(5369):1610-3.

Guiroy, D.C., Shankar, S.K., Gibbs, C.J., Jr., Messenheimer, J.A., Das, S., and Gajdusek, D.C. Neuronal degeneration and neurofilament accumulation in the trigeminal ganglia in Creutzfeldt-Jakob disease. Ann Neurol 1989 25:102-106.

Haass C, Koo EH, Mellon A, Hung AY, Selkoe DJ. Targeting of cell-surface beta-amyloid precursor protein to lysosomes: alternative processing into amyloid-bearing fragments. Nature 1992; 357: 500–3.

Haider L, Fischer MT, Frischer JM, Bauer J, Höftberger R, Botond G, Esterbauer H, Binder CJ, Witztum JL, Lassmann H. Oxidative damage in multiple sclerosis lesions. Brain. 2011 Jul;134(Pt 7):1914-24.

Han MH, Hwang SI, Roy DB, Lundgren DH, Price JV, Ousman SS, Fernald GH, Gerlitz B, Robinson WH, Baranzini SE, Grinnell BW, Raine CS, Sobel RA, Han DK, Steinman L. Proteomic analysis of active multiple sclerosis lesions reveals therapeutic targets. Nature. 2008 Feb 28;451(7182):1076-81.

Hanafy KA, Sloane JA. Regulation of remyelination in multiple sclerosis. FEBS Lett. 2011 Mar 30.

Haynes RL, Billiards SS, Borenstein NS, Volpe JJ, and Kinney HC. Diffuse axonal injury in periventricular leukomalacia as determined by apoptotic marker fractin. Pediatr Res 2008 63: 656-661.

Henderson AP, Barnett MH, Parratt JD, Prineas JW. Multiple sclerosis: distribution of inflammatory cells in newly forming lesions. Ann Neurol. 2009 Dec;66(6):739-53.

Herrero-Herranz E, Pardo LA, Gold R, Linker RA. Pattern of axonal injury in murine myelin oligodendrocyte glycoprotein induced experimental autoimmune encephalomyelitis: implications for multiple sclerosis. Neurobiol 2008. Dis 30:162–173.

Hill KE, Zollinger LV, Watt HE, Carlson NG, Rose JW. Inducible nitric oxide synthase in chronic active multiple sclerosis plaques: distribution, cellular expression and association with myelin damage. J Neuroimmunol. 2004 Jun;151(1-2):171-9.

Hsieh S-T, Crawford TO, Bouldin TW, Griffin JW. Influence of demyelination and remyelination on axonal organization. Brain Pathol 1993;3:307-307

Iarlori C, Gambi D, Lugaresi A, Patruno A, Felaco M, Salvatore M, Speranza L, Reale M. Reduction of free radicals in multiple sclerosis: effect of glatiramer acetate (Copaxone). Mult Scler. 2008 Jul;14(6):739-48.

Irvine KA, Blakemore WF. Remyelination protects axons from demyelination-associated axon degeneration. Brain. 2008 Jun;131(Pt 6):1464-77.

Izycka-Swieszewska E, Zoltowska A, Rzepko R, Gross M, and Borowska-Lehman J. Vasculopathy and amyloid beta reactivity in brains of patients with acquired immune deficiency (AIDS). Folia Neuropathol 2000 38:175-182.

Jack C, Antel J, Brück W, Kuhlmann T. Contrasting potential of nitric oxide and peroxynitrite to mediate oligodendrocyte injury in multiple sclerosis. Glia. 2007 Jul;55(9):926-34.

Jellinger KA. Cell death mechanisms in Parkinson's disease. J Neural Transm 2000 107:1-29.

Jones MV, Nguyen TT, Deboy CA, Griffin JW, Whartenby KA, Kerr DA, Calabresi PA. Behavioral and pathological outcomes in MOG 35-55 experimental autoimmune encephalomyelitis. J Neuroimmunol. 2008 Aug 13;199(1-2):83-93.

Kato T, Kurita K, Seino T, Kadoya T, Horie H, Wada M, Kawanami T, Daimon M, and Hirano A. Galectin-1 is a component of neurofilamentous lesions in sporadic and familial amyotrophic lateral sclerosis. Biochem Biophys Res Commun 2001 282:166-172.

Kikuchi, S., Shinpo, K., Ogata, A., Tsuji, S., Takeuchi, M., Makita, Z., and Tashiro, K. Detection of N epsilon-(carboxymethyl)lysine (CML) and non-CML advanced glycation end-products in the anterior horn of amyotrophic lateral sclerosis spinal cord. Amyotroph Lateral Scler Other Motor Neuron Disord 2002 3:63-68.

Kobayashi A, Arima K, Ogawa M, Murata M, Fukuda T, and Kitamoto T. Plaque-type deposition of prion protein in the damaged white matter of sporadic Creutzfeldt-Jakob disease MM1 patients. Acta Neuropathol 2008 116:561-566.

Koo EH, Park L, Selkoe DJ. Amyloid beta-protein as a substrate interacts with extracellular matrix to promote neurite outgrowth. Proc Natl Acad Sci U S A. 1993 May 15;90(10):4748-52.

Kornek B, Storch MK, Bauer J, Djamshidian A, Weissert R, Wallstroem E, Stefferl A, Zimprich F, Olsson T, Linington C, Schmidbauer M, Lassmann H. Distribution of a calcium channel subunit in dystrophic axons in multiple sclerosis and experimental autoimmune encephalomyelitis. Brain. 2001 Jun;124(Pt 6):1114-24.

Kremenchutzky M, Rice GP, Baskerville J, Wingerchuk DM, Ebers GC. The natural history of multiple sclerosis: a geographically based study 9: observations on the progressive phase of the disease. Brain. 2006 Mar;129(Pt 3):584-94.

Kriss A, Francis DA, Cuendet F, Halliday AM, Taylor DS, Wilson J, Keast-Butler J, Batchelor JR, McDonald WI. Recovery after optic neuritis in childhood. J Neurol Neurosurg Psychiatry. 1988 Oct;51(10):1253-8.

Kuhlmann T, Lucchinetti C, Zettl UK, Bitsch A, Lassmann H, Brück W. Bcl-2-expressing oligodendrocytes in multiple sclerosis lesions. Glia. 1999 Oct;28(1):34-9.

Kurihara T, Tsukada Y. The regional and subcellular distribution of 2',3'-cyclic nucleotide 3'-phosphohydrolase in the central nervous system. J Neurochem. 1967 Dec;14(12):1167-74.

Kutzelnigg A, Lucchinetti CF, Stadelmann C, Brück W, Rauschka H, Bergmann M, Schmidbauer M, Parisi JE, Lassmann H. Cortical demyelination and diffuse white matter injury in multiple sclerosis. Brain. 2005 Nov;128(Pt 11):2705-12.

Lappe-Siefke C, Goebbels S, Gravel M, Nicksch E, Lee J, Braun PE, Griffiths IR, Nave KA. Disruption of Cnp1 uncouples oligodendroglial functions in axonal support and myelination. Nat Genet. 2003 Mar;33(3):366-74.

Letournel F, Bocquet A, Dubas F, Barthelaix A, Eyer J. Stable tubule only polypeptides (STOP) proteins co-aggregate with spheroid neurofilaments in amyotrophic lateral sclerosis. J Neuropathol Exp Neurol 2003 62:1211-1219.

Liberski PP, and Budka H. Neuroaxonal pathology in Creutzfeldt-Jakob disease. Acta Neuropathol 1999 97:329-334.

Lo AC, Black JA, Waxman SG. Neuroprotection of axons with phenytoin in experimental allergic encephalomyelitis. Neuroreport. 2002 Oct 28;13(15):1909-12.

Lovas G, Szilagyi N, Majtenyi K, et al. Axonal changes in chronic demyelinated cervical spinal cord plaques. Brain 2000;123:308–17.

Lucchinetti C, Brück W, Parisi J, Scheithauer B, Rodriguez M, Lassmann H. Heterogeneity of multiple sclerosis lesions: implications for the pathogenesis of demyelination. Ann Neurol. 2000 Jun;47(6):707-17.

Ma Y, Haynes RL, Sidman RL, Vartanian T. TLR8: an innate immune receptor in brain, neurons and axons. Cell Cycle. 2007 Dec 1;6(23):2859-68.

Ma Y, Li J, Chiu I, Wang Y, Sloane JA, Lü J, Kosaras B, Sidman RL, Volpe JJ, Vartanian T. Toll-like receptor 8 functions as a negative regulator of neurite outgrowth and inducer of neuronal apoptosis. J Cell Biol. 2006 Oct 23;175(2):209-15.

Mahad D, Ziabreva I, Lassmann H, Turnbull D. Mitochondrial defects in acute multiple sclerosis lesions. Brain. 2008 Jul;131(Pt 7):1722-35.

Manning PT, Johnson EM Jr, Wilcox CL, Palmatier MA, Russell JH. MHC-specific cytotoxic T lymphocyte killing of dissociated sympathetic neuronal cultures. Am J Pathol. 1987 Sep;128(3):395-409.

Matthews PM, Pioro E, Narayanan S, De Stefano N, Fu L, Francis G, Antel J, Wolfson C, Arnold DL. Assessment of lesion pathology in multiple sclerosis using quantitative MRI morphometry and magnetic resonance spectroscopy. Brain. 1996 Jun;119 (Pt 3):715-22.

Matzinger P. An innate sense of danger. Ann N Y Acad Sci. 2002 Jun;961:341-2.

Medana I, Martinic MA, Wekerle H, Neumann H. Transection of major histocompatibility complex class I-induced neurites by cytotoxic T lymphocytes. Am J Pathol. 2001 Sep;159(3):809-15.

Medana, I.M., and Esiri, M.M. Axonal damage: a key predictor of outcome in human CNS diseases. Brain 2003 126:515-530.

Mews I, Bergmann M, Bunkowski S, et al. Oligodendrocyte and axon pathology in clinically silent multiple sclerosis lesions. Multiple Sclerosis 1998;4:55–62.

Mi S, Hu B, Hahm K, Luo Y, Kam Hui ES, Yuan Q, Wong WM, Wang L, Su H, Chu TH, Guo J, Zhang W, So KF, Pepinsky B, Shao Z, Graff C, Garber E, Jung V, Wu EX, Wu W. LINGO-1 antagonist promotes spinal cord remyelination and axonal integrity in MOG-induced experimental autoimmune encephalomyelitis. Nat Med. 2007 Oct;13(10):1228-33.

Miller DH, Leary SM. Primary-progressive multiple sclerosis. Lancet Neurol. 2007 Oct;6(10):903-12. Review. Erratum in: Lancet Neurol. 2009 Aug;8(8):699.

Nakazato, Y., Sasaki, A., Hirato, J., and Ishida, Y. Immunohistochemical localization of neurofilament protein in neuronal degenerations. Acta Neuropathol 1984 64:30-36.

Nave KA, Trapp BD. Axon-glial signaling and the glial support of axon function. Annu Rev Neurosci. 2008;31:535-61.

Neumann H, Medana IM, Bauer J, Lassmann H. Cytotoxic T lymphocytes in autoimmune and degenerative CNS diseases. Trends Neurosci. 2002 Jun;25(6):313-9.

Neumann H. Control of glial immune function by neurons. Glia. 2001 Nov;36(2):191-9.

Neumann M, Adler S, Schluter O, Kremmer E, Benecke R, Kretzschmar HA. Alpha-synuclein accumulation in a case of neurodegeneration with brain iron accumulation type 1 (NBIA-1, formerly Hallervorden-Spatz syndrome) with widespread cortical and brainstem-type Lewy bodies. Acta Neuropathol 2000 100:568-574.

Newell KL, Boyer P, Gomez-Tortosa E, Hobbs W, Hedley-Whyte ET, Vonsattel JP, Hyman BT. Alpha-synuclein immunoreactivity is present in axonal swellings in neuroaxonal dystrophy and acute traumatic brain injury. J Neuropathol Exp Neurol 1999 58:1263-1268.

Nikić I, Merkler D, Sorbara C, Brinkoetter M, Kreutzfeldt M, Bareyre FM, Brück W, Bishop D, Misgeld T, Kerschensteiner M. A reversible form of axon damage in experimental autoimmune encephalomyelitis and multiple sclerosis. Nat Med. 2011 Apr;17(4):495-9.

Nishizawa Y, Kurihara T, Masuda T, Takahashi Y. Immunohistochemical localization of 2',3'-cyclic nucleotide 3'-phosphodiesterase in adult bovine cerebrum and cerebellum. Neurochem Res. 1985 Aug;10(8):1107-18.

Noseworthy JH, Lucchinetti C, Rodriguez M, Weinshenker BG. Multiple sclerosis. N Engl J Med. 2000 Sep 28;343(13):938-52.

Ohgami T, Kitamoto T, Tateishi J. Alzheimer's amyloid precursor protein accumulates within axonal swellings in human brain lesions. Neurosci Lett. 1992 Feb 17;136(1):75-8.

Patel JR, McCandless EE, Dorsey D, Klein RS. CXCR4 promotes differentiation of oligodendrocyte progenitors and remyelination. Proc Natl Acad Sci U S A. 2010 Jun 15;107(24):11062-7.

Patrikios P, Stadelmann C, Kutzelnigg A, Rauschka H, Schmidbauer M, Laursen H, Sorensen PS, Brück W, Lucchinetti C, Lassmann H. Remyelination is extensive in a subset of multiple sclerosis patients. Brain. 2006 Dec;129(Pt 12):3165-72.

Peters G. Multiple sclerosis. In: Minckler J, editor. Pathology of the nervous system, Vol. 1. New York: McGraw-Hill, 1968: 821–43.

Peterson JW, Bö L, Mörk S, Chang A, Trapp BD. Transected neurites, apoptotic neurons, and reduced inflammation in cortical multiple sclerosis lesions. Ann Neurol. 2001 Sep;50(3):389-400.

Povlishock JT. Traumatically induced axonal injury: pathogenesis and pathobiological implications. Brain Pathol. 1992 Jan;2(1):1-12.

Prineas JW, Barnard RO, Kwon EE, Sharer LR, Cho ES. Multiple sclerosis: remyelination of nascent lesions. Ann Neurol. 1993 Feb;33(2):137-51.

Prineas JW, Wright RG. Macrophages, lymphocytes, and plasma cells in the perivascular compartment in chronic multiple sclerosis. Lab Invest. 1978 Apr;38(4):409-21.

Putnam TJ. Studies in multiple sclerosis. Arch Neurol Psychiatry 1936; 35: 1289–308.

Raine CS, and Cross AH. Axonal dystrophy as a consequence of long-term demyelination. Lab Invest 1989 60:714-725.

Raisanen J, Ghougassian DF, Moskvitch M, Lawrence C. Diffuse axonal injury in a rugby player. Am J Forensic Med Pathol 1999 20:70-72.

Raja F, Sherriff FE, Morris CS, Bridges LR, Esiri MM. Cerebral white matter damage in HIV infection demonstrated using beta-amyloid precursor protein immunoreactivity. Acta Neuropathol 1997 93:184-189.

Redford EJ, Kapoor R, Smith KJ. Nitric oxide donors reversibly block axonal conduction: demyelinated axons are especially susceptible. Brain 1997;120:2149–57.

Richards TL. Proton MR spectroscopy in multiple sclerosis: value in establishing diagnosis, monitoring progression, and evaluating therapy. AJR Am J Roentgenol. 1991 Nov;157(5):1073-8.

Sasaki S, and Iwata M. Immunoreactivity of beta-amyloid precursor protein in amyotrophic lateral sclerosis. Acta Neuropathol 1999 97:463-468.

Schwab C, Steele JC, and McGeer PL. Dystrophic neurites are associated with early stage extracellular neurofibrillary tangles in the parkinsonism-dementia complex of Guam. Acta Neuropathol 1997 94:486-492.

Sherriff FE, Bridges LR, Gentleman SM, Sivaloganathan S, Wilson S. Markers of axonal injury in post mortem human brain. Acta Neuropathol (Berl) 1994a; 88: 433–9.

Sherriff FE, Bridges LR, Jackson P. Microwave antigen retrieval of beta-amyloid precursor protein immunoreactivity. Neuroreport. 1994b May 9;5(9):1085-8.

Shibata N, Asayama K, Hirano A, Kobayashi M. Immunohistochemical study on superoxide dismutases in spinal cords from autopsied patients with amyotrophic lateral sclerosis. Dev Neurosci 1996 18:492-498.

Shindler KS, Ventura E, Dutt M, Rostami A. Inflammatory demyelination induces axonal injury and retinal ganglion cell apoptosis in experimental optic neuritis. Exp Eye Res. 2008 Sep;87(3):208-13.

Shintaku M, Hirano A, Llena JF. Increased diameter of demyelinated axons in chronic multiple sclerosis of the spinal cord. Neuropathol Appl Neurobiol. 1988 Nov-Dec;14(6):505-10.

Sloane JA, Batt C, Ma Y, Harris ZM, Trapp B, Vartanian T. Hyaluronan blocks oligodendrocyte progenitor maturation and remyelination through TLR2. Proc Natl Acad Sci U S A. 2010b Jun 22;107(25):11555-60.

Sloane JA, Blitz D, Margolin Z, Vartanian T. A clear and present danger: endogenous ligands of Toll-like receptors. Neuromolecular Med. 2010a Jun;12(2):149-63.

Smith KJ, Kapoor R, Hall SM, et al. Electrically active axons degenerate when exposed to nitric oxide. Ann Neurol 2001;49:470–9.

Smith KJ, Lassmann H. The role of nitric oxide in multiple sclerosis. Lancet Neurol. 2002 Aug;1(4):232-41. Review.

Smith, T.W., DeGirolami, U., Henin, D., Bolgert, F., and Hauw, J.J. (1990). Human immunodeficiency virus (HIV) leukoencephalopathy and the microcirculation. J Neuropathol Exp Neurol 1990 49:357-370.

Soulika AM, Lee E, McCauley E, Miers L, Bannerman P, Pleasure D. Initiation and progression of axonopathy in experimental autoimmune encephalomyelitis. J Neurosci. 2009 Nov 25;29(47):14965-79.

Steinman L, Zamvil SS. How to successfully apply animal studies in experimental allergic encephalomyelitis to research on multiple sclerosis. Ann Neurol. 2006 Jul;60(1):12-21.

Sternberger LA, Sternberger NH. Monoclonal antibodies distinguish phosphorylated and nonphosphorylated forms of neurofilaments in situ. Proc Natl Acad Sci U S A. 1983 Oct;80(19):6126-30.

Stewart WA, Alvord EC Jr, Hruby S, Hall LD, Paty DW. Magnetic resonance imaging of experimental allergic encephalomyelitis in primates. Brain. 1991 Apr;114 (Pt 2):1069-96.

Stokin, G.B., Lillo, C., Falzone, T.L., Brusch, R.G., Rockenstein, E., Mount, S.L., Raman, R., Davies, P., Masliah, E., Williams, D.S., et al. Axonopathy and transport deficits early in the pathogenesis of Alzheimer's disease. Science 2005 307:1282-1288.

Stys PK, Lesiuk H. Correlation between electrophysiological effects of mexiletine and ischemic protection in central nervous system white matter. Neuroscience. 1996 Mar;71(1):27-36.

Stys PK, Ransom BR, Waxman SG. Tertiary and quaternary local anesthetics protect CNS white matter from anoxic injury at concentrations that do not block excitability. J Neurophysiol. 1992b Jan;67(1):236-40.

Stys PK, Waxman SG, Ransom BR. Ionic mechanisms of anoxic injury in mammalian CNS white matter: role of Na+ channels and Na(+)-Ca2+ exchanger. J Neurosci. 1992a Feb;12(2):430-9.

Tourbah A, Stievenart JL, Iba-Zizen MT, Zannoli G, Lyon-Caen O, Cabanis EA. In vivo localized NMR proton spectroscopy of normal appearing white matter in patients with multiple sclerosis. J Neuroradiol. 1996 Sep;23(2):49-55.

Toyoshima, I., Sugawara, M., Kato, K., Wada, C., Hirota, K., Hasegawa, K., Kowa, H., Sheetz, M.P., and Masamune, O. Kinesin and cytoplasmic dynein in spinal spheroids with motor neuron disease. J Neurol Sci 1998 159:38-44.

Trapp BD, Nave KA. Multiple sclerosis: an immune or neurodegenerative disorder? Annu Rev Neurosci. 2008;31:247-69.

Trapp BD, Peterson J, Ransohoff RM, Rudick R, Mork S, Bo L. Axonal transection in the lesions of multiple sclerosis. N Engl J Med 1998; 338: 278–85.

Wakita H, Tomimoto H, Akiguchi I, Matsuo A, Lin JX, Ihara M, McGeer PL. Axonal damage and demyelination in the white matter after chronic cerebral hypoperfusion in the rat. Brain Res. 2002 Jan 4;924(1):63-70.

Wang D, Ayers MM, Catmull DV, Hazelwood LJ, Bernard CC, Orian JM. Astrocyte-associated axonal damage in pre-onset stages of experimental autoimmune encephalomyelitis. Glia. 2005 Aug 15;51(3):235-40.

Wang Y, Piao JH, Larsen EC, Kondo Y, Duncan ID. Migration and remyelination by oligodendrocyte progenitor cells transplanted adjacent to focal areas of spinal cord inflammation. J Neurosci Res. 2011 Jul 25. In press.

Waxman SG. Mechanisms of disease: sodium channels and neuroprotection in multiple sclerosis-current status. Nat Clin Pract Neurol. 2008 Mar;4(3):159-69..

Weiner HL. The challenge of multiple sclerosis: how do we cure a chronic heterogeneous disease? Ann Neurol. 2009 Mar;65(3):239-48.

Weiner JA, Hecht JH, Chun J. Lysophosphatidic acid receptor gene vzg-1/lpA1/edg-2 is expressed by mature oligodendrocytes during myelination in the postnatal murine brain. J Comp Neurol. 1998 Sep 7;398(4):587-98.

Weinshenker BG. Natural history of multiple sclerosis. Ann Neurol. 1994;36 Suppl:S6-11.

Wilkins A, Majed H, Layfield R, Compston A, Chandran S. Oligodendrocytes promote neuronal survival and axonal length by distinct intracellular mechanisms: a novel role for oligodendrocyte-derived glial cell line-derived neurotrophic factor. J Neurosci. 2003 Jun 15;23(12):4967-74.

Yasuhara O, Kawamata T, Aimi Y, McGeer EG, McGeer PL. Expression of chromogranin A in lesions in the central nervous system from patients with neurological diseases. Neurosci Lett 1994 170:13-16.

Young EA, Fowler CD, Kidd GJ, Chang A, Rudick R, Fisher E, Trapp BD. Imaging correlates of decreased axonal Na+/K+ ATPase in chronic multiple sclerosis lesions. Ann Neurol. 2008 Apr;63(4):428-35.

Zhou L, Miller BL, McDaniel CH, Kelly L, Kim OJ, and Miller CA. Frontotemporal dementia: neuropil spheroids and presynaptic terminal degeneration. Ann Neurol 1998 44:99-109.

Vascular Dementia and Alzheimer's Disease: Is There a Difference?

Said Ramdane
*Private Office of Neurology,
Algerian Society of Neurology,
Algeria*

1. Introduction

Dementia is a syndrome that can be caused by a number of progressive disorders that affect memory, thinking, behaviour and the ability to perform everyday activities, with increasing loss of function. Dementia mainly affects older people; after age 65, the likelihood of developing dementia roughly doubles every five years (Alzheimer's Association, 2011; Wimo & Prince, 2010). Patients with dementia usually survive 7-10 years after onset of symptoms, placing a tremendous burden not only on caregivers, but also on society (Alzheimer's Association, 2010; Wimo et al., 2010).

Due to increasing life expectancy the number of people suffering from dementia will increase rapidly in both developed and developing countries. As a result, the management of dementia patients is now becoming one of the most important public health problems (Wimo et al, 2003). It is estimated that 24.3 million people have dementia today, with 4.6 million new cases of dementia every year (one new case every 7 seconds). The number of people affected will double every 20 years to 81.1 million by 2040. Most people with dementia live in developing countries (60% in 2001, rising to 71% by 2040). Rates of increase are not uniform; numbers in developed countries are forecast to increase by 100% between 2001 and 2040, but by more than 300% in India, China, and their south Asian and western Pacific neighbours; i.e. the rate of increase in numbers of people with dementia is predicted to be three to four times higher in developing areas than in developed regions (Ferri et al., 2005). Hence, dementia is one of the most important public health problems.

The syndrome of dementia may be caused by various underlying diseases, each characterised by a specific constellation of signs and symptoms in combination with a presumed underlying substrate of neuropathology. Alzheimer's disease (AD) is the most prevalent cause of dementia. It is a neurodegenerative disorder, generally assumed to be caused by neuritic plaques and neurofibrillary tangles accumulating in the brain. The second most prevalent cause of dementia is vascular dementia (VaD), which may be caused by various types of vascular pathology in the brain, such as "large vessel"- large territorial or strategical infarctions, and "small vessel"- lacunes and white matter hyperintensities disease, (Van der Flier & Scheltens, 2005).

Current data from developing countries suggest that age-adjusted dementia prevalence estimates in 65 year olds are high (≥5%) in certain Asian and Latin American countries, but consistently low (1–3%) in India and sub-Saharan Africa (Kalaria et al., 2008). In 2000, prevalence data from 11 European population based studies were pooled to obtain stable estimates of prevalence of dementia in the elderly (> 65 years); age standardised prevalence was 6.4% for dementia (all causes), 4.4% for AD, and 1.6% for VaD (Berr et al., 2005; Lobo et al., 2000). The ratio between AD and VaD was similar in most studies of US, Europe and Africa. Alzheimer's disease is the most common etiology of dementia and accounts for 50-70% of total dementia cases. The second most common etiology is vascular dementia and account for 20-30% of total dementia (Fratiglioni et al., 1999).

Dementia syndrome develops over a long period of time characterized by progression from normal cognition defined as preclinical stage, through a transition phase of cognitive impairment defined as mild cognitive impairment- MCI, to full-scale dementia. Preventive strategies can be implemented before the onset of the process of dementia by eliminating or treating risk factors, as well as promoting protective factors (primary prevention). Secondary prevention relies on the identification of clinical or biological markers for disorders that lead to dementia in order to detect subjects early who will develop dementia within a few years. Tertiary prevention includes the identification of prognostic factors and the evaluation of the care provided to patients with dementia by comparing different care strategies in terms of specific individual and family outcomes (The Swedish Council SBU, 2008).

In that context, these two common etiology of dementia, i.e. Alzheimer's disease and vascular dementia have different characteristics, and there are diagnostic criteria for each of them. This article will focus on the difference between Alzheimer's disease and vascular dementia in light of recent development of research in each field.

2. Concepts of vascular dementia and Alzheimer's disease – Diagnosis criteria

2.1 Evolution of concepts

Since the 1970s, the concept of vascular dementia (VaD), a type of dementia secondary to stroke and vascular disease, has been distinguished from the purely neurodegenerative form of dementia, (AD). Since then, many clinical, neuropsychological, radiologic, and pathologic criteria have been proposed in an attempt to distinguish these entities in order to identify a homogenous group of patients who supposedly all share a common specific underlying mechanism of dementia; hence, allowing design of mechanism-specific therapies for this homogenous group of patients. The Diagnostic and Statistical Manual (DSM) of the *American Psychiatric Association* is the most influential classification of mental disorders worldwide. The third edition of this manual (DSM-III), published in 1980, was considered to be a major step forward in establishing a reliable diagnostic system based on evidence. The DSM has been revised periodically as new data have emerged, the last major revision having been in 1994 (DSM-IV), and a minor one in 2000 (DSM-IV-TR). The DSM-IV offers guidelines for diagnosis of one type of primary degenerative dementia - dementia of Alzheimer type (DAT) - and one type of VaD - multi infarct dementia (MID), now called VaD (*American Psychiatric Association*, 1994, 2000). ICD-10 offers four main categories of dementia, in which DAT is subclassified with respect to early versus late onset, typical versus atypical clinical features, and pure or combined with VaD; and VaD is described in terms of type of onset and predominant involvement. IDC-10 recognized 6 subtypes of "vascular (formerly arteriosclerotic) dementia", which includes such entities as "VaD of acute onset", "subcortical VaD", "mixed cortical and subcortical VaD", "other VaD" and "VaD unspecified" in addition to MID. Subcortical VaD with extensive diffuse demyelination and small focal infarctions was also referred to as "Binswanger's encephalopathy" (World Health Organization, 1992). The state of California Alzheimer Disease Diagnostic and Treatment Center (ADDTC) proposed the first set of criteria for the diagnosis of ischemic vascular dementia (IVD) in 1992, describing probable, possible, and definite IVD, as well as mixed dementia. VaD was also defined in terms of brain imaging, thereby extending the concept to include MID, single stroke dementia and Binswanger's disease (Chui et al., 1992). The criteria developed by the National Institute of Neurological Disorders and Stroke (NINDS) and the Association Internationale pour la Recherche et l'Enseignement en Neurosciences (AIREN) (Román et al., 1993), elaborated on the cause-effect relationship between cerebrovascular disease and symptoms of dementia; with the goal of facilitating treatment and epidemiological research, it emphasized the need of clinical and neuroimaging criteria for early and specific diagnosis of probable, possible and definite VaD. The NINCDS-ADRDA work group for standardization of clinical criteria for diagnosis of AD (McKhann et al., 1984) recommended the terms "possible AD" and "probable AD" and "definite AD", along with the pathologic criteria (Mirra et al., 1991). The introduction of MID was followed by the presentation of the Ischemic Score rating scale for differential diagnosis between AD and VaD (Hachinski et al., 1975). Differentiating among dementias presents many difficulties, especially at an early stage, and no single available diagnostic technique can solve all of these problems. The common clinical criteria (ICD-10, DSM-IV, ADDTC, NINDS-AIREN) for VaD are umbrella systems in that they do not consider the specific situation. Comparative studies show a lack of agreement among the systems; despite similarities, they identify different patients and patient groups. Not only do these differences affect prevalence and incidence estimates, but clinical management becomes more capricious. In order to promote the development of more effective pharmacological treatments and other improvements, the criteria systems need to be modified and made more specific. Thus, greater attention should be paid to vascular mechanisms and subtypes.

2.2 The DSM-V neurocognitive disorders cluster

In response to clinical and research developments since the publication of DSM-IV, the process to revise the classification for a DSM-V, to be published in 2012, started in 2006 with the establishment of a DSM-V Task Force, and a Work Group for neurocognitive disorders (Chair: Professor Dilip Jeste) in 2007. The draft proposed criteria from this Work Group was recently put on- line for general comments. The publication of DSM-V will have a major influence on the commonly used classification of neurocognitive disorders (Sachdev, 2010).

Among the major changes in structure and criteria for dementia and related disorders were: the term dementia is replaced with the more descriptive "Major Neurocognitive Disorder" (NCD); the criteria are reworded to reflect a focus on decline from a previous level of performance; also, the requirement for a deficit in memory is removed to better accommodate NCD due to other non-Alzheimer etiologies (Blacker, 2010). The field is moving towards earlier detection of the diseases underlying dementia, such that the disorder can be recognized, and possibly treatment started, before the dementia stage, e.g., the "mild cognitive impairment" stage of Alzheimer disease.

In other disorders, cognitive impairment may be static and not progress beyond the mild stage, but still be a focus for assessment and care. Hence, the category of Minor NCD (similar to Mild Cognitive Impairment) has been added given that this syndrome has become a major focus of research and clinical care (Ganguli, 2010).

The definitions of Major and Minor NCD are based on the primary cognitive disturbance, with a requirement for both cognitive symptoms elicited from the subject or an informant or observed by the clinician, and quantifiable deficits on cognitive assessments. At the Minor level, the cognitive symptoms may involve greater difficulty performing cognitive tasks (rather than inability), and the deficits are typically in the range of 1-2 SD below age- and education-adjusted means of neuropsychological tests. At the Major level, the deficits are typically >2 SD below the mean. The distinction between Minor and Major also rests on the preservation or loss of independence. Specific etiologic subtypes will also have specific criteria cutting across Major and Minor NCD (Blacker, 2010).

2.3 The new criteria for Alzheimer's disease

Criteria for the clinical diagnosis of Alzheimer's disease (AD) were established in 1984 (McKhann et al., 1984). Owing to clinical and research development, a broad consensus now exists that these criteria should be revised. The National Institute on Aging (NIA) and the Alzheimer's Association sponsored a series of advisory round table meetings in 2009 whose purpose was to establish a process for revising diagnostic and research criteria for AD. Two notable differences from the AD criteria published in 1984 are incorporation of biomarkers of the underlying disease state and formalization of different stages of disease in the diagnostic criteria. The recommendation from these advisory meetings was that three separate work groups should be formed with each assigned the task of formulating diagnostic criteria for one phase of the disease: the dementia phase, the symptomatic pre-dementia phase, and the asymptomatic preclinical phase of AD. A semantic and conceptual distinction is made between AD pathophysiological processes and clinically observable syndromes that result, whereas this distinction was blurred in the 1984 criteria. The new criteria for AD are presented in three documents. The core clinical criteria of the recommendations regarding AD dementia (McKhann et al., 2011) and MCI due to AD (Albert et al., 2011) are intended to guide diagnosis in the clinical setting. However, the recommendations of the preclinical AD workgroup (Sperling et al., 2011) are intended purely for research purposes.

2.4 Vascular dementia nosology

2.4.1 Historical overview

Modern history of dementia began in 1910 with Emil Kraepelin's influential textbook *Psychiatrie*. His work was based on clinical pathology studies by Otto Binswanger and Alois Alzheimer. The brain lesions that were assumed to be responsible for dementia consisted of arteriosclerotic brain atrophy (characterized by multiple lacunar strokes and " état criblé " - dilated perivascular spaces - associated with arteriosclerosis of small and large blood vessels), senile cortical atrophy (granular atrophy and laminar necrosis), periventricular white matter atrophy (Binswanger's disease), perivascular gliosis (wedgeshaped lesions resulting from severe stenosis of a large vessel), arteriosclerotic hemispheric foci (predisposing for "dementia postapoplexia") and the combined forms of dementia. In practice, arteriosclerotic dementia was synonymous with senile dementia. Successively impaired blood flow was thought to lead to neuron death (Roman, 1999). In the mid 1970s, AD was first regarded as the main cause of brain atrophy and dementia. The notion of chronic brain ischemia as an explanation of dementia was abandoned. Now vascular lesions in patients with dementia are receiving growing attention. Stroke-related dementia is increasingly in the spotlight, as is subcortical VaD with white matter damage and lacunae, regarded by some as the most common form of VaD (Roman et al., 2002).

2.4.2 Heterogeneity of vascular dementia

The increased percentage of elderly in the general population, along with changes in the cerebrovascular disease panorama in terms of reduced stroke mortality, has led to reevaluation and renewal in this field. Instead of using simplified disease categories, the assertion was that vascular mechanisms leading to cognitive impairment should form the basis of disease classification (Gorelick & Mangone, 1991; Hachinski, 1990). Among such vascular mechanisms are thromboembolism, vessel wall damage (Atherosclerosis, hyalinosis, amyloid angiopathy), cerebrovascular insufficiency (Disturbance of systemic circulation, vascular anatomy of the brain, disturbed regulation of cerebral blood flow), hyperviscosity, bleeding. Because several such mechanisms exist (Parnetti et al., 1994; Wallin & Blennow, 1993), there are also several types of VaD (Chui, 1989; Rockwood et al., 1999; Roman et al., 2002).

3. Mixed-type dementia

Mixed dementia is diagnosed when patients have evidence of Alzheimer dementia and cerebrovascular disease, either clinically or based on neuroimaging evidence of ischemic lesions. Growing evidence indicates that vascular dementia and Alzheimer dementia often coexist, especially in older patients with dementia (Langa et al., 2004). The occurrence of vascular risk factors and diseases are regarded as exclusion criteria for the diagnosis of AD. However, longitudinal epidemiological studies have shown that hypertension, diabetes, atrial fibrillation, and smoking are risk factors for AD as well as VaD. Ischemic processes have proven not only to co-exist with AD, but to potentiate its development (Cacabelos et al., 2003; Ravona-Springer et al., 2003; Skoog & Gustafson, 2003). Autopsy studies have shown an association between Alzheimer disease and vascular lesions (Snowdon et al., 1997). Toncosco et al. (2008) report autopsy findings from the Baltimore Longitudinal Aging Study among 122 men and 57 Women; macroscopic and microscopic infarcts contributed equally to dementia risk, and hemispheral infarcts, whether silent or clinically manifest, alone or in conjunction with AD pathology accounted for 35% of dementia cases. The findings support a synergism between AD and vascular pathology and the importance of burden and location of infarcts.

Vascular pathology in the aging brain and AD includes ischemic infarcts, lacunes, cerebral hemorrhages, white matter lesions, blood-brain barrier (BBB) dysfunction, cerebral amyloid angiopathy (CAA), and microvascular degeneration (Jellinger & Attems, 2003). These pathologies are commonly seen in various vascular diseases and can contribute to cognitive impairment by affecting neuronal networks involved in cognition, memory, behavior, and executive functioning (Jellinger, 2007). The OPTIMA project showed that cerebrovascular disease impaired cognitive performance in early phases of AD but not later in the course of the disease (Esiri et al., 1999). At the same grade of dementia, fewer Alzheimer's lesions were required in patients who had cerebrovascular damage (Zekry et al., 2002a). Another study reported that the combination of Alzheimer's disease and vascular pathology was common in patients with cognitive impairment, however, no threshold effects for the various changes could be found (Neuropathology group - MRC CFAS, 2001).

Recent evidence from epidemiological, clinical, pathological, and Neuroimaging studies implicates neurovascular dysfunction as an integral part of AD. Data from these studies reveal a distinct association between vascular risk factors and AD (Dickstein et al., 2010). These include hypertension (Kivipelto et al., 2001), total cholesterol, type II diabetes mellitus (Ott et al., 1999), hypotension, smoking (Ott et al., 1998) and oxidative stress (Zhu et al., 2007). Furthermore, dysfunction of the endothelial cells that compose the BBB has also been demonstrated and correlates with AD severity (Dede et al., 2007). The degree to which these factors contribute to AD may be influenced by genetic factors such as apolipoprotein E, which has a role in both AD and vascular disease. Ischemia via vasoactive effects of amyloid, impaired blood flow, reduced metabolism, inflammatory mechanisms and changes in the blood-brain barrier are among the factors that have been regarded as the genesis of vascular tissue damage in AD. Some authors have even claimed that AD is primarily microvascular, for which degeneration of the capillaries in the hippocampus and other brain regions, including secondary neuronal hypometabolism, is the central pathophysiological chain of events (De la Torre, 2002).

Identifying patients with AD and concurrent cerebrovascular disease is not easy when the patient lacks markers for AD. That may be one reason for the rate of mixed dementia having been underestimated (Kalaria & Ballard, 1999). According to a relatively current review of clinical neuropathological studies, mixed dementia accounts for 20 to 40% of dementia cases (Korczyn, 2002; Zekry et al., 2002b). Alzheimer's disease pathology occurs frequently in asymptomatic elderly individuals and clinical dementia is more likely to be present when AD is accompanied by strokes and cerebrovascular related brain changes (Riekse et al., 2004). The cognitive consequences of vascular lesions are cumulative. So VaD and perhaps also mixed dementia are potentially preventable if vascular risk factors are controlled and strokes do not recur. To better guide the treatment of patients with mixed dementia, future studies should similarly broaden their criteria to include patients with evidence for mixed causes of dementia, rather than identifying only pure AD and VaD (Langa et al., 2004).

4. Vascular cognitive disorders – Vascular cognitive impairment (VCI)

The term "vascular cognitive disorder" was proposed by Sachdev (1999) to define vascular cognitive deficits of sufficient severity to meet criteria for a diagnosable disorder. It was intended as an umbrella term to include the spectrum of impairment from mild vascular cognitive impairment to vascular dementia (Roman et al., 2002). Vascular cognitive impairment (VCI)) is the modern term related to vascular burden of the brain, reflecting all encompassing effects of cerebrovascular disease on cognition. VCI include all levels of cognitive decline from mild deficits in one or more cognitive domains to a broad dementia-like syndrome. VCI incorporates the complex interactions between vascular risk factors, cerebrovascular disease etiologies and cellular changes within the brain and cognition

(Chui, 2006; Erkinjuntti & Gauthier, 2009). The extent to which cognitive disturbance is progressive or non progressive is important to delineate, because it suggests initiation of a process for development of dementia, or instead a cognitive residual syndrome.

Vascular cognitive impairment (VCI) has continued to evolve over the past year. Much of the data has been confirmatory with further work on risk factors, silent strokes, leukoaraiosis and lesion volume and location. The importance of the interaction between cerebrovascular disease and other causes of cognitive impairment, most importantly Alzheimer disease (AD) remains a prominent theme (Bowler & Gorelick, 2009).

From a neuropathologic perspective, once irreversible parenchymal injury has occurred, there are downstream and retrograde effects in the central nervous system that result from the insult - as a function of Wallerian, trans-synaptic and other types of degeneration which almost certainly affect subsequent neurobehavioral morbidity (O'Brien et al., 2003; Vinters et al., 2000). Subcortical axonal injury and loss might be key elements in VaD pathogenesis and progression (Medana & Esiri, 2003). The identity of the neuropathologic substrates of leukoaraiosis, which also affects subcortical white matter, is still controversial, but might include apoptosis of oligodendroglia (Brown et al., 2000).

VCI represents a paradigm shift from vascular dementia towards a much earlier state, characterized most commonly by a subcortical frontal and executive pattern of cognitive impairment, as opposed to the previous concept of an Alzheimer-based amnestic syndrome. The principal object of VCI as a concept is to facilitate case identification in this early stage, because progression may be preventable through modification of vascular risk factors (Bowler, 2007). Data on VCI are still relatively limited, because much of the research done over the past two decades has been based now on the outdated criteria for vascular dementia. To help resolve this, the National Institute of Neurological Disorders and Stroke and Canadian Stroke Network have recently published comprehensive guidelines for research studies in VCI (Hachinski et al., 2006).

On the other hand, VCI is an evolving concept, and as our understanding grows, new questions arise (Chui, 2006; Merino, 2008). The development of a single, uniform set of criteria that apply to all subtypes of VCI has clearly been challenging, and some experts have recommended that separate criteria be developed for certain subtypes (Roman et al., 2002). (To be discussed in the next section).

5. Mild cognitive impairment (MCI) – Vascular cognitive impairment no dementia (VCIND)

Age-related cognitive change can be placed along a continuum from normal to severely demented, with intermediate stages of cognitive decline. To date, there is no consensus on where boundaries between disease and non-disease lie. Rather than a strict dichotomisation, the determination of impairment may instead be based on the likelihood or probability that ageing is not occurring in accordance with normative expectations (Stephan et al., 2009).

5.1 Mild cognitive impairment

The term mild cognitive impairment (MCI) broadly defines an intermediate state of cognitive decline, predominately linked to impaired memory function, which is thought to be predictive of dementia, primarily Alzheimer's disease. Various definitions have been proposed in the literature, each with differences in focus- age associated change versus pathological decline, and diagnostic criteria - memory versus non-memory impairment, (Morris, 2006; Winblad et al., 2004).

As a possible tool for identifying individuals at increased risk of dementia, MCI is an important concept. Indeed, in clinical samples, individuals with a case diagnosis of the anmestic subtype of MCI (a-MCI) have been found to progress to dementia at a rate of 10% to 15% per year compared with a progression rate of only 1% to 2% in normal controls (Bruscoli & Lovestone, 2004; Petersen et al., 2001). In contrast, in the general population, the positive predictive validity of a-MCI is poor (Matthews et al., 2008). Many incident dementia cases are found to be excluded from an a-MCI case diagnosis, and of persons with a-MCI, many remain stable or revert to normal cognitive status at follow-up (Matthews et al., 2007). These findings are consistent across all MCI definitions-amnestic versus nonamnestic, and single versus multiple domains MCI- (Matthews et al., 2008).

No MCI criteria can be recommended for population screening of individuals at high dementia risk (Stephan et al., 2008). Poor predictability possibly results from limitations in case findings due to a lack of clinical judgement and inflexibility in operationalisation of criteria when a diagnosis of MCI is made outside the clinical setting. However, it has been suggested that MCI predictability may be improved through consideration of the underlying pathogenesis of cognitive decline (Tervo et al., 2004). Subclassification of MCI with and without co-morbid vascular disease may therefore be important for discriminating individuals at high versus low dementia risk in the general population (Stephan et al., 2009). To better identify the link between vascular disease and cognitive impairment, the term vascular cognitive impairment (VCI) was introduced (Bowler, 2007; Bowler & Hachinski, 1995; Román et al., 2004; Selnes & Vinters, 2006).

5.2 Vascular cognitive impairment no dementia

As already mentioned, vascular cognitive impairment refers to cognitive decline attributable to vascular disease. However, unlike mild cognitive impairment which is a narrow term capturing a pre-clinical form of dementia, vascular cognitive impairment encompasses individuals affected with any degree of cognitive decline caused by or associated with vascular disease and its risk factors. As such, the level of impairment in vascular cognitive impairment ranges in severity from mild cognitive impairment to vascular dementia or mixed vascular dementia, in which cerebrovascular and AD pathologies co-occur. Calls for more specific staging have recently led to further subclassification of vascular cognitive impairment to capture vascular disease-related impairment not fulfilling criteria for dementia. This stage is defined using the term vascular cognitive impairment no dementia (VCIND). Whether within VCIND there is a state predictive of dementia is largely unknown. Where longitudinal outcome across the spectrum of vascular cognitive impairment has been investigated, progression is not always clinical -that is, decline/dementia, with many cases improving or remaining stable at follow-up (Hsiung, 2006; Rockwood et al., 2007; Wentzel et al., 2001). Predictive ability may depend on the nature of the vascular disturbance in addition to methodological factors- case description, sample and nature of cognitive impairment.

As with MCI, terminology and diagnostic criteria for VCIND have not been harmonised, making cross-study comparison of disease outcomes difficult. Generally, the differential diagnosis between MCI and VCIND is clinical and based on the distinction between Alzheimer's disease and Vascular dementia. Alzheimer disease is characterised by a steady and progressive loss of memory and cognitive faculties, including language deterioration, impaired visuospatial skills and poor judgement. In contrast, the disease course of Vascular dementia is highly variable, generally following a stepwise pattern of decline and fluctuating course. For a diagnosis of Vascular dementia , it is recommended that radiographic features of vascular disease, including evidence of an ischaemic lesion, white matter hyperintensities and/or hypometabolism, be confirmed (American Psychiatric Association, 2000). Frequently both pathologies co-occur (Neuropathology group- MRC CFAS, 2001; Snowdon et al., 1997). AD and VaD may share associated risk factors (stroke, arterial hypertension, increasing age and low educational attainment), structural changes, neuropathological profiles (white matter lesions and apoptosis) and neurochemical changes (that is, in the cholinergic system) (Small et al., 2002). In older people, multi-morbidity is common and a strict dichotomisation between degenerative and vascular dementing disorders at both pre-clinical and dementia stages is difficult to undertake, possibly artificial and perhaps not the most useful approach.

5.3 Cognitive, neuroimaging and neuropathological profiles of MCI and VCIND

5.3.1 Cognitive profile

Neuropsychological studies have identified attentional executive deficits and psychomotor slowing, with relatively preserved language and recognition memory in individuals with vascular disease (Hachinski et al., 2006). However, not all studies agree on the importance of each cognitive domain and no single deficit or pattern of deficits as yet accurately signals an underlying vascular cause (Graham at al., 2004). For example, cognitive impairment as a consequence of stroke would likely depend on not only timing and the anatomical location of the stroke, but also the laterality, severity and extent of the lesion.

The focus of MCI is predominantly impaired memory, but deficits in other cognitive domains will also be observed when, by definition, they are also included. Subdivisions between different cognitive subtypes of MCI, amnestic versus nonamnestic, and single versus multi-domain, have implications for inference about aetiology and outcomes. Indeed, while a-MCI (Petersen, 2007) is thought to be a precursor of AD, nonamnestic subtypes of MCI have been found to identify individuals at high risk of both AD and VaD (Rasquin et al., 2005).

Where the cognitive profile of individuals with MCI and comorbid vascular disease has been compared with that of individuals with MCI and no vascular disease, group differences have been reported in some (Hayden et al., 2005; Nordlund et al., 2007), but not all studies (Loewenstein et al., 2006). Where differences have been observed, the MCI vascular group shows more extensive cognitive impairment primarily in speed, attention and executive function, (Nordlund et al., 2007) consistent with the general pattern of cognitive difficulties resulting from vascular disease alone (Román et al., 2004).

The specific type of cognitive impairment associated with vascular disease needs to be defined and measures that are sensitive, specific and appropriate for longitudinal and observational assessment of cognition in the context of vascular disease (that is, memory versus non-memory domains) need to be identified in order to facilitate the development of diagnostic criteria for cognitive decline in the presence (VCIND) versus the absence (MCI) of vascular disease (Stephan et al., 2009).

5.3.2 Neuroimaging profile

Neuroimaging in VCIND shows a pattern of vascular lesions that are similar to, but less severe than, changes observed in VaD (Meyer et al., 2007). Pathology includes evidence of leukoaraiosis and white matter infarction (Vermeer et al., 2007), with mild hippocampal and entorhinal cortex atrophy relative to the level seen in MCI /AD (Meyer et al., 2007). In contrast, neuroimaging in MCI generally shows a pattern of changes similar to that observed in AD, namely temporal and hippocampal atrophy, reduction in whole-brain glucose metabolism and white matter degeneration, including hyperintensities and white matter lesions identified using diffusion tensor imaging (Assaf et al., 2008; Devanand et al., 2007; Johnson et al., 2006).

The severity and type of lesions required for a diagnosis of MCI and VCIND remain controversial. Vascular disease and its risks are associated with brain changes but the clinical relevance of such changes in the prediction of cognitive decline and dementia progression remains uncertain. Isolating unique disease effects from the effects of ageing and other risk factors (that is, genetic susceptibility) will be important in determining cellular/ molecular /functional vulnerability as a consequence of vascular disease as well as establishing with accuracy those changes that distinguish who will and will not develop cognitive decline and subsequent dementia (Stephan et al., 2009).

5.3.3 Neuropathology profile

MCI cases generally show an increase in neurofibrillary tangle pathology in memory-related cortical regions, including the entorhinal cortex, fusiform gyrus and temporal pole (Bennett et al., 2005). These changes are thought to represent one of the earliest pathological substrates of this condition and have been taken to suggest that many MCI cases are early or prodromal AD (Morris et al., 2001).

Whether there is a consistent neuropathological profile across the spectrum of vascular causes and severity levels of VCI is unknown but seems unlikely. Indeed, VCI is a multifactor disorder related to a wide variety of lesions and causes, and as such the pathological profile, similarly to the psychological and radiological profiles, would be expected to be heterogeneous. In autopsy studies, an increased prevalence of cerebral vascular pathology has been found in individuals with stroke, diabetes mellitus (Arvanitakis et al., 2006), angina with comorbid dementia (Andin et al., 2005) and hypertension (Petrovitch et al., 2000). Pathological features have included large- and small-vessel disease, gliosis, microvascular brain damage (severe cribriform change), white matter damage, microinfarction and haemorrhage (Kalaria et al., 2004). The profile of pathology across the different vascular disease factors is heterogeneous and the significance of such changes in the development of cognitive impairment is not known. Across the spectrum of age-associated brain changes, no neuropathological profile yet exists that reliably distinguishes impairment of different severity levels and causes. In the general population, currently identifiable pathological features have not been found to correlate well with observed clinical and cognitive profiles: many non-demented healthy controls also show evidence of pathological brain changes associated with both AD and VaD (Jagust et al., 2008). Techniques that better characterise the impact of vascular disease on brain structure and more sensitive measures for accurately staging cognitive status which incorporate known risk factors are needed for diagnostic differentiation between an at-risk and a "not at-risk" brain. However, as with AD, expecting neuropathology to be a gold standard at any given age for the diagnosis of VCI is an oversimplification (Brayne, 1993).

6. Disease manifestations of vascular dementia

6.1 Symptom profile

VaD is an heterogeneous disease group with symptoms that vary according to the type of tissue damage, location, size and number of lesions. The main subtypes of VaD included in current classifications are cortical VaD (or MID) and subcortical vascular dementia (or small vessel disease related dementia) (Brun, 1994; Cummings, 1994; Roman et al., 1993; Wallin et al., 2003). The clinical presentation of cortical and subcortical forms of VaD show remarkable differences. Large vessel occlusions resulting in large cortical infarcts produce cognitive and other deficits that depend on the location of the infarcts, while subcortical vascular dementia may have a relatively characteristic neuropsychological profile that includes early impairment of attention and executive function, with slowing of motor performance and information processing (O'Brien et al., 2003; Roman et al, 2002; Roman & Royall, 1999).

Selected original publications show that executive dysfunction was the key factor underlying functional impairment (Boyle et al., 2002). Disturbances in frontal lobe functions were found to be more pronounced in patients with VaD than AD. Memory disturbances proved to be less pronounced early in the course of the disease than for AD. However, once the disease had progressed to a moderately severe level, the disturbances were just as pronounced as in AD. Executive dysfunction may also appear in AD patients, but it more resembles attention deficit disorder. In VaD, executive dysfunction more involves a fundamental inability to work out strategies and carry out tasks (Cannata et al., 2002). To obtain a greater understanding of the clinical manifestations, many authors have recommended a subtype classification of VaD (Chui, 1989; Erkinjuntti, 1987).

6.2 Small vessel disease and subcortical vascular dementia

Subcortical vascular dementia is the current terminology for severe cognitive impairment associated with small vessel disease (Erkinjuntti et al., 2000). Given its strong vascular component, it is believed to be more preventable than dementia of the Alzheimer's type. Subcortical vascular dementia results from lacunar infarcts or multiple microinfarcts in the basal ganglia, thalamus, brainstem, and focal and diffuse ischaemic white matter lesions (WMLs), and are associated with more than 50% of the VaD cases (Kalaria et al., 2004; Kalaria & Erkinjuntti, 2006). It represents the most homogeneous and probably most common, subtype of VaD (Chui, 2001).

Clinically, subcortical vascular dementia is characterised by pure motor hemiparesis, bulbar signs and dysarthria, gait disorder, variable depressive illness, emotional lability, and deficits in executive functioning; however, these focal neurological signs are often subtle. Upon imaging, patients have multiple lacunes and extensive WMLs and often reveal clinical history of "prolonged transient ischemic attack" (TIA) or "multiple TIAs" which mostly are small strokes without residual symptoms and only mild focal findings (e.g. reflex asymmetry, gait disturbance). This supports the importance of neuroimaging requirements in the criteria (Erkinjuntti et al., 2000).

Most studies on stroke associated with small vessel disease focus on motor impairment and mortality. Few studies have investigated the frequency of differering severity levels of cognitive impairment. Mok et al. (2004) evaluated consecutive patients with or without previous stroke who were admitted to the acute stroke unit. In this hospital based study, half of the patients with stroke associated with small vessel disease had varying severity of cognitive symptoms 3 months after stroke. Pre-stroke cognitive decline and previous stroke predicted severe cognitive impairment. Their findings highlight the importance of cognitive impairment, and in particular, executive dysfunction, in affecting the functional outcome of patients with stroke associated with small vessel disease.

The early cognitive syndrome of subcortical vascular dementia is characterized by a dysexecutive syndrome with slowed information processing, usually mild memory deficit and behavioural symptoms (Kramer et al., 2002; Roman et al., 2002). The dysexecutive syndrome includes impairment in goal formulation, initiation, planning, organising, sequencing, executing, set-shifting and set-maintenance, as well as in abstraction (Desmond et al., 1999). The memory deficit is usually milder than in AD, and is specified by impaired recall, relative intact recognition, less severe forgetting and better benefit from cues. Episodic memory may be relatively spared, compared with AD.There is more learning impairment that can be partially corrected by providing salient cues to encourage learning and promote recognition. Therefore, memory deficits in VaD appear to be caused by problems in retrieval of information (Sachdev et al., 2004); in turn, memory retrieval deficits are due to aberrant frontal and subcortical mechanisms. In contrast, in AD involvement of the hippocampus by neurofibrillary tangles prevents storage of new information causing amnesic mild cognitive impairment.

Eventually, cognitive impairment in small vessel disease may progress from mild to severe cognitive impairment. Behavioural and psychological symptoms in subcortical vascular dementia include depression, personality change, emotional lability, apathy, incontinence, as well as inertia, emotional bluntness and psychomotor retardation. These may include greater tendencies of aggression and agitation. Such symptomatology is attributed to damage to the prefrontal subcortical circuits (Cummings, 1993).

Cerebral autosomal dominant arteriopathy with subcortical infarcts and leukoencephalopathy (CADASIL), is an example of familial subcortical vascular dementia that presents with recurrent subcortical strokes and slowly progressing course leading to cognitive impairment and dementia. This disorder is a rare cause of VaD, but is much more common than familial AD (Opherk et al., 2004).

Patients with subcortical VaD had more pronounced impairment than those with AD in their ability to deal with complex information, formulate strategies and exercise self-control.

The executive dysfunction of AD patients was mainly associated with attention deficit disorder and impaired working memory (Cannata et al., 2002). Patients with subcortical VaD have shown less pronounced episodic memory impairment, but more depressive symptomatology and greater variability in progress speed, than those with AD (Bennett et al., 1994). It has been suggested that patients with subcortical microvascular disease are the ones who later develop dementia that shows signs of mild cognitive impairment in the early phases of the disease (Meyer et al., 2002). A disturbance in the executive control function leads to global impairment of the ability to engage in everyday social activities and work, as well as the development of dementia. In addition to being a characteristic disturbance in VaD, there is much to suggest that executive dysfunction is the determining component in the dementia syndrome itself. Changes found by magnetic resonance imaging (MRI) in the subcortical area of patients with VaD showed an association with impairment of executive and psychomotor, but not global cognitive, capacity (Cohen et al., 2002; Libon et al., 2004).

6.3 Stroke

One way to obtain more specific information about VaD is to study cognitive ability in the course of the disease following an established stroke episode. In their recently published review, Leys et al. (2005) and Henon et al. (2006) summarized the previous studies that explored the impact of stroke on the risk of poststroke dementia. According to these studies, stroke increases the risk of dementia, with prevalence rates ranging from 6% to 32% within 3 months to 1 year after stroke, depending on the composition of the patient group and the choice of criteria for the dementia syndrome; and incidence rates of new-onset dementia after stroke ranging from 10% to 24% within 3 years and 15% to 33.3% within 5 years (Censori et al., 1996; Desmond et al., 2000; Kokmen et al., 1996; Tatemichi et al., 1992).

Studies that have examined the role of prestroke cognitive decline in the development of poststroke dementia have reported varying results. Pohjasvaara et al. (1998) found no difference in the proportion of demented and nondemented stroke patients with prestroke cognitive decline. However, Pohjasvaara et al. (1999) later reported that prestroke cognitive was positively correlated with poststroke cognitive decline. Barba et al. (2000) in a series of 251 consecutive unselected stroke patients found that 30% demonstrated dementia at 3-month follow up; and 10% had demonstrated dementia before the stroke. Reitz et al. (2008) in a prospective population-based study, with a mean follow-up time of 6.3 years between first assessment of cognitive function at baseline and time of incident first stroke, in which the slope of cognitive performance before stroke was also taken into account, and which had a nearly complete follow-up with respect to dementia, does not suggest that the prestroke level of cognitive function is a major determinant of the effect of stroke on the risk of poststroke dementia; an incident stroke doubled the risk of subsequent dementia independent of prestroke level of cognitive function and prestroke rate of cognitive decline. This finding contradicts previous studies reporting a higher risk of poststroke dementia in persons with prestroke cognitive impairment compared with persons with normal cognition before stroke (Gamaldo et al., 2006; Mok et al., 2004). In investigating patients during the acute phase, Henon et al. found signs of pre-stroke dementia in 15% of the cases. Gamaldo et al. (2006) study reported an increased risk of poststroke dementia in persons with prestroke mild cognitive impairment. Barba et al. (2000) commented that the frequency of post stroke dementia depends on various factors such as the exclusion of hemorrhage or recurrent stroke, age range, length of follow-up, and diagnostic criteria. Srikanth et al. (2006) in the first prospective data on long-term cognitive transitions in a population-based first-ever stroke cohort, found that stroke recurrence was associated with an increased rate of long-term global cognitive decline after a first-ever stroke; stroke recurrence, early poststroke cognitive impairment, and increasing age were independently associated with diagnosis of new clinical dementia two years after a first-ever stroke.

The influence of the location of the vascular lesion in the development of dementia remains to be determined. A role of the left hemisphere has been suggested (Lin et al., 2003; Zhou et al., 2004). Poststroke dementia was also found to be more frequent in patients with a hemispheric stroke compared to brainstem/posterior fossa lesions and in patients with a pooled anterior/posterior cerebral artery stroke compared to other locations (Desmond et al., 2000). Many studies did not find any relationship between stroke location and risk of poststroke dementia (Ivan et al., 2004; Madureira et al., 2001; Rasquin et al., 2004).

Strategic infarction dementia is sometimes characterized as a special variety of post-stroke dementia. Isolated bilateral infarctions in the hippocampus can lead to dementia, but milder cognitive disturbances are more common. Bilateral thalamic, unilateral thalamic and basal frontal infarctions, as well as infarctions in the angular gyrus, non-dominant parietotemporal region and dominant hemisphere, are other strategically localized infarctions that reportedly cause dementia (Schmahmann, 2003). In addition to memory impairment, bilateral thalamic lesions yield apathy, attention deficit, and disturbances in wakefulness. Thus, involvement of the thalamus and bordering brain areas is often found. Effects on the extensive reciprocal thalamus-frontal and frontal reticular nerve connections may explain the discrepancy between the relatively limited lesions and the extensive symptomatology. Strategic infarction dementia has been called into question as a disease entity, given that the influence of other lesions is generally ignored (Pantoni et al., 2001). Stroke cause, vascular risk factors, hypoxic-ischemic disorders, radiological data of silent infarcts, cerebral atrophy, white matter changes also play a role in the development of poststroke dementia (Reviewed, Henon et al., 2006). The variation in cognitive status prior to the stroke episode and the development of cognitive dysfunction after stroke, as well as the variation of stroke-related and lesion-related characteristics that contribute to the development of dementia, suggest that post-stroke dementia is a heterogeneous condition for which factors other than the infarction formation itself are of importance.

7. Biomarkers

One of the most important goals of current research in AD is to develop and validate biomarkers, which can detect at an early stage individuals who are likely to develop AD. Important advance in this field have been made recently by the workgroup under the auspice of the National Institute on Aging and the Alzheimer's Association (Sperling et al., 2011). Referring to evidence of the underlying brain disease process as AD-pathophysiological process (AD-P), a biomarker model - solely intended for research purposes at this time - adapted from the original graph proposed by Jack et al. (2010) has been recently proposed in which the most widely validated biomarkers of AD-P become abnormal and likewise reach a ceiling in an ordered manner. This biomarker model parallels the hypothetical pathophysiological sequence of AD, and is particularly relevant to tracking the preclinical stages of AD (Sperling et al., 2011). Biomarkers of brain Abeta amyloidosis include reductions in CSF Abeta 42 and increased amyloid tracer retention on positron emission tomography (PET) imaging. Elevated CSF tau is not specific to AD and is thought to be a biomarker of neuronal injury. Decreased fluorodeoxyglucose 18F (FDG) uptake on PET with a temporoparietal pattern of hypometabolism is a biomarker of AD-related synaptic dysfunction. Brain atrophy on structural magnetic resonance imaging (MRI) in a characteristic pattern involving the medial temporal lobes, paralimbic and temporoparietal cortices is a biomarker of AD-related neurodegeneration. Although solely intended for research purposes at this time, and pending the translation of research data into clinical practice, this biomarkers model represent an important step forward to advance the study of preclinical AD. Importantly, Lo et al. (2011) reported the result of a longitudinal study; a total of 819 research participants (229 with normal cognition, 397 with MCI, and 193 with AD) were enrolled for the Alzheimer's Disease Neuroimaging Initiative (ADNI) from 59 study sites in the United States and Canada during the period from 2005 to 2007. The authors concluded that trajectories of Abeta 42 level in CSF, FDG uptake, and hippocampal volume vary across different cognitive stages. The longitudinal patterns support a hypothetical sequence of AD pathology in which amyloid deposition is an early event before hypometabolism or hippocampal atrophy, suggesting that biomarker prediction for cognitive change is stage dependent.

For VaD, anatomical brain imaging helps determine the subtypes of VaD (hemorrhage versus ischemia, cortical versus subcortical, strategic infarction versus multi-infarction, large vessel disease versus small vessel disease) and thereby enhances our knowledge of vascular disease processes. Anatomical brain imaging has played a particularly large role in demonstrating small vessel-related white matter changes, evidence of leukoaraiosis and white matter infarction, with mild hippocampal and entorhinal cortex atrophy relative to the level seen in AD (Vermeer et al., 2007). Studies of neurochemical markers for VaD and its subtypes are considerably fewer than those on patients with AD. After acute ischemic stroke the CSF tau protein level is normal for one or two days, after which it increases and peaks after 2–3 weeks. The effect then subsides, and the values normalize after 3–4 months (Hesse et al., 2000). Several studies have shown a significant increase of phosphorylated tau in the fluid of AD patients, while the levels are normal in VaD patients (Blennow & Vanmechelen, 2003). Impaired BBB function occurs in patients with VaD, particularly subcortical VaD (Wallin et al., 2000). The impaired function probably reflects disorders in the arterioles, although the capillary level may also be compromised. Neurofilament, another cytoskeletal component, is concentrated in large myelinized neurons. The greatly increased neurofilament light subunit (NFL) in the CSF that has been found in patients with subcortical VaD has been associated with the presence of white matter changes (Wallin et al., 2001); while CSF-NFL has been shown to be normal in patients with pure AD. Knowledge of neurochemical markers may also be important to understanding mixed dementia (Rockwood et al., 2000).

8. Conclusions

The dominant view in the literature is that the symptom profile for vascular dementia differs from that of Alzheimer's disease. Vascular dementia is characterized by mental slowness; impaired initiative, planning, and executive function impairment; personality changes; and gait disorders. Thus, methodological advances aimed at identifying and measuring the severity of the cardinal symptoms of mental slowness and executive dysfunction and better clinical criteria, are needed for vascular dementia to help us reliably distinguish it from Alzheimer's disease.

Greater attention should be paid to vascular mechanisms and subtypes. The few studies that have attempted to consider the full range of cerebrovascular lesions have found them to be common, particularly the subcortical, small vessel disease and white matter damage that increasingly appears to be among the key factors underlying the origin of vascular dementia. Further studies are needed to identify the pathological changes that are most important in the disease and as a result, neuropathological criteria and examination methods need to be specified and standardized. Anatomic brain imaging is a good deal more reliable in helping to identify vascular lesions than Alzheimer's lesions, which is still under ongoing screening. The clinical criteria systems need to be modified and made more specific in the vascular dementia field.

Although much remains to be done, the ongoing process of revision of clinical criteria, the refinement of neuropathologic studies, the progress in biomarkers development with disease stage specificity including the preclinical one; along with identification, validation and refinement of predictors of cognitive decline and dementia, will pave the way for a very promising and hopeful future, in the prevention, treatment and management of Alzheimer's disease and vascular dementia. Earliest stage interventions may be the most efficacious.

9. Acknowledgments

Special thanks to my nephew, Madjid Ramdane, for his helpful technical assistance.

10. References

Alzheimer's Association. (2010). Alzheimer's Association Report. 2010 Alzheimer's disease facts and figures. *Alzheimer's & Dementia.* 6(2): 158-194.

Alzheimer's Association. (2011). Alzheimer's Association Report. 2011 Alzheimer's disease facts and figures. *Alzheimer's & Dementia.* 7(2): 208-244.

Albert, M.S., DeKosky, S.T., Dickson, D., Dubois, B., Feldman, H.H., Fox, N.C., Gamst, A., Holtzman, D.M., Jagust, W.J., Petersen, R.C., Snyder, P.J., Carrillo, M.C., Thies, B., & Phelps, C.H. (2011). The diagnosis of mild cognitive impairment due to Alzheimer's disease: Recommendations from the National Institute on Aging and Alzheimer's Association workgroup. *Alzheimer's & Dementia.* 7(3): 270-279

American Psychiatric Association. (1994). DSM-IV, Diagnostic and Statistical Manual of Mental Disorders. Washington DC: *American Psychiatric Association.* 1994.

American Psychiatric Association. (2000). *Diagnostic and Statistical Manual of Mental Disorders, Text Revision.* Washington, DC: *American Psychiatric Association. 2000.*

Andin, U., Gustafso, L., Passant, U., & Brun,A. (2005). A clinico-pathological study of heart and brain lesions in vascular dementia. *Dement Geriatr Cogn Disord.* 19(4): 222-228.

Arvanitakis, Z., Schneider, J.A., Wilson, R.S., Li, Y., Arnold, S.E., Wang, Z., & Bennett, D.A. (2006). Diabetes is related to cerebral infarction but not to AD pathology in older persons. *Neurology.* 67(11): 1960- 1965.

Assaf, Y., & Pasternak, O. (2008). Diffusion tensor imaging (DTI)-based white matter mapping in brain research: a review. *J Mol Neurosci.* 34(1): 51-61.

Barba, R., Martinez, E.S., Rodriguez, G.E., Pondal, M., Vivancos, J., & Del Ser, T. (2000). Poststroke dementia: clinical features and risk factors. *Stroke.* 31(7): 1494–1501.

Bennett, D.A., Gilley, D.W., Lee, S., & Cochran, E.J. (1994). White matter changes: neurobehavioral manifestations of Binswanger's disease and clinical correlates in Alzheimer's disease. *Dementia.* 5(3-4): 148-52.

Bennett, D.A., Schneider, J.A., Bienias, J.L., Evans, D.A., & Wilson, R.S. (2005). Mild cognitive impairment is related to Alzheimer disease pathology and cerebral infarctions. *Neurology.* 64(5): 834-841.

Berr, C., Wancata, J., & Ritchie, K. (2005). Prevalence of dementia in the elderly in Europe. *Eur Neuropsycho pharmacol.* 15(4): 463–471.

Blacker, D. (2010). Major Neurocognitive Disorder, and the case of AD. Session, classifying neurocognitive disorders in the 21st century - Toward DSM V. Presentation FT-01-03- ICAD 2010, Honolulu,HI, USA

Blennow, K., & Vanmechelen, E.. (2003). CSF markers for pathogenic processes in Alzheimer's disease: diagnostic implications and use in clinical neurochemistry. *Brain Res Bull.* 61(3): 235-242.

Boyle, P.A., Cohen, R.A., Paul, R., Moser, D., & Gordon, N. (2002). Cognitive and motor impairments predict functional declines in patients with vascular dementia. *Int J Geriatr Psychiatry.* 17(2): 164-169.

Bowler, J.V., Hachinski, V. (1995). Vascular cognitive impairment: a new approach to vascular dementia. *Baillieres Clin Neurol.* 4(2): 357-376.

Bowler, J.V. (2007). Modern concept of vascular cognitive impairment. *Br Med Bull.* 83: 291-305. Epub 2007 Aug 4.

Bowler, J.V., & Gorelick, P.B. (2009). Advances in Vascular Cognitive Impairment. *Stroke.* 40(5): e315-e318.

Brayne C. (1993). Clinicopathological studies of the dementias from an epidemiological viewpoint. *Br J Psychiatry.* 162: 439- 446.

Brown, W.R., Moody, D.M., Thore, C.R., & Challa, V.R. (2000). Apoptosis in leukoaraiosis. *AJNR Am J Neuroradiol.* 21(1): 79-82.

Brun, A. (1994). Pathology and pathophysiology of cerebrovascular dementia: pure subgroups of obstructive and hypoperfusive etiology. *Dementia.* 5(3-4): 145-147.

Bruscoli, M., Lovestone, S. (2004). Is MCI really just early dementia? A systematic review of conversion studies. *Int Psychogeriatr.* 16(2): 129-140.

Cacabelos, R., Fernandez-Novoa, L., Lombardi, V., Corzo, L., Pichel, V., & Kubota, Y. (2003). Cerebrovascular risk factors in Alzheimer's disease: brain hemodynamics and pharmacogenomic implications. *Neurol Res.* 25(6): 567-580.

Cannata, A.P., Alberoni, M., Franceschi, M., & Mariani, C. (2002). Frontal impairment in subcortical ischemic vascular dementia in comparison to Alzheimer's disease. *Dement Geriatr Cogn Disord.* 13(2): 101-111.

Censori, B., Manara, O., Agostinis, C., Camerlingo, M., Casto, L., Galavotti, B., Partziguian, T., Servalli, M.C., Cesana, B., Belloni, G., & Mamoli, A. (1996). Dementia after first stroke. *Stroke.* 27(7): 1205–1210.

Chui, H.C. (1989). Dementia. A review emphasizing clinicopathologic correlation and brain-behavior relationships. *Arch Neurol.* 46(7): 806-814

Chui, H.C., Victoroff, J.I., Margolin, D., Jagust, W., Shankle, R., & Katzman, R. (1992). Criteria for the diagnosis of ischemic vascular dementia proposed by the State of California Alzheimer's Disease Diagnostic and Treatment Centers. *Neurology.* 42(3): 473-480.

Chui, H.C. (2001). Dementia due to subcortical ischemic vascular disease. *Clin Cornerstone.* 3(4): 40-51.

Chui, H.C. (2006). Vascular cognitive impairment: Today and tomorrow. *Alzheimer's & Dementia.* 2(3): 185-194

Cohen, R.A., Paul, R.H., Ott, B.R., Moser, D.J., Zawacki, T.M., Stone, W., & Gordon N. (2002). The relationship of subcortical MRI hyperintensities and brain volume to cognitive function in vascular dementia. *J Int Neuropsychol Soc.* 8(6): 743-52.

Cummings, J.L. (1993). Fronto-subcortical circuits and human behavior. *Arch Neurol.* 50(8): 873-880.

Cummings, J.L. (1994). Vascular subcortical dementias: clinical aspects. *Dementia.* 5(3-4): 177-180

Dede, D.S., Yavuz, B., Yavuz, B.B., Cankurtaran, M., Halil, M., Ulger, Z., Cankurtaran, E.S., Aytemir, K., Kabakci, G., & Ariogul, S. (2007). Assessment of endothelial function in Alzheimer's disease: is Alzheimer's Disease a vascular disease? *J Am Geriatr Soc.* 55(10): 1613-1617.

De la Torre, J.C. (2002). Alzheimer disease as a vascular disorder: nosological evidence. *Stroke.* 33(4): 1152-1162.

Desmond, D.W., Erkinjuntti, T., Sano, M., Cummings, J.L., Bowler, J.V., Pasquier, F., Moroney, J.T., Ferris, S.H., Stern, Y., Sachdev, P.S., & Hachinski, V.C. (1999) The cognitive syndrome of vascular dementia: implications for clinical trials. *Alzheimer Dis Assoc Disord.* 13 (suppl 3): S21-29.

Desmond, D.W., Moroney, J.T., Paik, M.C., Sano, M., Mohr, J.P., Aboumatar, S.,Tseng, C.L., Chan, S., Williams, J.B., Remien, R.H., Hauser, W.A., & Stern, Y. (2000). Frequency and clinical determinants of dementia after ischemic stroke. *Neurology.* 54(5): 1124 - 1131.

Devanand, D.P., Pradhaban, G., Liu, X., Khandji, A., De Santi, S., Segal, S., Rusinek, H., Pelton, G.H., Honig, L.S., Mayeux, R., Stern, Y., Tabert, M.H., & de Leon, M.J. (2007). Hippocampal and entorhinal atrophy in mild cognitive impairment: prediction of Alzheimer disease. *Neurology.* 68(11): 828-836

Dickstein, D.L., Walsh, J., Brautigam, H., Stockton, Jr. S.D., Gandy, S., & Hof, P.R. (2010). Role of Vascular Risk Factors and Vascular Dysfunction in Alzheimer's Disease. *Mt Sinai J Med.* 77(1): 82–102.

Esiri, M.M., Nagy, Z., Smith, M.Z., Barnetson, L., & Smith, A.D. (1999). Cerebrovascular disease and threshold for dementia in the early stages of Alzheimer's disease. *Lancet.* 354(9182): 919-920.

Erkinjuntti, T. (1987). Types of multi-infarct dementia. *Acta Neurol Scand.* 75(6): 391-399

Erkinjuntti ,T., Inzitari, D., Pantoni, L., Wallin, A., Scheltens, P., Rockwood, K., Roman, G.C., Chui, H., & Desmond, D.W. (2000). Research criteria for subcortical vascular dementia in clinical trials.*J Neural Transm.* (Suppl.), 59: 23-30.

Erkinjuntti, T., & Gauthier, S. (2009). The concept of vascular cognitive impairment. *Front Neurol Neurosci.* 24: 79- 85. Epub 2009 Jan 26.

Ferri, C.P., Prince, M., Brayne, C., Brodaty, H., Fratiglioni, L., Ganguli, M., Hall, K., Hasegawa, K., Hendrie, H., Huang, Y., Jorm, A., Mathers, C., Menezes, P.R., Rimmer, E., Scazufca, M.; & ADI. (2005). Global prevalence of dementia: a Delphi consensus study. *Lancet.* 366 (9503): 2112–17.

Fratiglioni, L., De Ronchi, D., & Aguero-Torres, H. (1999). Worldwide prevalence and incidence of dementia. *Drugs Aging.* 15(5): 365-375.

Ganguli, M. (2010). Minor Neurocognitive Disorder in DSM V. Session, Classifying neurocognitive disorders in the 21st century - Toward DSM V. Presentation FT-01-02 - ICAD 2010, Honolulu,HI, USA

Gamaldo, A., Moghekar, A., Kilada, S., Resnick, S.M., Zonderman, A.B., & O'Brien, R. (2006). Effect of a clinical stroke on the risk of dementia in a prospective cohort. *Neurology.* 67(8): 1363–1369

Gorelick, P.B., & Mangone, C.A . (1991).Vascular dementias in the elderly. *Clin Geriatr Med.* 7(3): 599-615.

Graham, N.L., Emery, T., & Hodges, J.R. (2004). Distinctive cognitive profiles in Alzheimer's disease and subcortical vascular dementia. *J Neurol Neurosurg Psychiatry.* 75(1): 61-71.

Hachinski, V.C., Iliff, L.D., Zilhka, E., Du Boulay, G.H., McAllister, V.L., Marshall, J., Russell, R.W., & Symon, L. (1975). Cerebral blood flow in dementia. *Arch Neurol.* 32(9): 632-637.

Hachinski, V.C. (1990). The decline and resurgence of vascular dementia . *CMAJ.* 142(2): 107-111.

Hachinski ,V.C, Iadecola, C., Petersen, R.C., Breteler, M.M., Nyenhuis, D.L., Black, S.E., Powers, W.J., DeCarli, C., Merino, J.G., Kalaria, R.N., Vinters, H.V., Holtzman, D.M., Rosenberg, G.A., Wallin, A., Dichgans, M., Marler, J.R., & Leblanc, G.G. (2006). National Institute of Neurological Disorders and Stroke-Canadian Stroke Network vascular cognitive impairment harmonization standards. *Stroke.* 37(9): 2220-2241

Hayden, K.M., Warren, L.H., Pieper, C.F., Ostbye, T., Tschanz, J.T., Norton, M.C., Breitner, J.C.S., & Welsh- Bohmer, K.A. (2005). Identification of VaD and AD prodromes: the Cache County Study. *Alzheimer's & Dementia.* 1(1): 19-29.

Henon, H., Pasquier, F., & Leys, D. (2006). Poststroke dementia. *Cerebrovasc Dis.* 22(1): 61-70

Hesse, C., Rosengren, L., Vanmechelen, E., Vanderstichele, H., Jensen, C., Davidsson, P., & Blennow, K. (2000). Cerebrospinal fluid markers for Alzheimer's disease evaluated after acute ischemic stroke. *J Alzheimers Dis.* 2(3-4): 199-206

Hsiung, G.Y., Donald, A., Grand, J., Black, S.E., Bouchard, R.W., Gauthier, S.G., Loy-English, I., Hogan, D.B., Kertesz, A., Rockwood, K., & Feldman, H.H. (2006). Outcomes of cognitively impaired not demented at 2 years in the Canadian Cohort Study of Cognitive Impairment and Related Dementias. *Dement Geriatr Cogn Disord.* 22(5-6): 413-420.

Ivan, C.S., Seshadri, S., Beiser, A., Au, R., Kase, C.S., Kelly-Hayes, M., & Wolf, P.A. (2004). Dementia after stroke: the Framingham study. *Stroke.* 35: 1264-1268.

Jack, C.R. Jr., Knopman, D.S., Jagust, W.J., Shaw, L.M., Aisen, P.S., Weiner, M.W., Petersen, R.C., & Trojanowski J.Q. (2010). Hypothetical model of dynamic biomarkers of the Alzheimer's pathological cascade. *Lancet Neurol.* 9(1): 119–128

Jagust, W.J., Zheng, L., Harvey, D.J., Mack, W.J., Vinters, H.V., Weiner, M.W., Ellis, W.G., Zarow, C., Mungas, D., Reed, B.R., Kramer, J.H., Schuff, N., DeCarli, C., & Chui, H.C. (2008) Neuropathological basis of magnetic resonance images in aging and dementia. *Ann Neurol.* 63(1): 72-80.

Jellinger, K.A., & Attems, J. (2003). Incidence of cerebrovascular lesions in Alzheimer's disease: a post-mortem study. *Acta Neuropathol.* 105(1): 14–17.

Jellinger, K.A. (2007). The enigma of vascular cognitive disorder and vascular dementia. *Acta Neuropathol.* 113(4): 349–388.

Johnson, S.C., Schmitz, T.W., Moritz, C.H., Meyerand, M.E., Rowley, H.A., Alexander, A.L., Hansen, K.W., Gleason, C.E., Carlsson, C.M., Ries, M.L., Asthana, S., Chen, K., Reiman, E.M., & Alexander, G.E. (2006). Activation of brain regions vulnerable to Alzheimer's disease: the effect of mild cognitive impairment. *Neurobiol Aging.* 27(11): 1604- 1612.

Kalaria, R.N., & Ballard, C. (1999). Overlap between pathology of Alzheimer disease and vascular dementia. *Alzheimer Dis Assoc Disord.* 13 (Suppl 3): 115-123.

Kalaria, R.N., Kenny, R.A., Ballard, C.G., Perry, R., Ince, P., & Polvikoski, T. (2004).Towards defining the neuropathological substrates of vascular dementia. *J Neurol Sci.* 226(1-2): 75-80

Kalaria, R.N., & Erkinjuntti, T. (2006). Small Vessel Disease and Subcortical Vascular Dementia. *J Clin Neurol.* 2(1): 1-11.

Kalaria, R.N., Maestre, G.E., Arizaga, R., Friedland, R.P., Galasko, D., Hall, K., Luchsinger, J.A., Ogunniyi, A., Perry, E.K., Potocnik, F., Prince, M., Stewart, R., Wimo, A., Zhang, Z-X., Antuono, P., & The World Federation of Neurology Dementia Research Group. (2008). Alzheimer's disease and vascular dementia in developing countries: prevalence, management, and risk factors. *Lancet Neurol.* 7(9): 812–826.

Kivipelto, M., Helkala, EL., Hänninen, T., Laakso, MP., Hallikainen, M., Alhainen, K., Soininen, H., Tuomilehto,J., & Nissinen, A. (2001). Midlife vascular risk factors and late-life mild cognitive impairment: A population- based study. *Neurology.* 56(12): 1683-1989.

Kokmen, E., Whisnant, J.P., O'Fallon, W.M., Chu, C.P., & Beard, C.M.(1996). Dementia after ischemic stroke: a population-based study in Rochester, Minnesota (1960–1984). *Neurology.* 46(1): 154–159.

Korczyn, A.D. (2002). Mixed dementia - the most common cause of dementia. *Ann NY Acad Sci.* 977:129–134.

Kramer, J.H., Reed, B.R., Mungas, D., Weiner, M.W., & Chui, H.C. (2002). Executive dysfunction in subcortical ischemic vascular disease. *J Neurol Neurosurg Psychiatry.* 72(2): 217-220.

Langa, K.M., Foster, N.L., & Larson, E.B. (2004). Mixed dementia - Emerging Concepts and Therapeutic Implications. *JAMA.* 292(23): 2901-2908

Leys, D., Henon, H., Mackowiak-Cordoliani, M.A., & Pasquier, F. (2005). Poststroke dementia. *Lancet Neurol.* 4(11): 752–759

Libon, D.J., Price, C.C., Davis Garrett, K., & Giovannetti, T. (2004). From Binswanger's disease to leuokoaraiosis: what we have learned about subcortical vascular dementia. *Clin Neuropsychol.* 18(1): 83-100.

Lin, J.H., Lin, R.T., Tai, C.T., Hsieh, C.L., Hsiao, S.F., & Liu, C.K. (2003). Prediction of poststroke dementia. *Neurology.* 61(3): 343–348.

Lo, R.Y., Hubbard, A.E., Leslie M. Shaw, L.M., John Q. Trojanowski, J.Q., Petersen, R.C., Aisen, P.S., Weiner, M.W., & Jagust, W.J., for the Alzheimer's Disease Neuroimaging Initiative. (2011). Longitudinal Change of Biomarkers in Cognitive Decline. Arch Neurol. Published online June 13, 2011. doi:10.1001/archneurol.2011.123

Lobo, A., Launer, L.J., Fratiglioni, L., Andersen, K., Di Carlo, A., Breteler, M.M., Copeland, J.R., Dartigues, J.F., Jagger, C., Martinez-Lage, J., Soininen, H., & Hofman, A. (2000). Prevalence of dementia and major subtypes in Europe: a collaborative study of population-based cohorts. Neurologic diseases in the elderly research group. *Neurology.* 54 (11 suppl 5): S4–9.

Loewenstein, D.A., Acevedo, A., Agron, J., Issacson, R., Strauman, S., Crocco, E., Barker, W.W., & Duara, R.(2006). Cognitive profiles in Alzheimer's disease and in mild cognitive impairment of different etiologies. *Dement Geriatr Cogn Disord.* 21(5-6): 309-315.

Madureira, S., Guerreiro, M., & Ferro, J.M. (2001). Dementia and cognitive impairment three months after stroke. *Eur J Neurol.* 8(6): 621–627

Matthews, F.E., Stephan, B.C., Bond, J., McKeith, I., & Brayne, C. (2007). Medical Research Council Cognitive Function and Ageing Study: Operationalisation of mild cognitive impairment: a graphical approach. *PLoS Med.* 4(10): 1615-1619.

Matthews, F.E., Stephan, B.C., McKeith, I.G., Bond, J., & Brayne, C. (2008). Medical Research Council Cognitive Function and Ageing Study: Two-year progression from mild cognitive impairment to dementia: To what extent do different definitions agree? *J Am Geriatr Soc.* 56(8): 1424-1433

McKhann, G., Drachman, D., Folstein, M., Katzman R, Price, D., & Stadlan, E.M. (1984). Clinical diagnosis of Alzheimer's disease: report of the NINCDS-ADRDA Work Group under the auspices of Department of Health and Human Services Task Force on Alzheimer's Disease. *Neurology.* 34(7): 939-44.

McKhann, G.M., Knopman, D.S., Chertkow, H., Hyman, B.T., Jack, C.R. Jr., Kawas, C.H., Klunk, W.E., Koroshetz, W.J., Manly, J.J., Mayeux, R., Mohs, R.C., Morris, J.C., Rossor, M.N., Scheltens, P., Carillo, M.C., Thies, B., Weintraub, S., & Phelps, C.H. (2011). The diagnosis of dementia due to Alzheimer's disease: Recommendations from the National Institute on Aging and the Alzheimer's Association workgroup. *Alzheimer's & Dementia.* 7(3): 263-269.

Medana, I.M. & Esiri, M.M. (2003). Axonal damage: a key predictor of outcome in human CNS diseases. *Brain.* 126(3): 515-530

Merino, J.G. (2008). Untangling Vascular Cognitive Impairment. *Stroke.* 39(3): 739-740.

Meyer, J.S., Xu, G., Thornby, J., Chowdhury, M.H., & Quach, M. (2002). Is mild cognitive impairment prodromal for vascular dementia like Alzheimer's disease? *Stroke.* 33(8): 1981-1985

Meyer, J.S., Huang, J., & Chowdhury, M.H. (2007). MRI confirms mild cognitive impairments prodromal for Alzheimer's, vascular and Parkinson-Lewy body dementias. *J Neurol Sci.* 257(1-2): 97- 104.

Mirra, S.S., Heyman, A., McKeel, D., Sumi S.M., Crain, B.J., Brownlee, LM., Vogel, F.S., Hughes, J.P., van Belle, G., & Berg, L. (1991). The Consortium to Establish a Registry for Alzheimer's Disease (CERAD). Part II. Standardization of the neuropathologic assessment of Alzheimer's disease. *Neurology.* 41(4): 479–486

Mok, V.C.T., Wong, A., Lam, W.W.M., Fan, Y.H., Tang, W.K., Kwok, T., Hui, A.C.F., & Wong, K.S. (2004). Cognitive impairment and functional outcome after stroke associated with small vessel disease. *J Neurol Neurosurg Psychiatry.* 75(4): 560–566.

Morris, J.C., Storandt, M., Miller, J.P., McKeel, D.W., Price, J.L., Rubin, E.H., & Berg, L. (2001). Mild cognitive impairment represents early-stage Alzheimer disease. *Arch Neurol.* 58(3): 397-405.

Morris, J.C. (2006). Mild cognitive impairment is early-stage Alzheimer disease: time to revise diagnostic criteria. *Arch Neurol.* 63(1): 15-16.

Neuropathology Group of the Medical Research Council Cognitive Function and Ageing Study. (2001). Pathological correlates of late-onset dementia in a multicentre, community-based population in England and Wales. Neuropathology Group of the Medical Research Council Cognitive Function and Ageing Study (MRC CFAS).. *Lancet.* 357(9251): 169-175

Nordlund, A., Rolstad, S., Klang, O., Lind, K., Hansen, S., & Wallin, A. (2007). Cognitive profiles of mild cognitive impairment with and without vascular disease. *Neuropsychology.* 21(6): 706-712.

O'Brien, J.T., Erkinjuntti, T., Reisberg, B., Roman, G., Sawada, T., Pantoni, L., Bowler, J.V., Ballard, C., DeCarli, C., Gorelick, P.B., Rockwood, K., Burns, A., Gauthier, S., & DeKosky, ST. (2003). Vascular cognitive impairment. *Lancet Neurol.* 2(2): 89-98.

Opherk, C., Peters, N., Herzog, J., Luedtke, R., & Dichgans, M. (2004). Long-term prognosis and causes of death in CADASIL: a retrospective study in 411 patients. *Brain.* 127(11): 2533- 2539.

Ott, A., Stolk, R.P., van Harskamp, F., Pols, H.A., Hofman, A., & Breteler, M.M. (1999). Diabetes mellitus and the risk of dementia: The Rotterdam Study. *Neurology.* 53(9): 1937-1942.

Ott, A., Slooter, A.J., Hofman, A., van Harskamp, F., Witteman, J.C., Van Broeckhoven, C., van Duijn, C.M., & Breteler, M.M. (1998). Smoking and risk of dementia and Alzheimer's disease in a population-based cohort study: the Rotterdam Study. *Lancet.* 351(9119): 1840-1843

Pantoni, L., Basile, A.M., Romanelli, M., Piccini, C., Sarti, C., Nencini, P., & Inzitari, D. (2001). Abulia and cognitive impairment in two patients with capsular genu infarct. *Acta Neurol Scand.* 104(3): 185-90.

Parnetti, L., Mari, D., Mecocci, P., & Senin, U. (1994). Pathogenetic mechanisms in vascular dementia . *Int J Clin Lab Res.* 24(1): 15-22.

Petersen, RC., Stevens, JC., Ganguli, M., Tangalos, EG., Cummings, JL., & DeKosky, ST.(2001). Practice parameter: early detection of dementia: mild cognitive impairment (an evidence-based review). Report of the Quality Standards Subcommittee of the American Academy of Neurology. *Neurology.* 56(8): 1133-1142

Petersen, R.C. (2007). Mild cognitive impairment: current research and clinical implications. *Semin Neurol.* 27(1): 22- 31.

Petrovitch, H., White, L.R., Izmirilian, G., Ross, G.W., Havlik, R.J., Markesbery, W., Nelson, J., Davis, D.G., Hardman, J., Foley, D.J., & Launer, L.J. (2000). Midlife blood pressure and neuritic plaques, neurofibrillary tangles, and brain weight at death: the HAAS. *Neurobiol Aging.* 21(1): 57-62

Pohjasvaara, T., Erkinjuntti, T., Ylikoski, R., Hietanen, M., Vataja, R., & Kaste, M. (1998). Clinical determinants of poststroke dementia. *Stroke.* 1998; 29(1): 75- 81

Pohjasvaara, T., Mantyla, R., Aronen, H.J., Leskela, M., Salonen, O., Kaste, M., & Erkinjuntti, T. (1999). Clinical and radiological determinants of prestroke cognitive decline in a stroke cohort. *J Neurol Neurosurg Psychiatry.* 67(6): 742–748

Rasquin, S.M., Verhey, F.R., van Oostenbrugge, R.J., Lousberg, R., & Lodder, J. (2004). Demographic and CT scan features related to cognitive impairment in the first year after stroke. *J Neurol Neurosurg Psychiatry.* 75(11): 1562–1567

Rasquin, S.M., Lodder, J., Visser, P.J., Lousberg, R., & Verhey, F.R. (2005). Predictive accuracy of MCI subtypes for Alzheimer's disease and vascular dementia in subjects with mild cognitive impairment: a 2-year follow- up study. *Dement Geriatr Cogn Disord.* 19(2-3): 113-119

Ravona-Springer, R., Davidson, M., & Noy, S. (2003). The role of cardiovascular risk factors in Alzheimer's disease. *CNS Spectr.* 8(11): 824-833.

Reitz, C., Bos, M.J., Hofman, A., Koudstaal, P.J., & Breteler, M.M.B. (2008). Prestroke Cognitive Performance, Incident Stroke, and Risk of Dementia: The Rotterdam Study. *Stroke.* 39(1): 36-41

Riekse, R.G., Leverenz, J.B., McCormick, W., Bowen, J.D., Teri, L., Nochlin, D., Simpson, K., Eugenio, C., Larson, E.B., & Tsuang, D. (2004). Effect of vascular lesions on cognition in Alzheimer's disease: a community- based study. *J Am Geriatr Soc.* 52(9): 1442-1448.

Rockwood, K., Bowler, J., Erkinjuntti, T., Hachinski, V., & Wallin, A. (1999). Subtypes of vascular dementia. *Alzheimer Dis Assoc Disord.* 13; Suppl 3: 59-65.

Rockwood, K., Macknight, C., Wentzel, C., Black, S., Bouchard, R, Gauthier, S, Feldman, H, Hogan, D, Kertesz, A, & Montgomery, P. (2000). The diagnosis of "mixed" dementia in the Consortium for the Investigation of Vascular Impairment of Cognition (CIVIC*). Ann N Y Acad Sci*; 903: 522-528.

Rockwood, K., Moorhouse, P.K., Song, X., MacKnight, C., Gauthier, S., Kertesz, A., Montgomery, P., Black, S., Hogan, D.B., Guzman, A., Bouchard, R., & Feldman, H. (2007). Consortium to Investigate Vascular Impairment of Cognition (CIVIC) Cohort: Disease progression in vascular cognitive impairment: Cognitive, functional and behavioural outcomes in the Consortium to Investigate Vascular Impairment of Cognition (CIVIC) cohort study. *J Neurol Sci.* 252(2): 106-112.

Román, G. C., Tatemichi, T. K., Erkinjuntti, T., Cummings, J. L., Masdeu, J. C., Garcia, J. H., Amaducci, L., Orgogozo, J.M., Brun, A., Hofman, A., Moody, D. M., O'Brien, M. D., Yamaguchi, T., Grafman, J., Drayer, B. P., Bennett, D. A., Fisher, M., Ogata, J., Kokmen, E., Bermejo, F., Wolf, P. A., Gorelick, P. B., Bick, K. L., Pajeau,A.K., Bell, M. DeCarli, C., Culebras, A., Korczyn, A. D. Bogousslavsky, J., Hartmann, A., & Scheinberg, P. (1993). Vascular dementia: Diagnostic criteria for research studies: Report of the NINDS- AIREN International Workshop. *Neurology.* 43(2): 250-260

Roman GC. (1999). A historical review of the concept of vascular dementia : lessons from the past for the future. *Alzheimer Dis Assoc Disord.* 13 Suppl 3: 4-8.

Roman, G.C., & Royall, D.R. (1999). Executive control function: a rational basis for the diagnosis of vascular dementia. *Alzheimer Dis Assoc Disord.* 13 (Suppl 3): 69-80.

Roman, G.C., Erkinjuntti, T., Wallin, A., Pantoni, L. , Chui, H.C. (2002). Subcortical ischaemic vascular dementia. *Lancet Neurol.* 1(7): 426-436.

Roman, G.C., Sachdev, P., Royall, D.R., Bullock, R.A., Orgogozo, J.M., Lopez-Pousa, S., Arizaga, R., & Wallin, A. (2004). Vascular cognitive disorder: a new diagnostic category updating vascular cognitive impairment and vascular dementia. *J Neurol Sci.* 226(1-2): 81-87.

Sachdev, P. (1999). Vascular cognitive disorder. *Int J Geriatr Psychiatry.* 14(5): 402-403

Sachdev, P.S., Brodaty, H., Valenzuela, M.J., Lorentz, L., Looi, J.C.L., Wen, W., & Zagami, A.S. (2004). The neuropsychological profile of vascular cognitive impairment in stroke and TIA patients. *Neurology.* 62(6): 912-91

Sachdev, P. (2010). DSM-V neurocognitive disorders cluster. Session, Classifying neurocognitive disorders in the 21st century - Toward DSM V. Presentation, FT-01-01 - ICAD 2010 honolulu. HI, USA

Schamhmann, J.D. (2003). Vascular syndromes of the thalamus. *Stroke.* 34(9): 2264-2278.

Selnes, O.A., & Vinters, H.V. (2006). Vascular cognitive impairment. *Nat Clin Pract Neurol.* 2(10):538-47.

Skoog, I., & Gustafson, D. (2003). Hypertension, hypertension-clustering factors and Alzheimer's disease. *Neurol Res.* 25(6): 675-680.

Small, G.W. (2002).The role of neuroimaging in the diagnosis of vascular dementia. *Acta Neurol Scand* (Suppl). 178: 10-14

Snowdon, D.A., Greiner, L.H., Mortimer, J.A., Riley, K.P., Greiner, P.A., & Markesbery, W.R. (1997). Brain infarction and the clinical expression of Alzheimer disease. The Nun Study. *JAMA.* 277(10): 813-817.

Sperling, R.A., Aisen, P.S., Beckett, L.A., Bennett, D.A., Craft, S., Fagan, A.M., Iwatsubo, T., Jack, C.R., Kaye, J., Montine, T.J., Park, D.C., Reiman, E.M., Rowe, C.C., Siemers, E., Stern, Y., Yaffe, K., Carrillo, M.C, Thies, B., Morrison-Bogorad, M., Wagster, M.V., & Phelps, C.H. (2011). Toward defining the preclinical stages of Alzheimer's disease: Recommendations from the National Institute on Aging and the Alzheimer's Association workgroup. *Alzheimer & Dementia.* 7(3): 280-292.

Srikanth, V.K., Quinn, S.J., Donnan, G.A., Saling, M.M., & Thrift, A.G. (2006). Long-Term Cognitive Transitions, Rates of Cognitive Change, and Predictors of Incident Dementia in a Population-Based First-Ever Stroke Cohort. *Stroke.* 37(10): 2479-2483

Stephan, B.C., Brayne, C., McKeith, I.G., Bond, J., & Matthews, F.E. (2008). Medical Research Council Cognitive Function and Ageing Study: Mild cognitive impairment in the older population: Who is missed in classifications and does it matter? *Int J Geriatr Psychiatry.* 23(8): 863-871

Stephan, B.C.M., Matthews, F.E., Khaw, K.T., Dufouil, C., & Brayne, C. (2009). Beyond mild cognitive impairment: vascular cognitive impairment, no dementia (VCIND). *Alzheimer's Research & Therapy.* 2009; 1:4; Available online http://alzres.com/content/1/1/4

Tatemichi, T.K., Desmond, D.W., Mayeux, R., Paik, M., Stern, Y., Sano, M., Remien, R.H., Williams, J.B., Mohr, J.P., Hauser, W.A., & Figueroa, M. (1992). Dementia after stroke: Baseline frequency, risks, and clinical features in a hospitalized cohort. *Neurology.* 42(6): 1185–1193.

Tervo, S., Kivipelto, M., Hänninen, T., Vanhanen, M., Hallikainen ,M., Mannermaa, A., & Soininen, H. (2004). Incidence and risk factors for mild cognitive impairment: a population-based three-year followup study of cognitively healthy elderly subjects. *Dement Geriatr Cogn Disord.* 17(3): 196-203.

The Swedish Council on Technology Assessment in Health Care, SBU. Dementia - Etiology and Epidemiology. A Systematic Review. Report No 172E/1; Vol1. June 2008. ISBN 978-91-85413-23-2 ; ISSN 1400-1403

Toncosco, J.C., Zonderman, A.B., Resnick, S.M., Crain, B., Pletnikova, O., & O'Brien, R.J. (2008). Effect of infarcts on dementia in the Baltimore Longitudinal Study on Aging. *Ann Neurol.* 64(2): 168-176.

Van der Flier, W. M., & Scheltens, P. (2005). Epidemiology and risk factors of dementia. *Neurol Neurosurg Psychiatry.* 76(Suppl V): v2–v7.

Vermeer, S.E., Longstreth, W.T. Jr., & Koudstaal, P.J. (2007). Silent brain infarcts: a systematic review. *Lancet Neurol.* 6(7): 611-619.

Vinters, H.V., Ellis, W.G., Zarow, C., Zaias, B.W., Jagust, W.J., Mack, W.J., Chui, H.C. (2000). Neuropathologic substrates of ischemic vascular dementia. *J Neuropathol Exp Neurol.* 59(11): 931-945

Wallin, A., & Blennow, K. (1993). Heterogeneity of vascular dementia: mechanisms and subgroups. *J Geriatr Psychiatry Neurol.* 6(3): 177-188.

Wallin, A., Sjogren , M., Edman, A., Blennow, K., & Regland, B. (2000). Symptoms, vascular risk factors and blood-brain barrier function in relation to CT white matter changes in dementia. *Eur Neurol.* 44(4): 229-35.

Wallin, A., & Sjogren, M. (2001). Cerebrospinal fluid cytoskeleton proteins in patients with subcortical white- matter dementia. *Mech Ageing Dev.* 122(16): 1937-1949

Wallin, A., Milos, V., Sjogren, M., Pantoni, L., & Erkinjuntti, T. (2003). Classification and subtypes of vascular dementia. *Int Psychogeriatr.* 15(1): 27-37.

Wentzel, C., Rockwood, K., MacKnight, C., Hachinski, V., Hogan, D.B., Feldman, H., Østbye, T., Wolfson, C., Gauthier, S., Verreault, R., & McDowell, I. (2001). Progression of impairment in patients with vascular cognitive impairment without dementia. *Neurology.* 57(4): 714-716

Wimo, A., Winblad, B., Aguero-Torres, H., & von Strauss, E. (2003). The magnitude of dementia occurrence in the world. *Alzheimer Dis Assoc Disord.* 17(2): 63-67.

Wimo, A., & Prince, M. (2010). Alzheimer's Disease International World Alzheimer Report 2010. The Global Economic Impact of Dementia. London: Alzheimer's Disease International (ADI). 21 September 2010. www.alz.co.uk

Wimo, A., Winblad, B., & Jonson, L. (2010). The worldwide societal costs of dementia: Estimates for 2009. *Alzheimer's & Dementia.* 6(2): 98-103.

Winblad, B., Palmer, K., Kivipelto, M., Jelic, V., Fratiglioni, L., Wahlund, L.O., Nordberg, A., Bäckman, L., Albert, M., Almkvist, O., Arai, H., Basun, H., Blennow, K., de Leon, M., DeCarli, C., Erkinjuntti, T., Giacobini, E., Graff, C., Hardy, J., Jack, C., Jorm, A., Ritchie, K., van Duijn, C., Visser, P., & Petersen, R.C. (2004). Mild cognitive impairment - beyond controversies, towards a consensus: report of the International Working Group on Mild Cognitive Impairment. *J Intern Med.* 256(3): 240-246.

World Health Organization. (1992). ICD-10, World Health Organization Tenth Revision of the International Classification of Diseases. Geneva: WHO.

Zekry, D., Duyckaerts, C., Moulias, R., Belmin, J., Geoffre, C., Herrmann, F., & Hauw, J.J. (2002 a) Degenerative and vascular lesions of the brain have synergistic effects in dementia of the elderly. Acta Neuropathol. (Berl) 103(5): 481-487.

Zekry, D., Hauw, J.J., & Gold, G. (2002 b). Mixed dementia: epidemiology, diagnosis, and treatment. *J Am Geriatr Soc.* 50(8): 1431-1438

Zhou, D.H., Wang, J.Y., Li, J., Deng, J., Gao, C., & Chen, M. (2004). Study on frequency and predictors of dementia after ischemic stroke: the Chongqing stroke study. ***J Neurol.*** 251(4): 421-427

Zhu, X., Smith, M.A., Honda, K., Aliev, G., Moreira, P.I., Nunomura, A., Casadesus, G., Harris, P.L., Siedlak, S.L., & Perry, G. (2007). Vascular oxidative stress in Alzheimer disease. *J Neurol Sci.* 257(1-2): 240-246

10

Dictyostelium discoideum: Novel Insights into the Cellular Biology of Neurological Disorders

Michael A. Myre
Center for Human Genetic Research, Dept. of Neurology, Massachusetts General Hospital, Boston, Massachusetts, USA

1. Introduction

Here we will review the somewhat surprising, and novel emerging use of the classic model organism *Dictyostelium discoideum*, a species of soil-living amoeba, as a valuable biomedical tool to study the function of mutant genes implicated in human neurological disorders. Many neurodegenerative disorders, although related by their destruction of brain function, display remarkable cellular and/or regional pathogenic specificity most likely initiated through some deregulated aspect of the activity of the mutant protein. However, the expression of many neurodegenerative disease genes, including but not limited to *huntingtin* (*HTT*), the *ataxins*, the *presenilins* (*PSEN1/PSEN2*) are not simply localized to neurons but are found ubiquitously expressed throughout peripheral tissues. It is safe to say that when considering neurodegeneration, a term used to describe the progressive loss of function or death of neurons; it is paramount to properly understand the earliest precipitating events that lead to neuronal pathogenesis in order to ultimately develop long-term effective therapies. This means, in no unequivocal terms, that it is critical to understand the normal function of the disease-causing gene. Unfortunately, the normal function(s) of a large majority of mutant genes remain largely unknown which may in fact delay, and often precludes the development of assays for rapid and accurate assessment as to how the mutation initiates disease. As a result, a variety of lower and higher metazoan model systems have been established that range from worms to flies to mice, all designed to better understand neurological disease in humans. So the question arises: how reasonable is the use of simple organisms to study neurological disorders especially when the model of choice does not contain neurons? Historically, I believe the evidence suggesting the usefulness of using simple organisms to understand the etiology of cellular pathology cannot be denied. But using an organism without a central nervous system to understand diseases of the brain? The intrinsic complexity of the brain, without question, greatly complicates the accessibility to study the biochemical processes that contribute to pathology. Furthermore, functional genomic studies through the targeted deletion of genes may preclude their study due to essential cellular roles. As a consequence, determining the direct functional role and subsequent alteration of function by the mutation through phenotypic analysis is once again complicated further. Specifically, this has been true for huntingtin, the causative agent of Huntington's disease, and the beta-amyloid precursor protein (APP) and presenilins, responsible for the onset of Alzheimer's disease (AD) as well as a host of other neurological disorders where candidate mutant genes have been discovered but cannot readily be assigned a function. Reverse genetics in mice, the "gold standard" in human disease models, have shown that a number of disease genes including those mentioned previously are critical components involved in embryonic developmental. So again, the question might arise why *Dictyostelium*? The haploid life cycle of *Dictyostelium* is fascinating from a biological perspective, and provides unique opportunities to assess disease-related questions because it can be studied naturally as both single, dynamic independent cells and as a *bona fide* multicellular organism in a highly meaningful way with exceptional cellular clarity. Second, and importantly, unlike metazoans, growth precedes development in this eukaryotic organism. As such, targeted deletions of homologous disease genes that do not affect growth can be readily studied in great biochemical detail when the cells are induced to proceed through development with unparalleled synchronous timing and a robustly consistent pattern of gene expression even across evolutionarily divergent species (Parikh et al. 2010). Finally, since the completion of the *Dictyostelium* genome project a number of reviews on the use of this model system to elucidate mechanisms of disease including actin pathologies, mitochondrial disease, human lysosomal and trafficking disorders, host-pathogen interactions and anti-cancer drug action have been described (Carnell & Insall, 2011; Clark, 2010; Francione et al. 2011; Maniak, 2010; R.S. Williams et al. 2006). As will be reviewed below, the evolutionary conservation between *Dictyostelium* and human genes implicated in neurodegeneration, combined with the organisms genetic tractability and easy cellular accessibility, it can be argued that this model system, along side many other human diseases, also provides a fertile environment for discovering normal gene function(s) that cause neurodegeneration with the significant potential for translational and validation studies in higher eukaryotes including both mouse and human systems.

2. Contributions of *Dictyostelium* to neurodegenerative disease-gene function

When readers of this chapter pause to think about *Dictyostelium*, if at all, at least not since their Introductory Biology course back in University, I have a hunch that they might recollect faint memories of laboratory demonstrations involving cAMP-mediated chemotaxis or the observation of various developmental structures including fruiting bodies made up of spores and stalks that form from starved individual amoebae. Whereas bacteria, yeasts and several other invertebrate or vertebrate model systems are well known for their additions to our understanding of basic biology and human disease, *Dictyostelium*, unfortunately is rarely included among this list. However, quietly, over the last few years, primarily following the publication of the genome, public availability of RNA seq data and DNA microarray data, research conducted on the social amoeba has revealed some very common cellular features shared across various phyla, and almost uncannily, that many of its proteins are more similar to human orthologues than are those of *S. cerevisiae* (Eichinger et al. 2005). Moreover, unlike yeasts, the 34 Mb, *Dictyostelium* genome is densely populated with 12,646 genes and is surprisingly close in size to the 13,676 genes found in the *Drosophila* genome (Adams et al. 2000). I wish to suggest that, despite the wide evolutionary distance that separates humans and the social amoeba, mutations in *Dictyostelium* can provide direct insight into human neurological disease processes. In this chapter I will discuss in detail research using this organism on genes known to cause neurodegenerative disorders including Alzheimer's disease, Huntington's disease and Hirano bodies. However,

Dictyostelium also contain many other genes related to neurological disease including, but not limited to Adrenoleukodystrophy (*ABCD1*), Amyotrophic lateral sclerosis (*SOD1*), Miller-Dieker Lissencephaly (*LIS1*), Parkinson's disease (*UCHL1*) and Neuronal ceroid lipofuscinosis (*PPT1, CLN2, CLN3, CLN5*) (Eichinger et al. 2005). Later in this chapter I will introduce an emerging role for *Dictyostelium* in pharmacogenetics. More specifically, discoveries in *Dictyostelium* on the effects of valproic acid have uncovered common modes of action in mammalian neurons (R.S. Williams, 2005). Lastly, I will describe in detail *in vitro* studies using the unique small molecule DIF-1 (differentiation-inducing factor-1; 1-(3, 5-dichloro-2, 6-dihydroxy-4-methoxyphenyl) hexan-1-one), a morphogen produced by *Dictyostelium*, that has been shown to have anti-amyloid properties in a wide variety of mammalian cell types (Myre et al. 2009). DIF-1 selectively reduces the amyloidogenic processing of wild type and mutant APP (e.g., early onset mutations) which dramatically prevents production of Abeta40 and Abeta42, believed to be the causative agent of AD. Alzheimer's disease, the most common form of dementia among older adults, is nonreversible, and with the number of AD cases on the rise in the absence of effective treatments, it becomes even more urgent to explore and identify molecules with potential therapeutic potential. In essence, as a research community, what I hope to convince you of is that it is important we "leave no stone unturned".

2.1 *Dictyostelium* – Emergence of a classic model organism for the study of human disease

Dictyostelium discoideum is a species of soil-living amoeba belonging to the Kingdom Amoebozoa and phylum Mycetozoa. *Dictyostelium*, now commonly referred to as social amoeba, is a eukaryote that transitions from a collection of individual, self-sustainable phagocytic amoebae into a multicellular slug and then into a fruiting body within its life cycle (Figure 1a).

Upon starvation conditions, *Dictyostelium* transitions from a unicellular to a *bona fide* multicellular organism. During this period of multicellular development, the cells execute a series of morphological changes that proceed in defined stages over a 24 hour period. Within the first six hours of development, cells secrete, and undergo chemotaxis toward cyclic adenosine monophosphate (cAMP) to form aggregation territories. The secretion of cAMP promotes a G protein-coupled receptor signaling cascade that results in the formation of discrete mounds that may contain as many as 100,000 cells (Parent & Devreotes, 1996; Soderbom & Loomis, 1998). As development continues, cells within the mound remain motile and are directed to differentiate into either prestalk or prespore cells, leading to morphogenetic changes yielding a multicellular stalk, supporting a ball of encapsulated dormant spores (J.G. Williams et al. 1989). The entire process showing the various developmental structures is beautifully depicted in Figure 1b by scanning electron microscopy (SEM) and although the description of the life cycle appears simplistic, the process in actuality is quite complex with still many unresolved questions including the transition from growth to development, on how cells secrete cAMP, regulate organism size, and initiate cell-fate choices to name but a few. A PubMed search of the term *Dictyostelium* retrieves well over 7,000 articles with more than 600 reviews available to the reader that explore the life cycle in much greater detail than is presented here. It is now quite clear that *Dictyostelium* possesses signal-transduction pathways that are closely related to those of metazoa. Yet, with at least one major and exploitable fundamental difference: animals undergo embryogenesis, that is to say they develop from a single cell by a combination of cell division, morphogenetic movements and differentiation followed by growth of the organism. Whereas with *Dictyostelium*, growth precedes development, and in contrast, development requires no growth, and multicellularity is achieved by the concerted aggregation of many unicellular amoebae. This greatly simplifies the study of development and provides an exceptionally easier route to examine numerous cellular functions including cytokinesis, endocytosis, secretory pathways, protein trafficking, intracellular signaling, gene transcription and regulation, cell-cell communication and adhesion, differentiation and many molecular and biochemical aspects of random and directed cell motility. In addition, *Dictyostelium* cells undergo a relatively simple program of multicellular development, which in many ways resembles animal development. With the sequencing of the genome we are now entering a renaissance in the use of this model organism as a biomedical research tool.

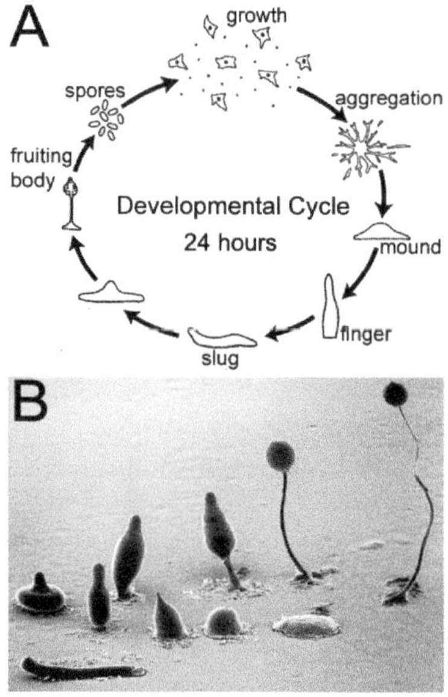

Fig. 1. The life cycle of *Dictyostelium discoideum*. (A) Most of its life exists in its growth phase, as a haploid social amoeba preying upon bacteria in the soil and dividing by mitosis. Once the food source is depleted cells enter into a 24 hour multicellular developmental program. During this transition, amoebae aggregate towards secreted cAMP by chemotaxis in the thousands to form a tight mound and then enter a stage where cells begin to differentiate. Cells within the mound remain motile and are directed to differentiate, by secreted morphogens, into either prestalk or prespore cells, culminating to form a fruiting body comprised of a multicellular stalk that supports a ball of encapsulated dormant spores. (B) Scanning electron microscopy showing the various structures formed during development. Permissions: CC Creative Commons Attribution - Share Alike 3.0, David Brown & Joan E. Strassmann. SEM courtesy of MJ Grimson & RL Blanton, Biological Sciences Electron Microscopy, Texas Tech University.

As will be discussed in more detail later, *Dictyostelium* offers numerous advantages as an experimental organism. Its haploid genome is gene dense, and where higher eukaryotes may express a large number of similar genes with redundant functions, *Dictyostelium* often carries only a single homologous or orthologous gene. In addition, GFP-fusions, expressed sequence tags, RNAi and just about all molecular biochemical experimentation can be performed using the organism with exceptional cellular clarity between differentiated cell types. Most importantly, genetic manipulation of *Dictyostelium* by targeted gene deletion using homologous recombination can be performed relatively quick and for a fraction of the cost of higher eukaryotic systems. In order to unveil the functions of homologous proteins by studying them in simple model systems, it is important that these functions retain a respectable level of conservation through the course of evolution. In many cases, it is possible to demonstrate directly, the conservation of function(s) of homologous proteins among species by expressing a recombinant version of the protein in a null genetic background and showing the restoration of phenotypic deficiencies. Importantly, to suggest the use of *Dictyostelium* as a model system to understand the normal function of human neurological disease genes, when the difficulty of using more complex eukaryotic models have either failed or provided only limited indirect information, there must, at the very least be a significant level of homology present. Sequencing of the *Dictyostelium* genome revealed that many genes encode proteins that meet this criterion of homology to their mammalian counterparts, and some have been shown to be extremely conserved throughout evolution at the amino acid level (>70%) (e.g., calmodulin has 88% identity, actin has 94% identity; see www. http://dictybase.org) and, are also functionally equivalent in an experimental setting. In *Dictyostelium*, some proteins that retain functional equivalence include but are not limited to Vmp1, a vacuolar membrane protein, involved in vesicle trafficking, autophagy, growth and morphogenesis in mammals but not yeast; Rbl1, retinoblastoma-like protein, which causes loss of retina structure/architecture, and ABP34, an actin-bundling protein that causes the formation of Hirano bodies in mammalian neurons (reviewed in Annesley & Fisher, 2009). Moreover, the sequencing of the *Dictyostelium* genome revealed, at a highly conservative and stringent threshold value of $e \leq 10^{-40}$, the presence of at least 64 proteins involved in a variety of human diseases that were similar in size and amino acid identity extending over 70% of the protein (Eichinger, et al. 2005). However, at this level of stringency, the number of orthologous *Dictyostelium* proteins involved in human diseases (e.g., PSEN1, PSEN2, HTT, Neurofibromatosis 1, LRRK2) are not as readily recognized, and so the actual number of predicted human disease proteins present in the genome is very likely to be much higher (Bosgraaf & Van Haastert, 2003; McMains et al. 2010; Myre et al. 2011; S. Zhang et al. 2008). Future biomedical research using this organism will undoubtedly continue to illuminate many more human disease genes with conserved function. Finally another strength that supports the use of this model are the multiple facets of the life cycle, where it can be observed at the organismal, cellular, biochemical and molecular level, all in the same system and with an extremely limited degree of artifact that is far more common among mammalian cell culture. This includes the issues of biological contamination of mammalian cell culture; between 11 percent and 15 percent of cultures in U.S laboratories have been or are infected with species of *Mycoplasma* (Lincoln & Gabridge, 1998), which affect the host cells' metabolism, morphology, cause chromosomal damage, and can provoke cytopathic responses, rendering any data from contaminated cultures unreliable. There are no reports that I am aware of detailing infection of *Dictyostelium* cultures with

Mycoplasma, or, surprisingly, no large DNA virus that infects *Dictyostelium* have been detected thus far. Taken together, the simplicity of its life cycle makes *Dictyostelium* a valuable model organism to study conserved genetic, cellular, and biochemical processes with a very high degree of translation in other model organisms from flies to zebrafish.

2.2 Alzheimer's disease

Dementia is an acquired condition typified by a severe decline in memory and other cognitive abilities. It represents a recession from an individuals established level of intellectual capacity that sufficiently interferes with their everyday ability to function. Alzheimer's disease (AD) is the most common cause of dementia, estimated to contribute to about 60 to 70% of cases (Barker et al. 2002). Estimates suggest that ~ 5.3 million Americans are afflicted with AD (http://www.alz.org), or ~1 in 8 people older than 65, with an estimated worldwide prevalence of AD approaching 30 million people and a quadrupling of numbers expected to occur over the next 40 years. The time course of AD averages 7 to 10 years, characterized by loss of specific neuronal populations and synapses in the cerebral cortex and certain subcortical regions that culminates in extreme atrophy of the diseased regions, including degeneration in the temporal lobe, parietal lobe, and parts of the frontal cortex and cingulate gyrus (Wenk, 2003). AD is a terminal disease that culminates in death. Impaired recent memory usually is an initial symptom of AD, but other cognitive deficits (e.g., changes in attention, problem-solving abilities) may also be present. Amyloid plaques and neurofibrillary tangles (NFTs), the characteristic pathological hallmarks of AD, are believed to be causative and accrue in the years preceding clinical symptoms.

2.2.1 The amyloid precursor protein and discovery of presenilin-dependent gamma-secretase activity

Amyloid plaques are accumulations of insoluble protein aggregates in the extracellular space of the brain. The principal proteinaceous component of plaques is the Abeta peptide, a 38- to 43-amino acid peptide derived from a much larger pre-cursor protein, the amyloid precursor protein (APP) (Golde et al. 2000; Hardy & Selkoe, 2002). APP is a type I integral membrane protein with a single-pass C-terminal transmembrane domain. Several isoforms of APP have been identified, the most common being comprised of 695, 751, or 770 amino acids, are highly expressed in the central nervous system and particularly enriched in neurons. Abeta peptides are derived from APP through the sequential enzymatic activity of two proteases, beta-secretase (BACE) and gamma-secretase, respectively. In addition to Abeta, these cleavage events also liberate an APP intracellular fragment (AICD) that has been suggested to have a transcriptional function (Cao & Sudhof, 2001). APP was identified as the first gene in which mutations in the coding sequence cause early-onset familial Alzheimer's disease (FAD) (Goate et al. 1991; Levy et al. 1990). The identification and location of mutations within the APP gene have provided important clues regarding the potential pathological mechanisms that lead to increased Abeta production in the brain in FAD, but have not been as insightful in the pathology of late-onset AD in which individuals do not contain mutant APP. The normal function of APP is not well understood. However, a review on the function and proteolytic processing of APP is beyond the scope of this chapter and can be thoroughly reviewed elsewhere (Y.W. Zhang et al. 2011).

In addition to APP, mutations in two other genes have been identified that when mutated result in the rare, autosomal dominant forms of early-onset FAD: presenilin-1 (*PSEN1*) (Levy-Lahad, 1995) and presenilin-2 (*PSEN2*) (Sherrington et al. 1995). These genes encode highly homologous, ubiquitously expressed multiple transmembrane domain proteins in which a vast number of mutations have been identified in FAD families. Several years passed before the AD field determined that PSEN1 and PSEN2 were integral parts of the elusive gamma-secretase (De Strooper et al. 1998). Finally, a series of seminal reports provided independent evidence supporting the hypothesis that presenilins provided the catalytic core of gamma-secretase (De Strooper et al. 1999, Struhl & Greenwald 1999, Wolfe et al. 1999). This was ultimately proven by the finding that transition-state, gamma-secretase inhibitors, targeted the presenilins (Esler et al. 2000, Li et al. 2000). The protein composition of the gamma-secretase complexes is now largely resolved (De Strooper 2003). The different gamma-secretases each consist of at least four proteins that are all required for proteolytic activity (Edbauer et al. 2003, Kimberly et al. 2003): APH-1, PEN2, and nicastrin (Edbauer et al. 2003; Yu et al. 2000). In contrast with this basic knowledge, tantalizing questions regarding the physiology, the cell biology, and the structure-function relation of these intriguing gamma-secretases will keep research groups around the world busy for several years largely because the normal function(s) of the presenilins, and other protein components that make up the gamma-secretase complex, remains unclear. *PSEN1* knockout mice die *in utero* and have a phenotype similar to that of Notch (another single-pass transmembrane domain protein) knockout mice (Thinakaran, 2002). However, what is clear is that the gamma-secretase complex directly cleaves the C-terminal transmembrane protein stubs of Notch, APP, APLPs and many other substrates. The mechanism by which gamma-secretase cleaves its substrates is not the focus of this chapter and the process has been described in great detail elsewhere (De Strooper & Annaert, 2010). Here we focus on the normal biological function of the presenilins which has been difficult to determine largely due to the fact that in mammals, it is an essential gene and knockout mice die *in utero*.

2.2.2 The role of presenilins in higher organisms

Notch is a protein involved in cell fate decisions during development and consequently the Notch field of research continues to provide novel insights into various cellular physiological processes, including the biology of the presenilins (Kopan & Ilagan 2009). Furthermore, the central role of presenilin-dependent gamma-secretase activity in Notch signaling has been unequivocally demonstrated in a long series of genetic experiments in various organisms including flies and worms (Levitan & Greenwald, 1995). In mammalian species, the situation is much more complicated because of gene duplication (*PSEN* and *APH-1*) and embryonic lethality of knocking out the *PSEN* and *Aph-1* genes (Ma et al. 2005). Moreover, in adult animals, partial or tissue-specific knockouts of PSEN-1 lead to gastrointestinal bleeding, hair-color changes, and immune problems (Tournoy et al. 2004). In addition, more than 60 other proteins have been proposed or identified as substrates for the gamma-secretases (McCarthy et al. 2009, Wakabayashi & De Strooper 2008). Almost all candidates are type I integral membrane proteins, and they obey the same consecutive-cleavage process as was outlined for APP and has suggested that in many cases, the whole PSEN1 process is aimed at clearance of transmembrane domain stubs from the cell membrane. Protein transport and turnover has also been suggested as a function of presenilin based upon work indicating that several members and/or effectors of the Rab family of small GTPases interact with PSEN (Dumanchin et al. 1999). Most recently it was suggested that PSEN1 is involved in the maturation of the V0a1 subunit and subsequent assembly of the V-ATPase proton pump, providing an explanation for the defects in acidification of cellular degradative compartments in *Psen* knockout cells (Lee et al. 2010). Despite a number of reports suggesting that PSEN mutations also affect Ca^{2+} signaling by disturbing the Ca^{2+} pool in the ER (Bezprozvanny & Mattson 2008), the origin of this disturbance is highly debated, contradictory and the literature remains confusing. What is true is that more is known about the function of presenilin substrates and their intracellular cleavage domains (ICDs) than presenilin itself (reviewed in Krishnaswamy et al. 2009). Of particular importance regarding this chapter, the function of PSEN-dependent gamma-secretase in more distantly related and unicellular species has not been demonstrated or explored to any comparable extent. PS-like components have been identified in moss (Khandelwal et al. 2007), but gamma-secretase activity could not be detected. Overall, a lot of difficult work is still needed in order to decipher the function of presenilin in different gamma-secretase complexes in mammals, but to also uncover the normal *in vivo* role of the protein in other readily available model systems including lower organisms.

2.2.3 The identification of presenilins and gamma-secretase activity in *Dictyostelium*

A recent development in *Dictyostelium* biomedical research was the identification of homologous genes to presenilin 1, presenilin 2, nicastrin, aph-1 and pen-2, the core components that constitute the gamma-secretase complex (McMains et al. 2010). As discussed in humans, mutations in the presenilins, which are integral for protease activity are intimately involved in the aberrant proteolytic processing of APP in a pathway that leads to the condition of early onset familial Alzheimer disease. How the defects cause disease, or more importantly the time course or precipitating events that lead to the pathogenesis of AD are not known, and as such, highlight the importance of uncovering the normal function of the gamma-secretase complex responsible for production of the toxic Abeta peptide. In this section, I discuss the importance of having a viable, organismal model, to aid in further understanding the normal physiological role of the presenilins and gamma-secretase from a conserved and evolutionary point of view in a system that has no Notch or APP equivalent (Eichinger et al. 2005). To study the gamma-secretase in *Dictyostelium* in great detail, strains were created containing single and/or double gene disruptions for *ps1*⁻, *ps2*⁻, *aph1*⁻, *ncst*⁻ and *ps1/ps2*⁻, *aph1/ps2*⁻, *ncst/ps2*⁻, and *aph/ncst*⁻ nulls. It is important to note that mutants of these genes in *Dictyostelium* are viable, unlike the embryonic lethality seen in mammalian systems, and that mutant amoebae show a variety of phenotypic defects during specific periods of development. Moreover, extensive sequence analysis reveals that the *Dictyostelium* presenilins are structurally similar to proteases in this family of proteins rather than the related signal peptidyl proteases (SPP) and that phylogenetic analysis firmly places them among this group (Figure 2A-D), and a majority of the mutations in the human PS1 gene associated with early-onset familial Alzheimer's disease alter residues (Kim & Kim, 2008) that are conserved in both *Dictyostelium* PS proteins (McMains et al. 2010).

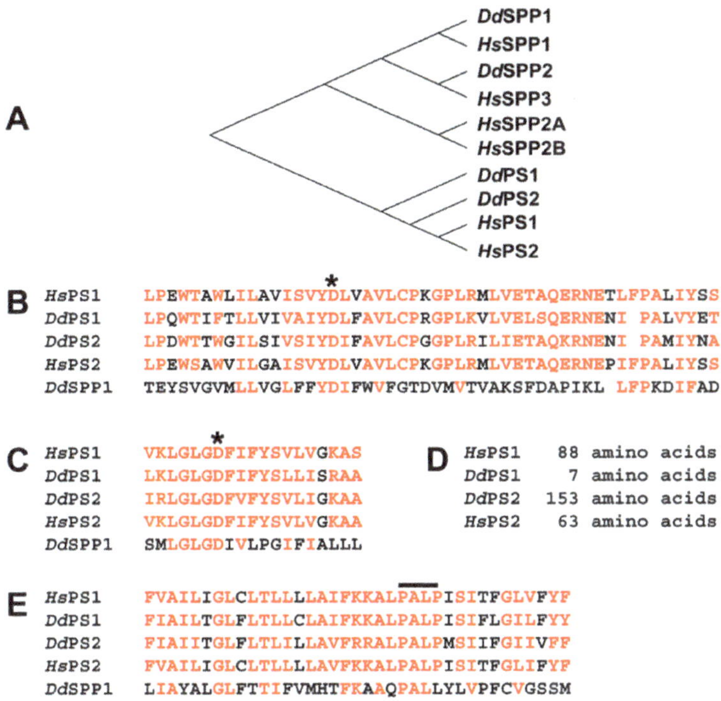

Fig. 2. *Dictyostelium* PS proteins align with human presenilins. (A) Phylogenic comparison of amino acid sequences of *Dictyostelium* and the human PS and signal peptidyl proteases (SPP) proteins. The *Dictyostelium* PS proteins cluster closely with human PS. (B-D) Sequence alignments of functional domains of PS and SPP proteins. Similar amino acid residues are indicated in red. Residue alignment surrounding the N-terminal enzymatic aspartate (*) is shown. Residue alignment surrounding the C-terminal enzymatic aspartate (*) is shown. Residue alignment within the conserved, *overlined* PALP domain region. Permissions: McMains, V.C. et al. (2010). *Dictyostelium* possesses highly diverged presenilin/gamma-secretase that regulates growth and cell-fate specification and can accurately process human APP: a system for functional studies of the presenilin/gamma-secretase complex. *Dis. Model. Mech.* 3, pp. 581-594.

2.2.4 The presenilin gamma–secretase complexes regulate cell differentiation and phagocytosis in *Dictyostelium*

Cells deficient for *ps1* did not show post-aggregative developmental defects compared to cells deficient for *ps2* suggesting that in *Dictyostelium*, PS1 gamma-secretase complexes may carry out different functional activities than PS2 gamma-secretase complexes during specific phases of the life cycle. This observation fits well with the suggestion that that there may be several distinct presenilin complexes that have different biological activities (Gu et al. 2004). Wild type and *ps1*- cells are able to complete development within 24 hours, whereas *ps2*-, *aph*1- and *ncst*- mutants not only form fewer fruiting bodies, but predominantly arrest as abnormal intermediate structures within the same time frame (McMains et al. 2010). It should be noted that the observed development defects were more pronounced in the double mutants and so PS1 might also contribute some functional activity during development. The authors also show that in *Dictyostelium* gamma-secretase complexes function to regulate cell differentiation as measured by cell-type specific gene expression and firmly establish that PS gamma-secretase activity is required in a cell-autonomous pathway that determines cell fate during development (McMains et al. 2010). Once again, these *in vivo* observations support a large body of suggestive evidence for presenilin gamma-secretase playing an essential role in cellular and neuronal differentiation during neural development and adult neurogenesis in mouse and zebrafish models (Baumeister, 1999; van Tijn, 2011). The authors also found that cells deficient for gamma-secretase display a reduced ability for phagocytosis. Quantification of phagocytic rates for the various mutant strains in comparison to wild type cells revealed that cells lacking PS1 had highly reduced rates of phagocytosis, but this was not the case for *ps2-* cells. The described phagocytosis defect supports observations that mammalian presenilins are present in lysosomal membranes, but also strengthens the argument that distinct presenilin complexes exist and have different biological activities. Further to this, when wild type amoeba were made to express a variant of human APP, the cells were clearly able to process APP in a manner identical to mammalian cells resulting in the differential production of C-terminal fragments and Abeta40/Abeta42, the toxic fragment believed to be the causative agent in AD (Figure3).

This work demonstrates the evolutionary conservation of this key regulatory enzyme and establishes the ability to now use the powerful molecular genetics of *Dictyostelium* to test a variety of biochemical predictions using an *in vivo* system. Therefore the most obvious value stemming from this work for the study of presenilin cellular functions and neurological disease falls into three categories. The first being the development of a viable organismal system to study both the ancient and conserved function(s) of the presenilin-dependent gamma-secretase complex, and the possibilities for elucidating presenilin-independent function(s) (Neely et al. 2011); secondly, the exciting prospects surrounding the finding that proteolytic processing of APP occurs in *Dictyostelium* exactly the same way as has been shown animal cells. This finding is important not only because it provides an excellent system in which to test therapeutic agents that target Abeta production *in vivo*, but it is remarkable that this enzyme, given the evolutionary distance between *Dictyostelium* and humans, is capable of cleaving a non-endogenous substrate to produce C-terminal fragments and ratios of secreted Abeta40/Abeta42 identical to mammalian systems. It should be mentioned that a survey of the *Dictyostelium* genome does not readily identify or predict the presence of either the known alpha-secretase or beta-secretase (BACE) (Eichinger et al. 2005) and suggests the presence of yet to be identified first-cleavage sheddases either unique to *Dictyostelium* or potentially conserved across metazoan species. Moreover, this model offers a biochemical clarity not offered by any other system to date to study gamma-secretase function directly, free from the multiple secondary effects that can arise from perturbation of proteolysis of more than 60 identified substrates (McCarthy et al. 2009). Experiments will need to be conducted to elucidate the mechanism by which *Dictyostelium* produces gamma-secretase targets from human APP in the absence of these characterized mammalian enzymes. Unfortunately, from the point of view of therapeutically targeting gamma-secretase it may also suggest that this enzyme is indeed a "membrane proteasome" with less stringent substrate requirements for target specificity than previously thought (Hemming et al. 2008). Clearly, this work further demonstrates the importance in understanding how gamma-secretase complexes recognize and differentiate between their many substrates which undoubtedly are essential for understanding the role of presenilins in biological processes. Lastly, this study provides strong *in vivo* evidence for presenilin function in regulating phagocytosis, only previously suspected in animal cell culture (Jutras et al. 2005). Further studies will be required to determine whether the mammalian *PSEN* gene can rescue *Dictyostelium ps1*-null phenotypes and proteolytic processing of human APP.

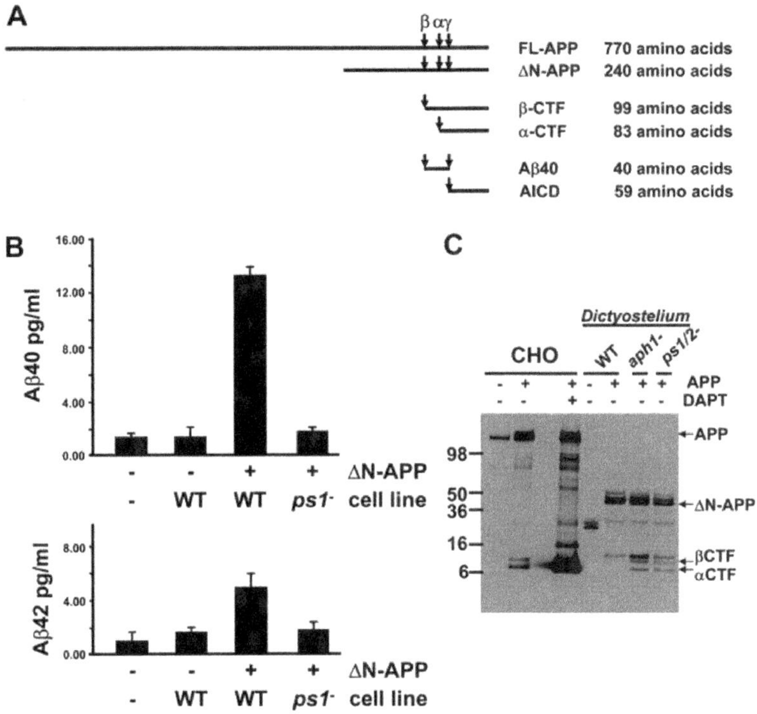

Fig. 3. *Dictyostelium* have PS-dependent gamma-secretase activity that processes human APP to release Abeta peptides. (A) Schematic showing various APP derived products and their respective sizes. (B) ΔN-APP, a truncated human APP expressed in transformed wild type (WT) and ps1-null cells were analyzed for secreted levels of Abeta40 and Abeta42 peptides by quantitative ELISA. Fresh media and media conditioned by native WT cells were used a negative controls. Bars indicate standard errors derived from two independent experiments, each with two replicates. (C) Protein samples were collected from native and APP-expressing CHO cells untreated or treated with DAPT, from growing WT *Dictyostelium* or WT, *aph1*-null and *ps1/2*-null *Dictyostelium* that express ΔN-APP. APP expression and processing was determined by immunoblot assay using anti-APP C-terminus antibodies. Permissions: McMains, V.C. et al. (2010). *Dictyostelium* possesses highly diverged presenilin/gamma-secretase that regulates growth and cell-fate specification and can accurately process human APP: a system for functional studies of the presenilin/gamma-secretase complex. *Dis. Model. Mech.* 3, pp. 581-594.

2.3 Huntington's disease

Huntington's disease (HD) is a fatal neurodegenerative disease (HD Collaborative Research Group, 1993) also known as Huntington's chorea, that affects muscle coordination and leads to cognitive decline, dementia and eventually death. The molecular mechanisms underlying the disease have been widely studied yet the normal function of the protein responsible for the disease remains largely unknown. HD is a monogenic neurological disorder that occurs because of a mutation in the huntingtin protein (HTT). The disease is caused by an unstable, but normally polymorphic, CAG trinucleotide repeat within the coding region of the *htt* gene that leads to the expansion (>35) of a homopolymer stretch of glutamine (Q) residues near the amino-terminus of the protein (HD Collaborative Research Group, 1993). Mutant HTT confers a gain-of-function property to some aspect of the protein, but recent evidence also suggests that mutant HTT impairs the ability of normal huntingtin protein to exert molecular activities that are fundamental for the survival and functioning of the neurons that predominantly degenerate in the disease (Cattaneo et al. 2005). Huntingtin is a large (350 kDa) alpha-solenoid HEAT (huntingtin, elongation factor 3, the A subunit of protein phosphatase 2A, and TOR1) repeat protein (Andrade & Bork, 1995) that bears little resemblance to any known protein. After almost 20 years of research and more than 13,000 research articles, the normal function of HTT, which is expressed in all cells, both neuronal and non-neuronal, still remains unclear for a number of reasons (reviewed in Zuccato et al. 2010).

The large size of HTT makes it challenging to perform biochemical experiments and develop robust structure/function assays. Manipulating such a large DNA fragment by conventional molecular cloning techniques is fraught with problems including sequence stability in bacterial hosts, expansion/contraction of the polyQ and deletions of the polyproline region. Consequently, few studies have been able to address the cellular function(s) of full-length HTT and its dysfunction(s) associated with the disease compared to the vast amount of literature on the amino-terminal fragment, which in essence, removes the mutation from the context of the full-length protein. One might be inclined to argue that studying N-terminal polyQ fragments is tantamount to research on polyQ disease rather than HD. However, the point of this chapter is not to create controversy as one cannot deny that much has been learned about HTT fragment toxicity in studies that utilize the N-terminal fragment. The few genetically precise mouse models for HD (knock-in mice that harbor the full-length mutant protein) have contributed significantly towards understanding HTT normal function, but these mice are laborious to create, expensive to maintain and the results expensive and difficult to validate. Moreover, sub-cellular localization, which often provides clues to protein function, has also been an arduous task due to conflicting reports between various antibodies and the effects that different immunocytological methods can have upon the apparent location of HTT in the cell (reviewed in Hughes & Jones, 2011). Lastly, a number of methods are available to map protein-protein interactions as a means to elucidate protein function. With each approach come strengths and weaknesses regarding specificity and/or sensitivity of the interaction, and again in the case with HTT, its large size and differential affinity for a variety of antibodies has made uncovering its normal function difficult to interpret. As such, a single large scale screening experiment identified at least 234 proteins that interact with mutant huntingtin (Kaltenbach et al. 2007). In this study, the authors assessed five different recombinant wild type and mutant HTT fragments spanning the length of the protein using yeast two-hybrid (Y2H) and affinity pull-down/mass spectrometry (MS) protein interaction screens. How these interacting partners ultimately contribute to understanding HTT normal function remains to be seen, and again, the interpretation of the results must be closely scrutinized as the screen used fragments and was not performed with full-length HTT, which when mutated, is the actual causal agent of HD.

2.3.1 Higher organism and cellular models of Huntington's disease

Genetic evidence in humans and mouse models of Huntington's disease suggests that the disease mutation acts through the deregulation of some aspect of the protein's normal function(s). Over time, the consequence of carrying the HD mutation is an extensive amount of neurodegeneration characterized by the preferential loss of efferent medium spiny neurons in the striatum of the basal ganglia. This massive amount of neuronal loss is primarily responsible for the typical HD symptoms (Reiner et al. 1988). However, it is now well known that as the disease progresses, a more widespread degeneration of the brain ensues and also involves cortical structures (Rosas et al. 2003, 2005). Thus, defining the disease-producing 'gain-of-function' - either a polyglutamine-length dependent increase or deregulation of a normal huntingtin activity or the introduction of a novel polyglutamine-length dependent activity, will without a doubt require an understanding of the protein's normal function(s) beyond what is currently feasible methodologically when using post mortem human brain samples.

I will now offer a brief look at the wide range of HD animal models currently available to the HD community. These models have been used to investigate pathological pathways, molecular targets, and potential therapeutics. A wide variety of species, including invertebrates such as *Drosophila melanogaster*, non-mammalian species (e.g., *Danio rerio*) and mammals, including mice, rats, sheep and non-human primates, have also been genetically engineered to model the HD mutation. Unfortunately, many of these models, that express either truncated or full-length human or mouse mutant huntingtin, display significant phenotypic discrepancies within species that are often attributed to differences in strains or protein context (HTT fragments vs full-length). However, with their size, organ capacity, and close resemblance to human physiology, these models are particularly well-suited for preclinical trials and long-term safety studies. The limitations associated with these models are often ethical concerns, the fact they take a considerable amount of time (e.g., years) to assess and are incredibly costly to maintain. Moreover, modeling the HD mutation, a human disease and without knowing the normal function of the protein, relies primarily on re-creating human symptoms in non-human systems. Although these systems are extremely important tools to understand HD, a large majority of studies focus upon the late end-stage disease symptoms and thus offer minimal insight into early manifestation including HTT normal function. An attempt to describe the phenotypic differences between these entirely different model systems is well outside the scope of this chapter and can be reviewed elsewhere (Zuccato et al. 2010). The existence of HD cell lines, which allow for the stable or inducible expression of wild-type or mutant huntingtin, have been, to a finite degree, useful for the dissection of huntingtin function and assessment of potential therapeutic compounds (Rigamonti et al. 2007; Varma et al. 2007). Further, *in vitro* cell lines often do not show overt defects suggesting they are unable to reproduce the pathophysiological mechanisms induced by the mutant gene.

I have established that the dominant nature of Huntington's disease (HD) and its tissue specificity relative to the fact that it is ubiquitously expressed indicate that the HD mutation may initiate pathogenesis through some unique characteristic activity of the huntingtin protein, making it critical that we understand the normal biochemical function(s) of huntingtin. This is true with respect to developing safe effective treatments. However, the truth is, we don't currently know the details of huntingtin's function nor do we have a ready assay for its rapid and accurate assessment. As mentioned earlier, many established model systems are based upon an amino-terminal fragment that results in perturbation of many cellular processes but these remove the polyglutamine tract from its normal protein context. Therefore, one cannot understate that strategies are badly needed to reveal full length huntingtin-dependent biochemical processes that contribute to HD pathology. Because of the evolutionary conservation of huntingtin, lower organism systems offer an attractive and affordable route that has yet to be exploited to understand huntingtin function. Consequently, we have used the model organism *Dictyostelium* to generate a viable huntingtin-null organism and have defined the various phenotypes.

2.3.2 The identification of *Dictyostelium* huntingtin

Use of the social amoeba *Dictyostelium* to uncover normal function(s) for HTT with a particular focus on the importance of how these functions might illuminate our total understanding of the early vulnerability of specific neuronal populations to mutant HTT is the long-term goal that requires validation in cross-species HTT-null mutants and *in vitro* cell lines. The *Dictyostelium* genome was screened and found to contain a single gene with sequence homology to human huntingtin. Bioinformatic and phylogenetic analysis of the primary amino acid sequence placed the protein firmly within the huntingtin family, including size, and the presence of numerous HEAT and HEAT-like repeats. In developing mutants' deficient for HTT we have determined that in *Dictyostelium*, cells are viable, unlike the embryonic lethality seen in higher eukaryotes. Moreover, *htt*$^{-}$ cells are fragile in that they display a number of subtle phenotypes which suggests that HTT is involved in a number of cellular processes (Myre et al. 2011). We show that huntingtin deficiency impacts upon growth, osmoregulation, cation homeostasis, cell motility, cell shape, chemotactic cAMP relay, homotypic cell-cell adhesion and cell fate determination in *Dictyostelium*. Importantly, these phenotypic deficits are greatly dependent upon the environment in which the cells are placed which suggests that HTT may serve as a multifunctional protein that aids in translating extracellular signals into cellular processes. These findings support the large body of evidence that suggest in metazoa, huntingtin is a multifunctional protein with suggested roles in embryogenesis, cell fate, cytoskeleton, apoptosis, BDNF production and signaling, vesicular and mitochondrial transport, iron homeostasis, autophagy, energy metabolism and transcriptional regulation (Cattaneo et al. 2005; Lumsden et al. 2007; reviewed in Imisario et al. 2008). Major issues of concern regarding HTT function is the inability to discern if these hypotheses correlate with each other, are mutually exclusive to one another, and which, if any, directly involve HTT or are secondary effects to HTT deficiency or mutant HTT activity. The power behind the *Dictyostelium* system is that it allows for the identification of different *in vivo* HTT functions at the level of both single cells and a multi-cellular environment all in the same organism and with a biochemical and cellular clarity that will identify functions that directly depend on HTT.

2.3.3 *Dictyostelium* cells deficient for huntingtin display cell shape and osmoregulatory defects

When *htt*- cells are induced to develop under non-nutrient, low ionic strength phosphate buffer (KK_2; ~40 mOsmol/L), the cells immediately elicit a round phenotype suggesting the presence of an actin-cytoskeleton defect, and a role for HTT in modulating the ability of cells to adapt to stress or changes in their ionic environment (Myre et al. 2011). Under these conditions and in large contrast to wild type cells, HTT-null cells show a disorganized cytoskeleton with a reduction of F-actin at the cortex of the cell (Figure 4A-D). This fits well with reports that mutant HTT in cells from HD patients or when normal huntingtin levels are reduced cells display defective actin-remodeling under conditions of stress (Munsie et al. 2011). *In vitro* binding of the HTT N-terminus to F-actin has been reported (Angeli et al. 2010). Together with our *in vivo* observations indicates a normal, perhaps transient, function for HTT in the regulation of the actin cytoskeleton. Considering the importance of extracellular tonicity to neuronal function, this model provides a valuable tool to uncover mechanisms by which HTT regulates intracellular ionic stores. The extreme cell rounding observed in low osmotic buffer also hinted at a potential defect in osmoregulation. In *Dictyostelium*, osmoregulation is maintained by a bladder-like intracellular membranous organelle called the contractile vacuole (CV) that also functions as a highly efficient acidic Ca^{2+}-store (Zhu & Clarke, 1992). When wild-type cells are placed in water, several small contractile vacuoles form within 30 minutes and, over time, the cells compensate for the sudden change in their osmotic environment, whereas *htt*- cells fail to form vacuoles, rapidly swell and undergo complete lysis within 5-6 hours (Myre et al. 2011) (Figure 4E). This finding is conducive with the role of the cortical cytoskeleton and F-actin crosslinking proteins that protect cells against osmotic stress ensuring both cell size and shape, and suggests a scaffolding role for HTT between the cytoskeleton, actin-remodeling proteins and the function of the CV system in *Dictyostelium*. These results are also consistent with mammalian studies that huntingtin regulates neurological processes including actin-rich dendritic spine formation and membrane branching (Dent et al. 2011; Ferrante et al. 1991). We suggest that the defective CV system in *htt*- cells renders cells not only sensitive to extreme hypoosmotic shock, but secondarily affects intracellular ion homeostasis. As a consequence, unless specific cations (Ca^{2+} or Mg^{2+}) are provided exogenously *htt*- cells appear unable to initiate cAMP-induced Ca^{2+}-transients that may act in a feedback loop to positively reinforce cAMP relay which impairs chemotaxis during *Dictyostelium* development. Although a role for HTT in chemotaxis has not been established in mammalian systems, a consensus is gradually emerging that the dyshomeostasis of Ca^{2+} is an important factor in the linkage of the HTT mutation to the onset and progression of the disease (reviewed in Bezprozvanny, 2007) and together suggest abnormal Ca^{2+} signaling and other Ca^{2+} signaling proteins should be explored further as an evolutionary conserved role for HTT.

2.3.4 Huntingtin regulates cell fate and differentiation during development in *Dictyostelium*

Furthermore, this study also provides compelling evidence to suggest HTT modulates cell fate and differentiation in *Dictyostelium* (Myre et al. 2011) (Figure 5). Using chimeras, we have shown that when *htt*- cells are challenged to differentiate in the presence of wild type cells, they fail to populate the prespore region of the slug, and as a consequence do not become spores. Differentiation defects in huntingtin deficient cells during development has also been observed in vertebrates. In zebrafish, reduced expression of huntingtin differentially targets development of telencephalic neurons compared to mid- and hind-brain (Henshall et al. 2009). In mouse chimeras, *Hdh-/-* cells also preferentially colonize the hypothalamus, midbrain, and hindbrain relative to the telencephalon and the thalamus during early development (Reiner et al. 2001). Thus, like these latter neuronal

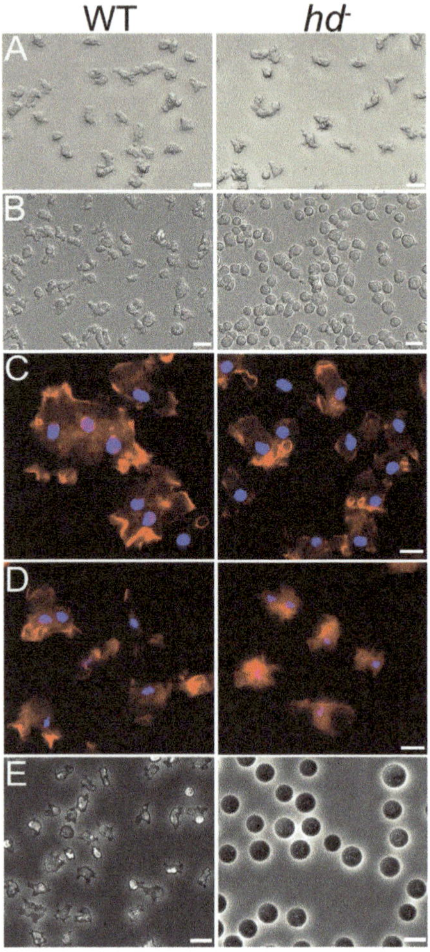

Fig. 4. *Htt-* cells round up under nutrient stress affecting F-actin localization and fail to osmoregulate. (A) The morphology of *htt-* cells as an adherent culture was similar to wild-type cells (left panel). (B) Removal of nutrients and replacement with starvation buffer caused rounding of *htt-* cells. (C) F-actin staining (*red*) in wild type and *htt-* cells is similar. (D) Aberrant localization of F-actin occurs in starved *htt-* cells. Nuclei are counterstained with Hoechst 33342 (*blue*) (E) Unlike WT cells (*left*) *htt-* cells are extremely sensitive to hypoosmotic shock, and begin to lyse after ~3 hours. Permission: Myre M.A. et al. (2009). Deficiency of huntingtin has pleiotropic effects in the social amoeba *Dictyostelium discoideum*. *PLoS Genetics*, 7(4), pp. e1002052.

populations, *Dictyostelium* cells require huntingtin for the proper development of viable spores in the presence of wild-type cells. Not surprisingly, the data thus far do not provide a simple definition for a single normal function for huntingtin, but, as huntingtin deficiency in *Dictyostelium* produces pleiotropic effects throughout the life cycle, the findings are consistent with the consensus from mammalian studies that huntingtin is a multifunctional protein that can impact upon many biochemical processes. Importantly, the existence of a *Dictyostelium* ortholog of human huntingtin, the viability of the null *htt-* mutant, and its discrete, readily assayed deficiency phenotypes indicate that this haploid organism provides an effective genetic model system to identify molecular and cellular processes affected by the loss of huntingtin function. Exciting new avenues of research have emerged in delineating which of these functions are conserved in mammals. Ultimately, determining to what degree these functions are altered by expansion of the polyglutamine tract in human huntingtin will also provide much needed insights into the mechanism by which mutant huntingtin triggers HD pathogenesis.

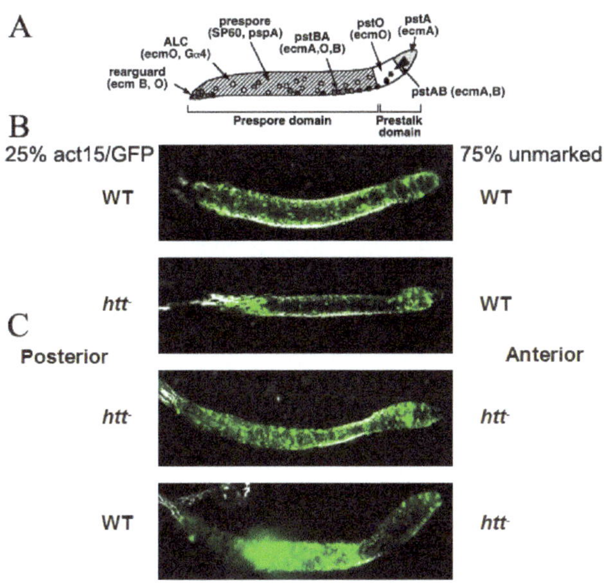

Fig. 5. Huntingtin regulates prespore/spore differentiation cell-autonomously. (A) Schematic representing the position and distribution of cell types in the slug. The prestalk (front) and prespore (rear) domains are *underlined*. Cell types within each region are shown. (B) GFP was expressed in htt- cells and their position in chimeras with unlabelled wild type cells was monitored. GFP:*htt-* cells fail to populate the prespore domain. (C) Reverse experiment in which GFP: WT cells in chimeras with unlabelled *htt-* cells occupy the prespore domain. Permission: Myre M.A. et al. (2009). Deficiency of huntingtin has pleiotropic effects in the social amoeba *Dictyostelium discoideum*. *PLoS Genetics*, 7(4), pp. e1002052.

2.4 Hirano bodies – *Dictyostelium* as the first available cultured cell model of Hirano bodies

Hirano bodies, first described more than 40 years ago, are bright eosinophilic intracytoplasmic inclusions/protein aggregates which have a highly characteristic crystalloid fine rod structures that occur preferentially in the neuronal processes of individuals with a number of neurodegenerative diseases including Alzheimer's disease, Creutzfeldt-Jacob disease, amyotrophic lateral sclerosis, parkinsonism-dementia and Pick's disease (Cartier et al. 1985; Hirano, 1995). Therefore, Hirano bodies are largely considered as a pathological hallmark of postmortem brain samples from patients suffering from neurodegenerative disorders and thus represent "tombstones" that mark neuronal cell death. Although Hirano bodies are most often encountered in neurons of the central nervous system, they have been reported in glial cells, in peripheral nerve axons, and in extraocular muscles of eyes (Tomonaga, 1983) suggesting that they may be more than products of cell death. It should be noted that Hirano bodies are also increasingly observed as a function of age in individuals without any obvious underlying neurodegeneration (Gibson & Tomlinson, 1977). The importance of these findings remains to be addressed. Hirano bodies are complex neuronal inclusions comprised of a variety of proteins including actin and actin-associated proteins (cofillin and alpha–actinin), tau, a C-terminal fragment of APP, microtubule associated bundling proteins (MAPs), and neurofilament proteins (Hirano, 1994). Moreover, they are not specific to humans and have been described in various experimental animals. Although their existence has been reported for decades, understanding the underlying pathological molecular mechanism responsible for their formation has been precluded by the lack of either an *in vitro* or *in vivo* experimental model system. In this section I highlight the development of *Dictyostelium* as the first available cultured cell model of Hirano bodies (Maselli et al. 2002). Of critical importance here is that research using *Dictyostelium* has shown that the formation of Hirano bodies is a pathological event and not simply related to cell death.

I have already established that abnormal protein aggregation results in formation of distinct types of protein assemblies frequently associated with neurodegenerative disease. Maselli et al. 2002 managed to show that expression in *Dictyostelium* of the CT fragment (amino acids 124-295) of the 34 kDa protein, a protein that exhibits activated actin binding and calcium-insensitive actin filament cross-linking activity induced cells to form ellipsoidal paracrystalline inclusions that contain ordered assemblies of F-actin, CT-myc, myosin II, cofilin and alpha-actinin that remarkably resembled the structure of Hirano bodies. They extended their findings to mammalian murine cells and discovered that F-actin rearrangements caused by a reduction in stress fibers accumulate as numerous punctate foci and large aggregates: Hirano bodies (Maselli et al. 2002). This suggested that the failure to regulate either the activity and/or affinity of an actin cross-linking protein can provide a signal for formation of Hirano bodies. Whereas wild type cells complete development in 24 hours, they found that CT-myc cells contained significantly higher amounts of F-actin, were able to form fruiting bodies, but displayed delayed developmental timing by ~6 hours. Further to this, an accumulation of F-actin was also shown to occur in murine cells expressing CT-myc. More importantly, this first report established for the first time that formation of Hirano bodies is not restricted to mammalian cells or nerve cells, occurs as a consequence of aberrant function of the actin cytoskeleton and demonstrated the physiological effects that Hirano bodies can exert on normal cell function. Because of the development of this system using *Dictyostelium*, the formation of Hirano bodies and induction of F-actin rearrangements in mammalian cell cultures by expression of the CT 34-kDa actin-bundling protein has now been shown to occur in HEK 293, HeLa, Cos7 cells, neuroblastoma and astrocytic cells, and in primary neurons (Davis et al. 2008).

The abundant detection of Hirano bodies in numerous neurodegenerative diseases suggest the complex aggregate might be involved in normal and neuronal disease processes. This prompted the study to determine how Hirano bodies are turned over in the cell. Hirano bodies in cultured mammalian cells are frequently observed within membrane-bound vesicles and therefore suggested they might be degraded by autophagosomes. Strains of *Dictyostelium* mutants with defects in autophagy and the use of proteasome inhibitors revealed that these aggregates are turned over by autophagic processes as well as the ubiquitin-proteasome pathway (Kim et al. 2009). Importantly, the authors were able to also show that Hirano bodies are also turned over in human H4 cells by both the proteasome and autophagy. These studies support the concept that the ability of clearance mechanisms to keep pace with accumulation of aggregates may have a major impact on disease progression and further showcase how the lower eukaryote *Dictyostelium* can be used to gain novel insight into mechanisms that potentially contribute to human neurodegenerative disease.

3. Pharmacogenetics

Pharmacogenetics is generally regarded as the study or clinical testing of genetic variation that gives rise to differing response to drugs, while pharmacogenomics is the broader application of genomic technologies to new drug discovery and further characterization of older drugs. Pharmacogenetics refers to genetic differences in metabolic pathways which can affect individual responses to drugs, both in terms of therapeutic effect as well as adverse effects. This section will discuss in detail, the discovery that *Dictyostelium* naturally produces small-molecules with anti-amyloidogenic properties and therefore serves as a valuable resource of novel compounds with the potential to become lead molecules in clinical trials with the long-term goal of treating neurodegenerative diseases such as AD. Importantly, *Dictyostelium* can serve as a high-throughput *in vivo* tool with the potential to identify common modes of action, toxic and therapeutic dosing and adverse effects with greater biochemical clarity than *in vitro* screening methods. One may even argue that in some cases, the use of this model system has the potential to rapidly and cost-effectively act as proof-of-principle for future validation studies to improve the safety of certain drugs. Very early during the development and clinical analysis of new pharmaceuticals, it is imperative to determine the teratogenic potential of promising drugs. *Dictyostelium* has successfully been used as a simple biological system to study the teratogenic effects of valproic acid (VPA) and valproic acid-analogues with results that are consistent with data obtained in mammalian teratogenicity assays (Dannat et al. 2003; Tillner et al. 1998). In keeping with this, *Dictyostelium* has also provided much needed detailed insight into the common mechanistic action of specific neuropsychiatric therapies for bipolar disorder including lithium and VPA, whose mode of action remains poorly understood (R.S. Williams et al. 2002). Early work was able to show that in *Dictyostelium*, drugs that provide a neuroprotective effect in individuals with bipolar disorder work through a common mechanism involving the activation of MAPK signaling and increased ERK2 phosphorylation by reducing protein kinase A (PKA) signaling (Eickholt et al. 2005). More recently, data from *Dictyostelium* models strongly suggest that VPA rapidly immobilizes phospholipid signaling through the modulation of phosphoinositide levels independent of inositol regulation which coincides with a reduction in endocytic trafficking and that VPA when tested in mammalian cells also abrogates this process as measured through depolarization-dependent neurotransmitter release in rat nerve terminals (Chang et al. 2011; Xu et al. 2007). The use of *Dictyostelium* as a model system to understand the common mechanism of action of drugs to treat bipolar disorders will not be discussed any further in this chapter as it has been recently and extensively reviewed (Ludtmann et al. 2011) but confirms the existence of conserved drug-sensitive signaling pathways between *Dictyostelium* and mammalian model systems.

3.1 Differentiation-Inducing Factor-1 from *Dictyostelium* has anti-amyloid properties

As discussed earlier in this chapter, many theories regarding the pathogenesis of AD resulting in abnormal Abeta production or clearance that include inflammation, oxidative stress, metal ion dysregulation and Ca^{2+}-dyshomeostasis, but the exact mechanisms leading to Abeta accumulation remain unclear (reviewed in Walsh & Selkoe, 2004). However, more and more evidence has suggested that irregular cell cycling in selective neuronal populations may contribute to the initiation of AD pathogenesis (reviewed in Herrup & Arendt, 2002; Nagy et al. 1998). Although a controversial area of AD research given the post-mitotic nature of neurons, a variety of cell cycle regulatory proteins, including proliferating cell nuclear antigen, cyclin

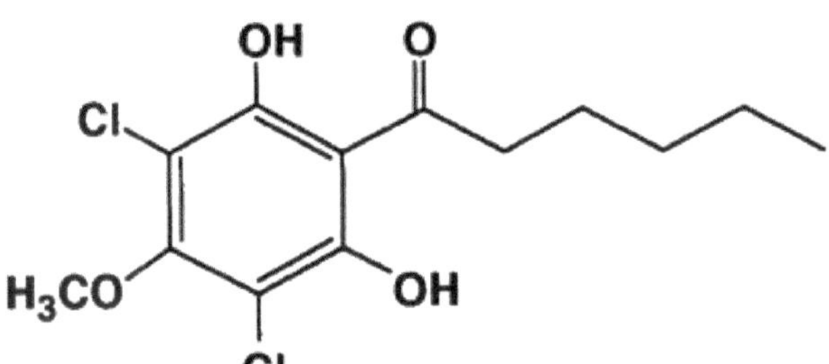

Fig. 6. Chemical structure of DIF-1. Differentiation-Inducing Factor-1 (DIF-1) (l-[3, 5-dichloro-2, 6-dihydroxy-4-methoxyphenyl]-l-hexanone) is a chlorinated alkyl phenone, isolated from the social amoeba *Dictyostelium discoideum*. Permission: Myre M.A. et al. (2009). Reduced amyloidogenic processing of the amyloid beta-protein precursor by the small-molecule Differentiation Inducing Factor-1. *Cellular Signalling*, 21(4), pp. 567-76.

D1, Cdk4, and cyclin B1, are often detected in animal models of AD well before the presence of plaques, and in human brain regions that display AD pathology (Khurana et al. 2006; Yang et al. 2006). Even though APP processing is clearly aberrant in neuronal signaling pathways, the relevance of neuronal cell cycle re-entry to this process remains unclear. Interestingly, APP processing is elevated in pancreatic cancer, oral squamous cell carcinomas and colon carcinomas, which strongly suggest that APP proteolysis is linked to physiological processes involving cellular proliferation and that treatment of cells with antisense oligonucleotides against APP reduced both secreted APP and proliferation

(Hanzel et al. 2003; Ko et al. 2004). Collectively, it would appear that genetic and/or environmental factors (e.g., oxidative and metabolic insults on brain aging) that impede upon the tight regulation of the cell cycle could indeed impact upon Abeta formation. I spoke earlier in this chapter on the various uses of *Dictyostelium* to understand eukaryotic cellular processes and the role that secretion of small chemical morphogens have on the coordinated cellular differentiation of amoeba into prestalk or prespore cells (J.G. Williams et al. 1989). One particular morphogen is a unique chlorinated alkyl phenone, (l-[3, 5-dichloro-2, 6-dihydroxy-4- methoxyphenyl]-l-hexanone) which has been termed Differentiation-Inducing Factor-1 (DIF-1) (Figure 6) (Kay & Jermyn, 1988). Even though the intracellular DIF-1 receptor(s) have yet to be identified in *Dictyostelium*, and no structural analogs of DIF-1 have been reported in mammalian systems, novel functions for DIF-1 in inhibiting the proliferation of mammalian tumors concomitant with decreased expression of specific cell cycle markers (e.g., cyclin D1 and beta-catenin) have been reported (Yasmin et al. 2005). Of particular interest and in support of the role of APP in cellular proliferation was the finding that mutant presenilin variants that bind beta-catenin significantly modify cell growth *in vivo* (Chevallier et al. 2005). Based on all of these lines of independent evidence, we hypothesized that DIF-1 might function as a novel small molecule with the ability to modulate APP catabolism in mammalian cells. Importantly, while there is no cure for Alzheimer's disease, the most common form of dementia, and no treatment to reverse or halt its progression, a small number of medicines are available that help treat symptoms in some people with the disease. These generally fall within the class of drugs known as cholinesterase inhibitors, but unfortunately are limited in their efficacy. At least 80 drugs, from vitamin E to Liptor™ to Abeta immunotherapies have been or are currently being tested in clinical trials. Unfortunately, the large majority of drugs fail or are discontinued from clinical trials, and to discuss the many drugs being tested is well beyond the scope of this chapter. However, it should be noted that *Dictyostelium* might also serve as a source of natural molecules with biomedical potential in the treatment of neurodegenerative disease.

3.1.1 DIF-1 reduction of APP secretion Abeta production in cultured mammalian cells is cell cycle-dependent

I will now discuss DIF-1, a unique, small-molecule from *Dictyostelium* and its ability to significantly reduce Abeta production in a large variety of mammalian cells from mouse embryonic fibroblasts to neuronally derived mouse N2a and human SH-SY5Y cells (Myre et al. 2009). In all cell types tested, DIF-1 inhibited cellular proliferation without inducing any detectable cytotoxic effects and simply washing the cells with phosphate buffered saline restored their rate of proliferation. Moreover, the cytostatic effect of DIF-1 was coupled with an average decrease of 82.41±0.74% in cyclin D1 levels and an increased number of cells in G0/G1 (Myre et al. 2009). Since healthy post-mitotic neurons are relatively locked in a G0/G1 state to prevent proliferation or migration (Arendt, 2003) and aberrant cyclin D1/cdk4 expression has been reported in AD-diseased brain regions suggesting entrance into S-phase (Khurana et al. 2006; Yang et al. 2006) one might speculate that as a consequence of aberrant cycling, associated with age-dependent, environmentally acquired insults, creates a biochemical state that results in increased APP processing. To see if cyclin D1 levels were correlated with either an increase or decrease in APP processing we treated cells with DIF-1 and monitored the levels of secreted APP and Abeta, and the proteolysis of APP into alpha- and beta-C-terminal fragments, respectively (Figure 7a-e).

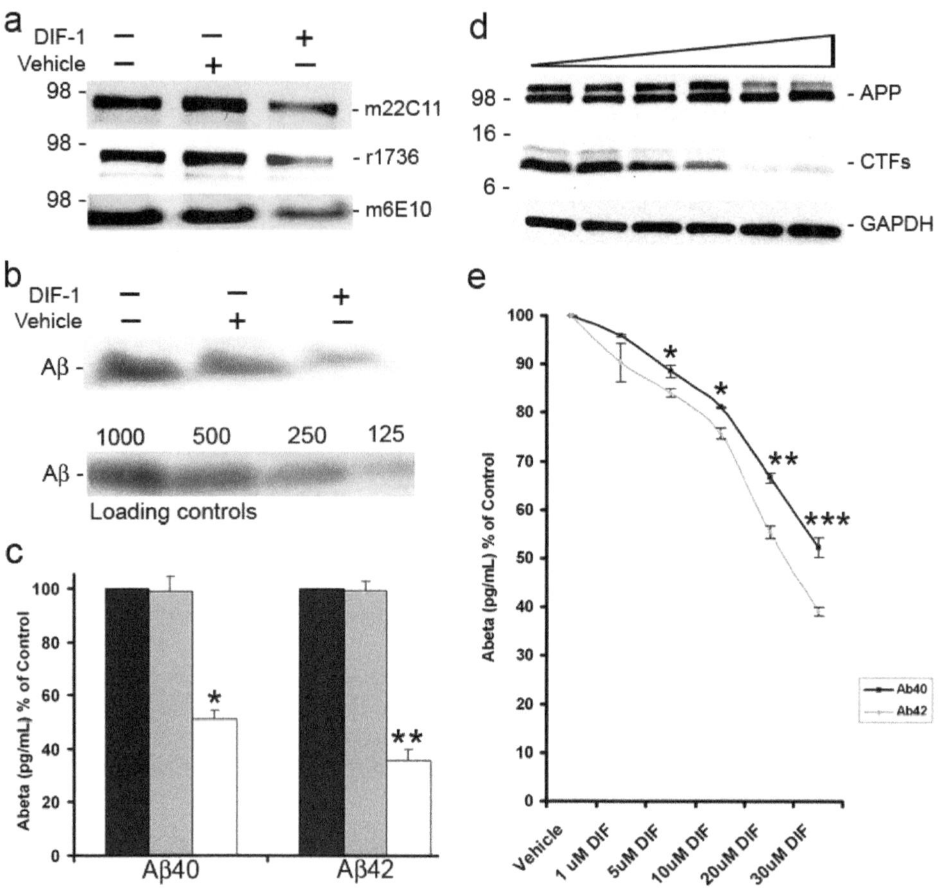

Fig. 7. DIF-1 reduces secretion of APP and inhibits Abeta production. (a) Western blot analysis shows CHO cells treated with DIF-1 show reduced levels of secreted APP into the media as analyzed using three different anti-APP N-terminus antibodies (*shown on right*). (b) Western blot analysis shows DIF-1 also reduced total secreted Abeta in conditioned media. (c) Levels of Abeta40 and Abeta42 were measured by sandwich ELISA. The graph represents the percent average reduction of Abeta (±S.D.) (n=3) compared to controls. Black bars = non-treated cells, grey bars = vehicle and white bars = DIF-1 treated CHO cells. One asterisk represents a P value < 0.003; two asterisks represent a P value < 0.001. (d) Extracts from CHO cells that stably overexpress BACE1 were treated with increasing concentrations of DIF-1 (0, 1, 5, 10, 20 and 30 µM) (*triangle*) show reduced proteolysis and CTF levels (e) The levels of secreted Abeta40 and Abeta42 is significantly reduced in conditioned media from CHO cells that stably overexpress BACE1 as measured by sandwich ELISA. One asterisk represents a P value < 0.003, two asterisks represent a P value < 0.001, and three asterisks represent a P value < 0.0005. Permission: Myre M.A. et al. (2009). Reduced amyloidogenic processing of the amyloid beta-protein precursor by the small-molecule Differentiation Inducing Factor-1. *Cellular Signalling*, 21(4), pp. 567-76.

As shown in figure 7, DIF-1, in a dose-dependent manner, decreased the level of secreted APP compared to controls, reduced APP maturation and beta-CTF levels and is associated with a differential reduction in the levels of Abeta40 (44.2±3.4%) and Abeta42 (66.9±2.6%). Taken together, the data suggests that in the presence of DIF-1, APP processing into Abeta either occurs less during the G0/G1 phase of the cell cycle or is directly affected by DIF-1. Importantly, these results were obtained from CHO cells with increased BACE1 expression and suggest that BACE1 activity is most likely not inhibited or targeted by DIF-1. The effect of DIF-1 on APP processing is also not a result of a general disruption in metabolic processing of type I transmembrane proteins, as when we investigated its effect on a highly related protein, APP-like protein 1 (APLP1), DIF-1 did not affect APLP1 maturation or CTF production.

3.1.2 The mechanism by which DIF-1 reduces of Abeta production involves APP phosphorylation at Thr668

Notably, APP that is phosphorylated at residue Thr668 appears to be a preferred substrate for amyloidogenic cleavage (Vingtdeux et al. 2005). We next assessed whether DIF-1 alters the level of APPT668 phosphorylation and found that in the presence of DIF-1, APP phosphorylation at Thr668 is drastically reduced (88.7± 3.16%) (Myre et al. 2009) and implies that the mechanism by which DIF-1 reduces amyloidogenic processing of APP is dependent upon the phosphor-state of this residue. In order to determine the importance of the Thr668 residue with respect to the effect of DIF-1 on APP metabolism, we generated constructs that result in changes of the Thr688 residue to either Thr688A or Thr688E which would result in the production of APP molecules that cannot be phosphorylated at Thr668. Unexpectedly, DIF-1 had no affect on the metabolic processing of either APPT668A or APPT668E as compared to wild type APP751. The APPT668E and APPT668A mutations abolished the effect of DIF-1 on APP maturation, CTF levels and total Abeta production. This result was surprising since the T668E mutation was expected to mimic a permanently phosphorylated form of APP. We then performed a bioinformatic analysis of the APP C-terminal sequence which predicts that mutating residue Thr668 to any other amino acid (with the exception of serine) in this region no longer meets the criteria as a potential group IV WW-binding motif (Ser/Thr-Pro). This form of WW domain is a small phosphoserine- or phosphothreonine-binding protein module found in various proteins that participate in cell signaling or binding regulation, including physiological substrates of enzymes, in a phosphorylation-dependent manner (Lu et al. 1999). We suggest that a glutamic acid residue cannot compensate for the actual phosphorylation of Thr668 with respect to the mechanism of DIF-1 action on APP processing. Future work on the mechanism of DIF-1 regarding APP processing and phosphorylation of Thr668 will hopefully elucidate how this residue functions in a modulatory manner in the production of Abeta.

The normal function of APP has remained elusive since its' initial discovery in 1987 and consequently, knowledge of the biology behind AD pathogenesis remains limited. This research is important because it has confirmed the importance of deregulated phosphorylation of APP and identification of cell-cycle markers in postmortem AD brains as important pathogenic mechanisms. Moreover, DIF-1 represents a novel small-molecule with the potential for therapeutic investigation into the pathological mechanisms that result in AD with the long-term possibility to serve as a lead molecule in the development of structural analogs in the pursuit of AD therapies. Further to this, DIF-1 serves as yet another compound the will help to realize the promise in the area of "chemical genomics." The goal of this application of genomics is to expand the universe of small molecules that can be used as probes for understanding biological pathways. While the human genome appears to contain more than 20,000 genes, the entire current pharmacopoeia targets only about 500 genes and their products (Drews, 2000). The use of chemical biological tools provides another resource that will compliment existing models and may allow for the discovery of alternative pathways that regulate Abeta production. We believe that our findings set the stage for the use of DIF-1 as a molecular probe to further elucidate cell cycle-dependent signaling mechanisms that regulate amyloidogenic processing of APP in mammalian systems and further suggest that *Dictyostelium* is a potential resource for unique molecules with biomedical relevance.

4. Future value and limitations of *Dictyostelium* as a biomedical model

All eukaryotic organisms share a cellular organization made up of functionally distinct, membrane-enclosed compartments such as the nucleus, endosome, mitochondria and endoplasmic reticulum/Golgi. In addition, similar, if not identical, mechanisms across diverse species control the cell cycle and division, the establishment of cell polarity (e.g., polarity and motility of chemotaxing *Dictyostelium*) in unicellular as well as multicellular eukaryotes. It is therefore important to not overlook the many basic molecular biological processes which are shared by all eukaryotes, of varying complexities, and in doing so exploit the strengths of each model system. It is my hope that this review exemplifies how the lower organism *Dictyostelium* fulfills the necessary scientific requirements that qualify its future use as an invaluable tool to understand the conserved cellular roles of genes implicated in neurodegenerative disorders. I believe most would agree that it is of fundamental importance to gain as much understanding about the earliest underlying pathogenic processes of any devastating human disease in order to increase drug efficacy and/or appropriate therapeutic targeting, but to also work towards a cure. This section will outline the cost-effectiveness of *Dictyostelium*, the rapid nature in which reverse genetics and genetic modifier screens can be employed to mine even the most subtle of phenotypes, and the recent discoveries of cell-cell signaling molecules that were previously thought to only exist in higher metazoan systems. Taken together, the genetic tractability of this model organism has the magnificent capacity in certain circumstances to illuminate protein function(s) and mechanisms that are conserved in higher organisms by careful, cross-species phenotypic analysis and biochemical structure/function studies.

4.1 *Dictyostelium* – A valuable model organism for biomedical research

For any model system to be of practical use, not only should it allow for the study of numerous basic and specialized physiological processes, but it must also do so in a cost-effective fashion. *Dictyostelium* undeniably offers great economic advantages over other eukaryotic systems as cells can grow in simple medium at room temperature effectively limiting the need for costly growth incubators. Furthermore, *Dictyostelium* cells can grow to very high cell density (10^{11} clonal cells) in a few days without the need for highly sophisticated equipment. The multicellular development is much shorter compared to mammalian systems and can be induced to proceed in a highly synchronous manner allowing for the rapid detection of developmental phenotypes. The haploid nature of the genome allows one to create gene deletions at a rate unparalleled in mammalian systems including the creation of strains that carry multiple gene deletions. Quite simply when all things are considered, the cell culture conditions are simple, inexpensive, less time consuming, and not as labor intensive as they are for mammalian cells, thereby making it a highly attractive, complementary biological system. As such, *Dictyostelium*, as a model system, has been chosen by the National Institutes of Health as part of its Model Organism Initiative.

Dictyostelium is a powerful molecular system as it offers most of the numerous molecular genetics techniques available for mammalian cells, including gene knock-out, gene knock-in, restriction enzyme-mediated mutagenesis (REMI), RNAi, and inducible gene expression, allowing a wide range of biological questions to be tested. The haploid nature of the genome clearly allows for the unbiased discovery of direct and indirect genetic modifiers of disease through comprehensive genetic screens. The successful use of cDNA complementation /multi-copy suppression strategies that correct phenotypic defects is well described and can be used in combination with the REMI technique to perform saturation screens aimed at recovering genetic modifiers (Kuspa & Loomis, 1994; Robinson & Spudich, 2000). REMI involves the transformation of cells with a mixture of plasmid DNA linearized with a restriction enzyme, along with a restriction enzyme capable of creating compatible cohesive ends in the genome (Kuspa, 2006). This powerful screening technique is not available in higher organisms, and in addition, makes it possible to carry out genetic selection schemes and screens in which greater than a billion progeny can be generated and tested. Genetic schemes of this kind are effective at isolating potential second-site intragenic suppressor loci as well as saturating for second-site mutations which modify the phenotype of a given mutant. Clearly this model system has no equal for establishing the networks of gene action involved in basic cell biological processes. However, one limitation of using unicellular organisms as models for assessing the function of genes involved in disease is that pathologies which affect specific organs cannot be as readily assessed as it might be in the relevant organism. This limitation may also apply to genes that are present in unicellular organisms but are required in a more stringent manner in specialized tissues, or expressed as a variety of different isoforms in specific cell types. Although *Dictyostelium* develops into a bona fide multicellular organism, it does present a limitation in the number of cell types that can be analyzed and therefore discoveries made using this organism must be rigorously assessed in the relevant mammalian cell type.

4.1.1 The surprising discovery of neurotransmitter homologues in *Dictyostelium*

Of the variety of mechanisms evolved that allow for cell-to-cell communication in animals, none maybe more complex than that within the mammalian brain. However, there is evidence to suggest that some of these mechanisms were already in use by pre-metazoan cells, prior to the development of nervous systems, and surprisingly, there exists a body of evidence for a functional role of neurotransmitter receptor homologues in the social amoeba *Dictyostelium*. Unlike the unicellular yeasts, *Dictyostelium* is not a confined immotile unicellular organism but a model system with a short life-cycle that comprises both cellular and multicellular developmental stages. Even in its amoeboid stage *Dictyostelium* can be considered a dynamic organism that is capable of carrying out many physiological processes once thought to only occur in higher metazoan systems. A prime example of this is the recent findings that the family of G-protein coupled receptors (GPCRs) linked to $GABA_B$ receptors, that are typically found in the central and peripheral autonomic nervous system that respond to a wide range of signals (e.g., main neurotransmitters glutamate, gamma-aminobutyric acid and for Ca^{2+}) were considered animal-specific and were not found outside the metazoan branch until the *Dictyostelium* genome was sequenced (Eichinger et al. 2005; Prabhu & Eichinger, 2006). In total, 17 genes encoding $GABA_B$ like receptors were identified based upon homology and are named GrlA through GrlR ($GABA_B$ or metabotropic glutamate - receptors like proteins) (Prabhu et al. 2007). *Dictyostelium* produces GABA in both growing and developing cells (Anjard & Loomis, 2006). Two genes exist in the *Dictyostelium* genome that encodes the enzyme glutamate decarboxylase which converts glutamate to GABA. Signaling in the central nervous system is mediated to a large extent by glutamate and GABA. These intercellular signaling molecules and their receptors have been found in *C. elegans, Drosophila* and all vertebrates but are not found in protists or yeasts. Glutamate and GABA activate ionotrophic and metabotropic receptors on the surface of neurons to initiate and modulate neurotransmission and also play roles in peripheral tissues. The generation of a *grlE*-null strain by homologous recombination found that *Dictyostelium* cells of this strain do not produce SDF-2, a secreted peptide similar to the mammalian neuropeptide diazepam binding inhibitor (DBI), and as a consequence, impairs the timing of sporulation in response to GABA (Anjard & Loomis, 2006). This suggests that GrlE is the GABA receptor in *Dictyostelium* and the findings have revealed that GABA functions not only as a neurotransmitter but has an early intercellular signaling role setting the stage for future studies on the molecular evolution of nervous systems.

Neurotransmitter homologues in *Dictyostelium* are not limited to glutamate and GABA signaling. Five genes homologous to animal P2X receptors have also been identified in *Dictyostelium* (named p2XA through p2XE) (Fountain et al. 2007; Fountain & Burnstock, 2009) and allows for the evolutionary study of purinergic receptors. In *Dictyostelium*, P2XA is an exclusively intracellular receptor, which is in contrast to the predominant cell surface expression of animal receptors, and localizes to the membrane of the contractile vacuole (Fountain et al. 2007). Deletion of the p2XA gene results in an osmoregulatory phenotype, where the cell volume decrease in response to hypoosmotic stress is abolished (Fountain et al. 2007). Although it is clear that the activity of this receptor is not entirely similar to the function of neuronal P2X receptors, these findings do imply that P2XA is absolutely required for the function of an intracellular compartment and has lead to the analysis of potential roles for P2X receptors in mammalian vacuoles (Qureshi et al. 2007). Glutamatergic, GABAergic and purinergic receptors are all present in *Dictyostelium* which represents a fascinating opportunity to garner insight into how these signaling molecules have evolved to function in neuronal signaling in animals and additionally, suggests neurotransmitters were in operation well before the development of the synapse.

The fact that *Dictyostelium,* the ancestor of vertebrate and invertebrate model organisms, appears as a highly evolved organism that had already invented complex interacting systems to control development, cellular physiology, and cellular behavior has profound implications for biomedical genetic research. The central points that I have explored in this chapter can be broadly put into two categories: (1) the great advantages of model organisms, specifically *Dictyostelium,* for identifying and understanding genes that are altered in heritable human diseases and (2) the functions of many of those genes and the evidence that they were present long ago and have remained largely intact in both vertebrate and invertebrate lineages during the course of evolution. New perspectives on disease pathologies are often a result of data collected from unbiased experimental approaches or saturation screens. Often, the identification of novel genetic modifiers then become prime targets of investigation in mammalian systems to explore their potential effects as players in the pathogenesis of disease and as possible alternative therapeutic targets. The logic behind using lower organisms to perform these screens is to partially cripple a process or pathway with a mutation which affects one component and then search for alterations in other genes encoding component functions in the same system. Importantly, one of the often overlooked but added values from studies using simple models is that they have the potential to open radically new perspectives in the study of a given pathology.

5. Conclusion

Several *Dictyostelium* genes are homologous or at the very least, retain a significant amount of structural conservation to human genes making the organism a useful biomedical model system. With the entire genome now sequenced and publicly available in a model organism database called dictyBase, these sequences will allow molecular and cellular biologists to examine with more clarity the complex multifunctional aspects of gene function. Coupled with translational experiments and validation in higher eukaryotes, research that utilizes *Dictyostelium* I believe, will expedite and contribute to our understanding of human neurological diseases. Individual cell behavior accounts for the many phases of health and pathogenic mechanisms that initiate disease. As described earlier, this has been elegantly portrayed in *Dictyostelium* with respect to the precise production of beta-amyloid from the heterologous expression of human APP. Chemotaxis is a critical cellular function with implications in immune health and embryogenesis and the discovery that *Dictyostelium* cells deficient for HTT show highly defective chemotactic behavior coupled to cytoskeletal/membrane deficits under conditions of low ionic conditions may reveal conserved mechanisms for this protein in axon guidance, neuritic extensions and embryogenesis. In this chapter I have provided a list of examples where studies in *Dictyostelium* have provided information that support, complement, or enhance the understanding of the defects that underlie human neurodegenerative diseases or trafficking disorders, or may do so in the future. Future endeavors with this organism that increase the amount of translational research conducted in higher organism or neuronal cell models will be beneficial for understanding both *Dictyostelium* cellular physiology and, more importantly, the cellular mechanisms of human disease. Indeed, bioinformatic analysis of the *Dictyostelium* genome reveals many homologies with animal genes associated with disease, drug targets, and the biosynthesis, storage and reception of neurotransmitters. I propose that multiple model systems can and should be employed in the cross-genomic analysis of human neurodegenerative disease genes to address multiple basic eukaryotic cellular functions (e.g., *Dictyostelium*), to their assembly into various types of more complex molecular pathways (e.g., flies and worms), and then validated and accurately assessed in models of human neurodegenerative disease (e.g., mice).

6. Acknowledgement

Funding: This study was funded by grants NINDS NS032765, Massachusetts HD Center Without Walls NS016367, Huntington's Disease Society of America Coalition for the Cure, and the CHDI Foundation. I also thank Dr. James Gusella for critical reading of the chapter.

7. References

Adams M.D., Celniker S.E., Holt R.A., Evans C.A., Gocayne J.D., Amanatides P.G., Scherer S.E., Li P.W., Hoskins R.A., Galle R.F., George R.A., Lewis S.E. et al (2000). The genome sequence of *Drosophila melanogaster*. *Science*. 287 (5461), pp. 2185-95.

Andrade M.A. & Bork P. (1995). HEAT repeats in the huntingtin protein. *Nature Genetics*, 11(2), pp. 115-116.

Angeli S., Shao J., &Diamond M.I. (2010). F-actin binding regions on the androgen receptor and huntingtin increase aggregation and alter aggregate characteristics. *PLoS One*, 5(2), pp. e9053.

Anjard C. & Loomis, W.F. (2006). GABA induces terminal differentiation of *Dictyostelium* through a $GABA_B$ receptor. *Development*, 133(11), pp. 2253-61.

Annesley S.J., & Fisher P.R. (2009). *Dictyostelium discoideum*--a model for many reasons. *Molecular and Cellular Biochemistry*, 329(1-2), pp. 73-91.

Barker W.W., Luis C.A., Kashuba A., Luis M., Harwood D.G., Loewenstein D., Waters C., Jimison P., Shepherd E., Sevush S., Graff-Radford N., Newland D., et al (2002). Relative frequencies of Alzheimer disease, Lewy body, vascular and frontotemporal dementia, and hippocampal sclerosis in the State of Florida Brain Bank. *Alzheimer Dis Assoc Disord*, 16(4), pp. 203-12.

Baumeister, R. (1999). The physiological role of presenilins in cellular differentiation: lessons from model organisms. *Eur. Arch Psychiatry Clin Neurosci.*, 249(6), 280-7.

Bezprozvanny I. (2007). Inositol 1,4,5-tripshosphate receptor, calcium signalling and Huntington's disease. *Subcell Biochem.*, 45, pp. 323-35.

Bezprozvanny I. & Mattson M.P. (2008). Neuronal calcium mishandling and the pathogenesis of Alzheimer's disease. *Trends in Neuroscience*, 31(9), pp. 454-63.

Bosgraaf L., & Van Haastert P.J. (2003). Roc, a Ras/GTPase domain in complex proteins. *Biochim Biophys Acta*, 1643, pp. 5-10.

Cao X., & Sudhof T. (2001). A transcriptionally active complex of APP with Fe65 and histone acetyltransferase Tip60. *Science*, 293(5527), pp. 115-20.

Carnell M.J., & Insall R.H. (2011). Actin on disease--studying the pathobiology of cell motility using *Dictyostelium discoideum*. *Semin Cell Dev Biol.*, 22(1), pp. 82-8.

Cartier, L., Galvez, S. & Gajdusek, D.C. (1985) Familial clustering of the ataxic form of Creutzfeldt-Jacob disease with Hirano bodies. *J.Neurol.Neurosurg.Psychiatry*, 48(3), pp. 234-238.

Cattaneo E., Zuccato C. & Tartari M. (2005). Normal huntingtin function: An alternative approach to Huntington's disease. *Nat Rev Neurosci*, 6(12), pp. 919-930.

Chang P., Orabi B., Deranieh R.M., Dham M., Hoeller O., Shimshoni J.A., Yagen B., Bialer M., Greenberg M.L., Walker M.C., & Williams RS. (2011). The antiepileptic drug valproic acid and other medium-chain fatty acids acutely reduce phosphoinositide levels independently of inositol in *Dictyostelium*. *Dis Model Mech.*, Sep 8. [Epub ahead of print].

Chevallier N.L., Soriano S., Kang D.E., Masliah E., Hu G., & Koo E.H. (2005). Perturbed neurogenesis in the adult hippocampus associated with presenilin-1 A246E mutation. *Am J Pathol.*, 167(1), pp. 151-9.

Clarke, M. (2010). Recent insights into host-pathogen interactions from *Dictyostelium*. *Cell Microbiol.*, 12(3), pp. 283-91.

Dannat K., Tillner J., Winckler T., Weiss M., Eger K., & Dingermann T. (2003). Effects of medicinal compounds on the differentiation of the eukaryotic microorganism *Dictyostelium discoideum*: can this model be used as a screening test for reproductive toxicity in humans? *Pharmazie.*, 58(3), pp. 204-10.

Davis R.C., Furukawa R., & Fechheimer M. (2008). A cell culture model for investigation of Hirano bodies. *Acta Neuropathol.*, 115(2), pp. 205-17.

Dent E.W., Merriam E.B., & Hu X. (2011). The dynamic cytoskeleton: backbone of dendritic spine plasticity. *Curr Opin Neurobiol.*, 21(1), pp. 175-81.

De Strooper, B., Saftig, P., Craessaerts, K., Vanderstichele, H., Guhde, G., Annaert, W., Von Figura, K. & Van Leuven, F. (1998). Deficiency of presenilin-1 inhibits the normal cleavage of amyloid precursor protein. *Nature*. 391, pp. 387-90.

De Strooper, B., Annaert, W., Cupers, P., Saftig, P., Craessaerts, K., Mumm, J. S., Schroeter, E.H., Schrijvers, V., Wolfe, M.S., Ray W.J., Goate A., & Kopan R. (1999). A presenilin-1-dependent gamma-secretase-like protease mediates release of Notch intracellular domain. *Nature*, 398, pp. 518-22.

De Strooper, B. (2003). Aph-1, Pen-2, and Nicastrin with Presenilin generate an active gamma-Secretase complex. *Neuron*, 38(1), pp. 9-12.

De Strooper, B. & Annaert, W. (2010). Novel research horizons for presenilins and gamma-secretases in cell biology and disease. *Annu Rev Cell Dev Biol*, 26, pp. 235-60.

Drews J. (2000). Drug discovery: a historical perspective. *Science*, pp. 287:1960

Dumanchin C., Czech C., Campion D., Cuif M.H., Poyot T., Martin C., Charbonnier F., Goud B., Pradier L., & Frebourg T. (1999). Presenilins interact with Rab11, a small GTPase involved in the regulation of vesicular transport. *Hum Mol Genetics*, 8(7), pp. 1263-9.

Edbauer, D., Winkler, E., Regula, J. T., Pesold, B., Steiner, H. & Haass, C. (2003). Reconstitution of gamma-secretase activity. *Nature Cell Biology*, 5, pp. 486-488.

Eichinger L., Pachebat J.A., Glöckner G., Rajandream M.A., Sucgang R., Berriman M., Song J., Olsen R., Szafranski K., Xu Q., Tunggal B., Kummerfeld S., et al (2005). The genome of the social amoeba *Dictyostelium discoideum*. *Nature*, 435, pp. 43-57.

Eickholt B.J., Towers G.J., Ryves W.J., Eikel D., Adley K., Ylinen L.M., Chadborn N.H., Harwood A.J., Nau H., & Williams R.S. (2005). Effects of valproic acid derivatives on inositol trisphosphate depletion, teratogenicity, glycogen synthase kinase-3 beta inhibition, and viral replication: a screening approach for new bipolar disorder drugs derived from the valproic acid core structure. *Mol Pharmacol*, 67(5), pp. 1426-33.

Esler W.P., Kimberly W.T., Ostaszewski B.L., Diehl T.S., Moore C.L., Tsai J.Y., Rahmati T., Xia W., Selkoe D.J., & Wolfe M.S. (2000). Transition-state analogue inhibitors of gamma-secretase bind directly to presenilin-1. *Nat Cell Biol*, 2(7), pp. 428-34.

Ferrante R.J., Kowall N.W., & Richardson E.P. (1991). Proliferative and degenerative changes in striatal spiny neurons in Huntington's disease: a combined study using the section-Golgi method and calbindin D28k immunocytochemistry. *J Neurosci.*, (12), pp. 3877-87.

Fountain S.J., Parkinson K., Young M.T., Cao L., Thompson C.R., & North R.A. (2007). An intracellular P2X receptor required for osmoregulation in *Dictyostelium discoideum*. *Nature*, 448(7150), 200-3.

Fountain S.J. & Burnstock, G. (2009). An evolutionary history of P2X receptors. *Purinergic Signal*, 5(3), pp. 269-72.

Francione L.M., Annesley S.J., Carilla-Latorre S., Escalante R., & Fisher P.R. (2011). The *Dictyostelium* model for mitochondrial disease. *Semin Cell Dev Biol.*, 22(1), pp. 120-30.

Gibson, P.H. & Tomlinson, B.E. (1977). Numbers of Hirano bodies in the hippocampus of normal and demented people with Alzheimer's disease. *J.Neurol.Sci.*, 33, pp. 199-206.

Goate, A., Chartier-Harlin, M.C., Mullan, M., Brown, J., Crawford, F., Fidani L., Giuffra L., Haynes A., Irving N., & James L. (1991). Segregation of a missense mutation in the amyloid precursor protein gene with familial Alzheimer's disease. *Nature*, 349, pp. 704-706.

Golde T.E., Eckman C.B., & Younkin S.G. (2000). Biochemical detection of Abeta isoforms: implications for pathogenesis, diagnosis, and treatment of Alzheimer's disease. *Biochim Biophys Acta*, 1502(1), pp. 172-87.

Gu Y., Sanjo N., Chen F., Hasegawa H., Petit A., Ruan X., Li W., Shier C., Kawarai T., Schmitt-Ulms G., Westaway D., St George-Hyslop P., & Fraser P.E. (2004). The presenilin proteins are components of multiple membrane-bound complexes that have different biological activities. *J Biol Chem.*, 279(30), pp. 31329-36.

Hardy, J & Selkoe, D.J. (2002). The amyloid hypothesis of Alzheimer's disease: progress and problems on the road to therapeutics. *Science*, 297(5580), pp. 353-6.

Hansel D.E., Rahman A., Wehner S., Herzog V., Yeo C.J., & Maitra A. (2003). Increased expression and processing of the Alzheimer amyloid precursor protein in pancreatic cancer may influence cellular proliferation. *Cancer Res.*, 63(21), pp. 7032-7.

Hemming M.L., Elias J.E., Gygi S.P., & Selkoe D.J. (2008). Proteomic profiling of gamma-secretase substrates and mapping of substrate requirements. *PLoS Biology*, 6(10), pp. e257.

Henshall T.L., Tucker B., Lumsden A.L., Nornes S., & Lardelli M.T. (2009). Selective neuronal requirement for huntingtin in the developing zebrafish. *Hum Mol Genet* , 18(24), pp. 4830-4842.

Herrup K., & Arendt T. (2002). Re-expression of cell cycle proteins induces neuronal cell death during Alzheimer's disease. *J Alzheimers Dis.*, 4(3), pp. 243-7.

Hirano, A. (1994). Hirano bodies and related neuronal inclusions. *Neuropath.Appl.Neurobiol.*, 20, pp. 3-11.

The Huntington's Disease Collaborative Research Group (1993). A novel gene containing a trinucleotide repeat that is expanded and unstable on Huntington's Disease chromosomes. *Cell*, 72, pp. 971-983.

Imarisio S., Carmichael J., Korolchuk V., Chen C.W., Saiki S., Rose C., Krishna G., Davies J.E., Ttofi E., Underwood B.R., & Rubinsztein D.C. (2008). Huntington's disease: from pathology and genetics to potential therapies. *Biochem. J.* 412(2), pp. 191-209.

Jutras I., Laplante A., Boulais J., Brunet S., Thinakaran G., & Desjardins M. (2005). Gamma-secretase is a functional component of phagosomes. *J Biol Chem*, 280(43) pp. 36310-7.

Kaltenbach LS, Romero E, Becklin RR, Chettier R, Bell R, Phansalkar A, Strand A, Torcassi C, Savage J, Hurlburt A, Cha GH, Ukani L., Chepanoske C.L., Zhen Y., Sahasrabudhe S., Olson J., Kurschner C., Ellerby L.M., Peltier J.M., Botas J., & Hughes R.E. (2007). Huntingtin interacting proteins are genetic modifiers of neurodegeneration. *PLoS Genetics*, 3(5), e82.

Kay R.R., & Jermyn K.A. (1983). A possible morphogen controlling differentiation in *Dictyostelium*. *Nature*, 303(5914), pp. 242- 4.

Khandelwal A., Chandu D., Roe C.M., Kopan R., & Quatrano R.S. (2007). Moonlighting activity of presenilin in plants is independent of gamma-secretase and evolutionarily conserved. *Proc Natl Acad Sci U S A*, 104(33), pp. 13337-42.

Khurana V., Lu Y., Steinhilb M.L., Oldham S., Shulman J.M., & Feany M.B. (2006). TOR-mediated cell-cycle activation causes neurodegeneration in a *Drosophila* tauopathy model. *Curr Biol.*, 16(3), pp. 230-41.

Kimberly W.T., LaVoie M.J., Ostaszewski B.L., Ye W., Wolfe M.S., & Selkoe D.J. (2003). Gamma-secretase is a membrane protein complex comprised of presenilin, nicastrin, Aph-1, and Pen-2. *Proc Natl Acad Sci U S A*, 100(11), pp. 6382-7.

Kim D.H., Davis R.C., Furukawa R., & Fechheimer M. (2009). Autophagy contributes to degradation of Hirano bodies. *Autophagy*, 5(1), pp. 44-51.

Kim, S.D. & Kim, J. (2008). Sequence analyses of presenilin mutations linked to familial Alzheimer's disease. *Cell Stress Chaperones*, 13, pp. 401-12.

Ko S.Y., Lin S.C., Chang K.W., Wong Y.K., Liu C.J., Chi C.W., & Liu T.Y. (2004). Increased expression of amyloid precursor protein in oral squamous cell carcinoma. *Int J Cancer.*, 111(5), pp. 727-32.

Kopan, R. & Ilagan, M.X. (2009). Gamma-secretase: proteasome of the membrane? *Nat Rev Mol Cell Biol.*, 5(6), pp. 499-504.

Krishnaswamy S., Verdile G., Groth D., Kanyenda L., & Martins R.N. (2009). The structure and function of Alzheimer's gamma secretase enzyme complex. *Crit Rev Clin Lab Sci.*, 46(5-6), pp. 282-301.

Kuspa, A. (2006). Restriction enzyme-mediated integration (REMI) mutagenesis. *Methods Mol Biol*, 346, pp. 201-9.

Kuspa, A. & Loomis, WF. (1994). REMI-RFLP mapping in the *Dictyostelium* genome. *Genetics*, 138(3), pp. 665-74.

Lee J.H., Yu W.H., Kumar A., Lee S., Mohan P.S., Peterhoff C.M., Wolfe D.M., Martinez-Vicente M., Massey A.C., Sovak G., Uchiyama Y., Westaway D., Cuervo A.M., & Nixon R.A. (2010) Lysosomal proteolysis and autophagy require presenilin 1 and are disrupted by Alzheimer-related PS1 mutations. *Cell*, 141(7), pp. 1146-58.

Levitan, D and Greenwald, I. (1995). Facilitation of lin-12-mediated signalling by sel-12, a *Caenorhabditis elegans* S182 Alzheimer's disease gene. *Nature*, 377(6547), pp. 351-4.

Levy, E., Carman, M.D., Fernandez-Madrid, I.J., Power, M.D., Lieberburg, I., van Duinen S.G., Bots G.T., Luyendijk W., & Frangione B. (1990). Mutation of the Alzheimer's disease amyloid gene in hereditary cerebral hemorrhage, Dutch type. *Science*, 248, pp. 1124-1126.

Levy-Lahad, E., Wasco. W., Poorkaj, P., Romano, D.M., Oshima, J., Pettingell, W.H., Yu, C.E., Jondro, P.D., Schmidt, S.D., Wang, K., Crowley, A.C., Ying-Hui, F., Guenette, S.Y., Galas, D., Nemens, E., Wijsman, E.M., Bird, T.D., Schellenberg, G.D. &Tanzi, R.E. (1995). Candidate gene for the chromosome 1 familial Alzheimer's disease locus. *Science*, 269, pp. 973–977.

Li Y.M., Lai M.T., Xu M., Huang Q., DiMuzio-Mower J., Sardana M.K., Shi X.P., Yin K.C., Shafer J.A., & Gardell S.J. (2000). Presenilin 1 is linked with gamma-secretase activity in the detergent solubilized state. *Proc Natl Acad Sci U S A*, 97(11), pp. 6138-43.

Lincoln, C.K. & Gabridge M.G. (1998). Cell Culture Contamination: Sources, Consequences, Prevention, and Elimination. *Methods in Cell Biology.*, Vol. 57, p. 49.

Ludtmann M.H., Boeckeler K., & Williams R.S. (2011). Molecular pharmacology in a simple model system: implicating MAP kinase and phosphoinositide signalling in bipolar disorder. *Semin Cell Dev Biol.*, 22(1), pp. 105-13.

Lumsden A.L., Henshall T.L., Dayan S., Lardelli M.T., & Richards R.I. (2007). Huntingtin-deficient zebrafish exhibit defects in iron utilization and development. *Hum Mol Genet*. 16(16), pp. 1905-20.

Ma G., Li T., Price D.L., & Wong P.C. (2005). APH-1a is the principal mammalian APH-1 isoform present in gamma-secretase complexes during embryonic development. *J Neurosci.*, 25(1), pp. 192-8.

Maniak, M. (2011). *Dictyostelium* as a model for human lysosomal and trafficking diseases. *Semin Cell Dev Biol.*, 22(1), pp. 114- 9.

Maselli A.G., Davis R., Furukawa R., & Fechheimer M. (2002). Formation of Hirano bodies in *Dictyostelium* and mammalian cells induced by expression of a modified form of an actin-crosslinking protein. *J Cell Sci.*, 115(Pt 9), pp. 1939-49.

McCarthy J.V., Twomey C., & Wujek P. (2009). Presenilin-dependent regulated intramembrane proteolysis and gamma- secretase activity. *Cell Mol Life Science*, 66(9), pp. 1534-55.

McMains V.C., Myre M.A., Kreppel L., & Kimmel A.R. (2010). *Dictyostelium* possesses highly diverged presenilin/gamma- secretase that regulates growth and cell-fate specification and can accurately process human APP: a system for functional studies of the presenilin/gamma-secretase complex. *Disease Models & Mechanisms*, 3(9-10), pp. 581-594.

Munsie L., Caron N., Atwal R.S., Marsden I., Wild E.J., Bamburg J.R., Tabrizi S.J., & Truant R. (2011). Mutant huntingtin causes defective actin remodeling during stress: defining a new role for transglutaminase 2 in neurodegenerative disease. *Hum Mol Genet.*, 20(10), pp. 1937-51.

Myre M.A., Washicosky K., Moir R.D., Tesco G., Tanzi R.E., & Wasco W. (2009). Reduced amyloidogenic processing of the amyloid beta-protein precursor by the small-molecule Differentiation Inducing Factor-1. *Cellular Signalling*, 21(4), pp. 567-76.

Myre M.A., Lumsden A.L., Thompson M.N., Wasco W., Macdonald M.E., & Gusella J.F. (2009). Deficiency of huntingtin has pleiotropic effects in the social amoeba *Dictyostelium discoideum*. *PLoS Genetics*, 7(4), pp. e1002052.

Nagy Z., Esiri M.M., & Smith A.D. (1998). The cell division cycle and the pathophysiology of Alzheimer's disease. *Neuroscience*, 87(4), pp. 731-9.

Neely K.M., Green K.N., & LaFerla F.M. (2011). Presenilin is necessary for efficient proteolysis through the autophagy- lysosome system in a gamma-secretase-independent manner. *J Neurosci.*, 31(8), pp. 2781-91.

Parent C.A., & Devreotes P. (1996). Molecular genetics of signal transduction in *Dictyostelium*. *Annu Rev Biochem*, 65, pp. 411- 440.

Parikh A., Miranda E.R., Katoh-Kurasawa M., Fuller D., Rot G., Zagar L., Curk T., Sucgang R., Chen R., Zupan B., Loomis W.F., Kuspa A., & Shaulsky G. (2010). Conserved developmental transcriptomes in evolutionarily divergent species. *Genome Biol.*, 11(3), R35.

Prabhu Y., & Eichinger L. (2006). The *Dictyostelium* repertoire of seven transmembrane domain receptors. *Eur Journal of Cell Biol*, 85, pp. 937-946.

Prabhu Y., Müller R., Anjard C., & Noegel A.A. (2007). GrlJ, a *Dictyostelium* $GABA_B$-like receptor with roles in post- aggregation development. *BMC Developmental Biology*, 14(7) pp. 44-58.

Qureshi O.S., Paramasivam A., Yu J.C., & Murrell-Lagnado R.D. (2007). Regulation of P2X4 receptors by lysosomal targeting, glycan protection and exocytosis. *Journal of Cell Sci*, 120(Pt 21), pp. 3838-49.

Reiner A., Albin R.L., Anderson K.D., D'Amato C.J., Penney J.B., & Young A.B. (1988). Differential loss of striatal projection neurons in Huntington disease. *Proc Natl Acad Sci U S A*, 85(15), pp. 5733-7.

Reiner A., Del Mar N., Meade C.A., Yang H., & Dragatsis I., (2001). Neurons lacking huntingtin differentially colonize brain and survive in chimeric mice. *J Neurosci*, 21(19), pp. 7608-7619.

Rigamonti D., Bolognini D., Mutti C., Zuccato C., Tartari M., Sola F., Valenza M., Kazantsev A.G., & Cattaneo E. (2007). Loss of huntingtin function complemented by small molecules acting as repressor element 1/neuron restrictive silencer element silencer modulators. *J Biol Chem*, 282(34), pp. 24554-62.

Rosas H.D., Koroshetz W.J., Chen Y.I., Skeuse C., Vangel M., Cudkowicz M.E., Caplan K., Marek K., Seidman L.J., Makris N., Jenkins B.G., & Goldstein J.M. (2003). Evidence for more widespread cerebral pathology in early HD: an MRI-based morphometric analysis. *Neurology*, 60(10), pp. 1615-20.

Rosas H.D., Hevelone N.D., Zaleta A.K., Greve D.N., Salat D.H., & Fischl B. (2005). Regional cortical thinning in preclinical Huntington disease and its relationship to cognition. *Neurology*, 65(5), pp. 745-7.

Sherrington, R., Rogaev, E. I., Liang, Y., Rogaeva, E. A., Levesque, G., Ikeda, M., Chi, H., Lin, C., Li, G., Holman, K. Tsuda T., Mar L,. et al (1995). Cloning of a gene bearing missense mutations in early-onset familial Alzheimer's disease. *Nature*, 375, pp. 754-60.

Soderbom F., & Loomis B. (1998). Cell-cell signaling during *Dictyostelium* development. *Trends Microbiol*, 6(10), pp. 402-406.

Struhl, G. & Greenwald, I. (1999). Presenilin is required for activity and nuclear access of Notch in *Drosophila*. *Nature*, 398 (6727), pp. 522-5.

Thinakaran, G. (2002). Metabolism of presenilins. *J Mol Neuroscience*, 17(2), pp. 183-92.

Tillner J., Nau H., Winckler T., & Dingermann T. (1998). Evaluation of the Teratogenic Potential of Valproic Acid Analogues in Transgenic *Dictyostelium discoideum* Strains. *Toxicol In vitro.*, 12(4), pp. 463-9.

Tomanaga, M. (1983). Hirano body in extraocular muscle. *Acta Neuropathol.*, 60, pp. 309-313.

Tournoy J., Bossuyt X., Snellinx A., Regent M., Garmyn M., Serneels L., Saftig P., Craessaerts K., De Strooper B., & Hartmann D. (2004). Partial loss of presenilins causes seborrheic keratosis and autoimmune disease in mice. *Hum Mol Genetics*, 13(13), pp. 1321-31.

van Tijn P., Kamphuis W., Marlatt M.W., Hol E.M., Lucassen P.J. (2011). Presenilin mouse and zebrafish models for dementia: focus on neurogenesis. *Prog Neurobiol.*, 93(2), pp. 149-64.

Varma H., Voisine C., DeMarco C.T., Cattaneo E., Lo D.C., Hart A.C., & Stockwell B.R. (2007). Selective inhibitors of death in mutant huntingtin cells. *Nat Chem Biology*, 3(2), pp. 99-100.

Vingtdeux V., Hamdane M., Gompel M., Bégard S., Drobecq H., Ghestem A., Grosjean M.E., Kostanjevecki V., Grognet P., Vanmechelen E., Buée L., Delacourte A., & Sergeant N. (2005). Phosphorylation of amyloid precursor carboxy- terminal fragments enhances their processing by a gamma-secretase-dependent mechanism. *Neurobiol Dis.*, 20(2), pp. 625- 37.

Wakabayashi, T & De Strooper, B. (2008). Presenilins: members of the gamma-secretase quartets, but part-time soloists too. *Physiology* (Bethesda), 23, pp. 194-204.

Walsh, D.M. & Selkoe, D.J. (2004). Deciphering the molecular basis of memory failure in Alzheimer's disease. *Neuron*, 44(1), pp. 181-93.

Wenk, G.L. (2003). Neuropathologic changes in Alzheimer's disease. *J Clin Psychiatry*, 64 Suppl 9, pp. 7-10.

Williams J.G., Duffy K.T., Lane D.P., McRobbie S.J., Harwood A.J., Traynor D., Kay R.R., & Jermyn K.A. (1989). Origins of the prestalk-prespore pattern in *Dictyostelium* development. *Cell*, 59(6), pp. 1157-1163.

Williams R.S., Cheng L., Mudge A.W., & Harwood A.J. (2002). A common mechanism of action for three mood-stabilizing drugs. *Nature*, 417(6886), pp. 292-5.

Williams R.S. (2005). Pharmacogenetics in model systems: defining a common mechanism of action for mood stabilisers. *Prog Neuropsychopharmacol Biol Psychiatry*, 29(6), pp. 1029-37.

Williams R.S., Boeckeler K., Gräf R., Müller-Taubenberger A., Li Z., Isberg R.R., Wessels D., Soll D.R., Alexander H., & Alexander S. (2006). Towards a molecular understanding of human diseases using *Dictyostelium discoideum*. *Trends Mol Med.*, 12(9), pp. 415-24.

Wolfe, M.S., Xia, W., Ostaszewski, B.L., Diehl, T.S., Kimberly, W.T. & Selkoe, D.J. (1999). Two transmembrane aspartates in presenilin-1 required for presenilin endoproteolysis and gamma-secretase activity. *Nature*, 398, pp. 513-7.

Xu X., Müller-Taubenberger A., Adley K.E., Pawolleck N., Lee V.W., Wiedemann C., Sihra T.S., Maniak M., Jin T., & Williams R.S. (2007). Attenuation of phospholipid signaling provides a novel mechanism for the action of valproic acid. *Eukaryot Cell.*, 6(6), pp. 899-906.

Yang Y., Varvel N.H., Lamb B.T., & Herrup K. (2006). Ectopic cell cycle events link human Alzheimer's disease and amyloid precursor protein transgenic mouse models. *J Neurosci*. 26(3), pp. 775-84.

Yasmin T., Takahashi-Yanaga F., Mori J., Miwa Y., Hirata M., Watanabe Y., Morimoto S., & Sasaguri T. (2005). DIF-1 suppresses gene expression of cyclin D1 in tumor cells. *Biochem Biophys Res Commun.*, 338(2), pp. 903-9.

Yu G., Nishimura M., Arawaka S., Levitan D., Zhang L., Tandon A., Song Y.Q., Rogaeva E., Chen F., Kawarai T., Supala A., Levesque L. et al (2000). Nicastrin modulates presenilin-mediated notch/glp-1 signal transduction and betaAPP processing. *Nature*, 407(6800), pp. 48-54.

Zhang S., Charest P.G., & Firtel R.A. (2008). Spatiotemporal regulation of Ras activity provides directional sensing. *Current Biology*, 18(20), pp. 1587-93.

Zhang Y.W., Thompson R., Zhang H., & Xu H. (2011). APP processing in Alzheimer's disease. *Mol Brain*, 4, pp. 3.

Zhu Q., & Clarke M. (1992). Association of calmodulin and an unconventional myosin with the contractile vacuole complex of *Dictyostelium discoideum*. *J Cell Biol* ,118(2), pp. 347-358.

Zuccato C., Valenza M., & Cattaneo E. (2010). Molecular mechanisms and potential therapeutical targets in Huntington's disease. *Physiol Reviews*, 90(3), pp. 905-81.

11

Neurofibromatosis – Diagnostic Assessment

Sónia Costa, Raquel Tojal and Ana Valverde
Neurology Department, Hospital Professor Dr. Fernando Fonseca EPE,
Amadora,
Portugal

1. Introduction

Descriptions of individuals supposed to have neurofibromatosis have been discovered in manuscripts dating from 1000 AD (Zanca, 1980). However, it was not until 1881 that Von Recklinghausen coined the term "neurofibroma" when he observed that this benign tumour arose from the peripheral nerve sheath. His colleagues honored his contribution by naming the condition Von Recklinghausen's disease. However, the different forms of neurofibromatosis were not separated and delineated until the latter part of the twentieth century (Ferner et al., 2007a). Neurofibromatosis is one of the called "neurocutaneous disorders" or "phakomatoses", genetic diseases that involve both skin and the nervous system. They share some features: hereditary transmission, involvement of organs of ectodermal origin and a tendency to develop certain types of central and peripheral nervous system tumours. Advances in clinical genetics allowed to separate neurofibromatosis in two diseases, each caused by a different gene, although recognition still requires an appreciation of the cutaneous and systemic symptoms. (Ferner 2007a, 2010)

2. Clinical manifestations and diagnostic criteria

2.1 Neurofibromatosis 1

Neurofibromatosis 1 (NF1) is an autosomal dominant disorder with an incidence of 1 in 3,500 live births. Half of all cases are spontaneous mutations. The gene was cloned on chromossome 17q11.2 in 1990. Neurofibrin, the protein product, is widely expressed with high levels in the nervous system. It acts as a tumour suppressor which explains why NF1 patients are prone to developing benign and malignant tumours (Ferner, 2010). Although recent advances in genetic testing may permit the laboratory diagnosis in as many as 95%, for the majority of patients the diagnosis is made on the basis of clinical manifestations. Diagnosis requires the presence of 2 or more major criteria: 6 or more *café au lait* spots, axillary or inguinal freckling, 2 or more cutaneous neurofibromas, 1 plexiform neurofibroma, characteristic bony lesions (pseudarthrosis, sphenoid wing hypoplasia), an optic glioma, 2 or more iris Lisch nodules, or a first-degree relative with NF1 (Table 1). Diagnosis can be made at birth in some cases, whereas others must be monitored for a few years for the presence of additional criteria (Ferner et al., 2007a, b, 2010; Tonsgard, 2006).

6 or more *café au lait* spots (>0,5 cm in prepubertal children, >1,5 cm in postpubertal individuals)
Axillary or inguinal freckling
2 or more cutaneous neurofibromas
1 plexiform neurofibroma
2 or more iris Lisch nodules
An optic glioma
Characteristic bony lesions (pseudarthrosis, sphenoid wing hypoplasia)
A first-degree relative with NF1

Table 1. Diagnostic Criteria for NF1

2.1.1 Cutaneous manifestations

Café au lait spots are generally the heralding feature of NF1. *Café au lait* spots are hyperpigmented flat spots that are oval or rounded with fairly smooth borders (Fig 1a). They are present at birth in many individuals and increase in size and number over the first 5 to 7 years of life. Most, but not all patients with NF1, have *café au lait* spots (Tonsgard, 2006).

Freckling is reported in children of about 3 years of age in the axillae, groins, around the neck, on the eyelids, and under the breasts. However it may not appear until 5 to 7 years of age (Tonsgard, 2006).

Cutaneous angiomas and hypopigmented maculaes are described, and xanthogranulomas (Fig1b) can appear fleetingly during childhood as orange papules. Cutaneous or dermal neurofibromas are tumors of the nerve sheath comprised of Schwann cells, fibroblasts, perineural cells, mast cells, axons, and blood vessels (Lott & Richardson, 1981). They may become visible in childhood but more commonly develop in adolescence or adulthood (Fig 1a). They may be purplish depressions in the skin or pedunculated lesions. Plexiform neurofibromas are histologically similar to cutaneous neurofibromas but have more extracellular matrix (Fig 1c). Often, they arise from the dorsal spinal roots, nerve plexus, large nerve trunks, or sympathetic chains. Plexiform tumours may be discrete, homogeneous, well circumscribed or diffuse, heterogeneous, and infiltrative. They may involve superficial skin or be entirely internal. They occur in at least 50% of patients and are probably present at birth. Many are asymptomatic (Tonsgard et al., 1998).

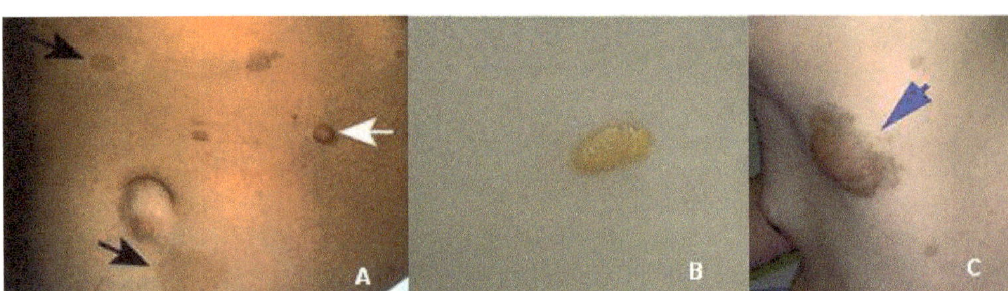

Fig. 1. A - *Café au lait* (black arrows) and pedunculated cutaneous neurofibromas (white arrow) B - Xanthogranuloma. C –Plexiform neurofibroma (blue arrow)

Individuals with NF1 harbor a 7–13% lifetime risk of developing malignant peripheral nerve sheath tumors (MPNST), which usually arises in a pre-existing plexiform or a focal subcutaneous neurofibroma. Cutaneous neurofibromas do not become malignant. MPNSTs metastasize widely and often presage a poor outcome. Vigilant monitoring is recommended for patients with a past history of malignancy or radiotherapy, a family history of MPNST, internal neurofibromas, lesions in the brachial or lumbosacral plexus, or neurofibromatous neuropathy. Individuals with neurofibromatous neuropathy have a mild axonal sensory and motor neuropathy with diffuse neurofibromatous change in the nerves. (Ferner, 2007a)

Diagnosis of MPNST is problematic within the context of NF1 because the emergence of a lump is not unusual. The clinical symptoms of malignancy are intertwined with the symptoms of benign tumours. Plexiform neurofibromas that are associated with persistent or nocturnal pain, rapid increase in size, change in texture, or new or unexplained neurological deficit require urgent assessment at a specialist unit. Targeted biopsy with 18-fluorodeoxyglucose (FDG) PET is the best method for diagnosis (Ferner et al., 2000).

2.1.2 Ocular/orbit manifestations

NF1 may affect the iris, retina, optic nerve, and the bony and soft tissue of the orbit. Lisch nodules are proliferations of melanocytes and fibroblasts that appear as reddish brown spots in the iris of blue- or green-eyed people and hypopigmented spots in brown eyed people. They are commonly found in the lower pole of the iris and have no effect on vision (Fig 2). Onset is usually in the teenage years. They are present in 90% of adults. Retinal hamartomas occur in a small percentage of patients. Optic gliomas (visual pathway tumors) are grade I pilocytic astrocytomas found in 15% of patients. They produce thickening of the optic nerve (Fig 3). Frequently bilateral and often involving the chiasm, they may extend to the optic tracts or inferiorly into the hypothalamus. They may present as decreased color vision or an afferent papillary defect and later with pallor of the optic disc or a decrease in visual acuity between 15 months to 7 years of age. Plexiform neurofibromas of the orbit are frequently found in patients with optic gliomas (Liternick et al., 1989; Tonsgard, 2006; Ferner, 2010).

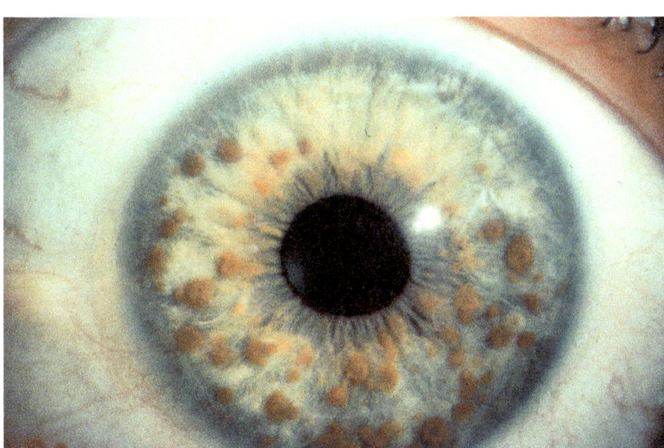

Fig. 2. Lisch Nodules

2.1.3 Bone abnormalities

Orthopedic problems arise in patients with NF1 from inherent abnormalities in the maintenance of bone structure and from reduction in bone mineral density. Individuals with NF1 have an increased risk of developing osteoporosis and osteopenia, which predominantly affect the load-bearing parts of the body (Crawford & Bagamery, 1986; Ferner, 2007).

Complications can also result from bony overgrowth or destruction caused by underlying plexiform neurofibromas. Bony dysplasia, bony erosion, demineralization, non ossifying fibromas, and scoliosis are all features of NF1. Dysplastic bony lesions include splayed ribs, vertebral anomalies, hypoplasia of the sphenoid or mandible, and pseudarthrosis. Pseudarthrosis most commonly involves the tibia and presents in early infancy with bowing of the affected limb followed by pathological fracture and impaired healing. The disorder represents thinning of the long bone cortex and the development of a false joint in a long bone (Crawford & Bagamery, 1986; Ferner, 2007).

Scoliosis affects 10% of those with NF1, most commonly involves the lower cervical and upper thoracic spine, and can be either idiopathic or dystrophic. The latter does not usually develop before 6 years of age and is rare after the first decade of life. Typically, there is a short curve with severe apical rotation, distortion of the vertebral bodies and ribs, and rapid disease progression (Crawford & Bagamery, 1986; Ferner, 2007).

2.1.4 Cardiovascular problems

An international database review identified cardiovascular malformations in 2% of patients with NF1 and most individuals had pulmonary stenosis. Hypertension occurs with increased frequency and is associated with premature death in adults with NF1. High blood pressure can be idiopathic or the result from dysplastic renal artery stenosis or pheochromocytoma. Dysplasia of blood vessels is usually multifocal and bilateral. The most common sites are kidney and brain (Lin et al., 2000; Ferner, 2007).

2.1.5 Neurological manifestations

Neurological complications affect both the peripheral and central nervous system, accounting for significant morbidity and mortality in NF1.

As already described, cutaneous neurofibromas are tumours of peripheral nerves, and plexiform neurofibromas can involve large nerves, plexus, spinal roots, sympathetic nerves, or small peripheral nerve fibers. Involvement of large nerves such as the sciatic may be asymptomatic or suggested only by hypertrophy of the affected extremity. When the sacral plexus is involved, there can be massive proliferation of tumor with infiltration of the bladder and compression of the ureters, rectum, and uterus. Plexiform tumours of the spinal roots may cause pain and erosion of the neural foramen or cord compression. High cervical nerve root neurofibromas are prone to compress the cord but the neurological deficit is frequently mild in comparison with the neuroimaging appearances. Involvement of the lumbar roots causes back pain that is aggravated by exertion (Tonsgard, 2006; Ferner, 2007).

Neurofibromatous neuropathy affects at least 1% of NF1 adults. They present with mild distal sensory and motor symptoms. Thickened peripheral nerves are infiltrated with neurofibromatous tissue. Although NF1 neurofibromatous neuropathy is not progressive, affected individuals require assiduous monitoring because they are at risk of developing malignant peripheral nerve sheath tumors (Ferner, 2010).

Cognitive disability is the commonest neurological symptom in children with NF1 and does not improve in adulthood. Characteristically, the intelligent quotient (IQ) is in the low-average range but mental retardation (IQ<70) is uncommon. Children with NF1 have specific learning difficulties that include visual spatial problems, impaired visual motor integration with abnormal ocular saccades, language deficits, and disorder of executive function. Problems that are typically associated with the NF1 phenotype include attention deficit hyperactivity disorder, which responds to methylphenidate medication, and poor socialization (Hyman et al., 2005).

Chiari 1 malformation and aqueduct stenosis due to subependymal glial cell proliferation are encountered in 1.5 % of NF1 patients (Valverde et al., 2007). Hydrocephalus is an uncommon complication. Sphenoid wing dysplasia is noticeable as pulsating exophthalmos without visual compromise; the absent sphenoid wing allows the temporal lobe to prolapse forwards into the orbit but surgical correction is not usually undertaken (Ferner et al., 2007a).

Epilepsy is diagnosed in about 6% of NF1 patients, it is frequently mild and it tends to start between childhood and middle age. There are several underlying causes, comprising brain trauma, infection unrelated to NF1, mesial temporal sclerosis, NF1 related gliomas and anecdotal reports of dysembryoblastic neuroepithelial tumours. All seizure types occur but complex partial seizures predominate.

Cerebrovascular problems have been reported in 2·5% of children with NF1 and include stenosis or occlusion of the internal carotid and cerebral arteries, aneurysms, and Moyamoya disease (Rosser et al., 2005).

Headaches occur in 20% of patients; most of these are consistent with migraine and respond well to prophylactic medications (Tonsgard, 2006).

Gliomas occur in all parts of the brain but have a predilection for the optic pathways, brainstem, and cerebellum. They are usually indolent pilocytic astrocytomas, but those that arise outside the optic pathways, which are symptomatic lesions or that release in adulthood, are more aggressive and are associated with a worse prognosis. About 15% of NF1 children have optic pathway gliomas but only 5% develop symptoms or signs (figure 3). They usually present before the age of 6 years and can cause impaired visual acuity and color vision, squint, proptosis, afferent pupillary defect, optic atrophy, visual field defects and precocious puberty. Adult onset or tumor progression, are unusual and visual screening is not required in adulthood. Young children rarely complain of visual loss and the best method of diagnosis is regular visual screening, at least until the age of 7 years. Grade III and IV astrocytomas occur in NF1 and require aggressive treatment. They are invariably symptomatic. The best outcome implies complete surgical removal coupled with chemotherapy. The outcome for malignant brain tumors in patients with NF1 is generally better than in not affected individuals (Liternick et al., 1989; Tonsgard, 2006; Ferner, 2010).

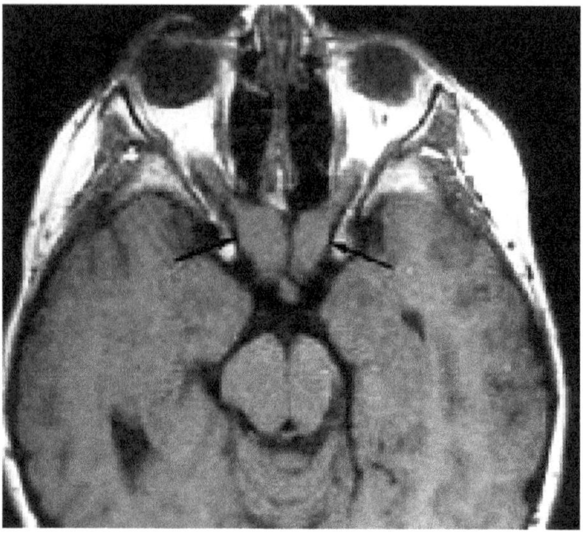

Fig. 3. Optic pathway gliomas involving both optic nerves (black arrows)

Primary progressive multiple sclerosis occurs with increased frequency in NF1 and relapsing remitting disease has also been reported. Although NF1 is a tumour suppressor condition, immunosuppressant therapy is not contraindicated and so far, there is no evidence of an increase in malignancy in NF1 patients with multiple sclerosis (Ferner, 2007b).

2.2 Neurofibromatosis 2

Neurofibromatosis type 2 (NF2), primarily known as acoustic neurofibromatosis or central neurofibromatosis is an autossomal dominant disorder caused by mutations on the NF2 gene, a tumour suppressor gene located on chromosome 22q12 that encodes a protein termed Merlin/Schwannomin, causing diminished or loss of function of these protein (Asthagiri et al, 2009; Ferner, 2007b; Gareth & Evans, 2009). It is less common than NF1, accounts for 5 to 10% of all cases of Neurofibromatosis and has an incidence of 1 in 25,000 livebirths and a prevalence of 1 in 60,000 (Asthagiri et al, 2009; Ferner, 2007b; Pérez-Grau et al, 2010). The average age of onset is 22 years of age (Asthagiri et al, 2009; Ferner, 2007b) (Gareth & Evans, 2009). There is a risk of 50% of an affected individual to transmit the mutation to their offspring and the penetrance will be complete at 60 years of age, however there is a high phenotypic variability between individuals, even within the same family(Asthagiri et al, 2009; Gareth & Evans, 2009). About one third of NF2 patients are mosaic, which means that the mutation took place after conception and that only certain cells of the body will be affected and these patients will have a milder form of the disease (Ferner, 2007b; Gareth & Evans, 2009; Pérez-Grau et al, 2010).

The characteristic feature is bilateral vestibular schwannomas (on cranial nerve VIII) that occur in 90-95% of patients. They present most commonly with progressive sensorineural hearing loss as the first sign, frequently unilateral at onset (Ferner, 2010; Gareth & Evans, 2009; Pérez-Grau et al, 2010). Since schwannomas usually do not develop before adolescence, in children the first manifestation, contrary to what occurs in adulthood, can be cranial, orbital or spinal meningioma, spinal or cutaneous schwannoma, mononeuropathy, focal amyotrophy or cataracts (Ferner, 2007b, 2010; Gareth & Evans, 2009; Pérez-Grau et al, 2010). Contrarily to tumours in NF1, schwannomas are benign tumours and the morbidity and early mortality rates are due to the multiple tumours in central and peripheral nervous system (Asthagiri et al, 2009; Ferner, 2007a; Pérez-Grau et al, 2010)

The efficiency of the set of existing criteria was compared in a study selecting 163 people from NF2 registry without bilateral vestibular schwannomas. (Baser et al., 1996) They evaluated the criteria for "definite NF2" and "probable NF2" at two points: initial assessment and the most recent clinical evaluation. (Baser et al., 1996) For both points, the Manchester criteria and the NNF (National Neurofibromatosis Foundation) criteria identified a higher proportion of people than with the NIH (National Institute of Health) criteria. The Manchester criteria identified an even higher number of people because they are based on the number of disease features of any types and a determined age is not necessary for diagnosis, contrary to NNFF which requires a certain number of different feature types and the existence of unilateral vestibular schwannomas with less than 30 years of age. The 1987 and the 1991 NIH Criteria each require a positive family history for the diagnosis of NF2 in people who do not have bilateral vestibular schwannomas, therefore, the proportion of these people identified with "possible NF2" is low and even lower with "definite NF2". (Baser et al., 1996) For people who do not have a family history of NF2 or bilateral vestibular schwannomas, a diagnosis can be made based on the Manchester and the NNFF criteria. (Baser et al., 1996) The Manchester criteria are more sensitive for identifying mosaics than all the other criteria. They considered that a new set of criteria should be created including the evidence of mononeuropathy (foot drop, wrist drop, facial palsy, or III nerve palsy) and the results of genetic testing.

2.2.1 Cutaneous manifestations

Three types of cutaneous tumours, all histologically schwannomas, are identified: cutaneous plaque-like lesions (raised, hyperpigmented and hairy), subcutaneous tumours (fusiform swelling) and intradermal tumours. (Asthagiri et al, 2009; Ferner, 2007b). These occur in about 70% of NF2 patients, though less prominent than in NF1 patients. (Gareth & Evans, 2009; Pérez-Grau et al, 2010)

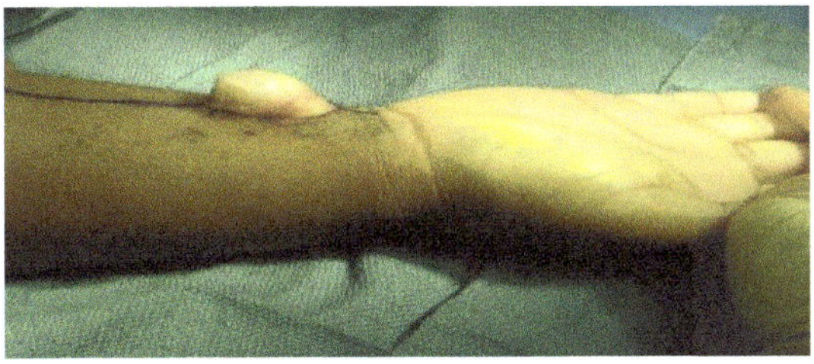

Fig. 4. Cutaneous schwannoma

Generally these tumours grow on or around a peripheral nerve (more frequently sensory nerves) and subcutaneous tumours usually cause pain and are sensitive to pressure. (McClatchey, 2007; Pérez-Grau et al, 2010) Rarely a cutaneous neurofibroma may appear or a dermal tumour may be confused with a neurofibroma. (Asthagiri et al, 2009; Ferner, 2007b; Gareth & Evans, 2009; McClatchey, 2007)

Café au lait patches are reported in almost 40% of patients with NF2, being more common than in the general population, but less numerous than in people with NF1 and generally they are singular and inconspicuous. (Asthagiri et al, 2009; Ferner, 2010)

2.2.2 Neurological manifestations

Although schwannomas on cranial nerve VIII are the cardinal feature of NF2, they can also grow on other cranial nerves (CN). The next most affected CN are III (oculomotor), V (trigeminal) and VII (facial), but they can affect IX-XII also (Ferner, 2010; Gutmann et al, 1997). When tumours arise in III and V CN, they are usually asymptomatic, opposite to tumours of the lower cranial nerves, mostly symptomatic (Asthagiri et al, 2009). The initial symptom associated with vestibular schwannomas usually is progressive sensorineural hearing loss, which can be preceded or accompanied by tinnitus (Ferner, 2010; Gareth & Evans, 2009). Other symptoms associated are: vertigo, gait instability, facial weakness, twitching, sensory deficit and headache (Ferner, 2010; Pérez-Grau et al, 2010). The growth rates of vestibular schwannomas are variable, but higher in patient under 30 years of age.

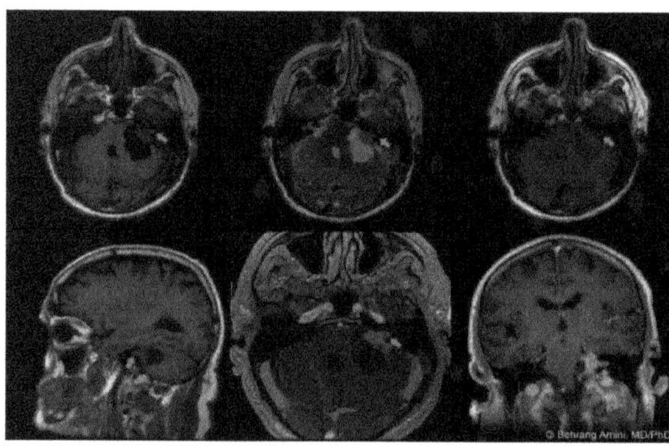

Fig. 5. Vestibular schwannoma (red arrows)

Meningiomas are the second most frequent tumour in NF2 patients. They are generally multiple, can occur in brain or spine, and the symptoms vary according to the location (Goutagny & Kalamarides, 2010). Cranial meningiomas have a high rate of neurological problems and mortality (Asthagiri et al, 2009; Ferner, 2010). Optic meningiomas may cause vision loss due to compression of the optic nerve, especially in children (Bosch et al, 2006).

Spinal schwannomas can occur and are regularly multiple (Ferner, 2010). These tumours and optic meningiomas can be found in about 90% of patients with NF2 (Ferner, 2010). For 20-30% of NF2 patients the initial symptoms have their origin in intracranial meningiomas, spinal or cutaneous tumours (Gareth & Evans, 2009).

Ependymomas (low-grade CNS malignancies) can be present, mostly in the brainstem and upper cervical cord and may be associated with a syrinx (fluid-filled cavity within spinal cord), with symptoms that could appear throughout life (Aguilera, 2011; Ferner, 2010; Gareth & Evans, 2009). For spinal cord ependymomas, the intramedullary lesions may present themselves as back pain, weakness or sensory disturbances (Asthagiri et al, 2009).

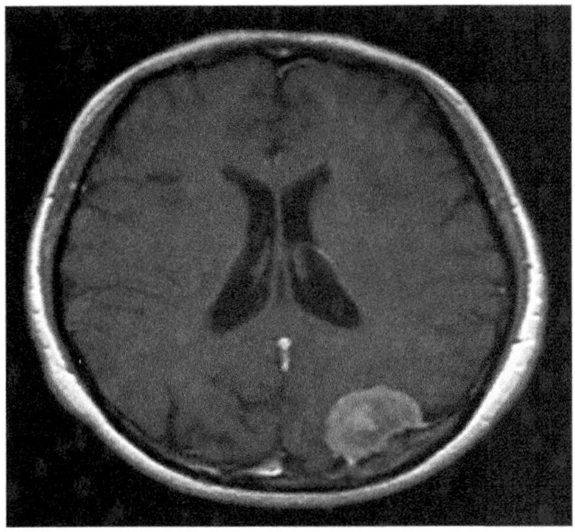

Fig. 6. Cranial meningiomas in NF2 patients

Also associated to NF2 is an axonal peripheral neuropathy (Asthagiri et al, 2009; Ferner, 2010). The majority of the cases are associated to tumours within or compressing the nerve, but in others the mechanisms are not yet fully understood as there is no evidence of a tumour and are probably related with compression from multiple Schwann cell tumourlets. (Asthagiri et al, 2009; Ferner, 2010). In children a clinical presentation with mononeuropathy (in particular facial nerve palsy) before the appearance of vestibular schwannomas is common, but also common is a polio-like illness (Ferner, 2007; Gareth & Evans, 2009). In both presentations full recovery is unusual. (Ferner, 2007a; Gareth & Evans, 2009).

2.2.3 Ocular manifestations

Usually lens changes appear in infancy or childhood (earlier than vestibular schwannomas) and most commonly include juvenile posterior subcapsular cataracts, cortical wedge cataracts and mixed cataracts and all can reduce visual acuity. (Gareth & Evans, 2009) They should be considered as specific of NF2 only in people younger than 50 years of age. They are present in about 60-80% of NF2 patients (Asthagiri et al, 2009; Gareth & Evans, 2009).

Other manifestations are epiretinal membranes and retinal hamartomas. The first, opposite to the second, don't usually affect visual acuity even in patients with severe disease, and may be present in more than a third of patients with NF2 (Asthagiri et al, 2009; Pérez-Grau et al, 2010).

The onset at a young age of ophthalmologic symptoms is a risk factor for marked disease progression. (Bosch et al, 2006) Therefore people at risk of developing NF2 should be screened for these abnormalities in infancy (Gareth & Evans, 2009; Baser, 1996).

Regarding diagnostic criteria, the National Institute of Health (NIH) Consensus Panel established in 1987 clinical guidelines for the diagnosis of Neurofibromatosis type 2, which were revised in 1991. However, these criteria were considered too rigid and leading to exclusion of patients that should be screened for NF2. Therefore, in 1997, a consensus review of published data was proposed by researchers in the neurofibromatosis field by the National Neurofibromatosis Foundation (NNF) (Gutmann et al., 1997; McClatchey, 2007). In order to promote higher specificity and sensitivity, in 2002 new diagnostic criteria were established, based on a comparison of this four different sets of criteria for NF2 (Table 2) (Baser et al., 1996; Ferner, 2007a).

1987 NIH criteria A. Bilateral vestibular schwannomas B. First-degree family relative with NF2 *and* unilateral vestibular schwannoma *or* any two of: meningioma, schwannoma, glioma, neurofibroma, juvenile posterior subcapsular lenticular opacity
1991 NIH criteria A. Bilateral vestibular schwannomas B. First-degree family relative with NF2 *and* unilateral vestibular schwannoma *or* any one of: meningioma, schwannoma, glioma, neurofibroma, juvenile posterior subcapsular lens opacity
Manchester criteria A. Bilateral vestibular schwannomas B. First-degree family relative with NF2 *and* unilateral vestibular schwannoma *or* any two of: meningioma, schwannoma, glioma, neurofibroma, posterior subcapsular lenticular opacities C. Unilateral vestibular schwannoma *and* any two of: meningioma, schwannoma, glioma, neurofibroma, posterior subcapsular lenticular opacities D. Multiple meningiomas (two or more) *and* unilateral vestibular schwannoma *or* any two of: schwannoma, glioma, neurofibroma, cataract
NNF criteria A. Confirmed or definite NF2 1. Bilateral vestibular schwannomas 2. First-degree family relative with NF2 *and* unilateral vestibular schwannoma at less than 30 y of age *or* any two of: meningioma, schwannoma, glioma, juvenile lens opacity (posterior subcapsular cataract or cortical cataract) B. Presumptive or probable NF2 1. Unilateral vestibular schwannoma at less than 30 y of age *and* at least one of: meningioma, schwannoma, glioma, juvenile lens opacity (posterior subcapsular cataract or cortical cataract) 2. Multiple meningiomas (two or more) *and* unilateral vestibular schwannoma at less than 30 y of age *or* at least one of: schwannoma, glioma, juvenile lens opacity (posterior subcapsular cataract or cortical cataract)

Table 2. Clinical diagnostic criteria for NF2 (Baser ME, 2002)

3. Differential diagnosis

The differential diagnoses of NF1 includes other forms of neurofibromatosis, conditions with *café au lait* patches or with pigment changes confused with *café au lait* patches. Likewise, tumors or localized body overgrowth can be mistaken for neurofibromas (table 3). It should be emphasized that one or two *café au lait* patches occur in 10% of the general population. Children with 3–5 *café au lait* patches but no other signs of NF1 should be followed up in a specialist neurofibromatosis clinic as they might have mosaic NF1 or NF2 (Ferner., 2007b).

Mosaic NF1 occurs as a result of a somatic mutation in the NF1 gene. The body's proportion affected depends on mutation's timing in embryonic development. The importance of making the diagnosis is that NF1 complications are relatively infrequent in segmental NF1 and there is a much lower risk of recurrence in offspring. Homozygotes for one of the genes causing hereditary non-polyposis cancer of the colon have *café au lait* patches and an affected first degree relative. However, the affected relative is a sibling and the parents are normal (Ruggierei & Huson, 2001).

The only subtype of NF1 that is distinct and has a uniform phenotype in families is Watson syndrome. It is characterized by pulmonary stenosis, cognitive impairment, *café au lait* patches and few, if any, cutaneous neurofibromas (Korf & Huson, 2006).

There is no clear evidence that neurofibromatosis–Noonan syndrome exists as a distinct phenotype with features of both syndromes. It is likely that some individuals with NF1 simply have facial features similar to those of Noonan syndrome and these characteristics are not consistent within families. Molecular studies indicate that neurofibromatosis–Noonan syndrome is caused by mutations of the NF1 gene, some of which have been identified in patients with classical NF1 (De Luca et al., 2002).

Other forms of neurofibromatosis: Segmental/mosaic NF1 Watson syndrome Autossomal dominant multiple *café au lait* alone Neurofibromatosis 2 Schwannomatosis
Other conditions with *café au lait* patches: McCune-Albright syndrome DNA repair syndromes Homozigoty for one of the genes causing hereditary non-polyposis cancer of the colon
Conditions with pigmented macules confused with NF1: LEOPARD syndrome Neurocutaneous melanosis Peutz-Jehers syndrome Piebaldism
Localized overgrowth syndrome: Klippel-Trenauny-Weber syndrome Proteus syndrome
Conditions causing tumors confused with neurofibromas: Lipomatosis Banaya-Riley-Ruvalcuba syndrome Fibromatoses Multiple endocrine neoplasia type 2B

Table 3. Differential diagnosis of neurofibromatosis 1

NF2 is clinically and genetically distinct from NF1, and is characterized by bilateral vestibular schwannomas. Affected individuals also develop schwannomas on other cranial, spinal, peripheral and cutaneous nerves. *Café au lait* patches are less numerous than in NF1, and the skin lesions are predominantly schwannomas. Central nervous system meningiomas and gliomas are observed, and slit lamp examination reveals juvenile subcapsular lens opacities in the majority of patients. Subcutaneous, peripheral nerve and spinal schwannomas lead to schwannomatosis without vestibular schwannomas or the ophthalmological features of NF2 (Ferner, 2007a).

Multiple lipomas occur primarily on the trunk, proximal thighs and distal arms, and are inherited in an autosomal dominant fashion. Biopsy is sometimes necessary to differentiate cutaneous neurofibromas from schwannomas and lipomas (Ferner et al., 2007a).

4. Diagnostic workup

The diagnosis of NF 1 is mainly clinic and (Baser et al, 1996; Ferner, 2007b), as explained before, two of the major criteria based on the modified NIH criteria must be fulfilled. Given the variety of clinical symptoms and the fact that these are age-dependent, it is sometimes difficult to make the diagnosis of NF1 at an early age because children might have, for example, the typical "café au lait" spots but only develop other features of the disease years later (Korf, 2011). Therefore, a complete physical and neurological exam together with a family history, ocular and cognitive (addressing learning skills) assessment and appreciation of bone deformities and cardiovascular alterations (with measurement of blood pressure) should be performed when a hypothesis of NF1 is considered or in an at-risk descendent.

Brain MRI is considered important at an early age for the exclusion of optic pathway glioma but for some aspects as sedation, costs and parents anxiety must be beared in mind. Bones imaging to look for bone dysplasia must also be assessed whenever a pain complaint occurs (Korf, 2011).

Because half the cases are familial, genetic counseling is very important in NF1 due to the high morbidity and mortality associated to this disease. Parents of affected children should know that a 50% risk of NF1 mutation transmitting is associated to each pregnancy (Tonsgard, 2006). Attention should be paid to the possibility of the subject being a mosaic, because a simple blood sample may miss the affected cells. A tissue sample from a tumour must be ideally collected in these situations.

For NF2 diagnosis the Manchester Criteria are the most commonly used. Therefore, as presented in Table 2, patients do not need to have a family history of NF2 or bilateral vestibular schwannomas but may have multiple other related lesions. Peripheral neuropathy and the presence of a constitutional NF2 mutation are not yet included in the diagnostic criteria of NF2 (Asthagiri et al, 2009; Baser et al., 1996; Gareth & Evans, 2009). Genetic testing could aid to rule out mutations in individuals from families with NF2 avoiding additional exams (Baser et al., 1996; Gareth & Evans, 2009).

The diagnostic evaluation as well, should always incorporate a thorough clinical and family history, a physical (including cutaneous), neurologic and as in NF1, ophthalmologic examination and a brain and spinal MRI with and without gadolinium (Gareth et al, 2009). MRI is the ideal imaging method when vestibular schwannomas are suspected but also to explore the presence of other cranial nerve tumours or meningiomas (Gutmann et al., 1997). The median age of NF2 diagnosis is 20-30 years with hearing loss as initial symptom. However, the clinical manifestations are age dependent and about 30% of children begin with other symptoms (Asthagiri et al, 2009; Gareth & Evans, 2009).

The screening of children with NF2 suspicion from an affected parent should include ophthalmologic examination (in the first ten years of life), neurologic examination (annually), audiology with auditory brainstem evoked potentials yearly from infancy (annually) and presymptomatic genetic testing (not before 10 years of age) (Evan et al., 1995; Gareth & Evans, 2009). MRI screening should be performed every 2 years when younger than 20 years of age and every 3 to 5 years when older than 20 years of age. However, if tumours are present screening should be done annually. For spinal MRI, the frequency should be every 3 years (Baser et al, 1996; Gareth & Evans, 2009).

5. Molecular genetic diagnosis of neurofibromatosis

5.1 Neurofibromatosis type 1

NF1 is an autosomal dominant genetic disorder. The gene locus discovered by linkage analysis and subsequently positional cloning in 1990, is found on chromosome 17 (Barker et al., 1987; Viskochil et al 1990; Wallace et al, 1990). It is a large gene that spans greater than 350-kb of genomic DNA, and it is composed of 60 individual exons (Gutmann et al 1999). The gene locus has a spontaneous mutation rate that is 100 times greater than average, and approximately half of NF1 cases appear to represent new mutations (Lewis and Riccardi 1981). The reason for the unusually high mutation rate and the mechanism of mutation are unknown. However, the vast majority of new mutations occur on the paternally derived chromosome. This phenomenon does not appear to be linked to paternal age as in other genetic diseases (Jadayel et al., 1990), and it is known as "genomic imprinting" (Hall, 1990). The mechanism by which genomic imprinting may play a role in the spontaneous mutation rate, may involve hypermethylation of the sperm genome, which is then at higher risk for mutations through the spontaneous deamination of 5-methylcytosine (Rodenhiser et al., 1993).

The most common gene product is a polypeptide of 2,818 amino acids, called neurofibromin (Gutmann & Collins 1992; Danglot et al 1995; Li et al., 2002). Neurofibromin is expressed in neurons, oligodendrocytes, Schwann cells, the adrenal medulla and white blood cells (Daston et al 1992; Gutmann, 1998). Sequence analysis of the full length NF1 gene cDNA revealed a portion that codes for a 360 amino acid peptide with structural and functional similarities to some guanosine triphosphatase activating proteins (GAP) in other mammalian and yeast cells (Xu et al 1995). The portion of the gene that codes for this protein interacts with the protooncogene, p21ras (Martin et al., 1990; Shen et al., 1996). The abovementioned proteins have the ability to accelerate hydrolysis of ras-guanosine triphosphate to ras-guanosine diphosphate, thus, activating the proto-oncogene. In some sporadic tumors of non-NF1 patients, ras activating mutations are implicated in malignant transformation (Reed & Gutmann 2001). This was the first hypothesis to the possible function of neurofibromin (Gutmann & Collins 1992). Loss of neurofibromin activity through mutation could lead to cellular proliferation, and thus to some of the disease expression of NF1. The NF1 gene is thus considered a tumor-suppressor gene as loss-of-function mutations have been associated with benign and malignant tumors in neural-crest-derived tissues in patients with NF1 (Coleman et al 1995; Serra et al 1997), being neurofibromin a tumor suppressor by down-regulating or inhibiting intracellular ras activity (Gutmann and Collins 1992). But beyond ras regulation, important intracellular signaling pathways are probably regulated by neurofibromin as cAMP generation that modulates cell growth and differentiation in the brain (Tong et al 2002). On the other hand, neurofibromin is highly expressed in Schwann cells, and may play a critical role in the formation of neurofibromas (Rutkowski et al., 2000).

There may be basic differences in how NF1 gene expression influences the development of tumors or the cognitive manifestations. Some tumors occur when both copies of the gene are functionally inactivated or defects in growth regulation are caused by reduced protein expression.

Some of the non-tumor features, including cognitive and learning problems, may be related to microenvironmental interactions between haploinsufficient astrocytes and neurons (Gutmann et al., 1999).

Finally, neurofibromin has been shown to play a crucial role on modulating mesenchimal stem and progenitor cell differentiation into osteoblasts, and this effect may contribute to the osseous abnormalities seen in NF1 (Wu et al 2006)

The factors that determine the genotype/phenotype correlations are not well understood (Ainsworth et al., 1993; Shen et al., 1996), and the discordance for several defining features of NF1 among pairs of monozygotic twins suggest that some manifestations are not entirely genetically controlled (Huson, 1994).

Cloning of the NF1 gene brought hope for routine prenatal diagnosis, but the large size of the gene and large number of potential mutations make this unlikely for at least several years (Marchuk & Collins 1994).

Genetic diagnosis is sometimes possible in NF1 families with two or more affected individuals by linkage analyses. Available polymorphic DNA markers, however, do not always have sensitivity enough to achieve it in all families (Marchuk & Collins, 1994). Conventional approaches to the identification of disease-causing mutations in individuals with NF1 have been limited because of the large size of the gene and the wide diversity of mutations, no clustering in any one region of the gene (Gutmann et al., 1999). For these reasons, identification of a mutation in a suspect case requires a variety of techniques to thoroughly examine DNA for mutations, most of them point mutations or small lesions leading to premature termination codons (Upadhyaya & Cooper, 1998). Some tests as the protein truncation test (in-vitro transcription-translation of the whole NF1 coding sequence (Heim et al., 1995) have been used to identify mutations, but it seems that a combination of approaches will be necessary (Gutmann et al., 1999). In addition, even when a mutation is identified, an individual risk is confirmed, but not how severely he will be affected. This point limits the usefulness of currently available technology for prenatal test.

5.2 Neurofibromatosis type 2

NF2 is now well characterized as an autosomal dominant inherited disease caused by mutation of a gene located on the long arm of chromosome 22(q11-13.1), distinct from NF1 (Rouleau et al., 1987; Wertelecki et al., 1988).

The abnormal gene product for NF2, merlin or Schawannomin identified in 1993 (Rouleau et al., 1993; Trofatter et al., 1993), functions as a tumor suppressor gene (Rouleau 1994). Unlike protooncogenes, which cause tumors by producing a protein that stimulates cellular proliferation and requires only one abnormal copy of the gene to produce the abnormal gene product, a tumor suppressor gene requires a critical mutation of both copies (alleles) of the gene for the normal suppressor gene product to be absent or inactive. As with other tumor suppressor genes, the germ-line mutation produces 1 abnormal allele in all the cells of an affected individual, and presumably, a "second hit" of the other allele occurs later, in the tissue from which a tumor arises (Knudson 1985). Indeed, evidence for somatic inactivation of both NF2 alleles is found in the majority of schwannomas and meningiomas thar arise in these patients (Hung et al., 2000; Lamszus et al., 2000).

The protein product, merlin, has a high degree of homology with a family of cytoskeletal proteins (ERM proteins) that link the actin skeleton of the cell to cell adhesion membrane proteins important for cellular remodelling and growth regulation (Trofatter et al., 1993). These proteins function looks like essential for the formation of specialized subcellular structures as well for adhesion and migration activities (McClatchey et al., 1998). Schwann cell cultures isolated from schwannomas of NF2 patients with identified germ-line mutations have shown striking differences in morphology, cell-cell contacts, and growth compared to normal control Schwann cells (Rosenbaum et al 1998). These findings permit to theorize that disruption of cytoskeletal organization by alteration in NF2 gene and protein product is involved in the genesis of tumors. Another approach to determine merlin functions, has involved molecules that interact with it and potentially transduce its growth suppressive signal. Merlin, like the ERM proteins, has an amino-terminal cell surface glycoprotein-binding domain (called FERM domain) with 3 subdomains that may mediate specific interactions with critical protein binding partners (Kang et al 2002; Shimizu et al 2002). Several candidate proteins include: CD44 (Herrlich et al., 2000; Morrison et al., 2001), actin (Xu & Gutmann, 1998), beta II-spectrin (Scoles et al., 1996), SCHIP-1 (Goutebroze et al., 2000), HRS (Scoles et al., 2000), NHE-RF (Gonzalez-Agosti et al., 1999) and beta1-integrin (Obremski et al., 1998). The merlin-actin association is tightly regulated by protein phosphorylation (Morrison et al 2001; Kissil et al 2002), and it is important for localizing merlin to the proper subcellular location (Fernandez-Valle et al., 2002). The association of merlin with CD 44 raises the possibility that merlin could function as a molecular switch. The merlin's ability to associate with CD44 may be influenced by merlin's phosphorylation state, intramolecular complex formation, and its interactions with other binding partners. With these influences, merlin may determine whether it traduces a growth stimulatory or inhibitory signal (Pearson et al 2000). Merlin also associates with other Schwann cell growth regulators. Hepatocyte growth factor-regulated tyrosine kinase substrate binds through residues in the C-terminal domain not shared with ERM proteins (Scoles et al 2000). This factor is one of the most potent stimuli for Schwann cell proliferation and motility (Gutmann et al 2001).

Approximately half of the cases of NF2 appear to be the result from a new gene mutation (Evans et al., 1992a) although the mutation rate is lower than of NF1. The mechanism of mutation is currently unknown, but has been shown to be related to increased paternal age (Evans et al., 1992a). Further analysis has shown a clearer link between the risk of mosaicism inheritance by offspring and age of vestibular schwannoma diagnosis (Evans & Wallace, 2009). Patients who inherit NF2 from their mothers generally have an earlier age of presentation and a more rapidly progressive course (Eldridge, 1990; Evans et al., 1992a).

This suggests the possibility of gene modification by a mechanism of maternal imprinting (Hall, 1990). On the other hand, different NF2 mutations result in varying disease courses. Point mutations are found in about 55% of cases clinically diagnosed, and genotype-phenotype correlations have been established based on the relationship between NF2 mutations and clinical severity (Parry et al., 1996; Evans et al., 1998a) Patients with constitutional mutations that produce a truncated protein with loss of merlin expression (generally nonsense or frameshift mutations) have an earlier onset, number and rate of growth of CNS tumors (Selvanathan et al 2010). Missense, in-frame mutations or large deletions result in the generation of merlin proteins defective in their negative growth regulatory ability (Gutmann et al., 1998b), with milder disease (Parry et al., 1996; Evans et al., 1998). However, exception to these correlations have been reported (Scoles et al 1996), suggesting that other factors different to the class of mutation are likely to be responsible for a portion of the clinical symptoms (Welling 1998).

Currently, linkage analysis using tightly-linked genetic markers has been available to determine NF2 mutations carrier status in at-risk individuals in families with this disease from at least two generations. The relatively low detection rate of mutations (55%) may be partially related to somatic mosaicism in sporadic cases (Bijlsma et al., 1997; Evans et al., 1998; Kluwe et al., 1998), as well as a significant number of gene deletions observed.

The child of a parent with NF2 has a 50% risk of having the disease (Evans et al 1992a), and even no mutation was detected due to the common gonosomal mosaicism found, penetrance is thought to be complete, with initial symptoms until age 35 to 60 (Evans et al 1992b; Eldridge 1990). Newer techniques for detection of protein truncations have been developed, but they are not still validated for NF2 patients without bilateral vestibular schwannomas, and its ability to detect mosaic mutations remains untested (Gutmann et al, 1998b). Since RNA mismatch cleavage method is available, tumors mutations are detected with higher sensitivity, so this technique could be used as a convenient method for germline NF2 mutations screening (Faudoa et al 2000; Hung et al 2000)

These and possibly other streamlined methods may eventually make the genetic diagnosis of NF2 in suspected cases, including sporadic ones in the future (Bourn et al 1994; Rouleau, 1994; Merel et al 1995; Legoix et al 1999). At present, in most families with more than one affected individual, linkage analysis still remains the test of choice, as this will provide a greater than 99% certainty of NF2 diagnosis.

6. References

Ainsworth PJ, Rodenhiser DI, Costa MT. Identification and characterization of sporadic and inherited mutations in exon 31 of the neurofibromatosis gene. Hum Genet 1993; 9; 151-6

Aguilera DG, Mazewski C, Schniederjan MJ, et al. Neurofibromatosis-2 and spinal cord ependymomas: Report of two cases and a review of the literature. Childs Nerv Syst 2011;27:757-76

Asthagiri AR, Parry DM, Butman JA, et al. Neurofibromatosis Type 2. Lancet 2009;373:1974-86

Barker D, Wright E, Nguyen K et al. Gene for von Recklinghausen NF in the pericentric region of chromosome 17. Science 1987; 236: 1100-2.

Baser ME, Mautner VF, Ragge NK, et al. Presymptomatic diagnosis of neurofibromatosis 2 using linked genetic markers, neuroimaging, and ocular examinations. Neurology 1996;47;1269

Bijlsma EK, Wallace AJ, Evans DJ. Misleading linking results in an NF2 presymptomatic test owing to mosaicism. J Med Genet 1997;34(11):934-7.

Bourn D, Carter SA, Mason S, Gareth D, Evans R, Strachan T. Germline mutations in the neurofibromatosis type 2 tumor suppressor gene. Hum Mol Genet 1994;3: 813-6

Bosch MM, Wichmann WW, Boltshauser E, et al. Optic nerve sheath meningiomas in patients with neurofibromatosis type 2. Arch Ophthalmol 2006;124(3):379-85

Coleman SD, Williams CA, Wallace MR. Benign neurofibromas in type 1 neurofibromatosis (NF1) show somatic deletions on NF1 gene. Nat Genet 1995;11:90-2.

Crawford AH Jr, Bagamery N. Osseous manifestations of neurofibromatosis in childhood. J Pediatr Orthop 1986;6:72–88

Danglot G, Regnier V, Fauvet D, Vassal G, Kujas M, Bernheim A. Neurofibromatosis 1 (NF1) mRNAs expressed in the central nervous system are differentially spliced in the 5′ part of the gene. Hum Mol Genet 1995;4:915-20.

Daston MM, Scrable H, Nordlund M, Sturbaum AK, Nissen LM, Ratner N. The protein product of the neurofibromatosis type 1 gene is expressed at highest abundance in neurons, Schwann cells and oligodendrocytes. Neuron 1992;8:415-28.

De Luca A, Bottiloo I, Sarkozy A, Carta C, Neri C, Bellacchio E, Schirinzi A, Conti E, Zampino G, Battaglia A, Majore S, Evans DG, Baser ME, McGaughran J, et al. Malignant peripheral nerve sheath tumours in neurofi bromatosis 1. J Med Genet 2002;39:311–14.

Eldrigde R. Neurofibromatosis type 2. In. Rubenstein AE, Korf BR, editors. Neurofibromatosis. A handbook for patients, families and health-care professionals. New York: Thieme Medical Publ, 1990:29-39.

Evans DG, Huson SM, Donnai D, et al. A genetic study of type 2 neurofibromatosis in the United Kingdom. I. Prevalence, mutation rate, fitness and confirmation of maternal transmission effect on severity. J Med Genet 1992;29(12):841-6.

Evans DG, Wallace AJ. An update on age-related mosaic and offspring risk in neurofibromatosis 2 (NF2). J Med Genet 2009;46:792.

Evans DG, Trueman L, Wallace A, Collins S, Strachan T. Genotype/phenotype correlations in type 2 neurofibromatosis (NF2): evidence for more severe disease associated with truncating mutations. J Med Genet 1998;35:450-5.

Evans DG, Bourn D, Wallace A, Ramsden RT, Mitchell JD, Strachan T. Diagnostic issues in a family with late onset type 2 neurofibromatosis. J Med Genet 1995;32(6):470-4.

Evans DG, Huson SM, Donnai D, et al. A clinical study of type 2 neurofibromatosis. Q J Med 1992;304:603-18.

Faudoa R, Xue Z, Lee F; Basser ME, Hung G. Detection of novel NF2 mutations by an RNA mismatch cleavage method. Hum Mutation 2000;15:474-8.

Fernandez-Valle C, Tang Y, Ricard J, et al. Paxillin binds schwannomin and regulates its density-dependent localization and effect on cell morphology. Nat Genet 2002;31(4):354-62.

Ferner R, Lucas JD, O'Doherty MJ, et al. Evaluation of 18-fluorodeoxyglucose positron emission tomography (18FDGPET) in the detection of malignant peripheral nerve sheath tumours arising from within plexiform neurofi bromas in neurofibromatosis 1. J Neurol Neurosurg Psychiatry 2000;68:353–57

Ferner RE, Huson SM, Thomas N, et al. Guidelines for the diagnosis and management of individuals with neurofibromatosis 1. J Med Genet 2007a;44:81–88

Ferner RE. Neurofibromatosis 1 and neurofibromatosis 2: a twenty first century perspective. Lancet Neurol 2007b;6:340-51

Ferner RE. The neurofibromatoses. Practical Neurology 2010;10:82-93

Gareth D, Evans R. Neurofibromatosis type 2: A clinical and molecular review. Orphanet Journal of Rare Diseases 2009; 4:16

Gonzalez-Agosti C, Wiederhold T, Herndon ME, Gusella J, Ramesh V. Interdomain interaction of merlin isoforms and its influence on intermolecular binding to NHE-RF. J Biol Chem 1999;274(48):34438-42.

Goutagny S, Kalamarides M. Meningiomas and neurofibromatosis. J Neurooncol 2010; 9:341-347

Goutebroze L, Brault E, Muchardt C, Camonis J, Thomas G. Cloning and characterization of SCHIP-1, a novel protein interacting specifically with spliced isoforms and naturally occurring mutant NF2 proteins. Mol Cell Bol 2000;20(5):1699-712.

Gutmann DA, Collins FS. Recent progress toward understanding the molecular biology of von Recklinghausen neurofibromatosis. Ann Neurol 1992;31:555-61.

Gutmann DH, Aylsworth A, Carey JC, et al. The diagnostic evaluation and multidisciplinary management of neurofibromatosis 1 and neurofibromatosis 2. JAMA 1997;278(1):51-8

Gutmann DH, Loehr A, Zhang Y, Kim J, Henkemeyer M, Cashen A. Haploinsufficiency for the neurofibromatosis 1 (NF1) tumor suppressor results in increased astrocyte proliferation. Oncogene 1999;18:4450-9.

Gutmann DH. Recent insights into neurofibromatosis type 1: clear genetic progress. Arch Neurol 1998a;55:778-80.

Gutmann DH, Geist RT, Xu HM, Kim JS, Saporito-Irwin S. Defects in neurofibromatosis 2 protein function can arise at multiple levels. Hum Mol Genet 1998b;7:335-45.

Gutmann DH, Hirbe AC, Haipek CA. Functional analysis of neurofibromatosis 2 (NF2) missense mutations. Hum Mol Genet 2001;10:1519-29.

Hall JG. Genomic imprinting: review and relevance to human diseases. Am J Hum Genet 1990; 46: 857-73.

Heim RA, Kam-Morgan LW, Binnie GG, et al. Distribution of 13 truncating mutations in the neurofibromatosis gene. Hum Mol Genet 1995;4:975-81.

Herrlich P, Morrison H, Sleeman J, et al. CD44 acts as both a growth- and invasiveness-promoting molecule and as a tumor-suppressing cofactor. Ann N Y Acad Sci 2000;910:106-18; discussion 118-20.

Hung G, Faudoa R, Baser ME, et al. Neurofibromatosis 2 phenotypes and germ-line NF2 mutations determined by an RNA mismatch method and loss of heterozygosity analysis in NF2 schwannomas. Cancer Gen Cytogen 2000;118(2):167-8.

Huson SM. Neurofibromatosis 1: a clinical and genetic overview. In: Huson SM, Hughes RAC, editors. The neurofibromatosis. A pathogenic and clinical overview. London: Chapman and Hall, 1994: 160-203.

Hyman SL, Shores A, North KN. The nature and frequency of cognitive deficits in children with neurofibromatosis type 1.Neurology. 2005;65:1037–44.

Jadayel D, Fain P, Upahyaya M, et al. Paternal origin of mutations in von Recklinghausen neurofibromatosis. Nature 1990;343:558-9.

Kang BS, Cooper DR, Devedjiev Y, et al. The structure of the FERM domain of merlin, the neurofibromatosis type 2 gene product. Acta Crystallogr 2002;58:381-91.

Kissil JL, Johnson KC, Eckman MS, Jacks T. Merlin phosphorylation by p21-activated kinase 2 and effects of phosphorylation on merlin localization. J Biol Chem 2002; 277: 10394-9.

Kluwe L, MacCollin M, Tatagiba M, et al. Phenotypic variability associated with 24 splice-site mutations in the NF2 gene. Am J Med Genet 1998;77:228-33.

Knudson AG. Hereditary cancer oncogenes and antioncogenes. Cancer Res 1985;45:1437-43.

Korf BR, Huson SM. The Phakamatoses. In: Rimoin D, Connor JM, Pyeritz RE, Korf BR, eds. Principles and practice of medical genetics, 5th edn. Edinburgh: Churchill Livingstone 2006;2817–50.

Korf BR. Diagnosis and management of Neurofibromatosis type 1. Current Neurology and Neuroscience Reports 2011;1:162-167

Lamszus K, Vahidiek F, Mautner VF, et al. Allelic losses in neurofibromatosis 2-associated meningiomas. J Neuropathol Exp Neurol 2000; 59: 504-12.

Legoix P, Legrand MF, Ollagnon E, Lenoir G, Thomas G, Zucman-Rossi J. Characterization of 16 polymorphic markers in the NF2 gene: application to hemizygosity detection. Hum Mutat 1999; 13(4): 290-3

Lewis RA, Riccardi VM. Von Recklinghausen neurofibromatosis; incidence of iris hamartoma. Ophtalmologica 1981; 88: 348-54.

Li Y, Velasco-Migual S, Vass WC, et al. Epidermal growth factor receptor signaling pathways are associated with tumorigenesis in the NF1: p53 mouse tumor model. Cancer Res 2002; 62: 4507-13.

Lin AE, Birch PH, Korf BR, et al. Cardiovascular malformations and other cardiovascular abnormalities in neurofibromatosis 1. Am J Med Genet 2000;95:108–17.

Listernick R, Charrow J, Greenwald MJ, et al. Optic gliomas in children with neurofibromatosis type 1. J Pediatr 1989;114:788-792

Lott IT, Richardson EP: Neuropathologic findings and the biology of neurofibromatosis. Adv Neuron 29:23-32, 1981

Marchuk DA, Collins FS. Molecular genetics of neurofibromatosis 1. In: Huson SM, Hughes RAC, editors. The neurofibromatosis. A pathogenic and clinical overview. London: Chapman and Hall, 1994:23-49.

Martin GA, Viskochil D, Bollag G, et al. The GAP-related domain of the neurofibromatosis type 1 gene product interacts with ras p21. Cell 1990;63:843-9.

McClatchey AI, Saotome I, Mercer K, et al. Mice heterozygous for a mutation at the NF2 tumor suppressor locus develop a range of highly metastatic tumors. Genes Dev 1998;12:1121-33.

McClatchey AI. Neurofibromatosis. Annu Rev Pathol Mech Dis 2007; 2:191-216

Merel P, Khe HX, Sanson M, et al. Screening for germline mutations in the neurofibromatosis 2 gene. Genes Chromosomes Cancer 1995;12:117-21.

Morrison H, Sherman LS, Legg J, et al. The NF2 tumor suppressor gene product, merlin, mediates contact inhibition of growth through interactions with CD44. Genes Dev 2001;15(8):968-80.

North KN, Riccardi V, Samango-Sprouse C, et al. Cognitive function and academic performance in neurofi bromatosis. 1: consensus statement from the NF1 Cognitive Disorders Task Force. Neurology 1997;48:1121–27.

Obremski VJ, Hall AM, Fernandez-Valle C. Merlin, the neurofibromatosis type 2 gene product, and beta 1 integrin associate in isolated and differentiating Schwann cells. J Neurobiol 1998;37(4):487-501.

Parry DM, MacCollin MM, Kaiser-Kupfer MI, et al. Germ-line mutations in the neurofibromatosis 2 gene: correlations with disease severity and retinal abnormalities. Am J Hum Genet 1996;59(3):529-39.

Pearson MA, Reczek D, Bretscher A, Karplus PA. Structure of the ERM protein moesin reveals the FERM domain fold masked by an extended actin binding tail domain. Cell 2000; 101(3): 259-70.

Pérez-Grau M, Miró N, Prades J, et al. Neurofibromatosis type 2. Acta Otorrinolaringológica Esp 2010;61(4):306-311

Reed N, Gutmann DH. Tumorigenesis in neurofibromatosis: new insights and potential therapies. Trends Molec Med 2001;7:157-62

Rinaldi MM, Carella M, Marino B, Pizzuti A, Digilio MC, Tartaglia M, Dallapiccola B. NF1 gene mutations represent the major molecular event underlying neurofibromatosis–Noonan syndrome. Am J Med Genet 2005;77:1092–1101.

Rodenhiser DI, Coulter-Mackie MB, Singh SM. Evidence of DNA methylation in the neurofibromatosis type 1 (NF1) gene region of 17q11.2. Hum Mol Genet 1993;2:439-44.

Rosembaum C, Kluwe L, Mautner VF, Friedrich RE, Muller HW, Hanemann CO. Isolation and characterization of Schwann cells from neurofibromatosis type 2 patients. Neurobiol Dis 1998;5:55-64.

Rosser TL, Vezina G, Packer RT. Cerebrovascular abnormalities in a population of children with neurofi bromatosis type 1. Neurology 2005;64:553–55.

Rouleau GA, Wertelecki W, Haines JL, et al. Genetic linkage of bilateral acoustic neurofibromatosis to a DNA marker on chromosome 22. Nature 1987;329:246-8.

Rouleau GA, Merel P, Lutchman M, et al. Alteration in a new gene encoding a putative membrane-organizing protein causes neurofibromatosis type 2. Nature 1993;363:515-21.

Rouleau GA. Molecular genetic studies of neurofibromatosis 2. In: Huson SM, Hughes RAC, editors. Neurofibromatosis: a pathogenetic and clinical overview. London: Chapman and Hall, 1994:50-61.

Ruggierei M, Huson SM. The clinical and diagnostic implications of mosaicism in the neurofibromatoses. Neurology 2001;56:1433–43.

Rutkowski JL, Wu K et al. Genetic and cellular defects contributing to benign tumor formation in neurofibromatosis type 1. Hum. Mol. Genet. (2000) 9 (7): 1059-1066.

Scoles DR, Baser ME, Pulst SM. A missense mutation in the neurofibromatosis gene occurs in patients with mild and severe phenotypes. Neurology 1996;47:544-6.

Scoles DR, Huynh DP, Chen MS, Burke SP, Gutmann DH, Pulst SM. The neurofibromatosis 2 tumor suppressor protein interacts with hepatocyte growth factor-regulated tyrosine kinase substrate. Hum Mol Genet 2000;9(11):1567-74.

Selvanathan SK, Shenton A, Ferner R, et al.. Further genotype-phenotype correlations in neurofibromatosis 2. Clin Genet 2010; 77(2):163-7.

Serra E, Puig S, Otero D, et al. Confirmation of a double-hit-model for the NF1 gene in benign neurofibromas. Am J Hum Genet 1997;61:512-9.

Shen MH, Harper PS, Upadhyaya M. Molecular genetics of neurofibromatosis type 1. J Med Genet 1996; 33: 2-17.

Shimizu T, Seto A, Maita N, et al. Structural basis for neurofibromatosis type 2. Crystal structure of the merlin FERM domain. J Biol Chem 2002;277:10332-6

Tong J, Hanna F, Zhu Y, et al. Neurofibromin regulated G-protein-stimulated adenyl ciclase activity. Nat Neurosci 2002;5:95-6.

Tonsgard JH. Clinical Manifestations and Management of Neurofibromatosis Type 1. Semin Pediatr Neurol 2006;13:2-7

Tonsgard JH, Kwak SM, Short MP, et al: CT imaging in adults with neurofibromatosis-1: frequent asymptomatic plexiform lesions. Neurology 1998;50:1755-1760

Trofatter JA, MacCollin MM, Rutter JL, et al. A novel moesin-, ezrin-, radixin-like gene is a candidate for the neurofibromatosis 2 tumor suppressor. Cell 1993;72:791-800.

Upadhyaya M, Cooper DN. The mutational spectrum in neurofibromatosis 1 and its underlying mechanisms. In: Upadhyaya M, Cooper DN, editors. Neurofibromatosis type 1: from genotype to phenotype. Oxford: BIOS Scientific Publishers, 1998:65-88

Valverde AH, Simões R, Campillo J. Cefalea en paciente con neurofibromatosis tipo I. Neurología 2007; 22(10):11-14.

Viskochil D, Buchberg AM, Xu G, et al. Deletions and a translocation interrupt a cloned gene at the neurofibromatosis type 1 locus. Cell 1990;62:187-92.

Wallace MR, Marchuk DA, Andersen LB, et al. Type 1 neurofibromatosis gene: identification of a large transcript disrupted in three NF1 patients. Science 1990;249:181-6.

Welling DB. Clinical manifestations of mutations in the neurofibromatosis type 2 gene in vestibular schwannomas (acoustic neuromas). Laryngoscope 1998;108:178-89.

Wertelecki W, Rouleau G, Superneau DW, et al. Neurofibromatosis 2: clinical and DNA linkage studies of a large kindred. N Engl J Med 1988;319:278-83.

Wu X, Estwick SA, Chen S, et al. Neurofibromin plays a critical role in modulating osteoblast differentiation of mesenchymal stem/progenitor cells. Hum Mol Genet 2006;15:2837-45.

Xu G, O'Conell P, Viskochil D, et al. The neurofibromatosis type 1 gene encodes a protein related to GAP. Cell 1995; 62:599-608.

Xu HM, Gutmann DH. Merlin differentially associates with the microtubule and actin cytoskeleton. J Neurosci Res 1998;51(3):403-15

Zanca A. Antique illustrations of neurofibromatosis. Int J Dermatol 1980;19:55–8.

12

The Time Onset of Post Stroke Dementia

Gian Luigi Lenzi[1], Giorgio De Benedetto[2] and Marta Altieri[1]
[1]*Clinica Neurologica A, Department of Neurology and Psichiatry,*
[2]*Department of Cardiovascular, Respiratory, Nephrological and Geriatric Sciences,*
"Sapienza" University, Rome,
Italy

1. Introduction

In a population of 1 million inhabitants, 2400 patients will have a stroke every year, of whom fewer than 50% will be independent 1 year later (Hankey & Warlow, 1999). Many independent survivors have residual physical or cognitive deficits, or behavioural changes which can affect family life and have professional consequences (Leys et al. 2002). Post Stroke Dementia (PSD), that includes any dementia after stroke, irrespective of its cause, is therefore a clinical syndrome - and not a disease - and it appears to be one of the main causes of dependency in stroke survivors.

An huge increase in prevalence and burden of PSD is likely to happen (Mackowiak-Cordolani et al. 2005) because of the decline in mortality after stroke (Rothwell et al. 2004) and ageing of populations.

Therefore, stroke has been found to be a strong predictor of dementia. This association is present both for clinically apparent strokes as well as for subclinical strokes. More than 25% of patients develop dementia after their first or recurrent stroke. The prevalence is slightly lower when patients with pre stroke cognitive impairment are excluded. On the other hand, the diagnosis of vascular dementia (VaD) remains a controversial issue in many aspects and concepts. These nosologic problems are caused both by the methods, insufficient to ascertain the diagnosis, as well as by the weak consistency of the clinical concept of VaD itself. VaD is defined as a combination of clinical and neuropathological manifestations characterized by dementia in association with variegated brain lesions of vascular or circulatory origin (Ferrer, 2010); PSD obviously includes all cases of VaD but also these cases where stroke adds to an already clinically evident neurodegenerative cognitive impairment. One of the most intriguing issues on VaD, and in particular on PSD, is related to the time of development of cognitive decline.

In clinical practice, the 3-month time threshold is usually chosen to enable resolution of a possible acute post-stroke delirium, and to obtain a more reliable cognitive assessment with a complete regression of acute neuropsychological stroke-related deficits. As a matter of fact, it has been found that most cognitive impairments after stroke, in particular visual memory and visuospatial construction, resolve beyond the subacute time period. Moreover, as the time after stroke increases, so does the likelihood that an individual might have other cerebrovascular injuries that could further contribute to impair cognition.

The time course of PSD is strictly related to its pathophysiology: it may be 1) the direct consequence of a vascular lesion; 2) due to the additive effect of recurrent strokes and white matter lesions; 3) the result of pre-existing neuropathological Alzheimer's Disease (AD) or similar neurodegenerative dementias, such as Lewy Body Dementia (LBD) or Fronto-Temporal Dementia (FTD). Concerning these neurodegenerative conditions, it is not clear if the effect of stroke on dementia is due to a direct increase in neuropathological changes associated with AD-LBD-FTD, or to the synergic effect of AD-LBD-FTD pathology and vascular pathology.

Another relevant issue is the possibility to predict which patient will develop PSD. In this regard, recent data indicate an overlap between AD-LBD-FTD and PSD, which seems to share risk factors and neuropathology. In most population samples these disorders appear together, and the consensus is growing that a degenerative component has a more important role in determining PSD onset shortly after stroke than previously recognized. Therefore, anamnestic data have a fundamental role in this prognostic approach.

In this chapter, the authors try to clarify the "mystery" of the time onset of PSD. They will start with an overview concerning the new pathogenetic determinants of PSD. Later, they will attempt to offer a systematic analysis of the amount of data concerning PSD itself. PSD and its onset time really are a dilemma; aim of this chapter is to suggest a new potential approach to make clarity in this puzzled question.

2. Timing of Vascular Dementia (VaD) and Post Stroke Dementia (PSD)

One of the most intriguing issues on VaD, and in particular on PSD, is the time course of the development of cognitive decline. In other words, what is the "correct" timing to define "demented" a stroke patient? Tatemichi 21 years ago was the first to put VaD in a temporal context, by observing that 3 months after stroke about one fourth of the patients developed PSD (Tatemichi et al., 1990). Several subsequent studies confirmed this finding, so the time relationship between stroke and cognitive decline was included in the diagnostic criteria for VaD.

Nevertheless, this time interval has been variously faced by different diagnostic criteria. In the ADDTC criteria the diagnosis of ischemic vascular dementia is "probable" when in addition to dementia there is "evidence of two or more ischemic strokes by history, neurologic signs, and/or a single stroke with a clearly documented temporal relationship to the onset of dementia" (Chui et al., 1992).

In the NINDS–AIREN criteria the relationship between stroke and dementia is "within 3 months after a recognized stroke"; however, this time relationship is not mandatory. In fact, a diagnosis of VaD is also probable when a patient presents "abrupt deterioration of cognitive functions after stroke or fluctuating, stepwise progression of cognitive deficits" (Roman et al., 1993). In the ICD-10 criteria for VaD, subdivided into ethiologic subtypes, VaD with acute onset is a dementia developing rapidly (i.e. usually within 1 but no longer than 3 months) after a succession of strokes, or (rarely) after a single large infarction. The diagnosis of VaD due to multi-infarcts is even more vague, being the onset of dementia "more gradual (i.e. within 3–6 months) and following a number of minor ischemic episodes" (WHO, 1989).

In clinical practice, the 3-month time threshold is usually chosen to enable resolution of a possible acute post-stroke delirium and to obtain a more reliable cognitive assessment with a complete regression of acute neuropsychological stroke-related deficits. On the other hand, about 50% of acute stroke patients may show some improvement in global cognition up to 1 year after stroke (Ballard et al., 2003). Long-term improvement in generalized cognitive function seems to occur more frequently in patients who have experienced left hemisphere infarctions or very severe hemispheric stroke syndromes.

On the contrary, diabetes mellitus seems to compromise the ability to achieve long-term improvement in cognitive function after stroke, both ischemic and hemorrhagic, suggesting that management of this important vascular risk factor should be performed with care and consistency (Desmond et al., 1996; Tham et al., 2002). Recent data show evidence for an overlap between Alzheimer's disease (AD) and PSD, which appear to share risk factors and neuropathology (Snowdon et al., 1997; O'Brien et al., 2003). Whether the relationship between AD and PSD in determining cognitive decline is "additive" or due to a "cause-effect" mechanism remains to be determined. In most population samples, these two disorders appear together, and the consensus is growing that a degenerative component has a more important role in determining the PSD onset shortly after stroke than previously recognized (Roman & Royall, 2004; Rockwood et al., 1999). Substantial data indicate that comorbid ischemic cerebrovascular disease may contribute to convert patients with "preclinical AD" to a clinical form, thus unmasking, and anticipating, a previous pathological process (de la Torre, 2002).

What is said for AD probably is true for the other degenerative dementias as well, therefore in this Chapter we will use the definition of AD-LBD-FTD to indicate the main group of these neurodegenerative processes. Clinicians rarely diagnose AD until pathology has reached the cortical regions related to executive functions (Royall, 2002). If executive impairment caused by sub-cortical vascular disease is superimposed on AD pathology, then clinical AD is likely to be diagnosed earlier (Roman & Royall, 2004).

In this view, the occurrence of a new vascular lesion might unbalance a previous equilibrium thus revealing a "clinical" dementia syndrome. Therefore, anamnestic data have a fundamental role in the prognostic approach. Clinically, previous cognitive status and post-stroke delirium show an important correlation with the future development of PSD (Rothwell et al., 2005; Henon et al., 1999). Anatomical location of the lesion and its volume are also important (Gold et al., 2005). All the other risk factors for VaD and for stroke show a correlation, but this is probably due to the chance of new vascular events, including the silent strokes (Vermeer et al., 2003). Whether PSD represents the same clinical and pathological entity from the early phase up to the following years remains to be determined.

2.1 Post Stroke Dementia: A misleading definition

The comprehension of the pathophysiological phenomena influencing the time onset of cognitive decline after stroke is very complex, and involves researchers in different fields, such as pathologists, neuroradiologists, molecular biologists and physicians.

The term PSD includes all kinds of dementia developing after stroke, independently of the intrinsic features of the stroke itself. This term is probably become outdated, because its concept was conceived when researchers supposed that just the occurrence of stroke could be responsible of the cognitive impairment and, subsequently, of dementia. Now, data show that this is a quite uncommon eventuality

In fact, in the largest number of cases, the occurrence of stroke seems to be only the clinical sign of an underlying vessels' disease. Nevertheless, it has been suggested that this vessels' disease could have a key role in the pathogenesis of vascular and neurodegenerative dementias.

Perhaps, VaD and sporadic AD-LBD-FTD could have a common origin, like a vascular disorder that affects the vessel wall (particularly the two inner layers), and that may have a wide range of clinical presentations. This heterogeneity is probably related to genetic differences between individuals; in fact, the genotypic variety allows the existence of different phenotypes. Because of those aforementioned concepts, epidemiological studies are not designed with uniform criteria (Pendlebury, 2009), since it is difficult to create a consensus concerning which kind of demented stroke patient deserves to be enrolled. In addition, many factors can influence the prevalence and incidence of PSD such as: the mean age of the study population, the exclusion or not of patients with aphasia or severe physical disability, the mortality rates, the delay between stroke onset and the cognitive assessment, the criteria used for the diagnosis of dementia, the presence of a previous cognitive impairment or dementia (Pendlebury, 2009).

Currently, we can safely affirm that: 1) the occurrence of stroke doubles the risk of PSD; 2) the attributable risk is the highest within the first year after stroke, then declines, while the relative risk of dementia remains stable around 2; 3) the risk of delayed dementia, including Alzheimer's disease (AD) and the other neurodegenerative dementias (LBD, FTD), also remains doubled 10 years and more after stroke. Researchers tried to fill this knowledge gap through the identification of the cause-effect relationship between specific pathological conditions and PSD. In particular, considerable efforts have been made in the attempt of understanding the role of specific cardiovascular risk factors determining PSD itself. In the Authors' opinion, the basic issues of this intense research activity are five, at least. They are: 1) What are the pathophysiological mechanisms of PSD?; 2) What are the risk factors more related to the development of PSD? 3) And which of them are more related to time onset of PSD? 4) Is it possible to create homogeneous groups of patients in order to perform a risk stratification of PSD? 5) Would it be possible to create a risk stratification also with regard to the time onset of PSD?

Obviously, it seems almost superfluous to say that no one has been able to give a satisfying answer to these fundamental questions. Until now, at least. However, it is precisely from these facts, apparently in conflict with each other, that we can draw the starting point not only to give a unified view of PSD, but also to explain the dilemma related to its onset time.

2.1.1 Role of risk factors

Currently, the state of affairs is quite garbled and there are no definitive data on this topic. However, scientific evidence allowed to set aside the idea that PSD is just the result of the occurrence of stroke. In fact, if the acute cerebrovascular event was the only responsible for the development of cognitive impairment, we would not be able to explain why not all stroke patients develop PSD.

In addition, we would not even have any plausible elucidation for the different time of onset of dementia in some patients than in others. Reported risk factors for pre- and post-stroke dementia are not always consistent between studies, probably owing to small sample sizes. To overcome this problem, available data was combined in a meta-analysis to attempt to determine the most significant factors involved in the development of PSD (Pendlebury et al., 2009).

All but one study addressed to the risk factors associated with pre-stroke dementia include patients with first ever and with recurrent stroke, so many of the patients will have had a past history of stroke. Patients with pre-stroke dementia are significantly older (weighted mean difference = 9.1, 8.4–9.8 years $p < 0.0001$) than those without pre-stroke dementia. Rates are also significantly higher in women and in those with little education, and in patients with medial temporal lobe atrophy, family history of dementia, previous stroke or TIA, leukoaraiosis, multiple infarcts, diabetes, atrial fibrillation, hypertension, and global cerebral atrophy (Pendlebury et al., 2009). Post-stroke dementia, like pre-stroke dementia, is associated with older age (weighted mean difference = 5.1, 4.6–5.7, years $p < 0.0001$) and low educational attainment, and also prior cognitive decline and premorbid disability (Pendelbury et al., 2009).

Associated vascular risk factors include diabetes and atrial fibrillation but not hypertension, ischemic heart disease, cholesterol, prior TIA or smoking. However, the majority of factors associated with post-stroke dementia are related to the stroke itself, and include hemorrhagic stroke, left hemisphere stroke, dysphasia, stroke severity, infarct volume, and the presence of multiple strokes separated in space and time (previous stroke, multiple infarcts, and recurrent stroke). Certain complications of stroke including incontinence, early seizures, acute confusion, hypoxic ischemic episodes and hypotension are also strongly associated with post-stroke dementia.

Being Caucasian is protective in comparison to black or Hispanic. It is unlikely that all the factors listed in are independent predictors of post-stroke dementia. Non-stroke-related risk factors that tend to remain significantly predictive of post-stroke dementia in multivariate analyses are age, low educational attainment, diabetes, atrial fibrillation, and leukoaraiosis (Pendlebury et al., 2009).

Therefore, although these risk factors are statistically independent, they could still be confounded by stroke-related factors. For example, atrial fibrillation and diabetes are associated with symptomatic stroke, asymptomatic stroke on imaging, recurrent stroke, multiple stroke lesions, and severity of stroke; and leukoaraiosis is associated with stroke severity and stroke recurrence. The factors associated with pre-stroke dementia are broadly similar to those for post-stroke dementia, perhaps unsurprisingly, since all but one study on the predictors of pre-stroke dementia include patients with recurrent as well as first-ever stroke. In pre-neuroimaging era, Fazio and Loeb frequently affirmed that in the past history of demented patients, the occurrence of TIAs was more frequent that in the general population. Medial temporal lobe atrophy, female sex and family history of dementia are much stronger predictors of pre- than post-stroke dementia, suggesting a more important role for primary degenerative pathology in pre-stroke dementia. Interestingly, hypertension, ischemic heart disease and prior TIA were associated with pre- but not post-stroke dementia. The fact that hypertension was not associated with post-stroke dementia may also be explained by the fact that hypertension is very common in both patients with and without post-stroke dementia. Atrial fibrillation is associated with both pre- and post-stroke dementia, presumably since its prevalence increases with age, and it is linked to multiple and recurrent strokes and increased stroke severity. There is also some evidence that atrial fibrillation is associated with cognitive impairment and hippocampal atrophy in the absence of symptomatic stroke or even silent infarction (Ott, 1997; Knecht, 2008). Diabetes is a known risk factor for dementia and mild cognitive impairment and is associated with both pre- and post-stroke dementia. In addition to age-related physiological decline, diabetes disturbs microvascular functions through mechanisms including activation of protein kinase C, excess production of reactive oxygen species and cellular activation of the receptor for advanced glycation endproducts (RAGE). Further, animal studies show that diabetes exacerbates post-stroke brain damage (Zhang et al., 2009) and there is evidence that diabetes is associated with reduced recovery of cognitive function after stroke (Nys et al., 2005).

As a matter of fact, it is difficult to give an accurate image of the role that every risk factor could have in the pathogenesis of PSD. This syndrome seems to be a real complex phenomenon, and each of them could probably determine PSD with a power that is different for every patient.

In conclusion, stroke could be the acute event that reveals an underlying cognitive impairment. Probably, it would be essential to read between the lines, understanding the limits of research and the restricted margins of our classifications criteria. In the future, scientific evidences will maybe force us to give a new interpretation of these elements, that could be viewed like various components of the same pathological process.

Four major determinants deserve to be mentioned, in order to better clarify what it has been said. They are: 1) demographic and medical characteristics of the patient with PSD and their influence on stroke outcome, 2) neuroimaging characteristics, 3) stroke characteristics, 4) pre-existing pathological alterations. (Pendelbury et al., 2009).

These elements are crucial for the understanding of the most accredited theories about the ethiology of PSD, but especially to recognize the state of knowledge on its onset time.

2.1.2 Demographic and medical characteristics of the patient with PSD and their influence on stroke outcome

The most important demographic predictors of dementia after stroke, in sufficiently powered studies, are increasing age and low education level, but not gender, when the analysis is adjusted for age (Zhu et al., 2000).

The risk of dementia after stroke is higher in patients who were already dependent before stroke (Zhu et al., 2000). Pre-stroke cognitive decline without dementia, assessed by standardized questionnaires, is obviously associated with a higher risk of dementia after stroke (Zhu et al., 2000; Snowdon et al., 1997).

Diabetes mellitus, atrial fibrillation and myocardial infarction were also independent risk factors for dementia after stroke in several studies. (Zhu et al., 2000). Arterial hypertension, a risk factor for VaD and AD, has not been clearly identified as a risk factor for PSD. Epileptic seizures (Esiri et al., 1999), sepsis, cardiac arrhythmias and congestive heart failure are independently associated with an increased risk of dementia after stroke (Zhu et al., 2000).

However, the statistical relationship found between these disorders and dementia does not mean a causal relationship: it is also possible that dementia increases the risk of such events (Zhu et al., 2000). The influence of hyperlipidemia, hyperhomocysteinemia, alcohol consumption and cigarette smoking on dementia after stroke remains unproven (Zhu et al., 2000). The results concerning cigarette smoking should be interpreted with caution, because smoking influences mortality and stroke recurrence. ApoE4 genotype is associated with an increased risk of dementia after stroke (de la Torre, 2002).

The most common causes of PSD are VaD, AD-BLD-FTD and mixed dementia (Leys et .al., 2005). AD-BLD-FTD, mixed AD-BLD-FTD and VaD account for 19-61% of patients with PSD. Vascular lesions have a prominent role in the development of PSD in the following circumstances: patients with stroke who are too young to have AD-BLD-FTD, and who have dementia just after stroke; when cognitive functions were normal before stroke, impaired immediately after, and did not worsen or improve over time; when a specific vascular condition known to cause stroke and dementia is proven by a specific marker; and when the lesion is located in a strategic area (Alexander & Freedman, 1984; Benson & Cummings, 1982; Bhatia & Marsden, 1994; Ott & Saver, 1993).

Even when vascular lesions, Alzheimer's pathology and white matter changes do not lead to dementia by themselves, their cumulative effect can reach the threshold of lesions required to produce dementia (Pasquier & Leys, 1997); as well as when stroke, white matter changes, or both, occur in a patient with asymptomatic Alzheimer's pathology, the period of preclinical AD might be shortened (Pasquier & Leys, 1997). This hypothesis is supported by the results of several studies. In the Optima and in the Nun studies, among patients who met neuropathological criteria for AD, those with brain infarcts had poorer cognitive functions and a higher prevalence of dementia (Nagy et al., 1997; Snowdon et al., 1997). In the dementia substudy of the Systolic Hypertension in Europe Trial (SYST-EUR), nitrendipine decreased the incidence rate of stroke and AD (Forette et al., 1998), suggesting that stroke prevention reduces the risk of new-onset AD; previous cognitive decline and no dementia, likely to be degenerative in origin in most patients (Henon et al., 1995), is a risk factor for PSD (Henon et al., 2001). Most patients with previous cognitive decline and no dementia who developed PSD have a clinical presentation of AD, but it occurs months after a stroke.

The concept of mixed dementia might be useful for those patients because it emphasizes that these patients should be treated for AD but should also receive an appropriate therapy to prevent stroke. Treatment of these patients as thought they have AD, even if the time-course suggests AD, may make practitioners ignore the vascular component that is treatable, especially if the stroke occurs years before.

Moreover, both population-based studies (Aevarsson et al., 1995; Baldereschi et al., 1999; Woo et al., 1992; Tatemichi et al., 1994) and hospital based (Roth, 1955) studies have shown that patients with PSD have higher mortality rates than patients without dementia, independent of age and comorbidities (Aevarsson et al., 1995). The long term mortality rate is two to six times higher in patients with PSD, after adjustement for demographic factors, associated cardiac diseases, stroke severity and stroke recurrence (Desmond et al., 2002; Henon et al., 2003; Tatemichi et al., 1994). In patients with pre-existing dementia, mortality rates are two to five times higher (Barba et al., 2002; Henon et al., 2003). The increased mortality among patients with PSD might be the result of several factors; 1) patients with dementia of any cause have high mortality (Helmer et al., 2001); 2) Stroke mortality may be high in patients with dementia (Helmer et al., 2001); 3) Dementia is associated with more severe vascular diseases and a higher risk of complications (Tatemichi et al., 1994); 4) Dementia may worsen co-occuring disorders; patients with dementia may receive less aggressive stroke prevention (Rockwood et al., 1997; Gurwitz et al., 1997), and less appropriate treatment of associate disorders (Krumholz et al., 1996) although causes of death can be similar in patients with and without PSD and management was similar for both groups in the Lille Study (Barba et al., 2002; Henon et al., 2003); 5) Patients with PSD may be less compliant to treatments necessary for stroke prevention (i.e. antithrombotic agents and treatment of vascular risk factors), which could lead to less effective prevention of new vascular events and a higher mortality rate. Furthermore, the New York study (Moroney et al., 1997) has demonstrated that dementia diagnosed 3 months after stroke was associated with a three times greater increased risk of stroke recurrence (relative risk: 2.71; 95% CI 1.36 - 5.42).

Dementia might be a marker for a more severe vascular disease leading to an increased risk of recurrence, but also an indicator of a less intensive stroke prevention and lack of compliance that can contribute to the increased risk of recurrence (Moroney et al., 1997). White matter changes could also be a confounding factor because they are associated with an increased risk of stroke recurrence (Henon et al., 2001).

In addition, the few data on the influence of PSD on functional outcome suggest that patients with PSD are more impaired and more dependent in daily living activities than patients with stroke who do not develop PSD (Tatemichi et al., 1990; Tatemichi et al., 1992; Barba et al., 2000; Lin et al., 2003; Prencipe et al., 1997).

In conclusions, many efforts have been made to define which kind of patient is at increased risk of PSD, but there are no definitive data. For the majority of the patients, the occurrence of stroke is only the clinical expression of a just advanced pathological process, which affect the brain and will lead to the loss of cognitive functions.

In this context, time of onset of PSD is strictly related to the pre-stroke conditions of the patient's brain. Actually, all the evidences confirm that dementia will occur more rapidly in individuals with the worst cognitive and clinical status. The strict connection between cardiovascular risk factors and PSD and the overlapping between VaD, particularly PSD, and AD-BLD-FTD, corroborate the hypothesis about the existence of a common pathogenetic mechanism (a vessel's wall disease), responsible not only for the pathogenesis of the classical "cardiovascular" risk factors, but also for a chronic brain hypoperfusion, which could cause/increase/accelerate the neurodegeneration of specific genetically predisposed neuronal populations and represent the starting point for VaD.

Obviously, the matter is quite complex, and there are no definitive data. This happens for many reasons, mainly related to the differences in inclusion criteria for subjects enrolled in clinical trials. We must also remember that all involved variables, particularly cardiovascular risk factors, have a wide range of clinical presentations between individuals, with a degree of complexity that is difficult to describe with a statistical program. So, it is very difficult to define the correct role that each of them could have in causing the occurrence of PSD and its onset time.

Later, the authors will attempt to clarify these concepts, starting from the assumption that every risk factor should not be considered independently from the others, but that each of them can be considered the epiphenomenon of the abovementioned underlying vascular disease. This perspective is of considerable relevance, because it allows a unique view of the heterogeneous landscape described in this chapter.

2.1.3 Neuroimaging charateristics

To our best knowledge, there is no study with functional neuroimaging techniques such a SPECT, PET, functional MRI, or spectroscopy, addressed to identify predictors of PSD in large series of consecutive patients with stroke. Functional neuroimaging studies have provided a useful conceptual framework for the understanding of VaD, but were not addressed to PSD. Plain neuroimaging has shown the frequent occurrence of silent infarcts, that is cerebral infarcts seen on CT or MRI scans that have never been associated with a corresponding neurological deficit. One study found no relation between silent infarcts and PSD (Bornstein et al. 1996), but the assessment of the pre-existing cognitive status was not standardized, and the study was underpowered. Other studies clearly identified silent infarcts as independent predictors of PSD (Tatemichi et al., 1990; Desmond et al., 2000; Henon et al., 2001; Pohjasvaara et al., 2000).

The influence of silent infarcts is more important when the delay between stroke and cognitive assessment is longer. In the Lille study, silent infarcts were associated with PSD in the third year but not in the second (Corea et al., 2001), and in the Maastricht study silent infarcts were independently related to dementia after 1 year, but not after 1 month or 6 months (Rasquin et al., 2004).

Global cerebral atrophy is associated with a higher risk of PSD (Linden et al., 2004; Desmond et al., 2000; Tang et al., 2004; Altieri et al., 2004; Ivan et al., 2004; Tatemichi et al., 1993).

Medial temporal lobe atrophy (MTLA) is most common in patients with stroke who have preexisting dementia (Henon H et al., 1998), but it can also be present in patients with stroke and no dementia. In the Lille study the cumulative proportion of 3-year survivors free of dementia was significantly lower in patients with MLTA (57.6% vs 80.8%) (Cordoliani-Mackowak et al., 2003).

MLTA clearly differentiates patients with dementia from those who do not have dementia after a first-ever ischaemic stroke, even after exclusion of patients who have pre-stroke cognitive impairment (Pohjasvaara et al., 2000; Ballard et al., 2003). Patients with stroke with MLTA might have a pre-clinical AD, which is clinically revealed by stroke (Pasquier & Leys, 1997). However, MLTA is not specific to AD, as it has also been observed in VaD (Jobst et al., 1998; Fein et al., 2000). In elderly patients with stroke and no dementia (with moderate to severe MLTA) after adjusting for age, volume of infarcts and cortical atrophy, do notably worse in tests of learning, story recall, visual reproduction, block design, and mental speed (Jokinen et al., 2004), suggesting that, in elderly patients who have stroke but no dementia, MLTA is associated with poor memory and visuo-spatial functions, whereas verbal and executive functions are preserved (Jokinen at al., 2004).

Presence and severity of white matter changes are independent predictors of PSD (Tang et al., 2004). However, there are major potential confounding factors: cerebral atrophy, which is more frequent in patients with white matter changes; lacunar infarcts, which share a common pathogenesis with white matter changes than those with stroke alone (Tatemichi et al., 1990; Pasquier & Leys, 1997). In a study to determine the neuroimaging correlates of cognitive ability in patients with lacunar infarcts, left frontal lobe atrophy and presence of thalamic infarct were independent predictors of worse cognitive performances (Mok et al., 2005).

Finally, silent infarcts, global cerebral atrophy, medial temporal lobe atrophy and white matter changes are predictors of PSD. There might be a lot of reasons to explain the inconsistency of data listed before: in particular the heterogeneity and the confusion of the selection criteria; the study samples not uniform. The simple occurrence of stroke cannot represent a crystal clear inclusion criteria. Every stroke is different than others, because there are many discrepancies in the basal conditions of the patient, in the etiology, in the pathogenesis and in the further mechanisms and evolution of stroke itself.

Moreover, following the "vessels disease" theory, stroke and atherosclerosis are not the disease, but only an epiphenomenon of a more complex matter. In addition, PSD occur more rapidly in those patients with a larger number of brain injuries, independently from their nature (vascular or neurodegenerative). Obviously, the aforementioned vessels' wall disease is not demonstrable with current neuroimaging techniques, because our detection tools allow only the identification of the consequences that this pathology produces on patients' brain, like strokes, silent and micro-infarcts, small vessels disease (cortical and sub-cortical), and cerebral atrophy. In the last years, TC-PET and SPECT have achieved a key role in the early diagnosis of Mild Cognitive Impairment (MCI) and AD-LBD-FTD. TC-PET and SPECT are perfusion techniques, at first. So, a chronic hypoperfusion in the early stages of AD-LBD-FTD has been demonstrated (Liu et al, 2011; de La Torre, 2010; Pakrasi & O'Brien, 2005). Consequently, you can not only suggest a possible role of chronic hypoperfusion in determining AD-LBD-FTD, but also suppose that new technologies could allow innovative and surprising findings concerning this fascinating issue, in the next future.

2.1.4 Stroke characteristics

Most studies found that a more severe clinical deficit at the onset of stroke is associated with a higher risk of PSD (Tatemichi et al., 1990; Desmond et al., 2000; Henon et al., 2001; Pohjasvaara et al., 1997). Studies that did not find this association (Kolmen et al., 1996; Altieri et al., 2004; Desmond et al., 2002), are characterized by high mortality rates in patients with severe deficits that may have created recruitment bias (because of a short delay between stroke onset and recruitment).

The risk of PSD and its severity are not influenced by the type of stroke (ischemic or hemorrhagic) (Linden et al., 2004; Pohjasvaara et al., 1998; Barba et al., 2000; Henon et al., 2001; Madureira et al., 2001; Rasquin et al., 2004). However, differences in survival rates between stroke subtypes are making the results difficult to interpret.

In the Framingham study large artery infarcts, lacunar infarcts and infarcts of unknown origin were associated with a higher risk of PSD than cardioembolic infarcts (Ivan et al., 2004). In other studies, the risk of PSD was lower in patients with small vessel occlusion than in patients with large arterial stroke (Tatemichi et al., 1990; Desmond et al., 2000; Mok et al., 2004; Rasquin et al., 2004). Accordingly, a study evaluating stroke volumes showed a relationship between higher stroke volume and the risk of dementia (Sachdev & Brodaty, 1999).

However, all these results are influenced by the higher mortality rate in stroke subtypes associated with more severe deficits, in patients who are the most likely to develop PSD when they survive. Supratentorial lesions, left hemispheric lesions, anterior and posterior cerebral artery territory infarcts, multiple infarcts and so-called "strategic infarcts", i.e. cerebral infarcts that may lead to dementia on their own in the absence of any other lesion, have been found to be associated with an increased risk of dementia after stroke in at least two independent studies (Leys et al., 2005). However, strategic locations (left angular gyrus, inferomesial temporal and mesiofrontal locations, thalami, left capsular genu, caudate nuclei) were described more than 20 years ago, in single case reports, or in small series, usually without MRI, and without follow-up (Leys et al., 2005). Other vascular brain lesions interfering with the neuropsychological deficit cannot be excluded in the absence of MRI (Leys et al., 2005), and coexisting AD-LBD-FTD cannot be excluded in absence of follow-up (Leys et al., 2005). Therefore, the concept of strategic stroke should be revisited with large prospective studies, with MRI scans to exclude associate lesions, and a follow-up long enough to exclude associated AD-BLD-FTD (Leys et al., 2005). In conclusion, stroke itself is rarely the only responsible of PSD. The clinical experience and scientific data show that the occurrence of a "strategic" or "large" brain infarct is an unfrequent event. Only in these cases, in fact, the stroke could cause deterioration of patients' cognitive functions and subsequent PSD. As the authors said in the previous paragraphs of this chapter, stroke should be considered as the clinical expression of an underlying vascular disease, that could cause dementia through the synergistic and addictive effect of a large number of clinically unrevealed brain injuries. Stroke itself would be only able to anticipate the timing of dementia. However, stroke would not be the disease, but only one of its clinical signs. These concepts are supported by several data; in fact, apart from the previous cited strategic locations, PSD most likely occurs in patients with a "more severe clinical deficit at onset". The term "More severe clinical deficit" means the presence of a large number of previous brain injuries (vascular or neurodegenerative), together with a worse clinical condition, caused by a poorer detection and control of classical cardiovascular risk factors (hypercholesterolemia, diabetes, hypertension, heart failure and so on). In both of cases, the clinical landscape is dominated by the vascular disease, which is the responsible not only for the accumulation of these chronic damages, but also of the occurrence of stroke. Therefore, stroke is simply an epiphenomenon, that contributes to anticipate or to reveal an earlier cognitive impairment, causing PSD, which merely is another consequence of this complex pathological process. As matter of fact, it is not easy to predict which kind of stroke patient will develop dementia before from the others. Certainly, the onset of PSD will be more rapid in those patients with the worst degree of clinical and cerebral involvement.

2.1.5 Pre-existing brain lesions in stroke patients

Silent infarcts, i.e. cerebral infarcts seen on CT or MRI scans that have never been associated with a relevant neurological deficit, are associated with an increased risk of dementia after stroke (Leys et al., 2005).

Their influence seems to increase according to the duration of the follow-up: in the Lille study, silent infarcts were associated with dementia after stroke at year 3 but (Henon et al., 2001) not at year 2, and in the Maastricht study silent infarcts were independently related to dementia after 12 months, but not after 1 or 6 months (Rasquin et al., 2004).

Stroke patients with associated previous silent infarcts seem to have a steeper decline in cognitive function than those without, but this decline might be confined to those with additional silent infarcts after base-line. Global cerebral atrophy is associated with a higher risk of dementia after stroke (Leys et al., 2005). MTLA is more frequent in stroke patients who have pre-existing dementia but it may also be present in non-demented stroke patients. MTLA clearly differentiates demented from non-demented patients after a first-ever ischemic stroke, even after exclusion of patients who had pre-stroke cognitive impairment (Leys et al., 2005).

Stroke patients with MTLA may have pre-clinical AD-BLD-FTD that is clinically revealed by stroke (Leys et al., 2005; Pasquier & Leys, 1997; Firbank et al., 2007). However, MTLA is not specific for AD-BLD-FTD, as it has also been observed in VaD (Leys et al., 2005). The presence and severity of leukoaraiosis are independent predictors of dementia after stroke (Leys et al., 2005), but there are many potential confounders, such as cerebral atrophy, more frequent in patients with leukoaraiosis, lacunar infarcts, which share a common pathogenesis with leukoaraiosis, and stroke recurrence, which is more frequent in stroke patients with leukoaraiosis (Leys et al., 2005). Microbleeds are frequent in stroke patients and especially those with intracerebral arteriolopathies (Cordonnier et al., 2007) and in patients with VaD, and to a lower degree AD (Cordonnier et al., 2006).

However, the question of their influence on the risk of post stroke dementia has never been systematically addressed. All these data confirm that the presence of previous brain injuries (vascular or neurodegenerative) is related to a higher risk to develop PSD, and their severity related to a more rapidly onset time. However, this "severity" may be not the NIHSS score or similar, but from one side the underlying "vessel disease" and from the other side the presence of subclinical neurodegenerative processes, or both, that is the overlap between AD and VaD, that is another intriguing issue influencing the time of onset of PSD. Vascular and degenerative dementias might be closer than previously thought, being dementia a spectrum which has only at the two extremities a "pure" degenerative type or a"pure" vascular one, while the majority of cases are definitely the results of different combinations of the two, always present. VaD and AD may thus be considered supplementary over the cognitive decline landscape. In conclusion, the debate about the vascular and neurodegenerative components of non-genetic AD is ongoing (Ivan et al., 2004).

To solve the diagnostic dilemma "is "Alzheimer's dementia" Alzheimer's disease, vascular dementia, or both?" (Roman et al., 1993), the first much needed step is a revision of the current diagnostic criteria for vascular dementia, in which the description of mixed forms of dementia appear to be inadequate.

2.1.6 The onset of Post Stroke Dementia according to time

Individuals with PSD are patients in whom stroke is only the epiphenomenon of an underlying long-acting vascular disease. Accordingly, stroke patients younger than 45 years show very few instances of PSD. This long-acting vascular disorder, affecting in particular the two inner layers of the vessel wall, may clinically occur with a wide range of clinical presentations.

Nevertheless, the mechanism that determine these different patterns of disease are not yet completely understood. This heterogeneity in clinical expression is probably related to genetic differences between individuals. As a matter of fact, in patients suffering from stroke, PSD would be determined by an underlying chronic cerebrovascular disease.

As a consequence, the time of onset of PSD would originate from the degree of severity of the abovementioned vascular disorder. In patients who have advanced chronic cerebrovascular disease, stroke would trigger the cognitive impairment and the time of onset of PSD will be extremely fast. On the other hand, in stroke patients with mild degree of "underlying" cerebrovascular disease, the risk of PSD will gradually increase over time, or be accelerated by the occurrence of subsequent single or multiple cerebrovascular events. In conclusion, with regard to vascular dementia and its various forms, it seems appropriate to say that the time of onset of PSD is closely linked to the severity of the impairment of the cerebral circulation. It has been shown that patients with global cerebral atrophy and MTLA may have pre-clinical AD clinically revealed by stroke (Leys et al., 2005).

There are several other significant predictors of PSD that are not related directly to the stroke itself, including increasing age, female sex, low education, race (increased in blacks, Hispanics and south-east Asians, and lower in Caucasians and Chinese), and leukoaraiosis. Most of these factors are also associated with AD-LBD-FTD. This, along with the fact that pre-stroke cognitive decline increases the risk of PSD, suggests an interaction between pre-existing degenerative pathology and stroke.

Neuropathological studies confirm that patients with AD pathology and cerebrovascular disease have a greater severity of cognitive impairment than those with similar severity of either pathology. Indeed, such "mixed" pathology is more common than either pure vascular or degenerative pathology. Vascular mechanisms may be important in the development of AD-BLD-FTD pathology: vascular risk factors are risk factors for AD-BLD-FTD also and cerebral hypoperfusion and microcirculatory changes may be a precursor of the neuropathological and clinical changes. In fact, it has been argued that there might be a pathogenic role of vascular disease in the basic phenomena of neuronal degeneration. The synthesis of these assumptions is called "Vascular Hypothesis of Alzheimer's disease" (de La Torre, 2011). According to this theory, AD would be primarily a vascular disease. Thus, "classical" cardiovascular risk factors would also be risk factors for AD, and neuronal degeneration would only be the result of an "energy crisis" of genetically predisposed neuronal populations. Several studies suggest that cerebral hypoperfusion is one of the earliest pathological signs in the development of cognitive failure (de la Torre, 2000). This phenomenon is more evident in the elderly, having already a dwindling cerebrovascular reserve due to advancing age. Other vascular risk factors may contribute to further decline in cerebral blood flow, resulting in unrelenting brain hypoperfusion. Brain hypoperfusion, in turn, can reach a critical threshold giving rise to a neuronal energy crisis via reduced ATP synthesis (Lassen et al., 1991). The ensuing metabolic energy crisis initially carves up ischemic-sensitive neurons in the hippocampus and posterior parietal cortex setting up cognitive meltdown and progressive neurodegenerative and later atrophic changes in the brain. Neuronal energy compromise accelerates oxidative stress, excess production of reactive oxygen species, aberrant protein synthesis, ionic membrane pump dysfunction, signal transduction impairment, neurotransmitter failure, abnormal processing of amyloid precursor protein resulting in beta-amyloid deposition and axonal microtubule disruption from tau hyperphosphorylation (de La Torre, 2002). Lenzi and Altieri investigated factors that might contribute to the development of delayed PSD and to the definition of its clinical presentation. 191 patients who were dementia-free 6 months after stroke were enrolled (Altieri et al., 2004). Dementia was diagnosed according to the ICD-10 criteria (Altieri et al., 2004), while ethiologic diagnoses followed the National Institute of Neurological and Communicative Disorders and Stroke and the Alzheimer's Disease and Related Disorders Associations (NINCDS–ADRA) for AD (McKhann et al., 1984), and the NINDS–AIREN group for VaD (Altieri et al., 2004). About 21% of patients developed delayed PSD during the 4-year follow up. This finding confirmed data reported in previous studies showing that dementia is a frequent consequence of stroke and that the risk of dementia development, though higher in the very short period after stroke, remains important in the long term (Desmond et al., 1996 ; Desmond et al., 2000 ; Barba et al., 2004 ; Henon et al., 1997). Further, Lenzi and Altieri (Lenzi & Altieri, 2007) excluded patients with pre-stroke dementia, known to markedly increase the incidence of PSD (Barba et al., 2004; Henon et al., 1997).

The clinical differentiation of delayed PSD yielded some intriguing results. Although the incidence of new cases of dementia was constant throughout the 4-year follow up, the cognitive pattern shifted from a predominant AD-BLD-FTD with cerebrovascular disease type in the first 2 years, and to a typical VaD type later on.

In this view, the time interval between stroke and dementia onset might be crucial as a means of differentiating between its ethiopathological subtypes: PSD which develops up to 15–20 months after stroke onset might present the clinical characteristics of the so-called "mixed dementia" arising from the unmasking effect of the vascular lesion on a previous degenerative process; subsequently, PSD may be due to the anatomical disruption of cortical relays and connections with other cortical or deeper structures, or to the cumulative effect of the new lesion which disrupts a previous functioning equilibrium (Tatemichi et al., 1990; Mungas et al., 2001 ; Mungas et al., 2002 ; Fein et al., 2000).

Let us remember that functional studies have shown that vascular patients may compensate for cognitive impairments by increasing both the number and the regional perfusion of activated areas. This last mechanism seems to be less effective and may, consequently, become inadequate after a new vascular event (Di Piero et al., 2001).

Both these mechanisms need a background of unimpaired neuronal network, and cannot be fully operative in presence of initial neurodegenerative processes. At present, is unclear if the interaction between stroke and degenerative pathology develop the unmasking previous degenerative changes, or whether there is a synergistic effect of stroke, perhaps through widespread synaptic or perfusional changes, that accelerates existing degenerative processes.

We can intuitively conclude that the presence of an underlying AD-BLD-FTD can dramatically influence the time onset of PSD. Therefore, individuals with AD-BLD-FTD will develop PSD much faster than those without AD-BLD-FTD. This event will occur both if the AD-BLD-FTD neuropathological changes are already evident, or when stroke represents the triggering event of an undiagnosed pathological condition.

3. Conclusion

Until recently, the term vascular disease was considered synonymous of atherosclerosis. Nowadays, scientific evidences show that atherosclerosis and its acute and chronic consequences could be only one of the possible manifestations of a more complex vascular disorder.

Probably, genetic differences allow the existence of a wide range of clinical expressions, in the context of a similar pathological process. First of all, we can recognize some individuals with a predominant "classical" vascular disorder; in these patients, the classical cardiovascular risk factors such as hypercholesterolemia, diabetes, hypertension and so on could lead to the genesis and development of the atherosclerotic plaque, which is the major target for the current strategies of prevention and treatment of the aterosclerothic disease.

In fact, in the largest part of cases, the aim of the modern medicine is to decrease the prevalence and the incidence of the acute and chronic cardio-cerebro-vascular consequences of this pathological process. The cognitive impairment of these patients manifests as VaD. We can also recognize another group of patients without the aforementioned "classical" vascular disorder.

These individuals are probably affected by a silent but persistent vascular disease, which could similarly lead to dramatic consequences. In these individuals, cardiovascular risk factors don't determine the development of atherosclerosis, but could cause a chronic brain hypoperfusion, responsible for the beginning and the progression of neuronal degeneration. The cognitive impairment of these patients manifests as AD-BLD-FTD. It could be speculated that vascular and degenerative dementias might be closer than previously thought, being dementia a spectrum which has only at the two extremities a "pure" degenerative type or a "pure" vascular one, while the majority of cases are definitely the results of different combinations of the two, always present.

VaD and AD may thus be considered supplementary over the cognitive decline landscape. However, their borders show an extensive and variable representation.

Nowadays, PSD is not considered as a specific entity requiring specific treatment. Patients with PSD are together patients with dementia and with stroke. Current guidelines for stroke prevention should be applied, but the specific issue of secondary prevention of stroke in patients with dementia (either pre-existing or new-onset dementia) is not addressed in any guidelines.

It has been proposed that lowering of blood pressure could, in theory, reduce the incidence of cognitive decline because of reduction in stroke recurrence rates and indirect effects on the anticipation of the clinical onset of AD-BLD-FTD (Pasquier & Leys, 1997): accordingly several controlled trials showed a beneficial effect of lowering blood pressure on the risk of dementia (Tzourio et al., 2003; Forette et al., 1998).

A symptomatic approach to dementia syndrome is necessary, depending on the presumed cause (AD-BLD-FTD, VaD or mixed). There have been no trials specifically done in PSD. However, both AD-BLD-FTD and VaD share a cholinergic deficit, and both disorders show some improvement when treated with cholinesterase inhibitors. Patients with AD-BLD-FTD and with vascular risk factors receive greater symptomatic benefits than patients with pure AD after short term treatment with rivastigmine, an inhibitor of acetylcholinesterase and butyrilcholinesterase. The additional apparent benefits on disease progression detected in patients with hypertension and AD might be linked to drug effects on cerebrovascular factors. These findings could have an important effect on the way cholinesterase inhibitors are prescribed.

In conclusion, the time of onset may be an important variable in the evaluation of patients with PSD. Currently, together with other conventional diagnostic techniques, it will provide us some useful details on the degree of cerebral impairment in the subject under examination. In addition, it is a very attractive starting point for research. For these reasons, the authors suggest to give more consideration at the time of onset in PSD evaluation criteria, in order to better stratify patients' risk and to improve the state of knowledge regarding this dramatic pathology

4. Acknowledgment

The authors would like to thank all the the staff of the Clinica Neurologica A, Department of Neurology and Psychiatry and Department of Cardiovascular, Respiratory, Nephrological and Geriatric Sciences of "Sapienza" University of Rome. All authors were involved in the selection of relevant papers of this chapter and for the drafting of specific sections.

5. References

Aevarsson O., Svanborg A., Skoog I., (1998). Seven-year survival rate after age 85 years: relation to Alzheimer disease and vascular dementia. *Arch Neurol*; 55: 1226-32.

Alexander M., Freedman M., (1984). Amnesia after anterior communicating artery aneurysm rupture. *Neurology*; 34: 752-57.

Altieri M., Di Piero V., Pasquini M., et al., (2004). Delayed poststroke dementia: a 4 year follow-up study. *Neurology*; 62: 2193-97.

Baldareschi M., Di Carlo A., Maggi S., et al., (1999). Dementia is a major predictor of death among the Italian elderly: ILSA Working Group, Italian Longitudinal Study on Aging. *Neurology*; 52:709-13.

Ballard C., Rowan E., Stephens S., Kalaria R., Kenny RA, (2003). Prospective follow-up study between 3 and 15 months after stroke. *Stroke*; 34: 2440–5.

Ballard C.G., Burton E.J., Barber R. et al., (2004). NINDS AIREN neuroimaging criteria do not distinguish stroke patients with and without dementia. *Neurology*; 63: 983-88.

Barba R., Martinez-Espinosa S., Rodriguez-Garcia E., Pondal M., Vivancos J., Del Ser T., (2000). Poststroke dementia: clinical features and risk factors. *Stroke*; 31: 1494-501.

Barba R., Morin M.D., Caemillan C., Delgado C., Domingo J., Del Ser T., (2002). Previous and incident dementia as risk factors for mortality in stroke patients. *Stroke*; 33: 1993-98.

Benson D.F., Cummings J.L., (1982). Angular gyrus syndrome simulating Alzheimer's Disease (1992). *Arch Neurol*; 39: 616-20

Bhatia K.P., Marsden C.D., (1994). The behavioural and motor consequences of local lesions of the basal ganglia in the man. *Brain*; 117: 859-76.

Bornstein N.M., Gur A.Y., Treves T.A., et al., (1996). Do silent brain infarctions predict the development of dementia after first ischemic stroke? *Stroke*; 27: 904-05.

Chui H.C., Victoroff J.I., Margolin D., Jagust W., Shankle R., Katzman R., (1992). Criteria for the diagnosis of ischemic vascular dementia proposed by the State of California Alzheimer's Disease Diagnostic and Treatment Centers. *Neurology*; 42: 473 -80.

Cordoliani Mackowiak M.A., Henon H., Pruvo J.P., Pasquier F., Leys D., (2003). Poststroke dementia: influence of hippocampal atrophy. *Arch Neurol*; 60: 585-90.

Cordonnier C., van der Flier W.M., Sluimer J.D., Leys D., Barkhof F., Scheltens P., (2006). Prevalence and severity of microbleeds in a memory clinic setting. *Neurology*; 66: 1356–60.

Cordonnier C., Al-Shahi Salman R., Wardlaw J., (2007). Spontaneous brain microbleeds: systematic review, subgroup analyses and standards for study design and reporting. *Brain*; 130: 1988–2003.

Corea F., Henon H., Pasquier F., Leys D., (2001). Silent infarcts in stroke patients: patients characteristics and effect on 2-year outcome. *J Neurol*; 248: 271-78.

de La Torre J.C., (2000). Critically attained threshold of cerebral hypoperfusion: the CATCH hypothesis of Alzheimer's Disease. *Neurobiol Aging*; 21 (2): 331-42.

de La Torre J.C., (2002). Alzheimer disease as a vascular disorder: nosological evidence. *Stroke*; 33: 1152–62.

de La Torre J.C., (2010). Vascular risk factor detection and control may prevent Alzheimer's Disease. *Aging Res Rev*; 9: 218-25.

de La Torre J.C., (2011). The Vascular Hypothesis of Alzheimer's Disease: bench to bedside and beyond. *Neurodegener Dis.*; 7: 116-21.

Desmond D.W., Moroney J.T., Sano M., Stern Y., (1996). Recovery of cognitive function after stroke. Stroke; 27 (10): 1798–803.

Desmond D.W., Moroney J.T., Paik M.C., et al., (2000). Frequency and clinical determinants of dementia after ischemic stroke. *Neurology*; 54: 1124-31.

Desmond D.W., Moroney J.T., Sano M., Stern Y., (2002). Mortality in patients with dementia after ischemic stroke. *Neurology*; 59: 537-43.

Di Piero V., Giannini M., Bragoni M., Vicenzini E., Di Legge S., Altieri M., et al., (2001). Vascular dementia: a cognitive SPET–CBF activation study. *Cerebrovasc Dis*; 12: 52–8.

Esiri M.M., Nagy Z., Smith M.Z., Barnetson L., Smith A.D., (1999). Cerebrovascular disease and threshold for dementia in the early stages of Alzheimer's disease. *Lancet*; 354 (September 11 (9182)): 919–20.

Fein G., Di Sclafani V., Tanabe J. et al., (2000). Hippocampal and cortical atrophy predict dementia in subcortical ischemic vascular disease. *Neurology*; 55: 1626-35.

Ferrer I., (2010). Cognitive impairment of vascular origin: Neuropathology of cognitive impairment of vascular origin. *J Neurol Sciences*; 299: 139-149.

Firbank M.J., Burton E.J., Barber R., et al., (2007). Medial temporal atrophy rather than white matter hyperintensities predict cognitive decline in stroke survivors. *Neurobiol Aging*; 28: 1664–9.

Forette F., Seux M.L., Staessen J.A., et al., (1998). Prevention of dementia in randomized double-blind placebo-controlled systolic hypertension in Europe (Syst-Eur) trial. *Lancet*; 352: 1347-51.

Gold G., Kovari E., Herrmann F.R., Canuto A., Hof P.R., Michel J.P., et al., (2005). Cognitive consequences of thalamic, basal ganglia, and deep white matter lacunes in brain aging and dementia. *Stroke*; 36: 1184–8.

Gurwitz J.H., Monette J., Rochon P.A., Eckler M.A., Avorn J., (1997). Atrial fibrillation and stroke prevention with warfarin in long term care setting. *Arch Intern Med*; 157: 974-78.

Hankey G.J., Warlow C.P., (1999). Treatment and secondary prevention of stroke: evidence, costs and effects on individuals and population. *Lancet*; 354; 1457–63.

Helmer C., Joly P., Letenneur L., Commenges D., Dartigues J.F., (2001). Mortality with dementia: results from a French prospective community based cohort. *Am J Epidemiology*; 154: 642-48.

Henon H., Godefroy O., Leys D. et al., (1995). Early predictors of death and disability after acute cerebral ischemic event. *Stroke*; 26: 392-98.

Henon H., Pasquier F., Durieu I., Godefroy O., Lucas C., Lebert F., et al., (1997). Preexisting dementia in stroke patients. Baseline frequency, associated factors, and outcome. *Stroke*; 28: 2429–36.

Henon H., Pasquier F., Durieu I., Pruvo J.P., Leys D., (1998). Medial temporal lobe atrophy in stroke patients: relation to pre-existing dementia. *J Neurol Neurosurg Psychiatry*; 68: 641-47.

Henon H., Lebert F., Durieu I., Godefroy O., Lucas C., Pasquier F., et al., (1999). Confusional state in stroke: relation to preexisting dementia, patient characteristics, and outcome. *Stroke*; 30: 773–9.

Henon H., Durieu I., Guerouaou D., Lebert F., Pasquier F., Leys D., (2001). Poststroke dementia: incidence and relationship to prestroke cognitive decline. *Neurology*; 57: 1216-22.

Henon H., Vroylandt P., Durieu I., Pasquier F., Leys D., (2003). Leukoarariosis more than dementia is a predictor of stroke recurrence. *Stroke*; 34: 2935-40.

Ivan C.S., Seshadri S., Beiser A. et al., (2004). Dementia after stroke: the Framingham Study. *Stroke*; 35: 1264-68.

Jobst K.A., Barnetson L.P., Stephsone B.J., (1998). Accurate prediction of histologically confirmed Alzheimer's Disease and the differential diagnosis of dementia: the use of NINCDS-ADRDA and DSM-III-R criteria, spect, X-ray CT and Apo E4 in medial temporal lobe dementias. Oxford Project to Investigate Memory and Aging. *Int Psychogeriatr*; 10: 271-302.

Jokinen H., Kalska H., Ylikoski R., et al., (1996). Medial temporal lobe atrophy and memory deficits in elderly stroke patients. *Eur J Neurol*; 11: 825-32.

Kokmen E., Whisnant J.P., O'Fallon W.M., Chu C.P., Beard C.M., (1996). Dementia after ischemic stroke: a population-based study in Rochester, Minnesota (1960-1984). *Neurology*; 46: 154-59.

Knecht S., Oelschlager C., Duning T., et al. (2008). Atrial fibrillation in stroke-free patients is associated with memory impairment and hippocampal atrophy. *Eur Heart J*: 29.

Krumholz H.M., Radford M.J., Ellerbeck E.F., et al., (1996). Aspirin for secondary prevention after acute myocardial infarction in the elderly: prescribed use and outcomes. *Ann Intern Med*; 124: 292-98.

Lassen N.A., Lenzi G.L., Fieschi C., (1991). Ischemic penumbra and neuronal death comments on the therapeutic window. *Cerebovasc. Dis.* ; 1: 32-35.

Lenzi G.L., Altieri M., (2007). Short term evolution as a marker of vascular dementia versus Alzheimer's Disease. *J. Neurol. Sciences*; 257:182-184.

Leys D., Bandu I., Henon H., et al., (2002). Clinical outcome in 287 consecutive young adults (15 to 45 years) with ischemic stroke. *Neurology*; 59: 26-33.

Leys D., Henon H., Mackowiak-Cordoliani M.A., Pasquier F., (2005). Poststroke dementia. *Lancet Neurol*;4:752–9.

Lin J.H., Lin R.T., Tai C.T., Hsieh C.L., Hsiao S.F., Liu C.K., (2003). Prediction of post-stroke dementia. *Neurology*; 61: 343-48.

Linden T., Skoog I., Fagerberg B., Steen B., Blomstrand C., (2004). Cognitive impairment and dementia 20 months after stroke. *Neuroepidemiology*; 23: 45-52.

Liu H., Xing A., Wang X., Liu G., Li L., (2011). Regulation of Beta-amyloid level in the brain of rats with cerebrovascular hypoperfusion. *Neurobiol. Aging*; Aug.1 (Epub ahead of print).

Mackowiak-Cordoliani M.A., Bombois S., Memin A., Henon H., Pasquier F., (2005) Post stroke dementia in the elderly. *Drugs Aging*; 22: 483-93.

Madureira S., Guerreiro M., Ferro J.M., (2001). Dementia and cognitive impairment three months after stroke. *Eur J Neurol*; 8: 621-27.

McKhann G., Drachman D., Folstein M., Katzman R., Price D., Stadlan E.M., (1984). Clinical diagnosis of Alzheimer's disease: report of the NINCDS- ADRDAWork Group under the auspices of Department of Health and Human Services Task Force on Alzheimer's Disease. *Neurology*; 34: 939–44.

Moroney J.T., Bagiella E., Tatemichi T.K., Paik M.C., Stern Y., Desmond D.W., (1997). Dementia after stroke increases the risk of long-term stroke recurrence. *Neurology*; 48:1317-25.

Mok V.C., Wong A., Lam W.W., et al., (2004). Cognitive impairment and functional outcome after stroke associated with small vessel disease. *J Neurol Neurosurg Psychiatry*; 75: 560-66.

Mok V.C., Chang C., Wong A., et al., (2005). Neuroimaging determinants of cognitive performances in stroke associated with small vessel disease. *J Neuroimaging*; 15: 129-37.

Mungas D., Jagust W.J., Reed B.R., Kramer J.H., Weiner M.W., Schuff N., et al., (2001). MRI predictors of cognition in subcortical ischemic vascular disease and Alzheimer's disease. *Neurology*; 57: 2229–35.

Mungas D., Reed B.R., Jagust W.J., DeCarli C., Mack W.J., Kramer J.H., et al., (2002). Volumetric MRI predicts rate of cognitive decline related to Ad and cerebrovascular disease. *Neurology*; 59: 867–73.

Murray C.J., Lopez A.D., (1997). Global mortality, disability and the contribution of risk factors: Global burden of disease study; *Lancet*; 349: 1436–42.

Nagy Z., Esiri M., Jobst K.A., et al., (1997). The effects of additional pathology on the cognitive deficits in Alzheimer disease. *J Neuropathol Exp Neurol*; 56:165-70

Nys G.M.,Van Zandvoort M.J., De Kort P.L., et al., (2005). Domain-specific cognitive recovery after first-ever stroke: a follow-up study of 111 cases. *J Int Neuropsychol Soc*; 11(7): 795–806.

O'Brien J.T., Erkinjuntti T., Reisberg B., Roman G., Sawada T., Pantoni L., et al., (2003). Vascular cognitive impairment. *Lancet Neurol*; 2: 89–98.

Ott A., Breteler M.M., de Bruyne M.C., van Harskamp F., Grobbee D.E., Hofman A., (1997). Atrial fibrillation and dementia in a population-based study. The Rotterdam Study. *Stroke*; 28(2): 316–21.

Pakrasi S., O'Brien J.T., (2005). Emission Tomography in dementia. *Nucl Med Commun*; 26: 189-96.

Pasquier F., Leys D., (1997). Why are stroke patients prone to develop dementia? *J Neurology*; 244: 135-42.

Pendlebury S.T., (2009) Stroke-related dementia: Rates, risk factors and implications for future research. *Maturitas*; 64: 165–171.

Prencipe M., Ferretti C., Casini A.R., Santini M., Giubilei F., Culasso F., (1997). *Stroke*; 28:531-36.

Pohjasvaara T., Erkinjuntti T., Vataja R., Kaste M., (1997). Dementia three months after stroke: baseline frequency and effect of different definitions of dementia in the Helsinki Stroke Aging Memory Study (SAM) cohort. *Stroke*; 28: 785-92.

Pohjasvaara T., Erkinjuntti T., Ylikoski R., Hietanen M., Vataja R., Kaste M., (1998). Clinical determinants of poststroke dementia. *Stroke*; 29: 75-81.

Pohjasvaara T., Mantyla R., Salonen O. et al., (2000). MRI correlates of dementia after first clinical ischemic stroke. *J Neurol Sci*; 181: 111-17.

Rasquin S.M., Verhey F.R., van Oostenbrugge R.J., Lousberg R., Lodder J., (2004). Demographic and CT scan features related to cognitive impairment in the first year after stroke. *J Neurol Neurosurg Psychiatry*; 75: 1562-67.

Rockwood K., Ebly E., Hachinski V., Hogan D., (1997). Presence and treatment of vascular risk factors in patients with vascular cognitive impairment (1997). *Arch Neurol*; 54: 33-39.

Rockwood K., Cosway S., Carver D., Jarrett P., Standyk K., Fisk J., (1999). The risk of dementia and death after delirium. *Age Aging*; 28:551–6.
Roman G.C., Tatemichi T.K., Erkinjuntti T., Cummings J.L., Masdeu J.C., Garcia J.H., et al., (1993). Vascular dementia: diagnostic criteria for research studies. Report of the NINDS–AIREN International Workshop. *Neurology*; 43: 250–60.
The international classification of diseases, 10th revision (ICD-10) (1989). Geneva, Switzerland: *World Health Organization*; p. 25–31.
Roman G.C., Royall D.R., (2004). A diagnostic dilemma: is "Alzheimer's dementia" Alzheimer's disease, vascular dementia, or both? *Lancet Neurol*; 3: 141.
Roth M., (1955). The natural history of mental disorder in old age. *J Ment Sci*; 101:281-301.
Rotwell P.M., Coull A.J., Giles M.F., et al., (2004).Change in stroke incidence, mortality, case fatality, severity and risk factors in Oxfordshire, UK from 1981 to 2004: Oxford Vascular Study. *Lancet*; 363: 1925–33.
Rothwell P.M., Coull A.J., Silver L.E., et al., (2005). Population-based study of event-rate, incidence, case fatality, and mortality for all acute vascular events in all arterial territories (Oxford Vascular Study). *Lancet*; 366 (9499): 1773–83.
Royall D.R., (2002). Alzheimer disease as a vascular disorder: nosological evidence. *Stroke*; 33: 2147–8.
Snowdon D.A., Greiner L.H., Mortimer J..A, Riley K.P., Greiner P.A., Markesbery W.R., (1997). Brain infarction and the clinical expression of Alzheimer disease. The Nun Study. *JAMA*; 277: 813–7.
Tang W.K., Chan S.S., Chiu H.F. et al., (2004). Frequency an determinants of prestroke dementia in a Chinese court. *J Neurol*; 251: 604-08.
Tatemichi T.K., Foulkes M.A., Mohr J.P., Hewitt J.R., Hier D.B., Price T.R.,et al., (1990). Dementia in stroke survivors in the Stroke Data Bank cohort. Prevalence, incidence, risk factors, and computed tomographic findings. *Stroke*; 21: 858–66.
Tatemichi T.K., Desmond D.W., Mayeux R., et al., (1992). Dementia after stroke: baseline frequency, risks and clinical features in a hospitalized cohort. *Neurology*; 42: 1185-93.
Tatemichi T.K., Desmond D.W., Paik M., et al., (1993). Clinical determinants of dementia related to stroke. *Ann Neurol*; 33: 568-75.
Tatemichi T.K., Pail M., Bagiella E., et al., (1994). Risk of dementia after stroke in a hospitalized cohort: results of a longitudinal study. Neurology; 44:1885-91.
Tham W., Auchus A.P., Thong M., Goh M.L., Chang H.M., Wong M.C., et al., (2002). Progression of cognitive impairment after stroke: one year results from a longitudinal study of Singaporean stroke patients. *J Neurol Sci*; 15(203–204): 49–52.
Tzourio C., Anderson C., Chapman N. et al., (2003). Effects of blood pressure lowering with perindopril and indapamide therapy on dementia and cognitive decline in patients with cerebrovascular disease. *Arch Intern Med*; 163: 1069-75.
Vermeer S.E., Prins N.D., den Heijer T., Hofman A., Koudstaal P.J., Breteler M.M., (2003). Silent brain infarcts and the risk of dementia and cognitive decline. *N Engl J Med*; 27(348) :1215–22.
Woo J., Kay R., Yuen Y.K., Nicholls M.G., (1992). Factors influencing long-term survival and disability among three month stroke survivors. *Neuroepidemiology*; 11: 143-50.
Zhang T., Pan B.S., Zhao B., Zhang L.M., Huang Y.L., Sun F.Y., (2009). Exacerbation of poststroke dementia by type 2 diabetes is associated with synergistic increases of betasecretase activation and beta-amyloid generation in rat brains. *Neuroscience*: 17.
Zhu L., Fratiglioni L., Guo Z., Winblad B., Viitanen M., (2000). Incidence of stroke in relation to cognitive function and dementia in the Kungsholmen Project. *Neurology*; 54(11): 2103–7.

13

Stroke, Epidemiological and Genetical Approach

Sellama Nadifi and Khalil Hamzi
Laboratory of Genetics and Molecular Pathology,
Faculty of Medicine and Pharmacy,
University Hassan II Casablanca
Morocco

1. Introduction

Current knowledge in genetics has began increasingly to reveal the complexity of the interaction between various risk factors. The purpose of this chapter is to present knowledge about stroke, particularly the role of genetic components as risk factors.

Despite remarkable progress in the recent years in the field of the management and treatment of Cerebral Vascular Accident (stroke), the latter remains a major cause of mortality and morbidity in many countries. In fact, it is admitted that even though the majority of strokes has been not fatal sofar, it has often been responsible for functional deficits (motor, visual and cognitive). Stroke is very common in industrialized countries (Casas J et al, 2007) and is the third leading cause of death in North America, Japan and China (Xiao Yuxin et al, 2009) (Table 1). The annual incidence in Canada is about 1/1000, and soars to 10/1000 after age 65. This incidence is much higher in Europe, (7/1000 in France, 5.6/1000 in Portugal) (Roshan Ariyaratnam et al, 2007) (Table 2).

Population	Stroke deaths Per 100 000 Population	Year of Publication *
Spain	39.2	2005
France	27.7	2006
Italy	31.9	2006
Portugal	96.1	1999
Germany	34.5	2006
Japan	56.3	2007
China	160.1	2000
Korea	93.1	2006

Table 1. International Death Rates of Stroke (Donald Lloyd-Jones et al. 2009).

Population	Stroke Incidence Per 1000	Publication*
UK	1.8	Alexander H et al, 2000
France	7.6	Lemesle M et al, 1999
Italy	2.7	Carolei A et al, 1997
Portugal	5.6	Correia M et al 2004
Germany	3.5	Kolominsky-Rabas PL et al 1998
Sweden	3.1	Johansson B et al 2000

Table 2. Stroke incidence study in Europe (Truelsen T. et al, 2006.)

In developing countries, this incidence is less well known due to the lack of adequate management of stroke patients. However, the data currently available show a frequency similar to those reported in some industrialized countries (Fig 1). They illustrate clearly that stroke is a major public health problem (Table 3). In Morocco, the incidence of stroke is estimated to 0.4 /1000 with 25% of death cases *(Stroke colloquium 2009.*

Population	Incidence Per 1000
Kuwait	0.8
Saudi Arabia	0.9
Bahrain	0.4
Qatar	0.4
Libya	0.65
Tunisia	0.54

Table 3. Stroke incidence study in Arab countries. (Hani TS Benamer et al, 2009)

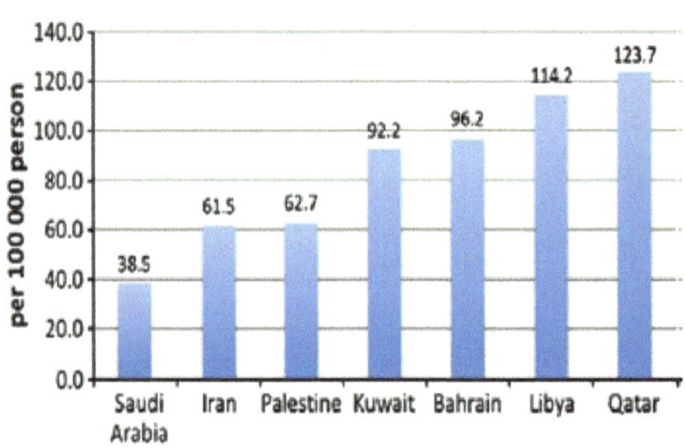

Fig. 1. Incidence rates of stroke in the Middle East and north of Africa (Tran J et al 2010)

1.1 Definition and types of stroke

Stroke is defined by the World Health Organization (WHO), on the basis of a clinical and pathophysiological approach, as "a rapid installation of neurological deficit, with symptoms lasting 24 hours or more, associated to focal or global cerebral dysfunction, that can be fatal, and the apparent cause of which is vascular" (Asplund et al, 1988). This definition encompasses a broad category of strokes:

Ischemic stroke: accounts for 80% of all strokes (M. Dichgans, 2007)
Hemorrhagic stroke (20% of all strokes) (AG Thrift, 2001),
Brain blood vessels disorders.
Ischemic strokes are related to a complete or incomplete lack of blood supply. They include ischemic stroke (AIC) and transient ischemic attack (TIA).

Stroke is thought of as a syndrome which represents a collection of disease processes all of which resulting in cerebral ischaemia. The different processes have different clinical phenotypes and different etiological mechanisms. Many symptoms can occur in stroke but not simultaneously. They depend on stroke localization in the brain and on vascular damage (Table 4).

SYMPTOMS	MANIFESTATIONS
Cognitive Disturbance	For many people, a clinical stroke elicits symptoms involving cognition. If one were to suffer a stroke, they may begin to feel dizzy or lightheaded. They may also suffer a loss of coordination, have trouble forming sentences or even lose consciousness.
Vocal Disturbance	Besides having a difficulty with words and sentences, it is also possible for a stroke to impede one's ability to speak, causing them to slur or garble their words.
Visual Disturbance	For others, a stroke causes some sort of visual disturbance, including a blurred, doubled or darkened vision. These may either be momentary or prolonged.
Mobility Issues	Sometimes, a stroke causes sudden mobility issues, triggering a paralysis or numbness to either the right or left side of the body.
Headaches	Though a headache alone is not a sure sign one is having a stroke, it is one of the common symptoms, especially when accompanied by pain or stiffness within the neck and face as well as digestive distress.
Digestive Distress	Often associated with the symptom of a headache, a stroke can cause one to experience a sudden nausea that often triggers vomiting.

Table 4. Clinical Stroke Symptoms (American Society of Neurology, 2007)

The International Classification TOAST (Table 5), classified strokes into five groups based on etiologic mechanisms (Adams et al, 1993). A subtype classification has been recommended for genetic association studies (Dichgans et al, 2005). Increasing evidence suggests that different subtypes of stroke may have both different degrees of heritability and genetic risk factor profiles.

Etiology	Caractéristique	REF
Atherosclerosis	The arteries of large and medium caliber seats of choice: the origin of the internal carotid artery, the carotid siphon, the origin and termination of the vertebral artery and the aortic arch.	(Markus et al 2001).
Lacunar Stroke	Occlusion of these arteries is responsible for brain deficiencies (small deep infarct <1.5 cm in diameter). They are located in the subcortical areas, mainly in the basal ganglia, capsules, and the brain stem). It has been suggested as an explanation to the thrombosis process, an overactive clotting in predisposed patients or an abnormality in blood vessels.	(Ward et Brown, 2002
Cardioembolic Stroke	Heart diseases that can cause embolic ischemic stroke are numerous. Atrial fibrillation is the heart disease most commonly involved (50% of cases), followed by ischemic heart disease and valvular heart disease.	(Warlow et al 2001
Indefined Stroke	Many other conditions may be responsible for stroke such as arterial dissection, arterial different nature dysplastic, inflammatory or infectious diseases or blood clotting abnormalities	(Milandre et al 1998).

Table 5. Stroke international Classification TOAST (Dichgans, 2004).

1.2 Stroke pathophysiology

In the medical literature, the term stroke refers to different events with a common pathophysiology, associated to subclinical atherosclerosis, or thromboembolic disease (MTE). As a multifactorial disease, stroke results from the synergistic combination of several risk factors, some of which are still unknown. (Fig 2)

In ischemic strokes, reduced blood flow causes a set of events that influence the severity of cerebral infarction (Lawrence R. Wechsler et al, 2011). These events are the result of interaction between vascular and cellular elements which lead to the release of amino acid neurotransmitters and to the increase in circulating calcium and free radicals. In addition, oxidative stress and inflammation contribute to the process of cellular damage and ischemia. These events have contributed to the emergence of the new concept "neurovascular unit" including astrocytes, neurons and vascular structure.

Studies of the experimental model and the analysis of brain imaging showed that brain damage depends on the infarction's duration. Thus, the areas affected by the infarct remain viable for 24 hours with the possibility of recovery after revascularization.

A phenotypic complexity is added with a gene-gene, gene-environment interactions component. The identification of environmental and genetic factors that predispose to stroke is a major research target for a better understanding of the pathophysiological mechanisms of the disease and for modulating its prevention and treatment.

1.3 Risk factors

1.3.1 The traditional risk factors

Age is the most important risk factor. The incidence of stroke doubles in men and women after 55 years of age (Wolfe 2000; Yannick Bejot, 2007). Smoking appears to increase the risk of stroke (MP Jones, 1990; Anthony Behin, 2002). However, this risk is reversible after 5 years of cessation. Tobacco may act through different mechanisms including endothelial cytotoxicity, mitogenic effect on the media, platelet activation, blood hyperviscosity, and lowering HDL blood rates (Bhat, VM, 2008). Alcohol increases the risk of hemorrhagic (relative risk × 6) or ischemic stroke (relative risk × 3) (Lowenfels, Albert B., 2000, Hart C, 1999). In addition, dietary factors play a role as well. A diet high in cholesterol, saturated fat and low in fruits, vegetables and fish increases the risk of stroke (Brigham and Women's Hospital. 2005), while a large consumption of vitamin C and folate would reduce its impact by an anti-oxidant effect and the reduction of homocysteine concentration. (Homocysteine Lowering Trialists' Collaboration, 1998). Studies, cohort and case-control, demonstrated that lack of exercise is associated with an increased risk of stroke. Such an effect could act, at least partially, by reducing blood pressure. (Chong Do Lee, 2003). Ethnicity: it is admitted that there is a genetic and environmental heterogeneity between races (Jun Z. Li, 2008, Neil Risch, 2002). Significant differences in incidence and stroke subtypes distribution have been reported among different ethnic groups (Dawn M. Bravata, 2005). The incidence is greater among African Americans and African Caribbeans versus Caucasians in the United Kingdom (Gillum et al, 1999). Personal or familial history is the best documented risk factor. In fact, the familial forms of stroke have been known since a long time (Voetsch B et al. 2003; Hassan A, 2002). The risk of stroke is higher in people with family history. (Duanping Liao, 1997). Hypertension is a major risk factor, it is present in 40-85% of patients with cerebral infarction and in 80% of those with a cerebral hematoma (Hu G, Sarti C, 2005) regardless of sex and age (Collins et MacMahon, 1994; Niclot P, 2003; HironoriImano, 2009) Similarly, diabetes mellitus increases by 2-5 the risk of stroke (B Stegmayr, 1995) (Mats Eliasson, 2003, Hu G, 2005, A Rautio, 2008). The increase in total cholesterol and low density lipoprotein (LDL-C) was strongly correlated with the risk of ischemic heart disease. (Toth PP , 2005).

1.3.2 The emerging risk factors

A number of case-control studies have shown an association between infection and acute ischemic stroke (Grau et al. 1995; IY Bova, 1996; Benoît Guillon, 2003; A. Paganini-Hill, 2003). The association is not specific to a particular type of infection resulting in a prothrombotic state and acute endothelial dysfunction (HC Emsley, 2008). Many cross-sectional and prospective studies have shown that chronic inflammation is a risk factor and suggest to assess this risk by measuring C-reactive protein and proteins of the inflammatory reaction (PIR), (Danesh et al. 2000, Ridker et al. 2000). This systematic search does not meet the consensus of professionals (Fifth Conference of the American Heart Association '(AHA) (Pearson et al, 2004). Other factors including psychosocial factors and some hormonal treatments have been implicated. Currently, there is a recent increasing interest in adhesion molecules such as the vascular endothelial growth factor (VEGF). It is one of the main factors controlling the development and maintenance of the vascular system in humans (angiogenesis). Indeed, high levels of circulating VEGF have been observed in cases of ischemic diseases such as stroke [Hojo et al. 2000; Blann et al, 2002). Currently targeted therapies, using VEGF, are undergoing clinical trials (Buysschaert et al, 2007).

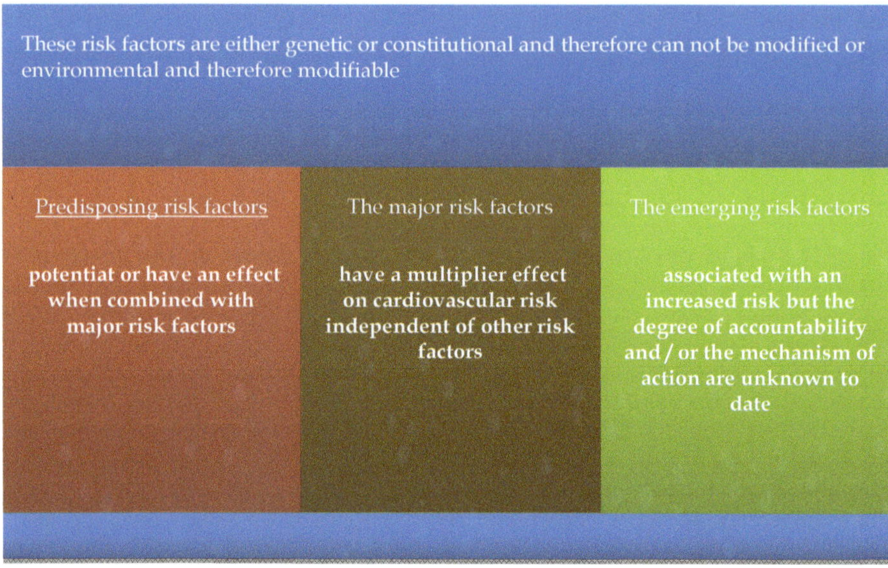

Fig. 2. Synthesis of stroke risk factors

2. Genetics of stroke

The genetics of complex diseases has known a great progress in recent years. The" Human Genome Project" is an international initiative that has enabled the sequencing of the human genome in its entirety as well as the discovery of SNP (Single nucleotide polymorphisms) which had a great success for association studies (Fig 3). The second initiative was the "HapMap project" which helped to develop a haplotype map of the human genome and allowed to describe the most common polymorphisms and the linkage disequilibrium blocks. It is currently a key for conducting further research on new genes and on both their association to disease and their response to drugs.

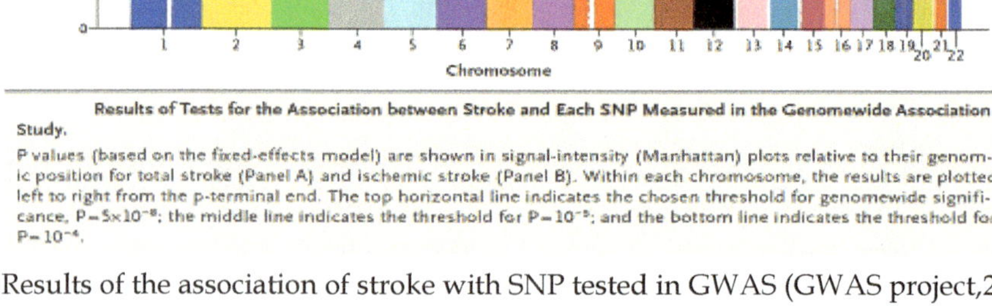

Fig. 3. Results of the association of stroke with SNP tested in GWAS (GWAS project,2009)

Apart from some rare Mendelian forms, most strokes are considered as multifactorial disease. The hypothesis of a genetic origin of stroke was based mainly on the observations of several family cases with a non-Mendelian transmission. In the Framingham project, the existence of a family history (paternal or maternal origin) of stroke was associated with an increased risk of this disease in the descendants (D. Kiely Ket al, 1993). This familial aggregation could be only the consequence of conventional risk factors like hypertension, diabetes and hypercholesterolemia. The strongest evidence has been reported by twins studies, and animal models (Rubattu S et al, 1996) (Table 6). These studies showed that the prevalence of stroke was multiplied by five in monozygotic twins compared to dizygotic (Flossmann E et al 2004, Jeff s Bet al 1997, Brass LM and al,1992).

Type of study (n)	Odds ratio (95% CI)	p-value	Stroke subclassified
Twin studies	1.65(1.2-2.3)	0.003	No
Cohort studies	1.30 (1.2-1.5)	<0.00001	2 studies
Case-control studies	1.76 (1.7-1.9)	<0.00001	15 studies

Table 6. Odds Ratios of a positive family history in different types of studies (Flossmann E et al 2004)

2.1 Rare Mendelian etiologies responsible for stroke

Many monogenic Mendelian diseases, be they autosomal dominant, autosomal recessive or X-linked, may be complicated by stroke in young patients without known risk factors (s Jeff B, 1997, Rolfs A et al, 2005, JA, Hess et al, 2006) (Table 7). Knowledge of these Mendelian forms is important. It helps in genetic counseling to identify patients at a presymptomatic stage in families with risk factors and, to discuss a preventive approach or treatment.

If expressed in the homozygous state, stroke may occur at an early stage (sometimes in infancy). Whereas, in the heterozygous state, the consequences of the genetic defect may be mild or even indistinguishable from conventional risk factors' effects. (Perry IJ et al. 1995.). Apart from this disease, cerebral autosomal dominant arteriopathy (CADASIL), sickle cell disease, Fabry disease (deficiency of lysosomal alpha-galactosidase) and mitochondrial diseases as MELAS syndrome are probably the most common metabolic causes of stroke.

CADASIL: The cerebral autosomal dominant arteriopathy with leukoencephalopathy and subcortical infarcts is a hereditary autosomal dominant cerebral arteriolopathy. Notch 3 gene was located on chromosome 19 (Tournier-Lasserve E, 1993), and the first mutations were identified in 1996 (Joutel A, 1996). The disease has been described in different families of European, African, North African, American (Arcos-Burgos OM, 2001), Indian, and Asian origin (Kotorii S, 2001). But its prevalence remains largely under-estimated, about 1 to 24,000. It occurs on an average of 42 years of age (Chabriat H, 1996, Chabriat H, 1997, Chabriat H, 1995), with extremes of 20 and 65 years (Chabriat H, 1995, Desmond DW, 1999, M Dichgans, 1998).

	diseases	Frequence	transmission	GENE
metabolic diseases	-Fabry disease (Neuropathic pain, cardiac failure, cataract, renal failure, reduction of α-Gal enzyme activity, mechanisms of ischemic stroke unknown -Mitochondrial diseases (MELAS, Development delay, sensorineural hearing loss, short stature, seizures, migraine. Pathophysiolog disruption of the blood-brain barrier a decrease in cerebral blood flow autoregulation of primary defects in neuronal oxidative metabolism - homocystinuria, -sulphite oxidase deficiency -aciduriesméthylmalonique, propionic	Frequent Frequent Frequent Frequent? Occasional	XL Mat. AR MT,AD ,AR AR	GAL Mitochondrial
Coagulopathies :	deficiency of factor V Leiden (resistance to activated protein C) Sneddon's syndrome (familial syndrome of antipholipides) fibrinogen deficiency deficiency of factor VIII, IX, X and VIII deficit in protein C, S	Frequent? Frequent Frequent Occasional	AD AD AR ARLX, AR AD	
neuro-cutaneous syndromes	Telangiectasies heorragic hereditary (Rendu-Osler-Weber) -syndrome de Bannayan-Zonana -sclérose tubéreuse de bourneville -neurofibromatose de type I -syndrome de Van Hippe I-Lindau	Frequent Occasional Rare Rare Rare	AD AD AD AD AD	
Primary disease of the cerebral vessels	fibromuscular dysplasia pseudo - xanthoma type I -Ehlers-Danlos disease (particularly type IV) cerebral-amyloidosis Icelandic type (deficiency cystatineC) Dutch type (B deficiency protein precursor amyloidal, APP B) cerebral vascular malformations, arterial dissection, familial forms of cavernous angioma adult polycystic kidney disease (APKD1 and APKD2) syndrome of arterial dissections and lentigines	Frequent Frequent Frequent Frequent Frequent Rare ? Rare Frequent	AD AD, AR AD, AR AD AD AD AD AD	

CADASIL	Migraine with aura is the principal sign, PATHOPHYSIOLOGY abnormal drainage of the portion of the Notch extramembranous 3 protein accumulation of the fragment extramembranous vessels	Frequent	AD	NOT CH3
Sickle-cell disease	Clinical feature Pain crisis, bacterial infection, VasoOclusive Crisis, pul Pathophysiology Deformation of red blood cell intimal hyperplasia proliferation of smooth muscle cells thrombosis. monary and abdominal crises, anaemia, myelopathy, seizure	Frequent	AR	HBB

Table 7. Etiologies responsible for rare mendelian stroke (Natowicz M et al, 1987)

Sickle cell disease is a common cause of stroke in children (JA Switzer, 2006), either in its homozygous or compound heterozygous form with hemoglobin C (HbC) or α-thalassemia (Old J. 2002). Hemoglobin S is due to a mutation by substitution of adenine for thymine in codon 6 of the β-globin gene on chromosome 11p15.4, resulting in the substitution of a valine by a glutamic acid in the protein chain. This alteration of the protein causes a deformation of the red cell that becomes sickle-shaped. Brain stroke appears to be a consequence of an abnormal interaction between sickle red blood cells and vascular endothelium (JA Switzer, 2006; Hebbel RP, 2004). The sickled red cells tend to clump together and adhere to the endothelium. The endothelial activation further promotes remodeling of the arterial wall and vascular disease. The typical atherothrombotic stroke is often located in the internal carotid artery and the proximal, middle and anterior portions of cerebral arteries. It is associated with hyperplasia of intima, fibroblasts proliferation and smooth muscle cells. (Stockman JA et al 1972). Many patients develop lacunar small-vessel disease (JA Switzer, 2006; J Schatz, 2002).

Fabry disease is a lysosomal disease, due to a deficiency of α-galactosidase A enzyme (GLA). Most patients are carriers of missense and nonsense mutations, large and small rearrangements or splicing defects in the coding region of α-galactosidase gene on the X chromosome (GLA) (Desnick et al 2001, Schaefer, 2005; Human Gene Mutation Database). Clinical signs include an acroparesthesia, angiokeratoma, and hypohidrosis, which often develop in childhood or adolescence before the systemic complications leading to heart and renal failure and ischemic stroke (Rolfs A et al 2005; Crutchfield KE et al 1998, Grewal RP et al 1994; Mitsias P et al, 1996). Ischemic stroke predominates in the vertebrobasilar circulation (Rolfs A, 2005).

MELAS syndrome: Mitochondrial Encephalomyopathy, Lactic Acidosis, and Stroke-like episodes, is a mitochondriopathy caused by many mutations, transmitted by maternal inheritance in mitochondrial DNA (Pavlakis SG, 1984, Martinez-Fernandez E, 2001). Over 80% of patients carry the A3243G mutation; an A to G transition at position 3243 of the gene MT-TL1. MELAS syndrome is associated with various symptoms. However, in monosymptomatic cases, ischemic stroke is the only existing expression (Martinez-

Fernandez E, 2001). In MELAS, the episodes of ischemic stroke are different from those of a typical cerebral infarction with the cortex being always involved.

Primitive genetic diseases of the cerebral vessels: an increasing number of genetic diseases of the cerebral vessels responsible for stroke have been identified in the last few years. Fibromuscular dysplasia is characterized by the presence of dilatations in small and medium arteries due to the destruction of the media, fibrosis and muscular hyperplasia. The occurrence of aneurysm rupture is a relatively common event in various forms of Ehlers-Danlos disease; especially type IV that is characterized by a deficiency of collagen type 3. Some forms of amyloidosis are characterized by a predominantly cerebral localization of amyloidal deposits in the vessels causing hemorrhagic or ischemic stroke. These disorders are genetically heterogeneous; some are due to mutations in cystatin C (an inhibitor of several cysteine proteinases), others are due to mutations in the precursor of the beta-amyloid protein (beta-APP) (Levy E et al. 1990, M. Abrahamson, 1992).

2.2 Stroke model of multifactorial disease with polygenic component

More than 2300 candidate polymorphisms are currently listed in association with stroke (Matthew B et al, 2010). These factors have been listed on the bases of their involvement in known metabolic pathways or through pangenomics studies. Most of them have been analyzed in different populations by association studies. The genes studied are typically those involved in the coagulation (Fig 4), homocysteine and lipid metabolism. Among those genes, the most explored with consensus were: FV, FII, MTHFR, ApoE, ACE (Fig 5) and fibrinogen, PAI1. Others have been explored without consensus (Enos, PON, LPL, FGA / FGB / FGG, F7, F13A1, vWF, F12, SERPINE1, ITGB3, PLA2, ITGA2B, ITGA2, GP1BA, AGT, NOS3, LPL, PON1, PDE4D, ALOX5AP, MTR, CBS, NINJ2) (Bersano et al. 2008). The results published today are often controversial depending on the population studied, the age of patients and stroke subtypes.

a- Factor V Leiden Mutation: is one of the most studied thrombotic variants. It is the main genetic risk factor for deep vein thrombosis. (JP Casas, 2004; Ye Z, 2006, Paluku T, 2011). Several meta-analyses were conducted to study the association between FVL and stroke. The results are controversial and are population age dependent; this Association was absent in Morocco (Paluku et al, 2011), weak in Asia (Jul K, 2002, Kim RJ, 2003). It is found highly significant with an OR of 1.33 (95% CI, 1.12 to 1.58) in the Caucasian population (Casas JP, 2004, Paul Bentley et al.).

The data published on the FV Leiden mutation showed a great diversity in geographical repartition. it is very common in Europeans, with a north-south gradient: 4.4% in the UK versus 1.7 % in Italy and is absent in sub-Saharian Africans and East-Asians. For Arab populations in the eastern basin of the Mediterranean, this mutation is high especially in Jordan (12.3%) (AWID, 1999), Syria (13.6%) (Irani-Hakim, 2000) and Lebanon (14.2%) (Irani-Hakim 2000, 2002 Tamim). Prevalence decreases as the distance from these regions of the Mediterranean basin increases. It is present in Tunisia, Algeria, and absent in Morocco (Mathonnet F, Nadifi S. et al, 2002). This geographical difference in the Maghreb could be explained by the region's history, including the presence of the Ottoman Empire (Turkish) since the XVIth century in Tunisia and Algeria (Cavalli et al, 1994), but not in Morocco (Mathonnet F, Nadifi S 2002). This mutation is probably due to a founder effect, which would have occurred in the eastern Mediterranean sea, 21000 to 34000 years ago (Zivelin 1997) and spread across the migration flows to other parts of the world (Castoldi 1997, Irani Hakim, 2000).

b- Mutation G20210A of prothrombin gene: Prothrombin G20210A mutation is considered as the second cause of inherited thromboembolic disease. This mutation is found at the heterozygous state in 4 to 8% of subjects with a first episode of venous thrombosis. The estimated relative risk is 2-7 times higher in carriers (De Moerloose, 2000, Emmrich 2001, Paluku et al, 2011). The homozygous forms are rarely observed (0.014% -0.0025%) (Poort SR, 1996) and risk associated with homozygosity is currently unknown. The mechanism of hypercoagulability is due to an increase in the formation of thrombin. However, there are conflicting results in the role of the G20210A prothrombin gene in ischemic stroke pathogenesis.

c-: fibrinogen: Studies have shown a strong link between high plasma fibrinogen and stroke (Wilhelmsen L, 1984 Gregory W. Albers 2009). The relative risk was estimated to 2.06 (1.83-2.33) (CO Fibrinogen Studies, 2005). This relationship is controversial because the levels of fibrinogen are influenced by tobacco, obesity, diabetes, inflammation and infection (L Wilhelmsen, 1984, Rothwell PM, 2004).

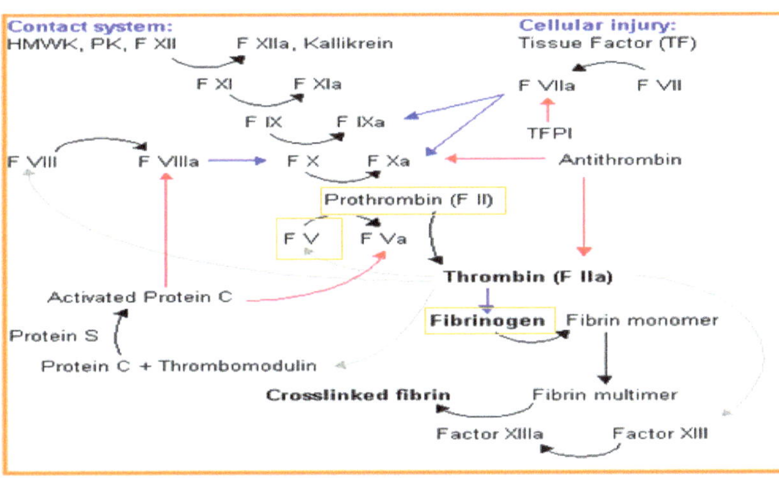

Fig. 4. Schema of cascade of coagulation with different factors

d- Mutations in the PAI1 gene: The Plasminogen activator inhibitor type 1 (PAI1) is a potent inhibitor of fibrinolysis (Dichgans et al, 2008). It was shown that a high activity of PAI1 is associated with an important cerebral risk and coronary vascular disease (Casas JP et al 2004). The 4G/5G polymorphism in the PAI1 gene promoter is most frequently studied in association with stroke (Roshan A et al, 2007). The data of association studies (Case-control) were not unanimous about the involvement of the 5G polymorphism in stroke (Dichgans, 2008).

e- Molecular mechanism of C667T Variant of MTHFR gene: The 5, 10-methylenetetrahydrofolate reductase (MTHFR) is an enzyme catalyzing the reduction of 5, 10 - methylenetetrahydrofolate (MTHF), to 5-MTHF, which is the predominant form of folate. The MTHFR gene is located in 1p36.3 (Goyette et al, 1994). It comprises 11 exons and extends over a length of 2.2 Kb (Goyette, 1998). The C667T mutation makes the protein thermolabile and its enzymatic activity is reduced by half (Frost, 1995). The presence of this mutation in the homozygous state affects folate metabolism and induces a moderate elevation of plasma homocysteine. The C677T mutation of the MTHFR gene has been extensively explored in association studies with stroke; based on strict criteria such as age, stroke subtypes. An association was found between the TT genotype and stroke; it was stronger when the subject is young, with significant OR (Corin 2005, Xiao2009, KT Moe, 2008, Paluku, Nadifi S. et al 2010). Subjects with the TT genotype had higher homocysteine levels and fewer circulating folate than those with CC genotype. (BM McQuillan, 1999; Deloughery TG, 1996, Ma J, 1996, Schwartz SM 1997, L Brattstrom, 1998))

f- Polymorphism insertion/deletion (I/D) ACE gene: The insertion/deletion polymorphism in the angiotensin-converting enzyme gene (ACE) is one of the most common genetic variants studied in relation with atherosclerotic vascular disease. A relative risk of 1.5 to 4 had been reported in association between this polymorphism and ischemic stroke (Cambienet al. 1992). However, other studies have failed to find significant association. This result can be explained by the high frequency of this polymorphism in the population (> 90%). (Catto A, 1996, Dikmen M, 2006, Doi Y, 1997, Pera J, 2006, Tuncer N, 2006, Gao X, 2006; Lin JJ, 2000, Pullicino P, 1996, Ueda S, 1995)

g-The gene for apolipoprotein E (ApoE): The apolipoprotein E gene is one of the most widely studied in vascular and neurodegenerative disease (JE Eichner, 2002). Several meta-analyses reported controversial results between the ApoE4 allele and the risk of ischemic stroke. This association appears to be weak in Asian patients (Xi, 2009) (Benerje, 2007), absent in Italy and Turkey (Cerrato P, 2005, Duzenli S, 2004),). So, the exact role of Apo E4 polymorphism in ischemic stroke is uncertain probably due to the variability of its distribution in populations around the world.

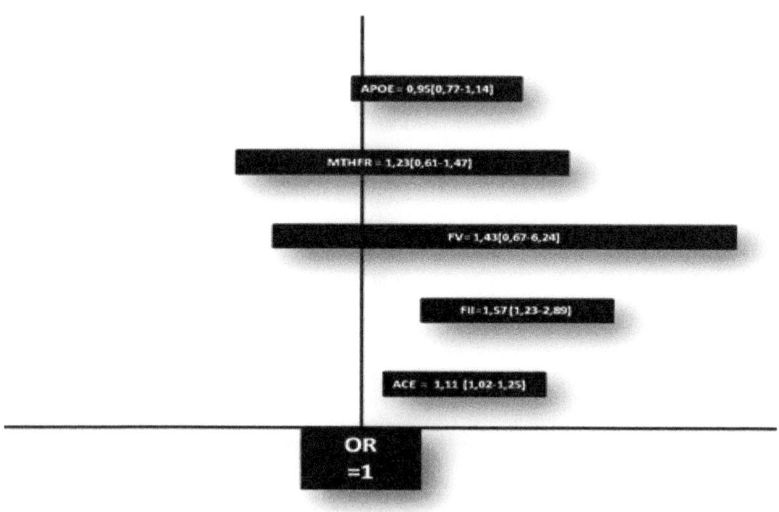

Fig. 5. Panel of 5 Genetic Factors with Degree of Association With Stroke. (Nadifi et al, 2011, Indian Journal of human genetics IJHG57-11)

h-the Phosphodiesterase 4D gene (PDE4D): The PDE4D is the first gene found by linkage in stroke Iceland patients; an association of SNPs of the PDE4D (83T / C) and (-889C / T) was reported, with an increased risk of developing stroke (Nan et al Li1. 2010). Other studies have led to conflicting results. There are few studies limited to a small number of patients. Thus, it is premature to conclude the association of PDE4D gene with stroke and its role in the stroke pathogenesis. In fact, it would be interesting to study larger series of different populations. Therefore, experimental studies on the function of PDE4D will help to unveil the mystery (E Lõhmussaar et al, 2005)

I-5-lipoxygenase-activating protein gene" gene: The locus13q12 ALOX5AP gene is involved in the metabolism of leukotrienes and atherosclerosis. HAPA is the most frequent polymorphism described. It has been associated with increased risk in stroke compared to controls (Helgadottir A, 2004). These results were found only in a Scottish study (Helgadottir A, 200, Meschia JF, 2005).

j-Other candidate genes and pathways have been studied for possible association with ischemic stroke. They are listed in the webtable (www.Genome.org) or discussed in reviews (Table 7). Those genes are involved in inflammation (interleukine 1, interleukin 6, TNF, Toll-like receptor 4, P-selectin and E-selectin, C-reactive protein), and lipid metabolism (apolipoprotein E, paraoxonase III; ApoA1, Apo A5…). (Table 8)

3. Conclusion and outlook

Stroke is an excellent research model for complex multifactorial disease; involving many risk factors (constitutional, environmental and genetic).

Historically, the epidemiological studies were based on a 'candidate gene' approach, defined by the knowledge of pathophysiology (table 9). The advent of Genome-Wide Scan (GWS) had permitted the emergence of new hypothesis in physiological pathways and novel biomarkers. The Genome Wide Association Studies had revolutionized the understanding of disease etiology and risk factors. However, they are still in their beginning and haven't yet incorporated complex statistical data that woul allow us to understand gene-gene (epistatsis) and gene-environment interactions.

These studies could be a major challenge that requires the collaboration of several centers and the elaboration of large clinical and epidemiological databases.

The genetic origin of stroke had been widely studied but many questions are still unsolved. Among them, the cumulative effect of identified mutations, the gene-gene, gene-environmental interactions that modulate the genetic effect represent a big mystery that still needs to be elucidated. The underestimated heritability of the risk factors is probably due to a deficiency in the clinical information and genetic modeling. The influence of all these factors is not only additive, or dominant/recessive, but also interactive. Epidemiological studies had largely explored the genetic mechanisms in a classical approach based on pathophysiology knowledge. But, there are probably other unknown mechanisms that could be explained by « pangenomics hypothesis free ». In this way, many metabolic pathways and novel variants involved in vascular diseases have been identified. Currently, only 12% of SNPs are located in coding regions. The majority of SNP (40% in intergenic regions, 40% in introns) may have a role in regulating the expression of these genes (Hardy et al. 2009, Hindorff et al. 2009]). In addition, gene-environment interactions are largely missed in the genome-wide approaches. The presence of functional genes is not sufficient to the occurring of a subject phenotype in the absence of environmental stimuli.

Type of factor	Factor	Gene	Polymorphisms	Association
Coagulation system	FactorV Leiden	F5	c.1691G>A	Possible
			c.4070A>G	Uncertain
	Prothrombin	F2	c.20210G>A	Possible
	Fibrinogen	FGA	c.4266A>G	Uncertain
		FGB	c.148C>T	Not demonstrated
			c.455G>A	Not demonstrated
	Factor VII	F7	A1/A2	Not demonstrated
			c.10976G>A	Not demonstrated
			c.323_324insCCTATATCT	Not demonstrated
			c.402G>A	Not demonstrated
			c.401G>T	Not demonstrated
	Factor XIII	F13A1	c.143G>T	Not demonstrated
			p.Pro564Leu	Not demonstrated
	Von Willebrand factor	VWF	Sma I	Uncertain
			c.1423C>T	Not demonstrated
			c.1793C>G	Not demonstrated
	Factor XII	F12	c.46C>T	Uncertain
Fibrinolytic system	Plasminogen activator inhibitor 1	SERPINE1	c.675_676delinsG	Possible
			c.1053 G>T	Not demonstrated
Platelet receptor	GpIIb–IIIa complex	ITGB3	GPIIIa PLA2	Not demonstrated
			GPIIIa c.1691G>A	Not demonstrated
		ITGA2B	GPIIb HPA-3	Not demonstrated
			GPIIb p.Ile843Ser	Not demonstrated
	Gp Ia-IIa Complex	ITGA2	GPIa c.807C>T	Not demonstrated
			GPIa c.873G>A	Not demonstrated
	GpIb/IX/V Complex	GP1BA	HPA2 c.3550C>T	Possible
			VNTR	Not demonstrated
			GPIb (–5) T/C Kozak	Possible
Renin-angiotensin-aldosterone system	ACE	ACE	g.11417_11704del287	Possible
	Angiotensinogen	AGT	p.Met174Thr	Not demonstrated
			p.Met235Thr	Not demonstrated
Homocysteine and eNOS metabolism	eNOS	NOS3	g.3726_3834insGAAGTCTAGACCTGCTGCGGGGGTGAG	Uncertain
			c.894G>T	Uncertain
			c.786T>C	Uncertain
	Hcy	MTHFR	MTHFR c.677C>T	Possible
			MTHFR c.1298A>C	Not demonstrated
		CBS	CBS c.844_845ins68	Not demonstrated
			CBS c.833T>C	Not demonstrated
		MTR	MTR c.275A>G	Not demonstrated
Lipoprotein metabolism	APOE		ε2, ε3, ε4	Possible
		APO ε2, ε3, ε4	p.Cys112Arg	Not demonstrated
			p.Arg158Cys	Not demonstrated
	LPL	LPL	S447X	Not demonstrated
			p.Asp9Asn	Not demonstrated
			c.1127A>G	Not demonstrated
			c. 93C>T	Not demonstrated
	PON1	PON1	p.Gln192Arg	Uncertain
			p.Leu55Met	Uncertain
			c.107C>T	Uncertain
Linkage-association studies	PDE4D	PDE4D	SNP 39-44-56-83-87-89	Uncertain
	5-lipoxygenase-activating-protein	ALOX5AP	HAPA	Uncertain
			SG13S106 - SG13S89	Uncertain

Table 8. Final panel of genetic factors with different degrees of association with stroke. (A. Bersano, et al 2008)

Finally, the understanding of stroke physiopathology and genetics requires developing more efficient tools:

Implementation of an epidemiological case-control study focusing on large populations in different ethnic groups.

Genotyping multiple deleterious polymorphisms in several genes.

In perspective, the development of pharmacogenetics has emerged recently as a promising area of research. For example, warfarine, an oral anticoagulant, is prescribed to millions of patients for cardiovascular problems and that causes many difficulties to determine the effective dose. The polymorphisms in the CYP2C9 and VKORC1 gene influence individual susceptibility response to warfarine. The genotyping of VKORC1 gene showed a strong association and researchers started treatment strategies according to individual patients genotypes.

Functional candidate gene approach
It takes into account their functions in physiological or metabolic pathways.
It starts with a hypothesis and the association between candidate gene and phenotype is sought. This approach involves a study of case-control association of unrelated individuals.
The study of association of a genotype or allele and complex disease with comparison of frequencies in patients and controls.
In SNP association studies in several stroke criticisms were made after many difficulties to reproduce the results published by other researchers (Hirchhorn et al.)
It is essential to apply strict criteria and standardized, as a good selection of genetic polymorphisms in which the candidate gene not only intervene in a pathophysiological pathway, but in which the SNP is real, supported by data on the function.
Finally, it should have large samples for the allele frequencies and odds ratios OR Dichgans and Marcus,

Positional candidate gene approach or positional cloning
is to locate regions of the genome containing susceptibility genes without prior knowledge of its function, except for certain diseases only. When a connection has been well identified, the gene will be cloned and lsa start function can be determined (Risch, N. and Merikangas, KR 1996). Linkage studies are most effective for identifying genes that have a significant effect (Lander, E. 1994).
The analysis of a link between two loci is tested by calculating the LOD score, a statistical analysis that compares the probability that the loci are linked
More than two loci are close to each other, the less likely it is that there is a recombination between the two during meiosis. If they are removed, the alleles of both loci will be sent randomly.
By convention, a LOD score above 3 states the obvious connections, while a LOD score less than -2 indicates no connection, and a score between -2 and 3 can never confirm or reject a bond in a single test.
When linkage analysis is done across the whole genome multipoint LOD score is used. This analysis is not limited only to enumerate all the markers genetically close but calculates allele frequencies of the markers used. This approach by mapping the entire genome suggests significant LOD scores exceeding + 3.3 (Lander, ES 1994).

Table 9. Design of studies on molecular genetics of stroke.

4. Conflicts

None.

5. Acknowledgments

Many thanks to Pr. FD Tiziano, in lab of Sacre Heart in Roma, Italy, Pr Zaki Abdellatif in The IAV-Rabat - Morocco, Dr.Afaf Benitto; Dr. Nadia Serbati in The Medical school of Casablanca - Morocco, for language revision.

Our work on stroke has been supported by the Hassan II Academy of Science and Technology, The Medical school and the Hassan II University.

6. References

A. Bersano, et al Genetic Polymorphisms for the Study of Multifactorial Stroke. Human mutation 2008;1-20.

Adams HP, Bendixen BH, Kappelle LJ, Biller J,Love BB, Gordon DL et al. Classification of subtypes of acute ischemic stroke. Definitions for use in a multicenter clinical trial. Stroke 1993;24(1):35-41.

Adams RW, Gandevia SC & Skuse NF. The distribution of muscle weakness in upper motoneuron lesions affecting the lower limb. Brain 1990;113:1459-76.

Adams, H.P., Jr., Bendixen, B.H., Kappelle, L.J., et al. (1993). Classification of subtype of acute ischemic stroke. Definitions for use in a multicenter clinical trial. TOAST. Trial of Org 10172 in Acute Stroke Treatment. Stroke, 24, 35–41.

American Stroke Association. [En ligne]. http://www.strokeassociation.org/ (Page consultée le 15mars 2010).

Annas, G.J. (2000). Rules for research on human genetic variation: lessons from Iceland. New England Journal of Medicine, 342, 1830–3.

Asplund K, Tuomilehto J, Stegmayr B, Wester PO & Tunstall-Pedoe H. Diagnostic criteria and quality control of the registration of stroke events in the MONICA Project. Acta Med Scand Suppl 1988:26-39.

Atkinson, J.L., Sundt, T.M. Jr.,Houser, O.W. & Whisnant, J.P. (1989). Angiographic frequency of anterior circulation intracranial aneurysms. Journal of Neurosurgery, 70, 551–5.

Bak, S., Gaist, D., Sindrup, S.H., Skytthe, A. & Christensen, K. (2002). Genetic liability in stroke: a long-term follow-up study of Danish twins. Stroke, 33, 769–74.

Bamford, J., Sandercock, P., Dennis, M., Burn, J., and Warlow, C. (1991). Classification and natural history of clinically identifiable subtypes of cerebral infarction. Lancet, 337, 1521–6.

Behin A et al Paraplegia disclosing an intracranial arterovenous fistula with perimedullary drainage Rev Neurol (Paris). 2002 Jan;158(1):70-3

Bener A et al The impact of air pollution on hospital admission for respiratory and cardiovascular diseases in an oil-rich country. East Afr J Public Health. 2009 Aug;6(2):124-7.

Bhat VM et al Dose-response relationship between cigarette smoking and risk of ischemic stroke in young women. Stroke. 2008 Sep;39(9):2439-43.

Bonita, R. (1992). Epidemiology of stroke. Lancet, 339, 342–4.

Brass, L.M., Page,W.F., and Lichtman, J.H. (1999). Stroke in Twins III: a follow-up study (abstract). stroke, 30, 256.

Braun, M.M., Haupt, R., and Caporaso, N.E. (1994). The National Academy of Sciences: National Research Council Veteran Twin Registry. Acta Geneticae Medicae et Gemellologiae (Roma), 43, 89–94.

Broderick, J.P., Brott, T., Tomsick, T.,Huster, G., and Miller, R. (1992). The risk of subarachnoid and intracerebral hemorrhages in blacks as compared with whites. New England Journal of Medicine, 326, 733–6.

Brown, R.D. Jr., Whisnant, J.P., Sicks, J.D., O'Fallon,W.M., Petty, G.W., and Wiebers, D.O. (2001). Subarachnoid hemorrhage and intracerebral hemorrhage: trends in incidence and survival in a population-based study (abstract). Neurology, 56 (Suppl), A86.

Brown, R.D.,Whisnant, J.P., Sicks, J.D., O'Fallon,W.M., and Wiebers, D.O. (1996). Stroke incidence, prevalence, and survival: secular trends in Rochester, Minnesota, through 1989. Stroke, 27, 373–80.

Buysschaert I et al Clinical and fundamental aspects of angiogenesis and anti-angiogenesis. Acta Clin Belg. 2007 May-Jun;62(3):162-9

Caicoya, M., Corrales, C., and Rodriguez, T. (1999). Family history and stroke: a community case–control study in Asturias, Spain. Journal of Epidemiology and Biostatistics, 4, 313–20.

Caplan, L.R. and Hennerici, M. (1998). Impaired clearance of emboli (washout) is an important link between hypoperfusion, embolism, and ischemic stroke. Archives of Neurology, 55, 1475–82.

Carmeliet P, Jain RK. Angiogenesis in cancer and other diseases. Nature. 2000 Sep 14;407(6801):249-57.

Casas JP, Hingorani AD, Bautista LE, Sharma P. Meta-analysis of genetic studies in ischemic stroke: thirty-two genes involving approximately 18,000 cases and 58,000 controls. Arch Neurol. 2004 Nov; 61 (11):1652-61.

Cavalli-Sforza, LL., Menozzi, P., Piazza, A., 1994, the History and Geography of Human Genes. Princeton University

Ceppa F et al Blood levels of homocysteine by high pressure liquid chromatography and comparison with two other techniques. Ann Biol Clin (Paris). 1999 Jul-Aug;57(4):474-80.

Chyatte, D., Chen, T.L., Bronstein, K., and Brass, L.M. (1994). Seasonal fluctuation in the incidence of intracranial aneurysm rupture and its relationship to changing climatic conditions. Journal of Neurosurgery, 81, 525–30.

Collins, R. and MacMahon, S. (1994). Blood pressure, antihypertensive drug treatment and the risks of stroke and of coronary heart disease. British Medical Bulletin, 50, 272–98.

Colloque international sur « l'épidémiologie des accidents vasculaires cérébraux » du 19-20 juin 2009, Université Mohamed V-Souissi Rabat M. Fouzi Mourji «Présentation des résultats Socio-démographiques de l'enquête d'épidémiologie des AVC au Maroc », Université Hassan II Aïn Chock - Casablanca M. El Mostafa El Alaoui Faris et al ; « Présentation des résultats médicaux de l'enquête épidémiologique des AVC au Maroc ».

Corwin, L.T.,Wolf, P.A., Kannel,W.B., and McNamara, P.M. (1982). Accuracy of death certification of stroke: the Framlingham Study. Stroke, 13, 816–8.
Danesh, J.,Whincup, P.,Walker, M., et al. (2000). Low grade inflammation and coronary heart disease: prospective study and updated meta-analyses. British Medical Journal, 321, 199–204.
De Boer, O.J., van der Wal, A.C., and Becker, A.E. (2000). Atherosclerosis, inflammation, and infection. Journal of Pathology, 190, 237–43.
De Braekeleer, M., Perusse, L., Cantin, L., Bouchard, J.M., and Mathieu, J. (1996). A study of inbreeding and kinship in intracranial aneurysms in the Saguenay Lac-Saint-Jean region (Quebec, Canada). Annals of Human Genetics, 60, 99–104.
De Faire, U., Friberg, L., and Lundman, T. (1975). Concordance for mortality with special reference to ischaemic heart disease and cerebrovascular disease: a study on the Swedish Twin Registry. Preventive Medicine, 4, 509–17.
Dichgans, M.,Holtmannspötter, M.,Herzog, J., Peters, N., Bergmann, M., and Yousry, T.A. (2002). Cerebral microbleeds in CADASIL: a gradient-echo magnetic resonance imaging and autopsy study. Stroke, 33, 67–71.
Dichgans M, Markus HS. 2005. Genetic association studies in stroke: methodological issues and proposed standard criteria. Stroke 36:2027–2031.
Dichgans M. 2007. Genetics of ischaemic stroke. Lancet Neurol 6:149–161.
Lloyd-Jones DM, Dyer AR, Wang R, Daviglus ML, Greenland P. Risk factor burden in middle age and lifetime risks for cardiovascular and non-cardiovascular death (Chicago Heart Association Detection Project in Industry). Am J Cardiol. 2007 Feb 15;99(4):535-40.
Donnan, G., Norrving, B., Bamford, J., and Bogousslavsky, J. (eds) (2002). Subcortical stroke, 2nd edn. Oxford University Press, Oxford.
Dunn, L.T., Stewart, E.,Murray, G.D., Nicoll, J.A., and Teasdale, G.M. (2001). The influence of apolipoprotein E genotype on outcome after spontaneous subarachnoid hemorrhage: a preliminary study. Neurosurgery, 48, 1006–10.
Eikelboom, J.W.,Hankey, G.J., Anand, S.S., Lofthouse, E., Staples, N., and Baker, R.I. (2000). Association between high homocyst(e)ine and ischemic stroke due to large- and small-artery disease but not other etiologic subtypes of ischemic stroke. Stroke, 31, 1069–75.
European Carotid Surgery Trialists' Collaborative Group. (1998). Randomised trial of endarterectomy for recently symptomatic carotid stenosis: final results of the MRC European Carotid Surgery Trial (ECST). Lancet, 351, 1379–87.
Fassbender, K.,Mielke, O., Bertsch, T., et al. (1999). Homocysteine in cerebral macroangiography and microangiopathy. Lancet, 353, 1586–7.
Feigin,V.L., Anderson, C.S., and Mhurchu, C.N. (2002). Systemic inflammation, endothelial dysfunction, dietary Fatty acids and micronutrients as risk factors for stroke: a selective review. Cerebrovascular Disease, 13, 219–24.
Feigin,V.L., Anderson, C.S., Anderson, N.E., et al. (2001). Is there a temporal pattern in the occurrence of subarachnoid hemorrhage in the Southern Hemisphere? Pooled data from 3 large, population-based incidence studies in Australasia, 1981 to 1997. Stroke, 32, 613–19.
Feldmann, E., Daneault, N., Kwan, E., et al. (1990). Chinese-white differences in the distribution of occlusive cerebrovascular disease. Neurology, 40, 1541–5.

Fisher, C.M. (1969). The arterial lesion underlying lacunes. Acta Neuropathologica (Berlin), 12, 1-15.

Fogelholm, R. (1992). Subarachnoid hemorrhage in Finland (letter). Stroke, 23, 437.

Gallerani, M., Portaluppi, F.,Maida, G., et al. (1996). Circadian and circannual rhythmicity in the occurrence of subarachnoid hemorrhage. Stroke, 27, 1793–7.

Gifford, A.J. (1966). An epidemiological study of cerebrovascular disease. American Journal of Public Health and the Nation's Health, 56, 452–61.

Gillum, L.A.,Mamidipudi, S.K., and Johnston, S.C. (2000). Ischemic stroke risk with oral contraceptives. A meta-analysis. Journal of the American Medical Association, 284, 72–8.

Gillum, R.F., Gorelick, P.B., and Cooper, E.S. (eds.) (1999). Stroke in Blacks. Karger, Basel.

Goldstein, L.B., Jones, M.R.,Matchar, D.B., Edwards, L.J.,Hoff, J., Chilukuri,V., Armstrong, S.B., and Horner, R. (2001). Improving the reliability of stroke subgroup classification using the Trial of ORG 10172 in Acute Stroke Treatment (TOAST) criteria. Stroke, 32, 1091–7.

Gorelick, P.B., Caplan, L.R., Langenberg, P., et al. (1988). Clinical and angiographic comparison of asymptomatic occlusive cerebrovascular disease. Neurology, 38, 852–8.

Gorelick, P.B., Caplan, L.R.,Hier, D.B., Parker, S.L., and Patel, D. (1984). Racial differences in the distribution of anterior circulation occlusive disease. Neurology, 34, 54–9.

Grau, A.J., Buggle, F., Steichen-Wiehn, C.,Heindl, S., Banerjee, T., Seitz, R., et al. (1995). Clinical and biochemical analysis in infection-associated stroke. Stroke, 26, 1520–6.

Gretarsdottir, S., Sveinbjornsdottir, S., Jonsson, H.H., et al. (2002). Localization of a susceptibility gene for common forms of stroke to 5q12. American Journal of Human Genetics, 70, 593–603.

Guillon B et al Infection and the risk of spontaneous cervical artery dissection: a case-control study.Stroke. 2003 Jul;34(7):e79-81.

Gulcher, J. and Stefansson, K. (1998). Population genomics: laying the groundwork for genetic disease modeling and targeting. Clinical Chemistry and Laboratory Medicine, 36, 523–7.

Gulcher, J.R. and Stefansson, K. (2000). The Icelandic Healthcare Database and informed consent New England Journal of Medicine, 342, 1827–30.

Haapanen, A., Koskenvuo, M., Kaprio, J., Kesaniemi, Y.A., and Heikkila, K. (1989). Carotid arteriosclerosis in identical twins discordant for cigarette smoking. Circulation, 80, 10–16.

Hackniski,V.C., Potter, P., and Merskey, H. (1987). Leukoaraiosis. Archives of Neurology, 44, 21–3.

Hankey, G., Jamorozik, K., Braodhurst, R., et al. (1998). Long-term risk of first recurrent stroke in the Perth community stroke study. Stroke, 29, 2491–500.

Hankey, G.J. and Eikelboom, J.W. (2001). Homocysteine and stroke. Current Opinion in Neurology, 14, 95–102.

Harvard University Press, Boston, MA. O'Sullivan, M., Lythgoe, D.J., Periera, A.C., Summers, P.E, Jarosz, J.M., Williams, S.C.R., and Markus, H.S. (2002). Patterns of cerebral blood flow reduction in patients with ischaemic leukoaraiosis. Neurology, 59, 321–6.

Hassan, A., Sham, P.C., and Markus, H.S. (2002). Planning genetic studies in human stroke: sample size estimates based on family history data. Neurology, 58, 1483–8.

Hassan, A., Hunt, B., O'Sullivan, M., Parmar, K., Bamford, J., Briley, D., Brown, M.M., Thomas, D., and Markus, H.S. (2003). The role of endothelial dysfunction in lacunar infarction and ischaemic leukoaraiosis. Brain. 126, 424–32.

Heart Protection Study Collaborative Group. (2002). MRC/BHF Heart Protection Study of

Homocysteine Lowering Trialists' Collaboration. (1998). Lowering blood homocysteine with folic acid based supplements: meta-analysis of randomised trials. British Medical Journal, 316, 894–8.

Inagawa, T. (2002). Seasonal variation in the incidence of aneurysmal subarachnoid hemorrhage in hospital- and community-based studies. Journal of Neurosurgery, 96, 497–509.

Ingall, T., Asplund, K.,Mahonen, M., and Bonita, R. (2000). A multinational comparison of subarachnoid hemorrhage epidemiology in the WHO MONICA stroke study. Stroke, 31, 1054–61.

Inzitari, D., Hachinski,V.C., Taylor, D.W., and Barnett, H.J. (1990). Racial differences in the anterior circulation in cerebrovascular disease: how much can be explained by risk factors? Archives of Neurology, 47, 1080–84.

Jakubowski, J. and Kendall, B. (1978). Coincidental aneurysms with tumours of pituitary origin. Journal of Neurology, Neurosurgery, and Psychiatry, 41, 972–9.

Jellinger, K. (1977). Pathology of intracerebral hemorrhage. Zentralblatt für Neurochirurgie, 38, 29–42.

Jerrard-Dunne, P.,Markus, H.S., Steckel, D.A., Buehler, A., von Kegler, S., and Sitzer, M. (2003). Early carotid atherosclerosis and family history of myocardial infarction and stroke—specific effects on arterial sites have implications for genetic studies: The Carotid Atherosclerosis Progression Study (CAPS). Arteriosclerosis, Thrombosis and Vascular Biology, 13, 302–6.

Jones, D.K., Lythgoe, D.,Horsfield, M.A., Simmons, A.,Williams, S.C.R., and Markus, H.S. (1999). Characterisation of white matter damage in ischaemic leukoaraiosis with diffusion tensor magnetic resonance imaging. Stroke, 30, 393–7.

Jousilahti, P., Rastenyte, D., Tuomilehto, J., Sarti, C., and Vartiainen, E. (1997). Parental history of cardiovascular disease and risk of stroke: a prospective follow-up of 14371 middle-aged men and women in Finland. Stroke, 28, 1361–6.

Juvela, S. (1996). Prevalence of risk factors in spontaneous intracerebral hemorrhage and aneurismal subarachnoid hemorrhage. Archives of Neurology, 53, 734–40.

Kagan A, et al Dietary and other risk factors for stroke in Hawaiian Japanese men. Stroke. 1985 May-Jun;16(3):390-6.

Kaposzta, Z., Young, E., Bath, P.M.W., and Markus, H.S. (1999). The clinical application of asymptomatic embolic signal detection in acute stroke: a prospective study. Stroke, 30, 1814–8.

Kaposzta, Z.,Martin, J.F., and Markus, H.S. (2002). Switching off embolisation from the

Kato, H., Izumiyama, M., Izumiyama, K., Takahashi, A., and Itoyama, Y. (2002). Silent cerebral microbleeds on T2*-weighted MRI: correlation with stroke subtype, stroke recurrence, and leukoaraiosis. Stroke, 33, 1536–40.

Kendler, K.S. and Holm, N.V. (1985). Differential enrollment in twin registries: its effect on prevalence and concordance rates and estimates of genetic parameters. Acta Geneticae Medicae et Gemellologiae (Roma), 34, 125–40.

Kiely, D.K.,Wolf, P.A., Cupples, L.A., Beiser, A.S., and Myers, R.H. (1993). Familial aggregation of stroke: the Framingham Study. Stroke, 24, 1366–71.

Kissela, B.M., Sauerbeck, L.,Woo, D., et al. (2002). Subarachnoid hemorrhage: a preventable disease with a heritable component. Stroke, 33, 1321-6.

Kunitz, S.C., Gross, C.R.,Heyman, A., Kasse, C.S.,Mohr, J.P., Proce, T.R., and Wolf, P.A. (1984). The pilot Stroke Data Bank: definition, design, and data. Stroke, 15, 740–6.

Kuwabara, Y., Ichiya, Y., Sasaki, M., Yoshida, T., Fukumura, T.,Masuda, K., Ibayashi, S., and Fujishima, M. (1996). Cerebral blood flow and vascular response to hypercapnia in hypertensive patients with leukoaraiosis. Annals of Nuclear Medicine, 10, 293–8.

Lammie, G.A. (2002). Pathology of lacunar infarction. In Subcortical stroke (eds G. Donnan, B.Norrving, J. Bamford, and J. Bogousslavsky), 2nd edn. pp. 37–46. Oxford University Press,Oxford.

Law, M. (1996). Commentary: evidence on salt is consistent. British Medical Journal, 312, 1284–5.

Lee CD et al Physical activity and stroke risk: a meta-analysis. Stroke. 2003 Oct;34(10):2475-81.

Leung, C.H., Poon,W.S., Yu, L.M.,Wong, G.K., and Ng, H.K. (2002). Apolipoprotein e genotype and outcome in aneurysmal subarachnoid hemorrhage. Stroke, 33, 548–52.

Liao, D.,Myers, R.,Hunt, S., et al. (1997). Familial history of stroke and stroke risk: the Family Heart Study. Stroke, 28, 1908–12.

Longstreth,W.T. Jr., Koepsell, T.D., Yerby, M.S., and van Belle, G. (1985). Risk factors for subarachnoid hemorrhage. Stroke, 16, 377–85.

Markus, H.S., Thomson, N., and Brown, M.M. (1995). Asymptomatic cerebral embolic signals in symptomatic and asymptomatic carotid artery disease. Brain, 118, 1005–11.

Markus,H. and Cullinane, M. (2001). Severely impaired cerebrovascular reactivity predicts stroke and TIA risk in patients with carotid artery stenosis and occlusion. Brain, 124, 457–67.

Marshall, J. (1971). Familial incidence of cerebrovascular disease. Journal of Medical Genetics, 8, 84–9.

McKusick,V.A. (2001). The anatomy of the human genome: a neo-Vesalian basis for medicine in the 21st century. Journal of the American Medical Association, 286, 2289–95.

Meschia, J.F., Brown, R.D. Jr., Brott, T.G., Chukwudelunzu, F.E.,Hardy, J., and Rich, S.S. (2002). The Siblings With Ischemic Stroke Study (SWISS) Protocol. BioMed Central Medical Genetics, 3, 1.

Meyer, F.B., Sundt, T.M. Jr., Fode, N.C.,Morgan, M.K., Forbes, G.S., and Mellinger, J.F. (1989). Cerebral aneurysms in childhood and adolescence. Journal of Neurosurgery, 70, 420–5.

Mhurchu C.N., Anderson, C., Jamrozik, K.,Hankey, G., Dunbabin, D. (2001). Hormonal factors and risk of aneurysmal subarachnoid haemorrhage: an international population-based, case-control study. Stroke, 32, 606–12.

Mohr, J.P., Thompson, J.L., Lazar, R.M., Levin, B., Sacco, R.L., Furie, K.L., Kistler, J.P.,Albers, G.W., Pettigrew, L.C., Adams, H.P., Jackson, C.M., and Pullicino, P. (2001).Warfarin–Aspirin Recurrent Stroke Study Group. A comparison of warfarin and aspirin for the prevention of recurrent ischemic stroke. New England Journal of Medicine, 345, 1444–51.

Molloy, J. and Markus, H.S. (1999). Asymptomatic embolization predicts stroke and TIA risk in patients with carotid artery stenosis. Stroke, 30, 1440–3.

Murray, C.J.L. and Lopez, A.D. (eds). (1996). The global burden of disease: a comprehensive assessment of mortality and disability from disease, injuries, and risk factors in 1990 and projected to 2020.

Mathonnet F, Nadifi S, Serazin-Leroy V, Dakouane M, Giudicelli Y. Absence of factor V Leiden mutation and low prothrombin G 20210 A mutation prevalence in a healthy Moroccan population. Thromb Haemost. 2002 Dec;88 (6):1073-4.

Olson, J.,Vongpunsawad, S., Kuivaniemi, H., et al. (1998). Genome scan for intracranial aneurysm susceptibility loci using Finnish families (abstract). American Journal of Human Genetics, 63, A17.

Paganini-Hill A, et al Infection and risk of ischemic stroke: differences among stroke subtypes. Stroke. 2003 Feb;34(2):452-7

Paluku, Nadifi S. et al Prothrombin G20210A and Factor V Leiden Polymorphisms in Stroke. J Mol Neurosci. 2011 Jun 24.

Petty, G.W., Brown, R.D.,Whisnant, J.P., Sicks, J.D., O'Fallon, M., and Wiebers, D.O. (2000). Ischaemic stroke subtypes. A population-based study of functional outcome, survival, and recurrence. Stroke, 31, 1062–8.

Polychronopoulos, P., Gioldasis, G., Ellul, J., et al. (2002). Family history of stroke in stroke types and subtypes. Journal of Neurologic Sciences, 195, 117–22.

Prospective Studies Collaboration. (1995). Cholesterol, diastolic blood pressure and stroke: 13,000 strokes in 250,000 people in 45 prospective cohorts. Lancet, 346, 1647–53.

Reduction of stroke events with pravastatin: the Prospective Pravastatin Pooling (PPP) Project. Circulation, 103, 387–92.

Ridker, P.M.,Hennekens, C.H., Buring, J.E., and Rifai, N. (2000). C-reactive protein and other markers of inflammation in the prediction of cardiovascular disease in women. New England Journal Medicine, 342, 836–43.

Rothwell, P.M., Gibson, R., and Warlow, C.P. (2000). Interrelation between plaque surface morphology and degree of stenosis on carotid angiograms and the risk of ischemic stroke in patients with symptomatic carotid stenosis. On behalf of the European Carotid Surgery Trialists' Collaborative Group. Stroke, 31, 615–21.

Roshan Ariyaratnam Genetics of ischaemic stroke among persons of non-European descent: a meta-analysis of eight genes involving approximately 32,500 individuals. PLoS Med. 2007 Apr;4 (4):e131.

Rudic, D.R. and Sessa,W.C. (1999). Nitric Oxide in endothelial dysfunction and vascular remodelling. American Journal of Human Genetics, 64, 673–7.

Rundek, T., Di Tullio, M.R., Sciacca, R.R., Titova, I.V.,Mohr, J.P.,Homma, S., and Sacco, R.L. (1999). Association Between Large Aortic Arch Atheromas and High-Intensity Transient Signals in Elderly Stroke Patients. Stroke, 30, 2683–6.

Sacco, R.L., Ellenberg, J.H.,Mohr, J.P., Tatemichi, T.K.,Hier, D.B., and Price, T.R. (1989). Infarcts of undetermined cause: the NINCDS stroke data bank. Annals of Neurology, 25, 382–90.

Sacco, R.L., Kargman, D.E., Gu, Q., and Zamanillo, M.C. (1995). Race-ethnicity and determinants of intracranial atherosclerotic cerebral infarction: the Northern Manhattan Stroke Study. Stroke, 26, 14–20.

Salamon, G. (1973). Atlas de la vascularisation arterielle du cerveau chez l'homme, 2nd edn. Sandoz, Paris.

Sankai, T., Iso, H., Shimamoto, T., et al. (2000). Prospective study on alcohol intakes and risk of subarachnoid haemorrhage among Japanese men and women. Alcoholism, clinical and experimental research, 24, 386–9.

Schievink,W.I., Schaid, D.J., Rogers, H.M., Piepgras, D.G., and Michels,V.V. (1994). On the inheritance of intracranial aneurysms. Stroke, 25, 2028–37.

Schievink,W.I., Schaid, D.J.,Michels,V.V., and Piepgras, D.G. (1995). Familial aneurismal subarachnoid hemorrhage: a community-based study. Journal of Neurosurgery, 83, 426–9.

Segal, J.B.,McNamara, R.L.,Miller, M.R., Powe, N.R., Goodman, S.N., Robinson, K.A., and Bass, E.B. (2001). Anticoagulants or antiplatelet therapy for non-rheumatic atrial fibrillation and flutter. Cochrane Database Systematic Reviews, 1, CD001938.

Siebler, M., Kleinschmidt, A., Sitzer, M., et al. (1994). Cerebral microembolism in symptomatic and asymptomatic high-grade internal carotid artery stenosis. Neurology, 44, 615-8.

Stefansson, K. (2001). Health care and privacy: an interview with Kari Stefansson, founder and CEO of deCODE Genetics in Reykjavik, Iceland. EMBO Reports, 2, 964–7.

Stewart, J., Dundas, R.,Howard, R., Rudd, A., and Wolfe, C.D.A. (1999). Ethnic differences in stroke incidence. The south London Stroke register. British Medical Journal, 318, 967–71.

Storrs, B.B.,Humphreys, R.P.,Hendrick, E.B., and Hoffman, H.J. (1982). Intracranial aneurysms in the pediatric age-group. Childs Brain, 9, 358–61.

The French Study of Aortic Plaques in Stroke Group. (1996). Atherosclerotic disease of the aortic arch as a risk factor for recurrent ischemic stroke. New England Journal of Medicine, 334, 1216–21.

The Stroke Prevention in Reversible Ischemia Trial (SPIRIT) Study Group. (1997). A randomized trial of anticoagulants versus aspirin after cerebral ischemia of presumed arterial origin. Annals of Neurology, 42, 857–65.

They-They TP, et al .Prevalence of angiotensin-converting enzyme, methylene tetra hydro folate reductase, Factor V Leiden, prothrombin and apolipoprotein E gene polymorphisms in Morocco. Ann Hum Biol. 2010 Nov;37(6):767-77

Thompson, S.G., Greenberg, G., and Meade, T.W. (1989). Risk factors for stroke and myocardial infarction in women in the United Kingdom as assessed in general practice: a case-control study.British Heart Journal, 61, 403–9.

Thorin, E., and Shreeve, S.M. (1998). Heterogeneity of vascular endothelial cells in normal and disease states. Pharmacology and Therapeutics, 78, 155–66.

Thorvaldsen, P., Asplund, K., Kuulasmaa, K., Rajakangas, A.M., and Schroll, M. (1995). Stroke incidence, case fatality, and mortality in the WHO MONICA project.World Health Organization Monitoring Trends and Determinants in Cardiovascular Disease. Stroke, 26, 361–7.

Thrift, A.G., Dewey, H.M.,Macdonell, R.A.,McNeil, J.J., and Donnan, G.A. (2001). Incidence of the major stroke subtypes: initial findings from the North East Melbourne Stroke Incidence Study (NEMESIS). Stroke, 32, 1732–8.

Tietjen, G.E. (2000). The relationship of migraine and stroke. Neuroepidemiology, 19, 13–9.

Truelsen T, Piechowski-Jóźwiak B, Bonita R, Mathers C, Bogousslavsky J, Boysen G.Stroke incidence and prevalence in Europe: a review of available data.Eur J Neurol. 2006 Jun;13(6):581-98.

Tunstall-Pedoe H. The World Health Organization MONICA Project (monitoring trends and determinants in cardiovascular disease): a major international collaboration. WHO MONICA Project Principal Investigators. J Clin Epidemiol 1988;41:105-14.

Tzourio, C., Kittner, S.J., Bousser, M.G., and Alperovitch, A. (2000).Migraine and stroke in young women. Cephalalgia, 20, 190–9.

van Exel, E.,Gussekloo, J., de Craen, A.J., Bootsma-van der Wiel, A., Frolich, M., and Westendorp, R.G. (2002). Inflammation and stroke: the Leiden 85-Plus Study. Stroke, 33, 1135–8.

Vitullo, F.,Marchioli, R., Di Mascio, R., Cavasinni, L., Pasquale, A.D., and Tognoni, G. (1996). Family history and socioeconomic factors as predictors of myocardial infarction, unstable angina and stroke in an Italian population: PROGETTO 3A Investigators. European Journal of Epidemiology, 12, 177–85.

Walton, J. (ed.) (1993). Brain's diseases of the nervous system, 10th edn. p. 203. Oxford University Press, Oxford, UK.

Wang, P.S., Longstreth,W.T. Jr., and Koepsell, T.D. (1995). Subarachnoid hemorrhage and family history: a population-based case-control study. Archives of Neurology, 52, 202–4.

Ward, N.S. and Brown, M.M. (2002). Leukoaraiosis. In Subcortical stroke (eds Donnan, G. Norrving, B. Bamford, J. and Bogousslavsky, J.), 2nd edn. pp. 4746–66. Oxford University Press, Oxford.

Warlow, C.P., Dennis, M.S., van Gijn, J.,Hankey, G.J., Sandercock, P.A.G., Bamford, J.M., and Wardlaw, J. (1996a).What caused this subarachnoid haemorrhage? In Stroke. A practical guide to management, pp. 322–59. Blackwell Science, Oxford, UK.

Warlow, C.P., Dennis, M.S., van Gijn, J.,Hankey, G.J., Sandercock, P.A.G., Bamford, J.M., and Wardlaw, J. (1996b).What caused this intracerebral haemorrhage? In Stroke. A practical guide to management, pp. 287-321. Blackwell Science, Oxford, UK.

Welin, L., Svardsudd, K.,Wilhelmsen, L., Larsson, B., and Tibblin, G. (1987). Analysis of risk factors for stroke in a cohort of men born in 1913. New England Journal of Medicine, 317, 521–6

White, R.,Vallance, P., and Markus, H.S. (2000). The effect of nitric oxide synthase inhibition on dynamic cerebral autoregulation in man. Clinical Science, 99, 555–60.

White, R.P., Deane, C.,Vallance, P., and Markus, H.S. (1998). Nitric oxide synthase inhibition in humans reduces cerebral blood flow but not the hyperaemic response to hypercapnia. Stroke, 29, 467–72.

WHO Collaborative Study of Cardiovascular Disease and Steroid Hormone Contraception. (1996). Haemorrhagic stroke, overall stroke risk and combined oral contraceptives; results of an international,multi centre, case-controlled study. Lancet, 348, 505–10.

Wolfe, C.D.A. (2000). The impact of stroke. British Medical Bulletin, 56, 275–86.

Wolfe, C.D.A., Rudd, A.G., Howard, R., Coshall, C., Stewart, J., Lawrence, E.,Hajat, C., and Hillen, T. (2002). The incidence and case fatility of stroke subtypes in a multi ethnic population. The South London Stroke Register. Journal of Neurology Neurosurgery and Psychiatry, 72, 211–6.

14

Idiopathic Parkinson's Disease, Vascular Risk Factors and Cognition: A Critical Review

Maxime Doiron and Martine Simard
École de Psychologie,
Université Laval & Centre de Recherche Université Laval-Robert Giffard, Québec, Canada

1. Introduction

Idiopathic Parkinson's disease (PD) is a neurodegenerative disorder of the central nervous system that affects 1.5 million of individuals in the United States (American Parkinson Disease Association, 2011). Although its etiology is still unclear, the degeneration of the dopaminergic neurons in the substantia nigra stands out as the prominent pathological feature (Hauser, 2010). It seems that the balance between the dopamine, acetylcholine and glutamate neurotransmitters is compromised in PD, which may play a role in the subcortical-frontal behaviour impairment (Dubois et al., 1990). Other classical features of PD include the presence of Lewy bodies in the brainstem pigmented neurons, typical characteristics of the α-synucloeopathy in PD (Jellinger, 2003, 2011), and neuronal losses in the *locus coeruleus* (Aarsland et al., 2009).

In addition, the incidence and prevalence of cognitive impairment and dementia, as well as the relative risk for dementia, are higher in PD than in healthy elderly (Aarsland et al., 2001; Aarsland et al., 2005; de Lau et al., 2005;); this is thus an important problem. Some clinical and demographical risk factors for cognitive impairment and dementia in PD (PDD) have consistently been reported. More severe motor features such as gait disturbance, rigidity and postural instability tend to predict a faster cognitive decline and thus, an earlier dementia diagnosis (Aarsland et al., 2005; Aarsland & Kurz, 2010). The association of extrapyramidal signs with cognitive impairment supports the hypothesis of a role for PD subcortical pathology in the development of dementia (Levy et al., 2002; Bancher et al., 1993). Older age, disease duration and older age at onset were also identified as prominent risk factors for cognitive impairment in PD (Aarsland et al., 2001; Aarsland & Kurz, 2010; Hughes et al., 2000). Other potential features likely to predict cognitive impairment and PDD include visual hallucinations and genetic factors (Aarsland et al., 2010). However, these risk factors and their impact on cognition will not be directly reviewed in the present chapter, as they are considered to be respectively neuropsychiatric and genetic risk factors.

As in Alzheimer's disease (AD) (Petersen, 2004), Mild Cognitive Impairment (MCI) is another potential predictive factor for PDD (Aarsland et al., 2010). In this context, a significant number of non-demented PD patients present with MCI (Aarsland et al., 2010;

Ebmeier et al., 1991; Muslimovic et al., 2005). Some cognitive deficits, notably on tests of memory and executive functions predicted a shorter evolution toward PDD in some studies (Levy et al., 2002; Janvin et al., 2005). Poor performances on tests involving posterior cortical areas such as the semantic fluency test and the copy of a figure test would be the most important predictors of cognitive decline according to some authors (William-Grays et al., 2007). However, the profile of cognitive impairment is heterogeneous, some patients presenting with memory impairment while others show more language, executive and visuospatial impairments (Elgh et al., 2009; Janvin et al., 2005; Uc et al., 2009). Identifying factors contributing to cognitive deterioration is a noteworthy goal because a diminution in quality of life and an augmentation of mortality are associated with cognitive impairment and dementia in PD. Vascular risk factors (VRF) are among those factors. Several studies support the contribution of VRF in elderly adults in the development of vascular dementia and of Alzheimer's disease (Gorelick et al., 2011, for a review; Wiederkehr et al., 2009). Indeed, in the statement for healthcare professionals from the American Heart Association/American Stroke Association, blood pressure, hyperglycemia/diabetes, hypercholesterolemia, stroke, heart disease, alcohol intake and smoking were some of the VRF pointed out as being involved in vascular cognitive impairment, a possible prodromal phase of dementia (Gorelick et al., 2011).

However, there is a controversy regarding the occurrence and impact of the VRF on cognition and on the clinical evolution in PD and there is a lack of systematic review on the topic (Aarsland & Kurz, 2010; Korczin, 2010). Only one review was found but it was strictly investigating the possible link between elevated (↑) homocysteinemia (Hcy), L-dopa treatment and cognitive dysfunction and dementia in PD but it did not question the possible involvement of other VRF in cognitive impairment in PD (Zoccolella et al., 2010). This article reviewed 16 studies on ↑Hcy and cognitive impairment, dementia and neurodegenerative markers in PD (Zoccolella et al., 2010). However, 5 of the studies were only available as abstracts of conference presentations. The current review will thus use more stringent inclusion criteria for articles and will update as well as build upon the data of Zoccolella et al. (2010) regarding hyperhomocysteinemia as a possible VRF for cognitive impairment and dementia in PD. The present work will also review the possible involvement of other VRF such as hypertension (HT), type 2 diabetes mellitus (DM), heart disease (HD), hypercholesterolemia (HCL), stroke history (SH) /transient ischemic attacks (TIA), alcohol intake (ALC) and smoking (SMO) in the development of cognitive impairment and dementia in PD.

In summary, there is currently no consensus regarding the presence of VRF and their impact on cognition in PD. Therefore, the first objective of the current chapter is to perform a critical literature review on the cognitive profile of patients with PD and VRF in order to clarify this issue. The second objective is to investigate the possible biological mechanisms underlying the presence of VRF and cognitive dysfunctions in PD. Finally, some recommendations will be made to improve future research in this area.

2. Method

A search in MEDLINE/PubMed, PsycINFO and AgeLine (EBSCO) databases was conducted using the following keywords: (1) "Parkinson" AND "cognition/cognitive" AND "vascular risk factors", (2) "Parkinson" AND "cognition" AND "smoking/tobacco smoking/cigarette" OR "hypertension" OR "hypercholesterolemia" OR "diabetes/diabetes mellitus" OR "homocysteine/hyperhomocysteinemia" OR "alcool" OR "heart disease. The search included articles published from 1990 to May 31st, 2011. A manual search in the references of the selected articles was also performed as a second step to identify other pertinent publications. The selected articles had to meet the following inclusion criteria: 1) articles had to be published in English or French in order to be reviewed. 2) While longitudinal controlled studies were prioritized, cross-sectional studies with controls and/or using between-patient or within-patient comparisons were also considered. 3) Studies had to not only report VRF in PD, but also had to assess cognition using at least one standardized cognitive measure; and the authors had to report the results of the cognitive assessment. The studies were excluded if they were only case reports. The articles were independently reviewed by the two co-authors and final data were registered following a consensus meeting.

3. Results

3.1 Search results

Eighteen articles published from 1990 to 2010 met the inclusion criteria of the review (Alves et al., 2004; Barone et al., 2008; Camicioli et al., 2009; Hassin-Baer et al., 2006; Haugarvoll et al., 2005; Kandiah et al., 2009; Levy et al., 2002; Marder et al., 1990; Matteau et al., 2010; O'Suilleabhain et al., 2006; Ozer et al., 2006; Rektor et al., 2009; Religa et al., 2006; Rodriguez-Oroz et al., 2009; Slawek et al., 2008; Weisskopf et al., 2007; Zoccolella et al., 2009; Zoccolella et al., 2005). Sixteen articles were rejected because: 5 were only abstracts (Antonini et al., 2006; Litvinenko et al., 2005; Menendez et al., 2007; Shin & Sohn, 2006; Stathis et al., 2006), 6 didn't report the results of the cognitive assessment or didn't assess cognition using at least one standardized cognitive measure (Blandini et al., 2001; Ebmeier et al., 1990; Kuhn et al., 1998; Muller et al., 1999; Nakaso et al., 2006; Yasui et al., 2000;) and 5 didn't assess the effects of vascular risk factors (Aarsland et al., 2004; de Lau et al., 2005; Hughes et al., 1992; Locascio et al., 2003; Papapetropoulos et al., 2006).

3.2 Design and sample size of the studies

Table 1 summarizes the study design and participant's characteristics in the 18 selected studies. Only 1 study had a randomized double-blind placebo-controlled design (R-DB-PC) since it was a clinical trial on rivastigmine, 1 study had a longitudinal (LON) case-control (CC) design (follow-up of 8 years), 4 studies were longitudinal with between-patient comparisons (BPC) with mean follow-ups ranging from 2.0 to 4.0 years, 6 studies had a case-controlled design, 5 studies were cross-sectional (CS) with between-patient comparisons, and 1 study was cross-sectional using within-patient comparisons (WPC).

The number of PD patients included in the studies ranged from 35 to 342, whereas the number of healthy controls (when applicable, n=7 studies) ranged from 28 to 1144. One study (Alves et al., 2004) had 2 control groups: 100 healthy controls and 100 patients with only diabetes mellitus. The mean (SD) sample size for the 18 selected studies is 124.7 (87.5) PD patients and 229.4 (405.8) healthy controls (HC). However, 9 studies (50%) had <100 PD patients in their samples; and these small sample sizes reduce statistical power.

The PD patient groups were often divided into comparison subgroups with VRF/no-VRF (n=7 studies), dementia/no dementia (n=3 studies), normal cognitive function/mild cognitive impairment/dementia (n=3 studies), cognitive decline/no cognitive decline (n=1 study) and levodopa treated/untreated (n=1 study).

3.3 Participants characteristics

The mean age of PD patients in the 18 studies varied from 59.0 to 75.5 years old. However, PD patients were usually older than 65 years old (11/18 studies). Regarding the gender of patients, only one study didn't report the gender of the subjects (Religa et al., 2006). In most studies (n=15 studies), the male/female ratio was equal. However, one study had a significant greater number of male patients in the VRF compared to the no-VRF group (Haugarvoll et al., 2005) and another study had a significantly greater number of male patients in the two elevated homocysteine groups (Hassin-Baer et al., 2006).

Out of the 18 selected articles, only 7 reported the level of education of the participants in mean years of schooling. Although one study reported education as the percentage of patients having completed primary school (Rodriguez-Oroz et al., 2009) and another study as the percentage of patients having completed an academic degree (Weisskopf et al., 2007), 11 studies didn't report the education level of the participants at all. Among the 7 studies reporting education as the number of years attending school, the mean years of education varied from 5.7 to 15.2 years. Nevertheless, PD patients had at least 10 years of education in 4/7 studies that reported the education level. Therefore, most patients were well-educated. PD patients were recruited in movement disorder centers/clinics (MDC) (9 studies), general hospitals (HOS) (3 studies), community (COM) (2 studies), movement disorder database (MDB) (2 studies) and in multiple centers from different North-American and European countries (MC) (1 study). Only one study didn't report clearly the recruitment location. Healthy controls (HC), when applicable, were recruited in general hospitals in 3 studies and in the community in 3 studies while the recruitment location was not clearly stated in 1 study.

Mean disease duration in PD patients (at baseline when applicable) varied from less than 2 years to 14.7 years. Only one study didn't report the disease duration directly, but specified that it was less than 2 years, because the study focused on newly diagnosed patients (Kandiah et al., 2009).

The Hoehn & Yahr stage (H&Y) is a simple scale to globally assess PD severity (Hoehn & Yahr, 1967): stage 0= no signs of disease; stage 1= very mild symptoms on only one side of the body; stage 1.5= symptoms on only one side of the body with axial involvement; stage 2= symptoms on both sides without balance impairment; stage 2.5= mild symptoms on both sides with recovery on pull test; stage 3= mild to moderate symptoms and potential postural instability with maintenance of independence; stage 4= severe symptoms (patient is severely debilitated and needs assistance but can walk and stand alone); and stage 5=very severe symptoms confining the patients to a wheelchair or a bed unless assisted.

Ten of the 18 selected articles reported the H&Y stage of the PD patients, and it ranged between 2.1 and 3.9. However, one study reported only that patients were equal to or below stage 3.0 (Religa et al., 2006). Another study (Barone et al., 2008) reported H&Y stages with the percentage of patients in each stage, including 54/342 patients in the 4.0-5.0 range, which was rare in the studies reviewed herein. Nonetheless, the mean H&Y stage was below 3.0 in 7 out of 9 studies; thus most studies included patients in the early stages of PD.

The Unified Parkinson's disease Rating Scale (UPDRS) is a tool designed to assess different clinical aspects of patients in the PD course (Fahn et al., 1987). It allows a comprehensive coverage of motor symptoms and was proved to be valid and reliable (Movement Disorder Society Task Force on Rating Scales for Parkinson's Disease, 2003). Higher scores are associated with greater disability. Section I (maximum=16 points) assesses mentation, behaviour and mood (4 items). Section II (maximum=52 points) evaluates the activities of daily living (ADL) with 13 items. Section III (maximum=108 points) consists in a motor examination (14 items). Section IV evaluates clinical signs. A total of 13/18 studies reported the UPDRS score of patients. Two studies reported the score for sections I-IV (ranging from 22.9 to 50.9) and only one study reported the total score (I-V). However, most studies (n=10) only reported the motor examination (section III) score. Motor scores ranged from 17.3 to 48.1 in these studies and most of them (n=8 out of 10) had PD patients with a score of 35.0 and lower. In other words, in most studies, patients had mild to moderate motor symptoms. Four studies assessed the UPDRS when patients were "ON", whenever ON-OFF fluctuations were present, while only one study assessed them in the OFF state, and 8 studies didn't specify the procedure.

Table 2 presents the three sets of PD diagnostic criteria that were used in the 18 articles. The United Kingdom Parkinson's Disease Society Brain Research Centre (UKPDSBRC) criteria (Gibb et al., 1988; Hughes et al., 1992) were the most commonly used (n=9 studies), followed by the National Institute of Neurological Disorders and Stroke (NINDS) criteria (Gelb et al., 1999) (n=3 studies) and the Norwegian criteria of Larsen et al. (1994) (n=2 studies). The diagnosis was made only using the clinical impression of neurologists in one study (Weisskopf et al., 2007) and 3 studies didn't specify the diagnostic criteria used.

3.4 Vascular risk factors

Table 3 summarizes the frequency of the different vascular risk factors in the selected studies, their measures and the medication taken by the participants.

3.4.1 Hyperhomocysteinemia (↑Hcy)

Homocysteine (Hcy) is a sulfur-containing amino acid found in blood plasma and naturally biosynthesized as an intermediate product from the demethylation of the amino acid methionine (Reutens & Sachdev, 2002; Stanger et al., 2003). Hcy is metabolized in three distinct pathways (Mattson & Shea, 2003). Two pathways involve remethylation: the first (via the enzyme betaine-homocysteine methyltransferase) occurs in the liver and kidneys while the second (via the enzyme methionine synthase), catalyzed by methylentetrahydrofolate reductase (MTHFR), occurs in all human tissue and requires vitamin B12 and folate as cofactors. A third metabolic pathway involves transsulfuration (via the enzymes cystathionine-β-synthase (CβS) and γ-cystathionase) with vitamin B6 as a cofactor. (Mattson & Shea, 2003; Reutens & Sachdev, 2002).

The American Society of Human Genetics and the American College of Medical Genetics (ASHG/ACMG, 1998) define normal blood plasma level of Hcy as ranging from 5.0 to 15.0

μmol/L and hyperhomocysteinemia as a fasting total plasma Hcy level of >15.0 μmol/L. Plasma Hcy level increases with age and is higher in men than in women. The effect of age is partly explained by the diminution of renal function with increasing age (Stanger et al., 2003).

Hyperhomocysteinemia(↑Hcy) is due to multiple etiologies. Genetic abnormalities in genes encoding for enzymes involved in Hcy metabolism could partially explain an increase in Hcy concentration. Carriers of a thermolabile variant of MTHFR at nucleotide position 667 (MTHFR 677C→T) present a reduced enzymatic activity of MTHFR by approximately 70%, which leads to an increased level of blood plasma Hcy (Stanger et al., 2003). Vitamin deficiencies are probably the main factors of acquired ↑Hcy and can be the consequences of insufficient dietary intake, reduced absorption, increased consumption and drug interactions (Stanger et al., 2003). Some other relevant acquired causes of ↑Hcy include older age, renal failure (impaired remethylation), hypothyroidism (enzyme induction), alcohol intake (interference with B6, B12 and folate + enzyme inhibition) and cigarette smoking (interference with B6, B12 and folate + redox) (Finkelstein, 1998; Reutens & Sachdev, 2002; Stanger et al., 2003).

Levodopa (L-dopa) intake in PD was associated with Hcy blood and plasma levels (Kuhn et al., 1998; Müller et al., 1999; Rogers et al., 2003; Yasui et al., 2000). Levodopa is a substrate for S-adenosyl methionine (SAM)-dependent methylation. In fact, levodopa O-methylation to 3-O-methyldopa by cathecol-O-methyltransferase (COMT) constitutes a main metabolic pathway (Müller et al., 2002). COMT converts S-adenosylmethionine to S-adenosylhomocysteine which will eventually become Hcy. Therefore, ↑Hcy in PD is most likely the consequence of S-adenosylhomocysteine formation during levodopa breakdown (Müller et al., 2001, 2002).

Some studies also support a genetic role in ↑Hcy in PD: blood plasma levels are elevated in levodopa-treated patients homozygous for the MTHFR C667T mutation (Kuhn et al., 2001; Todorovic et al., 2006; Yasui et al., 2000). Hcy has also been involved in multiple biological mechanisms and notably as a neurotoxin contributing to neurodegeneration. Hcy is linked to increased oxidative stress, excitotoxicity, promotion of cellular apoptosis and the promotion of the pathophysiological processes of Alzheimer's like disease (Sachdev, 2005).

A total of 9 studies reported total Hcy levels in the PD groups and the number of PD patients with ↑Hcy ranged from 17 to 247. Only two studies didn't report the number of hyperhomocysteinemic patients. Nevertheless, the number of PD patients with ↑Hcy was below 31 in 5/7 studies, which are rather small groups.

3.4.2 Smoking (SMO)

Smoking is associated with cardiovascular disease and is potentially a VRF for cognitive impairment because its pathological mechanisms are known to increase oxidative stress, to increase inflammation and to promote thrombosis and atherosclerotic processes (Ambrose & Barua, 2004; Swan & Lessov-Schlaggar, 2007). Cigarette smoking reduces blood circulation by narrowing the arteries and thus, puts tobacco users at higher risk of developing peripheral vascular disease. Light and heavy smoking also results in a detrimental effect on endothelial vasoregulatory activity, thus leading to increased cardiovascular risk (Barua et al., 2002).

A total of 9 studies reported smoking in the PD patients. The number of PD patients who ever smoked (past + current smokers) varied from 10 to 78. However, the number of smokers is unknown in 2/9 studies. Only one study included smoking HC (n=49) (Alves et al., 2004). The distinction between past smokers and current smokers is clear in only 2 studies.

3.4.3 Diabetes Mellitus – Type 2 Diabetes (DM)

Type 2 diabetes mellitus (DM) is a metabolic disorder characterized by high blood glucose in the context of insulin resistance and insulin deficiency. Hyperglycemia is associated with functional changes in cerebral blood flow (Cosentino et al., 2009). Although the mechanism underlying the link between DM and cognitive impairment and dementia is still not well understood, it likely involves several inter-related processes. DM is thus a risk factor for stroke (Stegmayr & Asplund, 1995) and it is also assumed to be a risk factor for vascular dementia (Skoog, 1994; Tatemichi et al., 1993). Some biological links have also been described between DM and AD, such as indications of advanced glycation end-products (AGE) and increased AGE receptor expression in brains of patients with AD. As AGEs are known to be involved in DM complications, diabetes might thus influence AD brain pathology (Yan et al., 1997), and AD pathogenesis can be present in PD and PDD.

A total of 8 studies reported DM in PD and the number of PD patients with DM varied from 3 to 16. Out of these, the number of PD patients with DM is unknown in 3/8 studies. Another study (Alves et al., 2004) had 100 control participants with DM but not with PD.

3.4.4 Arterial Hypertension (HT)

A normal blood pressure (nBP) is required to maintain cognitive functioning, because it contributes to adequate cerebral perfusion. Hypertension (HT) is not only an important risk factor for strokes and heart disease; it is also an immediate risk factor for cognitive impairment and vascular dementia (Breteler, 2000). Individuals suffering from HT have stiffer artery walls and increased blood vessel resistance. This requires the heart to work harder in order to pump the blood, thus increasing the pressure of the blood leaving the heart and consequently increasing the risk of cerebrovascular ischemic damage (Chobanian et al., 2003). Blood pressure is often classified in different stages. According to the American Heart Association (Chobanian et al., 2003), nBP is defined as systolic pressure (SP) of 90-119 mmHg and diastolic pressure (DP) of 60-79 mmHg. Prehypertension is characterized by SP=120-139 mmHg and DP=80-89 mmHg, stage 1 hypertension by SP=140-159 mmHg and DP=90-99 mmHg, and stage 2 hypertension as SP ≥160 mmHg and DP ≥100 mmHg (Chobanian et al., 2003).

A total of 10 studies reported arterial HT in PD. The number of PD patients with HT varied from 14 to 68, and was generally below or equal to 40 patients (n=6 studies). However, 3/10 studies didn't report the exact number of PD patients with HT.

3.4.5 Heart Diseases (HD)

Commonly included in the heart disease (HD) category are coronary heart disease, heart failure and atrial fibrillation (AF). Coronary heart disease consists in the narrowing by atherosclerosis of the blood vessels that supply blood, nutrients and oxygen to the heart. Therefore, the consequent limitation of the blood flow to the heart muscle is responsible for ischemia. Coronary heart disease is one of the most common causes of heart failure (American Accreditation Health Care Commission (A.D.A.M.) Medical Encyclopedia, 2011). Heart failure is a condition in which the heart can no longer pump enough blood to every body part (Jessup et al., 2009). Systolic heart failure is characterized by insufficient blood ejection out of the heart while diastolic heart failure consists in heart muscles harder to fill up with blood. AF consists in a problem with the contraction rhythm of the atria that causes the blood to be ineffectively pumped to the ventricles. Hence, the arrhythmia is responsible for irregular blood flow throughout the whole body. AF is also a risk factor for heart failure (National Collaborating Centre for Chronic Conditions, 2006). Moreover, some studies reported that atrial fibrillation is associated with a higher risk for conversion to dementia in MCI non-PD patients (Ravaglia et al., 2006).

A total of 6 studies reported heart diseases in PD. The number of PD patients with HD ranged from 14 to 28, but the number is unknown in 2/6 studies. Four out of 6 studies included coronary heart disease in the HD category with n of PD patients varying from 9 to 17 (unknown in 2 studies). Atrial fibrillation (AF) and heart failure were reported in 2 studies: in one of these studies, only one patient was affected by AF, and 9 patients had heart failure, whereas the numbers for AF and heart failure are unknown in the other study.

3.4.6 Hypercholesterolemia (HCL)

Hypercholesterolemia (HCL) is a form of dyslipidemia defined as an abnormal amount of lipids in the blood, and is an established VRF for dementia (Luschinger et al., 2005). The mechanisms underlying the role of HCL in the development of dementia are not clearly understood. However, there is evidence that cholesterol alters the degradation of amyloid precursor protein and shows an effect on amyloid fibril formation, which may play a role in the pathogenesis of AD (Sponne et al., 2004). Amyloid abnormalities were described in the brains of PD patients with cognitive impairment (Braak & Braak, 1990) as well as of PDD patients (Nobili et al., 2011). Therefore, HCL could be a VRF for cognitive impairment and PDD, via its possible contribution to amyloid aggregation.

Three studies reported HCL in PD patients but only 2 studies mentioned the number of patients presenting with this condition (n=16 and 34).

3.4.7 Stroke History (SH) / Transient Ischemic Attacks (TIA)

The link between stroke and cognitive impairment and dementia is very well known (Chui et al., 1992; Roman et al., 1993). A stroke in any higher processing cerebral area will inevitably cause cognitive dysfunctions. One of the strongest predictors of cognitive decline after an initial stroke is the occurrence of a second stroke (Gorelick et al., 2011).

Only 4 studies reported a stroke history (SH) or transient ischemic attacks (TIA) and the number of patients with this VRF varied from 2 to 5 in 3 studies; one study didn't indicate the number of patients with this VRF.

3.4.8 Alcohol (ALC)

Observational studies have shown that alcohol consumption might be related to Hcy in a J-shaped fashion: chronic consumers (alcoholics) have very high levels of Hcy and moderate alcohol consumers (≤ 4 glasses/day) have lower Hcy levels as compared to non-drinkers (De Bree et al., 2001). Therefore the rationale for considering alcohol as VRF for cognitive impairment in PD might be partly explained by its deleterious effect on Hcy levels. It also lowers vitamin B12 and folate levels (Gibson et al., 2008).

Only 3 studies reported alcohol intake and the number of PD patients consuming alcohol was unknown in one study, n=7 in another, and another study distinguished 44 former and 29 current consumers.

3.5 Medication

L-Dopa was the most common medication taken by PD patients (n=14 studies) and doses varied from 326.7 to 1028.0 mg/day with a mean of 589 mg/day. Other medications included dopamine agonists (n=5 studies) and anticholinergics (n=3 studies). Only one study reported the use of antipsychotic and antidepressant drugs. Thus the groups included in this review were generally neither depressed nor psychotic. Only 3/18 studies didn't report the medication taken by the PD patients.

3.6 Cognition and VRF

Results and tests of the neuropsychological assessment in the 18 studies are illustrated in Table 4. Cognitive tests are grouped under specific cognitive domains and are presented below, starting from the most prevalent to the least prevalent in the studies.

Global cognitive function was assessed in 17/18 studies and the most administered tests were the Mini-Mental State Examination (MMSE) (n=15 studies) and the Dementia Rating Scale (DRS) (n=3 studies). Intelligence (global cognitive function) was also evaluated in one study using the Wechsler-Bellevue Intelligence Scale (WBIS). However, no association with the VRF could be made, since the authors used the WBIS only to assess the premorbid cognitive state of the patients. The other tests assessing global cognitive function were only used once (see Table 4).

3.6.1 Association between VRF and risk for dementia (global measure of dementia)

Six studies investigated the association between VRF and the risk of incident dementia in PD. Dementia was generally assessed using MMSE in 5/6 studies (see Table 4). Zoccolella et al. (2009) found that Hcy levels were significantly higher in the PDD group compared to the PD group without dementia. The risk for dementia in the ↑Hcy group was significantly higher than in the <12.4 μmol/L (normal Hcy) group. A multivariate logistic regression showed that ↑Hcy was associated with presence of dementia. However, Rodriguez-Oroz et al. (2009) found that Hcy levels didn't predict the cognitive status of PD patients.

Levy et al. (2006) found that current and ever smoking were associated with a higher risk for PDD, but past smoking was not. They also reported that smokers who stopped smoking less than 8 years before PD onset had a higher risk for PDD. However, pack-years of smoking and smoking duration weren't associated with a higher risk for PDD.

Zoccolella et al. (2009) found that HT was significantly more frequent in the PDD group compared to the PD group without dementia. Haugarvoll et al. (2005) found that PDD had more heart failure than patients without dementia after a 4-year follow-up. Slawek et al. (2008) demonstrated that HD was significantly more prevalent in the PDD group compared to the cognitively normal PD patients, though it was only a weak predictive factor for dementia.

However, results of various regression analyses did not find heart failure, coronary HD, AF, stroke, TIA, HT, DM, HCL, ALC and SMO to be predictive of dementia (Haugervoll et al., 2005; Levy et al., 2006; Marder et al., 1990; Slawek et al., 2008; Zoccolella et al., 2009).

3.6.2 Association between VRF and a score of global cognition

↑Hcy in PD patients was associated with worse global cognition per the MMSE compared to patients with normal Hcy in only 2 studies (Religa et al., 2006; Zoccolella et al., 2005), but there was no difference between L-dopa-treated and non-L-dopa treated patients (Religa et al., 2006).

Six studies (Barone et al., 2008-at baseline only); Camicioli et al., 2009; Hassin-Baer et al., 2006; O'Suilleabhain et al., 2004, 2006; Ozer et al., 2006; Rodriguez-Oroz et al., 2009) found no association between ↑Hcy and worse global cognition as measured by the MMSE (n=5 studies), the ADAS-Cog (n=1), the BDS (n=1), the DRS (n=1) and the STMS (n=1 study). However, the R-DB-PC study of Barone et al. (2008) found that ↑Hcy-rivastigmine-treated patients significantly improved their performance after 24 weeks on the ADAS-Cog and the MMSE compared to ↑Hcy–placebo-treated-patients. This improvement wasn't present in the normal/low Hcy groups, suggesting a relationship between cognition, ↑Hcy and successful treatment with a cholinesterase inhibitor (rivastigmine). Interestingly, O'Suilleabhain et al. (2004, 2006) only found a significant difference between the PD group with Hcy ≥14 µmol/L compared to the PD with Hcy <14 µmol/L when they pooled together the results of all neuropsychological tests (14). However, ↑Hcy at baseline was not associated with a greater decline on the pooled scores 2 years later.

Two studies reported some kind of relationship between smoking in PD patients and poor cognition. Weisskopf et al. (2007) found that smoking was associated with worst global cognition (per the TICS), and the risk for cognitive impairment was significantly higher for current smokers compared to never smokers. In the study of Matteau et al. (2010), patients with VRF (smoking in the past 10 years, myocardial infarct, stroke, DM and HT) performed significantly more poorly on the MMSE compared with no-VRF patients, independently of disease duration. In this particular study, the most prevalent VRF (in 66% of PD patients) was a history of smoking in the past 10 years, suggesting a possible relationship between smoking and global cognition in PD.

However, smoking and global cognitive function were not associated together in 4 studies with cross-sectional analyses and at 4 and 8-year follow-ups in one study. In addition, there was no difference between PD non-smokers, all smokers and heavy smokers (20 pack-years and more) on cognition (Alves et al., 2004; Marder et al., 1990). In another study, the MMSE score of PD patients was associated with an increase of intimomedial thickness (an indicator of large vessel impairment) but not with smoking, HT, DM, ischemic HD and stroke (Rektor et al., 2009).

Finally, Slawek et al. (2008) found that coronary HD was associated with a lower score on the MMSE, whereas Kandiah et al. (2009) found that diabetes mellitus didn't predict cognitive decline as measured by the MMSE.

3.6.3 Episodic memory

Episodic memory was assessed in 10 studies and the most administered tests were the Benton Visual Retention Test (BVRT) (n=2 studies), the Rey Auditory Verbal Learning Test (RAVLT) (n=2 studies) and memory subtests of the Wechsler Memory Scale (WMS) (n=2 studies). All other tests assessing episodic memory were only used once (see Table 4).

Ozer et al. (2006) found significant lower scores on the Sozel Bellek Surecleri Test (SBST) - delayed recall (verbal memory) in the PD group with Hcy ≥14 µmol/L compared to PD with Hcy <14 µmol/L, but not on the visual memory subtest of the WMS. In the study of O'Suilleabhain et al. (2004, 2006), PD with Hcy ≥14 µmol/L significantly declined on the Rey-Osterrieth-Complex-Figure (ROCF)-immediate recall at 2-year follow-up, whereas PD with Hcy <14 µmol/L did not. However, the baseline performances of these patients were comparable on episodic memory measures.

Two studies assessing episodic memory did not find significant differences or correlations between patients Hcy levels and measures of episodic memory (Hassin-Baer et al., 2006; Rodriguez-Oroz et al., 2009).

Coronary heart disease was associated with a lower score on the RAVLT, a measure of verbal episodic memory (Slawek et al. 2008) whereas an increased intimomedial thickness and pulsatility index (an indicator of small vessel impairment) were correlated with the WMS-III- Recognition-word list II (Rektor et al., 2009).

There was no association between the presence of SMO (Rektor et al., 2009; Slawek et al., 2008; Weisskopf et al., 2007), HT, DM, ischemic heart disease, HCL, stroke, and alcohol intake and measures of episodic memory (Rektor et al., 2009; Slawek et al., 2008).

3.6.4 Executive functions

Executive functions were assessed in 10 studies and the most administered tests were the Stroop (n= 4 studies), the Frontal Assessment Battery (FAB) (n=4 studies) and the Trail Making Test (TMT) (n=2 studies). All other tests assessing executive functions were used only once (see Table 4).

Ozer et al. (2006) found significant lower scores on the Stroop and Wisconsin Card Sorting Test (WCST) in PD with Hcy ≥14 µmol/L compared to PD with Hcy <14 µmol/L. However, 4 studies registered no association between Hcy levels and executive functions: on the Stroop test (O'Suilleabhain et al. 2004; Rodriguez-Oroz et al., 2009), even after 2 years of follow-up (O'Suilleabhain et al., 2006); and on the TMT and the Raven Progressive Matrices (Hassin-Baer et al., 2006; Rodriguez-Oroz et al., 2009).

Slawek et al. (2008) found no association between the Tower of Toronto score and the presence of HT, DM, HCL, HD, smoking and alcohol intake. Haugarvoll et al. (2005), Levy et al. (2002) and Camicioli et al. (2009) didn't report results on tests of executive functions in relation with VRF.

3.6.5 Language

Language was assessed in 10 studies and the most administered tests were verbal fluency tests (VFT; category and letter; n=7 studies) and the Boston Naming Test (BNT) (n=2 studies). All other tests assessing language were used only once (see Table 4).

In the R-DB-PC study of Barone et al. (2008), ↑Hcy-rivastigmine-treated patients improved significantly on letter fluency after 24 weeks compared with ↑Hcy–placebo-treated patients, and this improvement wasn't present in the normal/low homocysteine groups. Moreover, O'Suilleabhain et al. (2004, 2006) found that PD patients with Hcy ≥14 µmol/L compared to those with Hcy <14 µmol/L had significantly lower score on verbal fluency at baseline, but the scores of the 2 groups were comparable at follow-up. However, other studies found no association between Hcy levels and scores of verbal fluency (Hassin-Baer et al., 2006; Ozer et al., 2006; Rodriguez-Oroz et al., 2009) and of the BNT (Rodriguez-Oroz et al., 2009).

Verbal fluency scores were significantly associated with an increase of intimomedial thickness and of the pulsatility index (Rektor et al., 2009), as well as with coronary HD (Slawek et al, 2008).

However, verbal fluency scores were not associated with presence of smoking, HT, DM, ischemic heart disease and stroke (Rektor et al., 2009). Levy et al. (2002) and Camicioli et al. (2009) didn't report results on language tests.

3.6.6 Attention and vigilance

Attention and vigilance were assessed in 5 studies and the most administered test was Digit Span (n= 4) while the CDR Computerized Assessment System Power of Attention test (CDR-PoA) was only administered once. The R-DB-PC study of Barone et al. (2008) found that ↑Hcy-rivastigmine-treated patients had a significant improvement on the CDR-PoA after 24 weeks compared to ↑Hcy-placebo-treated patients, and this improvement wasn't present in the rivastigmine and placebo-treated Hcy-normal groups.

However, in other studies, PD with Hcy ≥14 µmol/L and PD with Hcy <14 µmol/L had comparable performances on Digit Span at baseline (Hassin-Baer et al., 2006; O'Suilleabhain et al., 2004; Rodriguez-Oroz et al., 2009;) and 2 years later (O'Suilleabhain et al., 2006).

3.6.7 Visual perception

Visual perception was assessed in 3 studies using the Benton Judgment of Line Orientation (BJLO) test (n=2 studies), the Benton Face Recognition (BFR) test (n=1 study) and the matching part of the Benton Visual Retention Test (BVRT) (n=1 study).

Ozer et al., 2006 reported a significant negative correlation between the concentration of Hcy and the BFR. Results on the BVRT (Levy et al., 2002) and on the BJLO (Haugervoll et al., 2005) were not reported.

Authors	Design	FU (yrs)	n of participants: Total	n of participants: HC	n of participants: PD (main group and *subgroups*)		Participants' characteristics: Age (mean in yrs)	M/F	Education (mean in yrs)	Recruited in	PD duration (mean in yrs)	H&Y stage	UPDRS score	PD diagnostic criteria
Barone et al. (2008) & Emre et al. (2004) (same trial)	R-DB-PC	0.46 (24 weeks)	342	-	**Total PD=342**	→	-	-	?	MC	?	?	?	UKPDSBRC criteria & DSM-IV criteria (for dementia)
					Hcy levels (subgroups)									
					≥14 µmol/L (n= 247)	→	73.3	167/80	?	MC	10.2	1-3=83% 4-5=17%	34.0 ^{III}	
					<14 µmol/L (n=95)	→	71.3	56/39	?	MC	8.9	1-3=87% 4-5=13%	31.0 ^{III}	
Alves et al. (2004)	LON CC	8.0	439	100 HC + 100 DM	*(HC)*	→	72.8	51/49	?	HOS	-	-	-	Larsen et al. (1994)
					Total PD=239	→	73.4	117/122	?	HOS	?	?	?	
					SMO=78	→	71.9	60/18	?	HOS	9.5	2.7	46.0 $^{I-IV}$	
					no-SMO=161	→	74.1	57/104	?	HOS	9.0	2.9	50.9 $^{I-IV}$ (both on)	
Haugarvoll et al. (2005)	LON BPC	4.0	BL= 171 FU=130	- -	**Total PD=171**	→	?	84/87	?	COM	?	?	?	Larsen et al. (1994)
					VRF=100	→	72.0	56/44	9.5	COM	9.0	2.4	24.0 $^{I-IV}$	
					no-VRF=71	→	70.0	28/43	9.5	COM	9.0	2.4	22.9 $^{I-IV}$	
Kandiah et al. (2009)	LON BPC	2.8 (mean)	106	-	**Total PD=106**	→	61.2	62/44	7.1	MDD	?	2.1	19.8 ^{III}	NINDS criteria
					CD=33	→	65.0	15/18	5.0	MDD	?	2.2	20.0 ^{III}	
					no-CD=73	→	59.0	47/26	8.0	MDD	?	2.1	19.0 ^{III}	
Levy et al. (2002)	LON BPC	3.6 (mean)	180	-	**Total PD=180**	→	71.0	83/97	11.1	COM	6.3	?	25.0 ^{III}	UKPDSBRC criteria
					DEM=52	→	74.6	29/23	9.4	COM	7.3	?	32.0 ^{III}	
					no-DEM=128	→	69.5	54/74	11.8	COM	5.9	?	22.2 ^{III}	
O'Suilleabhain et al. (2004) [BL]	LON BPC	2.0	BL=97	-	**Baseline**									NINDS criteria
					Total PD= 97	→	65.0	68/29	?	MDC	3.6	?	?	
					Hcy<14 µmol/L; n=66	→	64.0	43/23	?	MDC	3.6	?	23.0 ^{III}	
&				-	*Hcy≥14 µmol/L; n= 31*	→	68.0	25/6	?	MDC	3.8	?	28.9 ^{III}	
					Follow-up									
O'Suilleabhain et al. (2006) [FU]			FU=79		**Total PD=79**	→	67.0	55/24	?	MDC	5.5	?	?	
					Hcy<14 µmol/L; n=54	→	?	?	?	MDC	?	?	22.9 ^{III}	
					Hcy≥14 µmol/L; n=25	→	?	?	?	MDC	?	?	31.0 ^{III}	

Table 1. Study Design and Participant's Characteristics

Authors	Design	FU (yrs)	n of participants: Total	HC	PD (main group and *subgroups*)		Participants' characteristics: Age (mean in yrs)	M/F	Education (mean in yrs)	Recruited in	PD duration (mean in yrs)	H&Y stage	UPDRS score	PD diagnostic criteria
Rodriguez-Oroz et al. (2009)	CC	-	119	30	*(HC)*	→	68.5	16/14	?	COM	-	-	-	UKPDSBRC criteria
					Total PD=89	→	?	?	?	MDC	?	?	?	
					CN=37	→	69.9	20/17	?	MDC	14.7	3.4	41.9 ^{III}	
					MCI=22	→	70.2	14/8	?	MDC	13.1	3.4	43.8 ^{III}	
					PDD=30	→	74.9	18/12	?	MDC	14.7	3.9	48.1 ^{III} (all off)	
Weisskopf et al. (2007)	CC	-	1430	1144	*(HC)*	→	72.2	466/678	?	COM	-	-	-	Clinical Impression/ Neurologists
					Total PD=286	→	71.9	137/149	?	COM	6.4	?	?	
Zoccolella et al. (2009)	CC	-	275	154	*(HC)*	→	68.7	97/57	?	HOS	-	-	-	UKPDSBRC criteria
					Total PD=121	→	67.4	72/49	?	MDC	?	?	?	
					PDD=42	→	71.2	27/15	5.7	MDC	10.0	?	32.3 ^{III}	
					no-PDD=79	→	65.4	45/34	7.9	MDC	10.0	?	26.8 ^{III} (all on)	
Religa et al. (2006)	CC	-	214	100	*(HC)*	→	71.2	?	?	HOS	-	-	-	NINDS criteria
					Total PD=114	→	?	?	?	COM	?	≤ 3.0	?	
					L-dopa= 99	→	70.5	?	?	MDC	6.1	?	?	
					Untreated= 15	→	66.0	?	?	MDC	1.9	?	?	
Ozer et al. (2006)	CC	-	67	28	*(HC)*	→	61.9	15/13	?	?	-	-	-	Not specified
					Total PD= 39	→	67.0	25/14	?	MDC	6.4	?	?	
					Hcy>14 *μmol/L; n=17*	→	68.5	?	?	MDC	?	?	29.4	
					Hcy<14 *μmol/L; n=22*	→	64.4	?	?	MDC	?	?	29.7	
Camicioli et al. (2009)	CC	-	101	50	*(HC)*	→	71.6	29/21	15.0	COM	-	-	2.1 ^{III}	UKPDSBRC criteria
					Total PD=51	→	71.5	30/21	13.9	MDC	8.7	2.2	17.3 ^{III} (all on)	
Hassin-Baer et al. (2006)	CS BPC	-	72	-	**Total PD=72**	→	68.7	46/26	12.0	MDC & Neurology Service	6.7	?	24.9 ^{III} (all on)	UKPDSBRC criteria
					Hcy <12.5 mol/L; n=23	→	69.9	10/12	10.9		5.0	?	22.4 ^{III}	
					12.5-16.7 μmol/L; n=24	→	67.0	18/6	13.2		6.0	?	21.7 ^{III}	
					Hcy >16.7 μmol/L; n=25	→	69.3	18/7	11.8		8.0	?	27.3 ^{III}	

Table 1. Study Design and Participant's Characteristics (continued)

Authors	Design	FU (yrs)	n of participants: Total	HC	PD (main group and *subgroups*)	Participants' characteristics: Age (mean in yrs)	M/F	Education (mean in yrs)	Recruited in	PD duration (mean in yrs)	H&Y stage	UPDRS score	PD diagnostic criteria
Matteau et al. (2010)	CS BPC	-	124	-	**Total PD=124** →	?	?	?	MDD	?	?	?	UKPDSBRC criteria
					VRF: 67 →	63.9	49/18	12.8	MDD	5.8	3.7	?	
					no-VRF: 57 →	61.3	39/18	15.2	MDD	8.9	3.8	?	
Sławek et al. (2008)	CS BPC	-	60	-	**Total PD=60** →	68.4	35/25	?	MDC	8.4	2.7	27.4 ^{III}	UKPDSBRC criteria
					CN: 17 →	64.5	?	?	MDC	6.8	2.3	20.9 ^{III}	
					MCI: 25 →	68.6	?	?	MDC	9.0	2.7	25.1 ^{III}	
					PDD: 18 →	71.7	?	?	MDC	9.0	3.1	36.7 ^{III}	
Zoccolella et al. (2005)	CS BPC	-	35	-	**Total PD=35** →	?	25/10	?	?	?	?	?	Not specified
					CogI: 14 →	67.8	10/4	?	?	10.5	?	?	
					CN: 21 →	63.7	15/6	?	?	9.3	?	?	
Marder et al. (1990)	CS BPC	-	71	-	**Total PD=71** →	?	53/18	?	HOS	?	?	?	Not specified
					PDD: 17 →	75.5	17/0	?	HOS	11.9	?	?	
					no-PDD: 54 →	64.0	36/18	?	HOS	8.8	?	?	
Rektor et al. (2009)	CS WPC	-	57	-	**Total PD=57** →	68.2	39/18	?	MDC	9.3	2.7	22.5 ^{III}	UKPDSBRC criteria

Legend: - (not applicable), ? (unknown or not clear), BL (Baseline), FU (Follow-Up);
Design: BPC (Between Patients Comparisons), CC (Case-Control Study), CS (Cross-sectional Study), LON (Longitudinal Study), R-DB-PC (Randomized Double-Blind Placebo-Controlled design), WPC (Within-Patient Comparisons);
Participants: CD (Cognitive Decline), HC (Healthy Controls), CN (Cognitively Normal), CogI (Cognitive Impairment), DEM (Dementia), Hcy (Homocysteine= hyperhomocysteinemia), MCI (Mild Cognitive Impairment), no-VRF (No Vascular Risk Factors), PD (Idiopathic Parkinson's Disease), PDD (Parkinson's disease with dementia), VRF (Vascular Risk Factors);
Participants' characteristics: COM (Community), H&Y (Hoehn and Yahr Stage), HOS (Hospitals), III-OFF (Section III : Motor Examination - OFF of the UPDRS), MC (Multicenter), MDC (Movement Disorder Center), MDD (Movement Disorder Database), M/F (Males / Females ratio), UPDRS (Unified Parkinson's Disease Rating Scale);
PD diagnostic criteria: DSM-IV (Diagnostic and Statistical Manual of Mental Disorders - 4th edition), NINDS (National Institute of Neurological Disorders and Stroke), UKPDSBRC (United Kingdom Parkinson's Disease Society Brain Research Centre).

Table 1. Study Design and Participant's Characteristics (continued)

UKPDSBRC criteria (Gibb et al., 1988)	NINDS criteria (Gelb et al., 1999)	"Norwegian" criteria (Larsen et al., 1992)
Step 1 - Diagnosis of Parkisonism Bradykinesia At least one: muscular rigidity, 4-6 Hz rest tremor, postural instability not caused by primary visual, vestibular or proprioceptive dysfunction. **Step 2 - Exclusion criteria for PD** History of repeated strokes with stepwise progression of parkinsonian features History of repeated head injury History of definite encephalitis Oculogyric crises Neuroleptic treatment at onset of symptoms More than one affected relative Sustained remission Strictly unilateral features after 3 years Supranuclear gaze palsy Cerebellar signs Early severe autonomic involvement Early severe dementia with disturbance of memory, language and praxis Babinski sign Presence of cerebral tumor or communicating hydrocephalus on CT scan Negative response to large doses of levodopa (if malabsorption excluded) MPTP exposure **Step 3 - Supportive prospective positive criteria for PD** (3 or more required for diagnosis of definite IPD) Unilateral onset Rest tremor present Progressive disorder Persistent asymmetry affecting side of onset most	Grouping of clinical features of Parkinson's disease according to diagnostic utility **Group A: characteristic of PD** - Resting tremor, Bradykinesia, Rigidity,Asymmetric onset **Group B: suggestive of alternative diagnoses** - Features unusual early in the clinical course: prominent postural instability in the first 3 years after symptoms onset, freezing phenomena in the first 3 years, hallucinations unrelated to medications in the first 3 years, dementia preceding motor symptoms or occurring in the first year - Supranuclear gaze palsy (other than restriction of upward gaze) or slowing of vertical saccades - Severe, symptomatic dysautonomia unrelated to medications - Documentation of a condition known to produce parkinsonism and plausibly connected to the patient's symptoms (such as suitably located focal brain lesions or neuroleptic use within the past 6 months) **1) Criteria for POSSIBLE diagnosis of PD** At least 2 of the 3 features in Group A are present and at least 1 of these is tremor or bradykinesia. **and** Either none of the feature in Group B is present Or symptoms have been present for less than 3 years, and none of the features in Group B is present to date **and** Either substantial and sustained response to levodopa or a dopamine agonist has been documented Or patients has not had an adequate trial of levodopa or dopamine agonist	**1) Criteria for POSSIBLE diagnosis of PD** - Presence of at least two of the following signs: resting tremor, akinesia/ bradykinesia, rigidity, postural abnormality - Moderate response to dopamine agonist - At onset of disease absence of significant changes on CT or MRI other than diffuse cortical atrophy or mild hyperintense periventricular foci on MRI. Mild/moderate dementia and autonomic failure which still may be compatible with Parkinson's disease. Absence of pyramidal and cerebellar signs, as well as environmental factors like drugs and toxic substances and a history of encephalitis that may cause a symptomatic parkinsonism. **2) Criteria for PROBABLE diagnosis of PD** **Type A:** Patients with bilateral onset of signs and who fulfill the following I, II and III criteria. **Type B:** Patients with unilateral onset and who fulfill criteria I, II and IV. **Type C:** Patients with unilateral onset and who fulfill criteria I, III and V. I. Presence of at least two of the following signs: resting tremor, akinesia/bradykinesia, rigidity, postural abnormality II. Good/excellent response to dopamine agonist. III. At onset of disease absence of significant changes on CT or MRI other than diffuse cortical atrophy or mild hyperintense

Excellent (70-100%) response to levodopa Severe levodopa-induced chorea Levodopa response for 5 years or more Clinical course of 10 years or more	**2) Criteria for PROBABLE diagnosis of PD** At least 3 of the 4 features in Group A are present **and** None of the features in Group B is present (symptom duration of at least 3 years is necessary to meet this requirement) **and** Substantial and sustained response to levodopa or a dopamine agonist has been documented **3) Criteria for DEFINITE diagnosis of PD** All criteria for POSSIBLE diagnosis of PD are met **and** Histopathologic confirmation of the diagnosis is obtained at autopsy **Proposed criteria for Histopathologic confirmation of Parkinson Disease** - Substantial nerve cell depletion with accompanying gliosis in the substantia nigra - At least 1 Lewy body in the substantia nigra or in the locus coeruleus (note: it may be necessary to examine up to 4 non-overlapping sections in each of these areas before concluding that Lewy bodies are absent) - No pathological evidence for other diseases that produce Parkinsonism (eg progressive supranuclear palsy, multiple system atrophy, cortical-basal ganglionic degeneration) (Note: in excluding other diseases that produce Parkinsonism, published consensus criteria should be used when available)	periventricular foci on MRI. Absence of clinical exclusion criteria like dementia, pyramidal and cerebellar signs and autonomic failure which may indicate another neurodegenerative disorder. Absence of environmental factors like drugs and toxic substances and a history of encephalitis that may cause a symptomatic parkinsonism. IV. Unilateral onset of symptoms and asymmetrical development of disease. Presence of mild dementia or autonomic failure. Otherwise, as in III. V. Unilateral onset of symptoms and asymmetrical development of disease. Moderate response to dopamine agonist. **3) Criteria for DEFINITE diagnosis of PD** Presence of resting tremor and at least two of the following signs: akinesia/bradykinesia, rigidity,postural abnormality Unilateral onset of signs and asymmetrical development of the disease. Good/excellent response to dopamine agonist. At onset of disease absence of significant changes on CT or MRI other than mild diffuse cortical atrophy or mild hyperintense periventricular foci on MRI. Absence of clinical exclusion criteria like dementia, pyramidal and cerebellar signs and autonomic failure which may indicate another neurodegenerative disorder. Absence of environmental factors like drugs and toxic substances and a history of encephalitis that may cause a symptomatic parkinsonism.

Table 2. The Diagnostic Criteria for PD

Authors	*n* of IPD patients presenting with this VRF								VRF Measures	Medication
	↑Hcy	SMO	DM	HT	HD	HCL	SH/TIA	ALC		
Barone et al. (2008) & Emre et al. (2004)	247	-	-	Yes; n=? + orthostatic hypotension; n=? (192 with vascular disorders)	-	-	-	-	- Blood plasma level: - *High: ≥ 14 µmol/L=↑Hcy* *-Low or normal: < 14 µmol/L=↓Hcy*	**Medication** / **Hcy level (group)** ≥14 µmol/L / <14 µmol/L L-dopa (mg/d) *727.3* *671.6* DAA (mg/d) *4.9* *5.3* Antipsychotics *30.0%* *24.2%* Antidepressants *29.6%* *34.7%* Benzodiazepines, sedatives & hypnotics *22.3%* *26.3%* - Mean exposures to rivastigmine and placebo= respectively 20.7 and 22.3 weeks - Rivastigmine: mean dose at week 24 = 7.8 mg/d
Alves et al. (2004)	-	PD: 78 HC: 49	-	-	-	-	-	-	- Pack-years of smoking *(average number of cigarette per day divided by 20 and multiplied by years of smoking)* - Medical examination & questionnaires	- L-dopa - *SMO: 491.0 mg/d* - *no-SMO: 505.0 mg/d*
Haugarvoll et al. (2005)	-	45	3	16	19	-	2	-	- Interviews with patients (cross-checked with medical records)	- L-dopa - *VRF : 494.0 mg/d* - *no-VRF : 532.0 mg/d*
Kandiah et al. (2009)	-	-	?	-	-	-	-	-	- *Not specified*	- L-dopa (n=78) [*? mg/d]* - DAA (n=49) [*? mg/d]* - Anti-ACh (n=14) [*? mg/d]*
Levy et al. (2002)	-	Curr.:10 Past: 69	16	68	-	-	-	Curr.: 29 Past: 44	- Pack-years of smoking - Smoking duration (in years) - Smoking cessation (in years before onset, if applicable) - Questionnaires (BL) & Interviews (FU)	- L-dopa - *Total: 354.1 mg/d* - *PDD: 326.7 mg/d* - *no-PDD: 364.2 mg/d* - Anti-Ach (n=28)
O'Suilleabhain et al. (2004, 2006)	31 25	BL: - FU: -	- 8	- 39	- 17	- -	- 5	- -	- Interviews (for HT, HS, HD, DM) - Blood plasma level: - *↑Hcy= > 1.89 mg/L or >14 µmol/L* - *B12, folate, creatinine and L-dopa* - Polymorphisms in MTHFR CC,CT,TT	- Baseline L-dopa (n=54) - *Total: 532.0 mg/d* - Follow-up L-dopa (n=57) - *nHcy: 377.0 mg/d* - *↑Hcy: 754.0 mg/d*
Rodriguez-Oroz et al. (2009)	?	-	-	-	-	-	-	-	- Hcy, B12 & B6 and folic acid plasma - MRI (n= 101)/CT scan (n= 18) looking for WMH *[Wahlund Scale]* - Polymorphisms in genes related to HCY metabolism *(MTHFR, MTR, MTRR & CBS)*	- L-dopa - *PD-CN : 786.1 mg/d* - *PD-MCI : 825.0 mg/d* - *PDD : 811.3 mg/* - DAA (n=53) [? mg/d] (n) - *Pramipexol (25),Ropinirol (14), Cabergoline (10), Pergolide (4)*
Weisskopf et al. (2007)	-	Curr.: 16 Past: 112	-	-	-	-	-	-	- Pack-years of smoking - Questionnaires	?

Zoccolella et al. (2009)	?	-	-	40	-	-	-	-	- Blood level of Hcy, B12 and folate	- L-dopa - *PDD: 636.0 mg/d* - *no-PDD: 592.0 mg/d*
Religa et al. (2006)	214	-	-	-	-	-	-	-	- Blood level of Hcy, B12 and folate	- L-dopa (treated group)= *681.2 mg/d*
Ozer et al. (2006)	17	-	-	-	-	-	-	-	- Blood level of Hcy, B12 and folate - *↑Hcy = > 14 μmol/L* - *Low or normal = < 14 μmol/L*	- L-dopa: Mean of 2 groups (↑Hcy + ↓Hcy or normal)= *338.5 mg/d*
Camicioli et al. (2009)	PD:21 HC:5	?	?	?	?	?	-	-	- Blood level of Hcy, B12, creatinine and folate - *↑Hcy= >14 μmol/L*	- L-dopa - *PD (n=47): 535.0 mg/d* - *21 of these also took DAA* - Other medication (n) - *DAA alone (3), Amantadine (6), Rasagiline (3), Entecapone (3), Trihexyphenidyl (1)*
Hassin-Baer et al. (2006)	28	-	-	-	-	-	-	-	- Blood plasma level of Hcy: 1st tertile (< *12.5 μmol/L*), 2nd tertile (*12.5-16.7 μmol/L*)and 3rd tertile (*>16.7 μmol/L*) - Common Carotid Artery Intima-media Thickness(*CCA-IMT*)	- L-dopa: - Low-dose < *376 mg/d* - Medium dose *376-750 mg/d* - High dose > *750 mg/d* - Other medications (?)
Matteau et al. (2010)	-	44	?	30	?	34	?	-	- History of smoking in the past 10 years (yes/no) - Interviews	- Rx (n VRF; n no-VRF) - *NSAID (n=15; n=6)* - *Aspirin (n=13; n=4)* - *DAA (n=65; n=56)* - *Statins (n=30; n =0)*
Sławek et al. (2008)	-	20	3	14	28	16	-	7	- Interviews - MRI: WMH *[Wahlund Scale]*	- L-dopa - *PD-CN : 623.5 mg/d* - *PD-MCI : 773.0 mg/d* - *PDD : 1028.0 mg/d*
Zoccolella et al. (2005)	24	-	-	-	-	-	-	-	- Blood level of Hcy, B12 and folate - *↑Hcy= >14 μmol/L*	- L-dopa - *PD-CI: 547.0 mg/d* - *PD-CN: 644.0 mg/d*
Marder et al. (1990)	-	?	-	?	-	-	-	?	- Interviews - Questionnaires	?
Rektor et al. (2009)	-	11	5	14	14	-	4	-	- Number of cigarettes and duration - Questionnaires and medical records - MRI - CCA-IMT, PI & RI	?

Legend: - (not applicable), ? (unknown or not clear); Vascular risk factors (VRF): ↑Hcy (Hyperhomocysteinemia), ALC (Alcoholism), DM (Type 2 Diabetes Mellitus), HCL (Hypercholesterolemia), HD (Heart Disease), HT (Hypertension), SMO (Smoking), HS/TIA (Stroke History & Transient Ischemic Attacks); VRF measures: ↓Hcy (Low/normal Level of Homocysteine), CCA-IMT (Common Carotid Artery Intima-Media Thickness), Hcy (Homocysteine), MRI (Magnetic Resonance Imaging), PI (Pulsatility Index), RI (Resistance Index), WMH (White Matter Hyperintensities); Medication: Anti-ACh (Anticholinergics), DAA (Dopamine Agonist), L-dopa (levodopa); Groups: PD (Parkinson's disease), PD-CN (Parkinson's disease-Cognitively Normal), PDD (Parkinson's disease with Dementia), PD-MCI (Parkinson's disease with Mild Cognitive Impairment).

Table 3. Vascular Risk Factors and their Measurements

Authors	Cognitive measures	Cognitive results	Other key results
Barone et al. (2008)	- **Global Cognition:** MMSE, ADAS-Cog, ADCS-CGIC - **Attention-Vigilance :** CDR-Computerized Assessment System PoA tests - **Speed of information processing :** CRT - **Language :** D-KEFS letter fluency score	- **BL ADAS-Cog:** ↑Hcy PD group= ↓Hcy or normal PD group - **BL MMSE:** ↑Hcy PD group= ↓Hcy or normal PD group - **BL dementia severity (per MMSE total scores):** ↑Hcy PD group= ↓Hcy or normal PD group - **ADAS-Cog at week 24: ITT-RDO, LOCF and OC analyses:** ↑Hcy- PD group treated with rivastigmine improved > ↑Hcy-PD group with placebo (p < .001) - **ADCS-CGIC at week 24: ITT-RDO and LOCF analyses:** ↑Hcy- PD group treated with rivastigmine improved > ↑Hcy- PD group with placebo (p = .003); **OC analysis** (p < .001) - **ADCS-CGIC (% of responders) at week 24: ITT-RDO analyses:** ↑Hcy PD group treated with rivastigmine > ↑Hcy PD group with placebo (p = .010) - **ADCS-CGIC (% of patients with mild, moderate or marked deterioration relative to baseline) at week 24: ITT-RDO analyses:** ↑Hcy- PD group treated with rivastigmine < ↑Hcy- PD group with placebo (p = .011) - **MMSE score at week 24: ITT-RDO analyses:** ↑Hcy- PD group treated with rivastigmine < ↑Hcy- PD group with placebo (p = .012) - **PoA at week 24: ITT-RDO analyses:** ↑Hcy-PD group treated with rivastigmine < ↑Hcy- PD group with placebo (p = .037) - **CRT at week 24: ITT-RDO analyses:** ↑Hcy- PD group treated with rivastigmine < ↑Hcy- PD group with placebo (p = .007) - **D-KEFS letter fluency score at week 24: ITT-RDO analyses:** ↑Hcy- PD group treated with rivastigmine < ↑Hcy- PD group with placebo (p = .006) - **On all cognitive measures at week 24:** ↓Hcy or normal PD group treated with rivastigmine = ↓Hcy or normal PD group with placebo (p = NS)	- **BL demographics** (gender; time since 1st symptoms of PD, since PD diagnosis, since 1st dementia symptoms and since PDD diagnosis; H & Y stages; UPDRS^{III} scores; L-dopa, DAA, antipsychotics, antidepressants, benzodiazepines, sedatives and hypnotic agents intake): ↑Hcy-PD group= ↓Hcy or normal PD group **-BL ADCS-ADL:** ↑Hcy- PD group < ↓Hcy or normal PD group *(p=.025)* **-BL hallucinations:** ↑Hcy- PD group > ↓Hcy or normal PD group *(p=.005)* **-ADCS-ADL at week 24: ITT-RDO analyses:** ↑Hcy- PD group treated with rivastigmine > ↑Hcy- PD group with placebo (p = .033) **-NPI-10 score at week 24: ITT-RDO analyses:** ↑Hcy- PD group treated with rivastigmine > ↑Hcy- PD group with placebo (p = .003) **-NPI-Caregiver distress at week 24: ITT-RDO analyses:** ↑Hcy- PD group treated with rivastigmine > ↑Hcy- PD group with placebo (p = NS) **-On ADCS-ADL, NPI-10 score and NPI-Caregiver distress at week 24:** ↓Hcy or normal PD group treated with rivastigmine = ↓Hcy or normal PD group with placebo (p = NS)

Alves et al. (2004)	- **Global Cognition:** MMSE	- **MMSE at BL: PD smokers= PD non-smokers**
		- **MMSE changes (4 & 8 yrs): PD smokers= PD non-smokers** ; and no difference between non-smokers, all smokers and heavy smokers (20 pack-years and more)
			- % PD smokers < % HC smokers & DM smokers *(p<.01)*
			- **Gender:** M > F in PD smokers *(p<.001)*
			- **Age at PD onset:** SMO (62.4) < non-SMO (65.1) *(p<.05)*
			- **H&Y changes (4 & 8 yrs):** SMO=no-SMO *(p= NS)*
			- **MADRS changes (4 & 8 yrs):** SMO=no-SMO *(p= NS)*
			- **S&E changes (4 & 8 yrs):** SMO=no-SMO *(p= NS)*
			
			- **UPDRS changes (4 & 8 yrs):** SMO=no-SMO *(p=NS)*
			- **Survival rate (8 yrs):** SMO=no-SMO *(p=NS)*
			  - *30 smokers still alive (38.5%)*
			  - *59 non-smokers still alive (36.6%)*

Haugarvoll et al. (2005)	- **Global Cognition :** GBS (BL), MMSE, DRS (FU), UPDRS (intellectual item) - **Episodic Memory (visual) :** BVRT - **Executive Functions :** Stroop - **Visual perception :** BJLO	- **PD-D at FU :** VRF (35% with PDD) = no-VRF (31% with PDD) (p= *n.s.)* - **Heart failure: PDD > PD (p<.05)** *[univariate analysis only] . This association was not found in the logistic regression controlling for age, H & Y, low MMSE, gender.*	- **Atrial fibrillation & Smoking:** men > women respectively *(p<.05) and (p<.001)* - **Mortality:** VRF (24%) > no-VRF (16.9%) *(p=NS)* - **Mortality:** 36/171 deceased at FU (21%)

Kandiah et al. (2009)	- **Global Cognition:** MMSE	- **CD group :** -2.39 points/year on MMSE - **Cox proportional hazards model:** - **Univariate analysis:** Education (p=.003), age (p=.008) and depression (p=.043) but not DM predicted CD - **Multivariate analysis: Only (low) education predicted CD [HR=.91, 95% CI (.82-.99), P=.047]**	- **Severity of motor symptoms (UPDRS) and H & Y stage did not influence CD.**
Levy et al. (2002); Stern et al. (1992)	- **Orientation:** Items from MMSE, - **Language:** COWAT and category; BNT, BDAE (some subtests) - **Episodic memory (verbal):** SRT - **Episodic memory (visual):** BVRT - **Executive functions:** Similarities (WAIS-R); DRS (Identities and Oddities) - **Visual perception:** BVRT-Matching part	- **Current smoking & risk for PDD:** (RR 4.5; 95% CI, 1.2-16.4; P=.02) - **Ever smoking & risk for PDD:** (RR 2.0; 95% CI, 1.0-3.;9*P=.05*) - **Past smoking & risk for PDD: : NS** - **Smoking (cessation):** < 8 yr before PD = ↑ Risk for *PDD (RR 2.3; 95% CI, 1.1-4.9; P=.03)* - **Smoking:** ↑ pack-year ≠ ↑ RR for PDD - **Smoking:** ↑ smoking duration ≠ ↑ RR for PDD - **Alcohol, DM & HT ≠ development of PDD**	- **BL Age:** PDD > PD (*p<.05*) - **BL Education:** PDD < PD (*p<.05*) - **BL motor signs (UPDRS):** PDD > PD (*p<.05*) - **FU:** ApoE-ε4 ≠ Incident PDD (*P=NS*)

O'Suilleabhain et al. (2004, 2006)	- **Global cognition:** MMSE
	- **Attention:** Digit span (WAIS-III),
	- **Language:** Verbal Fluency Tests (COWAT)
	- **Episodic memory (verbal):** HVLT-Revised
	- **Episodic memory (visual):** ROCF (immediate & delayed recall)
	- **Executive functions:** Stroop
	- **Construction Praxis:** Block Design (WAIS-III), ROCF (copy)
		BASELINE (2004)
		- **Cognition (averaged Z scores of 14 tests) worse in Hcy >14 μmol/L than in Hcy < 14 μmol/L (*p<.01*)**
		- **Cognitive results (analysis of variance):**
		- **PD with Hcy>14 μmol/L < PD with Hcy < 14 μmol/L only on** Block design, animal fluency, ROCF-copy (p<.05)
		
		FOLLOW-UP (2006)
		- **Cognitive results (decline):** ↑HCY = nHcy (NS) on all cognitive measures except for ROCF-immediate recall on which PD with ↑Hcy declined significantly compared to 2004 (p=.035) whereas nHcy did not.
			BL&FU
			- **Age:** ↑Hcy > nHcy (*p=.06*)
			- **L-Dopa dose:** ↑Hcy > nHcy (*p=.003*)
			
			BL (2004)
			- **Age ↔ Hcy (*r=.28, p=.006*)**
			- **Mood:** ↑Hcy [>14 μmol/L] (worst) < nHcy (*p=.02*)
			- **Creatinine ↔ Hcy (*r=.32, p=.001*)**
			- **Higher L-dopa dose ↔ higher Hcy level (*r=.35, p<.01*)**
			- **Hcy levels:** L-dopa users > non-users (*p=.01*)
			- **Plasma L-dopa ↔ Hcy (*r=.42, p<.002*)**
			- **MTHFR:** Hcy level the same with or without T alleles
			- **Plasma B12 ↔ Hcy**
			  - *r= -.34, p=.04 among L-Dopa non-users*
			  - *r= -.04, p=NS among L-Dopa users*
			- **UPDRS ↔ Hcy >14 μmol/L (*p=.20*)**
			
			FU (2006)
			- **HT, HS, HD, DM:** ↑Hcy = nHcy (P= *NS*)
			- **Mortality (n):** ↑Hcy (n=4) > nHcy (n=1) (*p=.03*)
			- **Hcy concentrations :** 2004 ↔ 2006 (*r^2=.53, p=.0001*)
			- **Hcy:** ↑ with L-dopa dose (*p=.0001*) and age (*p=.02*)

Rodriguez-Oroz et al. (2009)	- **Global Cognition:** MMSE, BDS
	- **Episodic Memory:** CERAD Word List, FCSRT, Copy & delayed recall of 2 simple figures
	- **Language:** BNT; Verbal Fluency Tests
	- **Attention:** Digit Span (Forward and Backwards)
	- **Executive fonctions :** Stroop, TMT-A & B, Raven Progressive Matrices
		- **Hcy ≠ predict cognitive status (p=.403) (multinomial logistic regression)**
		- **Cognitive tests results ≠ Hcy levels (all correlation: *p=NS*)**
		- **Cognitive status ≠ polymorphisms studied (*p=NS*)**
		  - Genes (variants) = MTHFRC677T (CC, CT, TT), MTHFRA1298C (AA, AC, CC), , MTRA2756G (AA, AG, GG), & CBS844ins68(II, ID, DD)
		
		- WMH (per the Wahlund scale) : PD-CN = PD-MCI = PDD (*p=NS*)
			- **Age :** PDD > HC & PD-CN (*p=.0001*) & PD-MCI (*p=.02*)
			- **GDS :** PDD > PD-CN (*p=.001*)
			- **GDS :** PD-MCI > PD-CN (*p=.04*)
			- **Hcy levels ≠ depression (p=NS)**
			- **Hcy:** all PD patients > HC (*p=.0001*)
			  - *HC : 8.6 μmol/L*
			  - *PD-CN : 14.9 μmol/L*
			  - *PD-MCI : 15.1 μmol/L*
			  - *PDD : 15.4 μmol/L*

Weisskopf et al. (2007)	- **Global Cognition:** TICS - **Attention:** Digit span-backwards, - **Episodic Memory:** 10-word list delayed recall, EBMT - **Language:** Verbal Fluency Test (category)	- **PD < HC on all cognitive tests (*p<.0001*)** - **PD Current smokers < PD Never smokers on all cognitive tests but only significant for TICS** (*p=.002*) - **Logistic regression models:** current smokers odds ratio for cognitive impairment on global cognitive score: (OR=3.3 (95% CI: 1.1-10.4; P=.04)	- **PD smoked less than HC** - **Adjustments for alcohol and physical activity ≠** impact on relationship between current smoking and cognition
Zoccolella et al. (2009)	- **Global cognition:** MMSE - **Executive functions:** FAB	- **Hypertension:** PDD> PDnD (48% vs 25%; *p=.02*) - **Hcy:** PDD [20.7 µmol/L] > PDnD [15.8 µmol/L] (*p<.002*) - **Hcy:** PDD > PDnD even after restriction to highest quartile of age (>72 yrs) (p=.04) - **MTHFR genotype: PDD= PD (frequency of the T677T genotype)** - **Univariate logistic regression model:** **Risk for dementia** (Hcy >18.9 µmol/L vs Hcy < 12.4 µmol/L): - OR=5.0 (*95% CI: 1.87-13.60, p=.01*) **Presence of dementia** ↔ older age, lower educational level, more severe motor impairment, and HT - **Multiple linear regression model:** - Hcy ↔ age (*r=.10; p=.008; r²=.10*) for whole sample - Hcy ↔ L-dopa dose (*p= NS*) - **Multivariate logistic regression:** - ↑Hcy ↔ presence of dementia (*OR 3.68, 95% CI: 1.14-11.83, p=.03*) - Hypertension ↔ presence of dementia (*p= NS*)	- **Hcy:** all PD [17.5 µmol/L] > HC [11.0 µmol/L] (*p<.00001*) - **B12 and folate blood concentration:** PD = HC - **L-dopa dose:** PDD = PD (*p=NS*) - **L-dopa treatment duration:** PDD = PD (*p= NS*) - **UPDRS:** PDD > PD (*p=.04*) - **MTHFR (T677T):** PDD = PD (*p=NS*)
Religa et al. (2006)	**Global Cognition:** MMSE	- **↑Hcy:** Correlated (*r=?*) with cognitive impairment per MMSE (*p < .05*) - **MMSE:** L-dopa treated PD (27.1 ± 2.3)= L-dopa non-treated PD (26.2 ± 6.3)	- **Disease duration:** L-dopa Treated PD > L-dopa non-treated PD (*p= .03*) - **Hcy:** Correlation with duration of disease in 2 PD groups (*p < .001*) - **Hcy:** L-dopa Treated PD [17.25 ± 5.96 µmol/L] > Controls [14.42 ± 4.48 µmol/L] (*p < .05*) - **Hcy levels** unrelated to L-Dopa doses - **Hcy:** L-dopa non-treated PD [16.37 ± 5.53 µmol/L] = Controls (*p= NS*) - **B12:** L-dopa Treated PD < Controls (*p < .01*) - **B12:** L-dopa non-treated PD < Controls (*p < .05*) - **MTHFR (CC, CT and TT genotypes):** L-Dopa Treated PD = L-dopa non-treated PD= Controls
Ozer et al. (2006)	- **Global cognition:** STMS - **Language:** Verbal Fluency Test (Category) - **Episodic memory (verbal):** SBST - **Episodic memory (visual):** Visual memory subtest (WMS) - **Executive functions:** WCST, Stroop - **Visuoconstruction praxis:** CDT - **Visual perception:** BFR, BJLO	- **Mann-Whitney U-test analysis of variance:** - **PD with ↑Hcy < PD with ↓Hcy or normal on:** - WCST-failure score in the continuation of establishment (*p = .009*); - SBST-delayed recall (*p= .05*); - Stroop time (*p= .04*) - Controls and 2 patient groups were only compared on the CDT and STMS-total score (*p= NS*).	- **Hcy** higher in patients taking L-dopa > 300 mg/d compared with patients taking L-dopa < 300 mg/d - **B12:** Only PD with ↑Hcy < Controls (*p= .007*) - **Folate acid:** Only PD with ↑Hcy < Controls (*p= .04*)

Camicioli et al. (2009)	- **Global cognition:** MMSE, DRS - **Language: NART** - **Episodic memory:** BDS Orientation-Memory-Concentration - **Construction praxis:** CDT - **Executive functions:** FAB - **Visuoconstruction praxis:** CDT	- **Hcy, B12 and folate levels:** NO ↔ with cognitive results per the DRS (*p= NS*)	- **GDS:** PD > HC (*p=.001*) - **No ↔ of depressive symptoms per the GDS with Hcy, B12 and folate levels.** - **Hcy:** PD (13.6 µmol/L) > HC (10.5 µmol/L) (*p<.0005*) - In PD with L-dopa: no ↔ with L-dopa duration and L-dopa dose - No ↔ **between Hcy and B12.** - **Hcy level ↔ folate** (r=*.31, p=.035*) - **B12:** PD (299.0 pmol/L) < HC (379.0 pmol/L) (*p=.01*) - Use of vitamin B12 ↔ lower Hcy (*p=.02 for PD & HC*) - **Logistic regression model:** - ↑B12 ↔ lower risk of dyskinesias (*RR 0.99, 95% CI: 0.983-0.999, p=.027*) - **MTHFR genotype:** - ANOVA (PD versus HC): - Significant group difference for MTHFR 677 genotype and B12 use (F=13.8, p < .0005) but only significant association for B12 use (F=21.5, p < .0005). - Significant interaction between MTHFR genotype and B12 (*F= 5.2, p=.02*).
Hassin-Baer et al. (2006)	- **Global Cognition:** MMSE - **Attention:** Digit Span (Forward and Backwards - **Episodic Memory (verbal):** RAVLT - **Language:** Verbal Fluency Tests - **Executive fonctions :** TMT A-B, FAB	- **One-way analysis Kruskall-Wallis test of variance:** **All cognitive tests:** No differences between the 1st, 2nd and 3rd tertile of Hcy levels.	- Correlation between L-dopa treatment duration and Hcy level (*p= .036*) - No effect of L-dopa dose on Hcy levels. - No correlation between vascular comorbidity (coronary heart disease or with history of cerebrovascular disease, such as stroke or TIA) and Hcy levels.
Matteau et al. (2010)	- **Global Cognition:** MMSE	- **PD duration ↔ MMSE (*r= -.22; p=.02*)** - **PD-VRF < PD-noVRF on the MMSE total Z score** *F(2,115)=5.58, p=.005, d=.3*	- History of smoking in past 10 years was the most prevalent VRF (66%) - **Age (at dx):** VRF > no-VRF (*p=.003*) - **Age (at sx onset):** VRF > no-VRF (*p=.007*) - **Education:** VRF < no-VRF (*p=.005*) - **PD duration:** VRF < no-VRF (*p=.004*)
Sławek et al. (2008)	- **Global cognition:** MMSE - **Intelligence:** WBIS - **Language:** Verbal Fluency Test (Animals) - **Episodic memory:** RAVLT, DCS - **Executive functions:** Tower of Toronto	- **VRF (except HD) ≠ Cognitive status** PDD > PD-CN (p<.01): HD - **HD:** weak predictive factor of dementia - **HD** ↔ *MMSE, RAVLT , VFT all p<.05*	- PDD > PD-CN (*p<.05*): Age at examination, H & Y stage -HD ↔ Age and age at disease onset (*p<.05*) - PD-CN=PD-MCI=*PDD: Age at disease onset*, disease duration and BDI - PD-CN=PD-MCI=PDD: WMH (*per* the Whalund score)
Zoccolella et al. (2005)	- **Global cognition:** MMSE - **Executive functions:** FAB	- **Hcy : PD-**CogI (21.2 µmol/L) > PD-CN (15.8 µmol/L) (*p=.001*) - **Most common CI in PD-CI:** memory impairment (n=12), apraxia (n=8), dementia per DSM-III-R (n=5) - **Logistic regression** - Risk of CogI ↑ with ↑ Hcy (continuous variable): *OR=19.1 (95% CI: 1.5- 241.4; p=.02)* - Risk of CogI ↑ in the Hcy highest quartile compared to the lowest quartile: (*OR=19.0; 95% CI: 1.0-346.2, p=.004*) after adjustment for age, sex, B12 and folate status	- **Hcy ↔ Age** (*r^2=.03, p=.006*) - **Hcy ↔ Folate** (*r^2=.30, p=.006*)

Marder et al. (1990)	- **Global cognition:** mMMS	- **SMO:** PDD = PDnD (p=NS); Logistic regression: OR= 1.62 (95%CI: .484-4.127) - **ALC (beer): Logistic regression:** OR= 2.64 (95%CI: .712-7.073) - **HT(antihypertensive drugs):** PDD = PDnD (p=NS)	- **Age:** PDD > PD (*p<.001*) - **1st degree relative - history of DEM:** Logistic regression: OR=6.47 (*95%CI: 1.22-22.04*) - **Amateur sports:** Logistic regression: OR=2.73 (*95%CI: .614-7.892*)
Rektor et al. (2009)	- **Global cognition:** MMSE - **Orientation:** BTOT - **Language:** Verbal Fluency Test (Category) - **Episodic memory:** Word List I-II (*WMS-III*) - **Construction praxis:** CDT	- **Cognitive tests results** - **↑ CCA-IMT ↔ Cognitive tests results (*p< .05*):** - *MMSE(r= -.44, p=.004), CDT (r= -.42, p=.007), MMSE+ Clock (r=-.49, p=.001), BTOT (r= .42, p=.006), VFT (r= -.32, p=.043), WMS-III (recognition-word list II) (r=-.33, p=.037)* - **RI ↔ Cognitive tests results (*p<.05*)** - *BTOT (r= .32, p=.039)* - **PI ↔ Cognitive tests results (*p≤.05*)** - *CDT (r= -.35, p=.023), BTOT (r= .56, p=.0001), VFT (r=-.348, p=.05), WMS-III (delayed recall-word list II) (r=-.42, p=.007,), WMS- III (recognition-word list II) (r=-.35, p=.025)* - **Multiple regression analysis:** IMT ↔ with MMSE and MMSE+ Clock **& PI ↔ with** BTOT and *WMS-III (recognition-word list II)*	- **MRI:** n=30 PD with white matter lesions (volume < 10,000mm³ in n=25 and volume > 10,000mm³ in n=5) - **Atherosclerotic plaques:** n=27 PD patients (but haemodynamically not significant) - **Multiple regression analysis: IMT ↔ with** H & Y stage, IADL, Barthel Index

? =unknown or unclear / NS = Not Significant

Legend: ↑ (Increase), ↔ (Association), ADAS-Cog (Alzheimer's Disease Assessment Scale- Cognition), ADCS-ADL (Alzheimer's Disease Cooperative Study-Activities of Daily Living), ADCS-CGIC (Alzheimer's Disease Cooperative Study-Clinician's Global Impression of Change), BDS (Blessed Dementia Scale), BFR (Benton Face Recognition), BJLO (Benton Judgment of Line Orientation), BL (Baseline), BNT (Boston Naming Test), BTOT (Benton Temporal Orientation Test), BVRT (Benton Visual Retention Test), CCA-IMT (Common Carotid Artery Intima-Media Thickness), CD (Cognitive Decline), CDR (Cognitive Drug Research), CDT (Clock Drawing Test), CI (Confidence Interval), CogI (Cognitive Impairment), COWAT (Controlled Oral Word Association Test), CRT (Choice Reaction Time), DA (Dopamine), D-KEFS (Delis-Kaplan Executive Fonction System), DM (Diabetes Mellitus), DRS (Dementia Rating Scale), dx (Diagnosis), EBMT (East Boston Memory Test), FAB (Frontal Assessment Battery), FCSRT (Free & Cued Selective Reminding Test of Buschke), FU (Follow-up), GBS (Gottfried-Brane-Steen scale), GDS (Geriatric Depression Scale), H & Y (Hoehn and Yahr), HC (Healthy Controls), HT (hypertension), HVLT (Hopkins Verbal Learning Test), IADL (Instrumental Activities of Daily Living), ITT-RDO (Intention to treat-Retrieved drop-out), LOCF (Last Observation Carried Forward), MC (Multiple Centers), MMSE (Mini-Mental State Examination), nHcy (Normal homocysteine level), no-VRF (No Vascular Risk Factors), NPI (Neuropsychiatric Inventory), NSAID (Nonsteroidal Anti-Inflammatory Drug), OC (Observed Cases), OR (Odds Ratio), PD-CN(Parkinson's Disease – Cognitively Normal), PDD (Parkinson's Disease with Dementia), PD-MCI (Parkinson's Disease with Mild Cognitive Impairment), PDnD (Parkinson's disease, no dementia), PoA (Power of Attention tests), PI (Pulsatility Index), RAVLT (Rey Auditory Verbal Learning Test), RI (Resistance Index), ROCF (Rey-Osterrieth Complex Figure), RR (Risk Ratio), S&E (Schwab and England score), SBST (Sozel Bellek Surecleri Test), STMS (Short Test of Mental Status), sx (Symptoms), TMT (Trail Making Test), UPDRS (Unified Parkinson's Disease rating Scale), VFT (Verbal Fluency Task), VRF (Vascular Risk Factors), WBIS (Wechsler-Bellevue Intelligence Scale), WMH (White Matter Hyperintensities), WMS-III (Wechsler Memory Scale, 3rd version), WCST (Wisconsin Card Sorting Test), WMH (White Matter Hyperintensities), WS (Wahlund Scale).

Table 4. Cognitive Measures, Cognitive Results and Other Key Results

3.6.8 Construction praxis

Construction praxis was assessed in 4 studies using the Clock Drawing Test (CDT) (n=3 studies), the Block Design of the Wechsler Adult Intelligence Scale 3rd edition (WAIS-III) and the copy part of the ROCF. Only 1/4 studies reported a significant association between the presence of VRF and a decline in the construction praxis. O'Suilleabhain et al. (2004; 2006) found a significantly worse performance on Block Design (WAIS-III) and on ROCF-copy in the PD group with Hcy>14 μmol/L compared to PD with Hcy < 14 μmol/L at baseline, but not at 2-year follow-up.

Ozer et al. (2006) didn't find significant differences on the CDT score between PD ≥14 μmol/L, PD <14 μmol/L and healthy controls. Camicioli et al. (2009) didn't report results of specific analyses concerning the CDT. In addition, CDT was significantly associated with an increase of intimomedial thickness and of the pulsatility index, but not with the presence of smoking, HT, DM, ischemic HD and stroke (Rektor et al., 2009).

3.6.9 Orientation

Orientation was assessed in 2 studies using the Benton Temporal Orientation Test (BTOT) (1 study) and some MMSE items (1 study). Positive correlations between the BTOT and the increase of intimomedial thickness, the pulsatility index and the resistance index were found, but there was no correlation with smoking, HT, DM, ischemic HD and stroke (Rektor et al., 2009). Levy et al. (2002) didn't report results on the MMSE-orientation items.

3.6.10 Speed of information processing

Speed of information processing was assessed in only one study with the Choice Reaction Time (CRT) test. The R-DB-PC study of Barone et al. (2008) found that ↑Hcy patients treated with rivastigmine had a significant improvement on the CRT after 24 weeks compared to ↑Hcy-placebo-treated patients, and this improvement wasn't present in the < 14 μmol/L group.

4. Conclusion

The main objective of this review was to determine whether there is a relationship between VRF and cognition in PD or not. Consequently, a thorough search in several relevant databases was conducted, and 18 studies were found. After a comprehensive analysis of the articles content, a relationship was evidenced between cognition and ↑Hcy, but the link between heart disease, smoking and cognition was more controversial. There was no evidence of any relationship between cognition and diabetes mellitus, hypertension, alcohol intake, stroke history/transient ischemic attack and hypercholesterolemia.

4.1 Homocysteine and cognition

Hyperhomocysteinemia in PD was associated with worse cognition and/or dementia in 6/9 studies of this review; 3/9 studies found no association. This finding is partly supported by the results of a previous review of 16 articles by Zoccolella et al. (2010) who reported significant associations in 9 publications investigating cognition or dementia in relationship with ↑Hcy. Nine out of 16 studies of Zoccolella and colleagues overlapped some articles included in the current review. However, the inclusion criteria of the current review were more rigorous, and excluded published abstracts of conference presentations. Furthermore, the current review also collected more demographic and clinical data on PD patients and controls, and reported results in a more detailed fashion, hence allowing easier comparisons and exploration of possible interactions or co-occurrence between VRF. Nevertheless, the relationship between cognition/dementia and ↑Hcy remained relatively consistent.

Some of the divergent findings in the global cognitive outcomes of the 9 studies that investigated Hcy may be explained by several factors. For instance, in all these studies, those with greater sample size and using a longitudinal design were more likely to find a significant association compared to the studies that didn't find a significant association. In brief, studies that found significant associations possibly presented a more robust design, greater statistical power and also possibly a higher dosage of L-dopa. Among the 3 studies that didn't find an association with Hcy and cognition, one didn't clearly report medication dosages. Other possible explanations involve the use of different technologies to measure Hcy levels (high performance liquid chromatography with fluorescence detection, fluorescence polarization immunoassay, chemiluminescent enzyme immunoassay) and the measurement of Hcy levels under different fasting conditions (food and drugs).

Interestingly, the Hcy studies demonstrated that ↑Hcy may affect episodic memory (O'Suilleabhain et al., 2004, 2006; Ozer et al., 2006), executive functions (Ozer et al., 2006), language (Barone et al., 2008; O'Suilleabhain et al., 2004, 2006), attention/vigilance (Barone et al., 2008), construction praxis (O'Suilleabhain et al., 2004, 2006) and speed of information processing (Barone et al., 2008). This could reflect a vascular contribution to cognitive impairment since executive functions, attention and some aspects of episodic memory are linked to frontal-subcortical loops (Sachdev et al., 2005). Indeed similar results were found in studies performed in elderly with VRF, some even found poorer performance with ↑Hcy for specific cognitive domains like episodic memory (Morris et al., 2001), executive functions (Duthie et al., 2002) and attention (Duthie et al., 2002). However, this cognitive profile is prominently found in PD patients with cognitive impairment (without VRF), since the alteration of the frontal-striatal system could cause a similar executive dysfunction (Zgaljardic et al., 2003). Hence, it could be hypothesized that: 1) ↑Hcy amplifies the severity of the executive impairment already present in PD patients; and/or 2) that ↑Hcy increases the susceptibility of some cerebral regions to vascular impairment (i.e. ischemic lesions in these specific regions); and/or 3) that ↑Hcy accelerates the neurodegenerative process of PD in some aspects, because of its acknowledged neurotoxicity (Sachdev, 2005). Nonetheless, further research is required to clarify these hypotheses.

4.1.1 What could explain the link between Hcy and cognition?

Elevated Hcy is associated with brain atrophy by several vascular mechanisms (for a review on the question, see Sachdev, 2005) such as promoting endothelial cell injury (formation of atherosclerosis in the blood vessel walls and reduced thrombo-resistance), increasing platelet aggregation (by increasing thromboxane A2 synthesis and decreasing postacyclin), affecting factors of the clotting cycle (and inhibition of the natural anticoagulants), and favors the adhesion of platelets to the endothelium. Hence, these results may support a possible vascular contribution to cognitive impairment by ↑Hcy. As mentioned in section 3.4.1, L-dopa intake in PD patients induces increased levels of Hcy (Kuhn et al., 1998; Müller et al., 1999; Rogers et al., 2003; Yasui et al., 2000) because L-dopa breakdown interferes with Hcy metabolism. Since Hcy also has been associated with hypertrophy of the intima-media complex of the carotid artery, a marker of atherosclerotic disease (Megnien et al., 1998), L-dopa-induced ↑Hcy may promote systemic atherosclerosis processes, thus compromising vascular health. This is supported by the findings of Nakaso et al. (2003) who reported that patients treated with L-dopa for longer duration had increased hypertrophic changes in the intima-media complex of the carotid artery, and that ↑Hcy promoted by both longer L-dopa treatment and MTHFR T/T genotype may amplify atherosclerotic processes.

4.1.2 Neurotoxicity of homocysteine

In the current review, the study conducted by Barone et al. (2008) brought indirect support for a neurotoxic effect of Hcy on brains cells. As mentioned above, ↑Hcy causes increased oxidative stress, excitotoxicity, promotes cellular apoptosis and accumulation of amyloid β-peptide and abnormal tau phosphorylation. The brain is particularly vulnerable to ↑Hcy, because it lacks two major Hcy metabolic pathways (via methionine synthase and via cystathionine-β-synthase)(Finkelstein, 1998). The R-DB-PC study of Barone et al. (2008) successfully demonstrated that global cognitive function, verbal fluency, attention, and speed of information processing of hyperhomocysteinemic PD patients benefited from rivastigmine treatment. These results may support the hypothesis of the contribution of a cholinergic system imbalance in cognitive impairment and dementia in PD. Indeed, rivastigmine inhibits acetycholinesterase (AChE) and butyrylcholinestersase (BuChE) (Darreh-Shori et al., 2002), two enzymes that catalyze the hydrolysis of acetylcholine (ACh) in neurons (Lane et al., 2006). Hyperhomocysteinemia could be deleterious to the ACh system of PDD because a metabolite of homocysteine (*homocysteine thiolactone*) is known to increase the enzymatic activity of BuChe (Darvesh et al., 2007). Since the BuChE highest activity is reported in deep gray and white matter brain regions, hyperhomocysteinemia may be linked to subcortical atrophy and white matter lesions (Darvesh et al., 2007; Sachdev et al., 2005). Apart from the compensation for ACh deficiencies, another hypothesis for the benefit of rivastigmine treatment could be that rivastigmine may reduce inflammation and oxidative stress in neurons (Schulz et al., 2002; Tanaka et al., 1995). These pathological phenomena are promoted by ↑Hcy (Sachdev et al., 2005) and could be involved in PDD. Nevertheless, the underlying mechanisms of rivastigmine treatment effects on cognition in hyperhomocysteinemic patients are still hypothetical (Barone et al., 2008).

4.2 Smoking and cognition in PD

The question of whether smoking is a protective factor for PD or a factor promoting cognitive impairment and dementia is very controversial. A significant relationship between cognition and smoking in PD was found in 3/8 studies of this review: a higher risk for dementia in current smokers (Levy et al., 2006), and a worse performance on a global cognitive measure in patients with history of smoking (indirectly in Matteau et al., 2010; and directly in Weisskopf et al., 2007). Nevertheless, the data extracted from the 8 articles were conflicting since 5/8 studies didn't find a significant association between cognition and smoking in PD. However, most of these 5 studies only reported smoking as present or not in the sample. Consequently, comprehensive analyses between different smoking status and cognitive results were not conducted. In fact, Haugarvoll et al. (2005), Rektor et al. (2009)

and Slawek et al. (2008) didn't report results specific to smoking. Moreover, the number of PD smokers in the samples was very small, thus making it difficult to draw any conclusion on the definitive impact of smoking on cognition in PD. It could be argued that studies that found significant associations had a larger sample size of smokers and thus more statistical power. In addition, when specified, the number of current smokers compared to past smokers was relatively small. Although some studies assessed smoking in a more detailed fashion, cognition was only assessed with brief global measures that could potentially mask effects on specific cognitive domains. Hence, it is justified to doubt if cognitive deficits, when found in association with smoking, were present at the time of diagnosis or reflected a faster decline after PD onset. Nevertheless, an early study evaluating the risk of dementia in PD smokers compared to non smokers (Ebmeier et al., 1990) found that the odds ratio for dementia in smokers was 4.0 (95% CI:1.4 -12.0) compared to non smokers, which clearly indicates a risk for cognitive deterioration in PD smokers.

The controversy regarding the association between smoking and greater cognitive decline in PD patients stems from the fact that tobacco use has been quite consistently reported as a dose-dependent protective factor for PD development in several studies as evidenced in the pooled analysis of Ritz et al. (2007). Although the current review couldn't draw definitive conclusions on smoking as a VRF for cognitive decline in PD, some hypotheses can be made over the conflicting results. Animal studies hypothesized that nicotine delivered through cigarette smoke may exert a protective effect on dopaminergic (DA) neurons in the substantia nigra, thus enhancing the survival rate of animals. In fact, Parain et al. (2003) examined the effects of cigarette smoke and nicotine in an animal model of PD provoked by 1-methyl-4-phenyl-1,2,3,6-tetrahydropyridine (MPTP) intoxication in mice. They found that the loss of DA neurons in the substantia nigra was significantly less severe in the group treated with injections of nicotine and in the group with low exposure to cigarette smoke, compared to the groups treated with placebo and highly exposed to cigarette smoke.

Moreover, the study of Park et al. (2007) with microglia cultures demonstrated that nicotine had a neuroprotective effect on DA neurons due to an anti-inflammatory action. Supporting the results of animal studies, Kelton et al. (2000) reported improvements in reaction time, central processing speed and tracking in 15 non-demented PD patients after they received an acute administration of nicotine (phase I). Several motor measures also improved after chronic administration of nicotine patches (phase II), thus reinforcing the aforementioned hypothesis. This is particularly interesting for PD, since alterations of the nicotinic binding sites in the pars compacta of the substantia nigra were associated with PD (as well as in AD and in Lewy body disease) (Perry et al., 1995). In fact, abnormalities of the nicotinic receptors may precede DA neurodegeneration.

On the other side, while nicotine may protect against nigral neuronal losses, side effects from the other compounds of cigarette smoke may be deleterious for the vascular system and for brain cells health even in non PD elderly. A diminution of gray matter density in the posterior cingulate cortex, the precuneus, the right thalamus and the frontal cortex were found in elderly smokers (otherwise healthy) compared to non-smokers. These cerebral regions are associated with incipient AD (Almeida et al., 2008). Some neuroimaging studies associated smoking with increased cerebral infarcts, white matter hyperintensities, subcortial atrophies and elevated amyloid plaques (Swan & Lessov-Schlaggar, 2007; Tyas et al., 2003). Furthermore, some studies conducted in non-demented elderly reported that smoking increased difficulties in psychomotor and information processing speed (Hill, 1989; Kalmijn et al., 2002), verbal learning, cognitive flexibility (Kalmijn et al., 2002), distracters inhibition and global executive functions (Paul et al., 2006; Razani et al., 2004). However, some authors didn't find any deleterious effect of smoking on cognitive measures (Schinka et al., 2002). These findings highlight the controversy regarding the impact of cigarette smoking on cognition. Nonetheless, the results of the current review cannot draw a specific cognitive profile in PD associated with smoking as a VRF, because significant effects were only reported on global cognitive measures. In fact it is possible that cigarette smoking – especially nicotine in cigarette smoke – could affect PD brains differently than healthy elderly, probably because of PD-related changes.

4.3 Heart disease and cognition in PD

The data of the current review associated the presence of HD in PD with dementia (Haugarvoll et al., 2005; Slawek et al., 2008), and impairment in episodic memory and language (Slawerk et al., 2008). However, these associations were weak and controversial, since another study did not report any association (Rektor et al., 2009). Yet the association between HD and cognition in PD is at least partly supported by the literature in non-PD elderly. For instance, Ylikoski et al. (2000) reported that non-PD elderly with heart failure and showing white matter changes and central atrophy had significantly worse cognitive performance in tests measuring visuoconstruction, attention and cognitive flexibility compared to healthy individuals. Interestingly, several studies strongly associated ↑Hcy with a higher risk of HD in healthy individuals. For instance, a meta-analysis by Wald et al. (2002) evidenced a causal relationship between Hcy levels and ischemic HD and found that lowering Hcy levels from current level by 3µmol/L could reduce the risk of ischemic HD by 11% to 20%. Nonetheless, none of the articles investigating Hcy in this review reported the cardiac health condition of the ↑Hcy patients and none of the studies reporting heart diseases assessed Hcy levels, so this relationship wasn't reported in the 9 articles.

4.4 Diabetes mellitus, hypertension, hypercholesterolemia, alcohol and cognition in PD

None of the studies of this review reported a significant association between DM, HT and HCL and cognition in PD. However, in most cases, these VRF were considered only as secondary variables and the potential relations with cognition were not always thoroughly assessed. In addition, these results don't reflect those obtained in non-PD populations, because several studies associated type 2 DM with cognitive impairment. A literature review showed that type 2 DM is cross-sectionally associated with cognitive impairment in healthy elderly and is considered as a risk factor for both vascular dementia and AD in several studies (Stewart & Liolitsa, 1999). Moreover, higher risk of poor performance on verbal episodic memory and concept formation with longer DM duration was demonstrated in a large prospective cohort of non-PD individuals with DM followed during nearly 30 years (Elias et al., 1997).

A possible explanation for the difficulty to draw specific conclusions regarding the presence of HT, DM and HCL in PD and their impact on cognition could be that some studies found inverse associations with these VRF and the risk for PD. In fact, a significant inverse relation/lower odds ratio for PD was shown in individuals with HT (Herishanu et al., 2001;

Miyake et al., 2010; Scigliano et al., 2006), DM (Herishanu et al., 2001; Miyake et al., 2010; Scigliano et al., 2006) and HCL (Miyake et al., 2010 Scigliano et al., 2006). The study of Scigliano et al. (2006) suggested that the reduced risk for vascular disorders in untreated PD patients could stem from a reduced autonomic activity in PD. While sympathetic hyperactivity is known to exacerbate high blood pressure, diabetes and dyslipidemia, PD patients present with cardiac sympathetic denervation and parasympathetic dysfunction (Buob et al., 2010; Shibata et al., 2009), thus possibly reducing HT and other VRF related to it. In addition, the reduction in sympathetic activity may be relevant for postural hypotension reported in 70% of PD patients (Appenzeller & Goss, 1971; Shindo et al., 2003). The fact that patients were untreated in the study of Scigliano et al. (2006) could be a key factor since L-dopa-treated patients are more susceptible to have higher Hcy levels (see section 3.4.1), they are also at an increased risk for cerebrovascular and cardiovascular disorders. Yet, Jellinger (2003) found that the frequency of brain lesions associated with vascular disease such as white matter lesions, ischemic infarcts, hemorraghes and lacunes, was higher in PD patients compared to controls, but more severe ischemic and hemorrhagic strokes often leading to death were less frequent in PD patients. The findings of Jellinger thus mitigate the impact of cerebrovascular lesions in PD patients.

4.5 Limitations of the reviewed articles

The studies included in the review presented several limitations. There was a small number of studies for some VRF such as DM, HCL, HT, HD, SH/TIA and as a consequence, there was a lack of analyses on these variables in link with cognitive measures. For instance, although HT didn't seem associated with cognition in 6/9 studies, 3/9 did not report if there was any association or not, thus suggesting that these analyses were not even realized, probably because these VRF weren't the main focus in these studies. Moreover, it is rather difficult to draw a conclusion regarding the impact of some VRF such as SH, TIA, alcohol intake and HCL because only a few studies assessed their links with cognition. As explained previously, PD patients are less susceptible than controls to be diagnosed with HT, DM and HCL, thus making it difficult to perform a comprehensive assessment of the relation between these VRF, cognitive impairment and PDD.

The cross-sectional design of the studies could also have influenced the cognitive profile of PD patients with and without VRF. For instance, two studies with a longitudinal component (Barone et al.,2004; O'Suilleabhain et al., 2004; 2006) found a significant association with elevated Hcy and worse cognitive performance, but inconsistencies were found in the case-control studies. Thus, an important limitation of the review data concerns the lack of longitudinal and cohort studies on most VRF.

While most studies used comparable diagnostic criteria (see Table 2), a considerable number of studies reported severe exclusion criteria for PD participants, such as the exclusion of cognitively impaired or demented patients (see Table 1). Since demented and cognitively impaired PD patients were systematically excluded in 7 studies, it is possible that an association between VRF and cognition was missed in these particular studies.

Several studies (n=11) didn't report education levels of the participants, and this may have had an impact on cognitive evaluation. Education is an important variable to consider when cognition is assessed because it is strongly correlated with cognitive performance on neuropsychological tests, and this is the reason why good standardized cognitive tests are normalized according to age and education (Lezak et al., 2004). For the reasons stated above, it is delicate to compare results of patients with low-levels of education with those of patients with higher levels of education as Weisskopf et al. (2007) and Rodriguez-Oroz et al. (2009) did in their respective study.

Only a few studies reported the use of magnetic resonance imaging (MRI) to correlate the cognitive deficits with objective brain changes and lesions. Apart from plasma measures of Hcy, the only biological measures used in the 18 articles that could without a doubt confirm a vascular disease or impairment were the measures of intimomedial thickness of the common carotid artery, as well as the pulsatility and resistance index in the studies of Rektor et al. (2009) and Hassin-Baer et al. (2006).

Another important point to consider is the fact that the treatment of vascular conditions such as HT with antihypertensive medications could have mitigate the effects of some VRF, thus creating some kind of "false" at risk groups. It is particularly hard to estimate the consequences of such an effect, because most studies only reported PD-related drugs, and not the VRF treatment. Conversely, some medications such as beta-blockers, administered to control HT, are known to have deleterious effects on cognition (Gliebus and Lippa, 2007). Unfortunately this is also true for benzodiazepines (Kleykamp et al., 2010) often prescribed in PD as a muscle relaxant. Therefore it would be a good idea in the future to include information regarding medications in studies investigating the relationship between VRF and cognition in PD.

Finally, the current review had specific inclusion criteria for the articles and thus, studies that didn't report cognitive measures were not selected. However, other kinds of studies may bring some support to the effect of vascular disease and VRF on the clinical course of PD. For instance, Papapetropoulos et al. (2004) studied the impact of HT, DM, ischemic HD and stroke in late-onset PD patients and found that H&Y stages were significantly higher in patients with stroke, ischemic HD and DM compared to those without those VRF, thus suggesting some impact of VRF on disease severity and mechanisms.

4.6 Recommendations for future studies

Considering the outcomes of this review, some recommendations to improve research in this area can be formulated. Since the current review showed important inconsistencies in the neuropsychological assessment of PD patients, the development of a standardized and comprehensive assessment of cognition especially adapted for PD is mandatory. In fact, apart from the study of Weisskopf et al. (2007) that reported no changes in cognitive results after removing the results of one test that could be affected by bradykinesia, no study mentioned the use of motor controls for the neuropsychological assessment. Although some tests didn't have a motor component, others, such as the CDT and ROCF, did. Since motor impairment is a prominent feature of PD, obtaining pure cognitive measures can be challenging in tests requiring motor manipulations.

In addition, studies assessing the impact of the interaction of several VRF (such as ↑Hcy and HD; ↑Hcy and smoking) on cognition should also be performed as well as studies comparing the VRF and cognitive functions in *de novo* untreated patients versus patients treated with L-dopa (e.g. for 5, 10 and 15 years). In all these studies, structural and functional imaging data shall be provided in order to perform correlations with the cognitive and clinical measurements.

Finally, future studies shall investigate indirectly the role of VRF in cognition by evaluating the impact of some VRF treatment like nicotine patch or antihypertensive/anti-HCL medication on the cognitive functions in PD patients.

5. References

Aarsland, D., Bronnick, K., Williams-Gray, C., Weintraub, D., Marder, K., Kulisevsky, J., Burn, D., et al. (2010). Mild cognitive impairment in Parkinson disease: a multicenter pooled analysis. *Neurology, 75*(12), 1062-1069.

Aarsland, D., & Kurz, M. W. (2010). The epidemiology of dementia associated with Parkinson disease. *Journal of the Neurological Sciences, 289*(1-2), 18-22. doi:10.1016/j.jns.2009.08.034

Aarsland, D., Londos, E., & Ballard, C. (2009). Parkinson's disease dementia and dementia with Lewy bodies: different aspects of one entity. *International psychogeriatrics,* 21(2), 216-219.

Aarsland, D., Zaccai, J., & Brayne, C. (2005). A systematic review of prevalence studies of dementia in Parkinson's disease. *Movement Disorders, 20*(10), 1255-63. doi:10.1002/mds.20527

Aarsland, D., Andersen, K., Larsen, J. P., Perry, R., Wentzel-Larsen, T., Lolk, A., & Kragh-Sørensen, P. (2004). The rate of cognitive decline in Parkinson disease. *Archives of Neurology, 61*(12), 1906-1911.

Aarsland, D., Andersen, K., Larsen, J. P., Lolk, A., Nielsen, H., & Kragh-Sørensen, P. (2001). Risk of dementia in Parkinson's disease: a community-based, prospective study. *Neurology, 56*(6), 730-736.

Almeida, O. P., Garrido, G. J., Lautenschlager, N. T., Hulse, G. K., Jamrozik, K., & Flicker, L. (2008). Smoking is associated with reduced cortical regional gray matter density in brain regions associated with incipient Alzheimer disease. *The American Journal of Geriatric Psychiatry, 16*(1), 92-98.

Alves, G., Kurz, M., Lie, S. A., & Larsen, J. P. (2004). Cigarette smoking in Parkinson's disease: influence on disease progression. *Movement Disorders, 19*(9), 1087-1092.

Ambrose, J. A., & Barua, R. S. (2004). The pathophysiology of cigarette smoking and cardiovascular disease: an update. *Journal of the American College of Cardiology, 43*(10), 1731-1737.

American Accreditation Health Care Commission (A.D.A.M.) (2011). Coronary heart disease, In: *A.D.A.M. Medical Encyclopedia,* accessed 15-08-2011, Available from: http://www.ncbi.nlm.nih.gov/pubmedhealth/PMH0004449/

American Parkinson Disease Association (APDA). (2011). About Parkinson: To ease the burden and to find the cure, In: *Basic information about Parkinson 's disease,* accessed 02-04-2011, Available from:
http://www.apdaparkinson.org/UserND/AboutParkinson.asp.

American Society of Human Genetics/American College of Medical Genetics Test and Technology Transfer Committee Working Group (1998). ASHG/ACMG STATEMENT: Measurement and Use of Total Plasma Homocysteine. *American Journal of Human Genetics,* 63:1541–1543.

Antonini A, Barone P, Abbruzzese G, Bonuccelli U, Righini SA & Vado S. (2006). How vascular disease affects parkinsonism. The VADO study. *Movement Disorders,* 21(Suppl. 15): S533

Appenzeller O, Goss JE. A (1971). Autonomic deficits in Parkinson's syndrome. *Archives of Neurology,* 24: 50-57

Bancher, C., Braak, H., Fischer, P., & Jellinger, K. A. (1993). Neuropathological staging of Alzheimer lesions and intellectual status in Alzheimer's and Parkinson's disease patients. *Neuroscience Letters, 162*(1-2), 179-182.

Blandini, F., Fancellu, R., Martignoni, E., Mangiagalli, A., Pacchetti, C., Samuele, A., & Nappi, G. (2001). Plasma homocysteine and l-dopa metabolism in patients with Parkinson disease. *Clinical Chemistry, 47*(6), 1102-1104.

Barone, P., Burn, D. J., van Laar, T., Hsu, C., Poewe, W., & Lane, R. M. (2008). Rivastigmine versus placebo in hyperhomocysteinemic Parkinson's disease dementia patients. *Movement Disorders, 23*(11), 1532-40. doi:10.1002/mds.21997

Barua, R. S., Ambrose, J. A., Eales-Reynolds, L.-J., DeVoe, M. C., Zervas, J. G., & Saha, D. C. (2002). Heavy and light cigarette smokers have similar dysfunction of endothelial vasoregulatory activity: an in vivo and in vitro correlation. *Journal of the American College of Cardiology, 39*(11), 1758-1763.

Braak, H., & Braak, E. (1990). Cognitive impairment in Parkinson's disease: amyloid plaques, neurofibrillary tangles, and neuropil threads in the cerebral cortex. *Journal Of Neural Transmission,* 2(1), 45-57.

Breteler, M. M. (2000). Vascular risk factors for Alzheimer's disease: an epidemiologic perspective. *Neurobiology of Aging, 21*(2), 153-160.

Buob, A., Winter, H., Kindermann, M., Becker, G., Möller, J. C., Oertel, W. H., & Böhm, M. (2010). Parasympathetic but not sympathetic cardiac dysfunction at early stages of Parkinson's disease. *Clinical Research in Cardiology,* 99(11), 701-706.

Camicioli, R. M., Bouchard, T. P., & Somerville, M. J. (2009). Homocysteine is not associated with global motor or cognitive measures in nondemented older Parkinson's disease patients. *Movement Disorders, 24*(2), 176-82. doi:10.1002/mds.22227

Chobanian, A. V., Bakris, G. L., Black, H. R., Cushman, W. C., Green, L. A., Izzo, J. L., Jones, D. W., et al. (2003). Seventh report of the Joint National Committee on Prevention, Detection, Evaluation, and Treatment of High Blood Pressure. *Hypertension,* 42(6), 1206-1252. National Heart, Lung, and Blood Institute.

Chui, H. C., Victoroff, J. I., Margolin, D., Jagust, W., Shankle, R., & Katzman, R. (1992). Criteria for the diagnosis of ischemic vascular dementia proposed by the State of California Alzheimer's Disease Diagnostic and Treatment Centers. *Neurology,* 42(3 Pt 1), 473-480.

Cosentino F, Battista R, Scueri A, De Sensi F, De Siati L, Di Russo C, Camici GG & Volpe M. (2009) Impact of fasting glycemia and regional cerebral perfusion in diabetic subjects: a study with technetium-99m-ethyl cysteinate dimer single photon emission computed tomography. *Stroke;* 40: 306-308.

Darreh-Shori, T., Almkvist, O., Guan, Z. Z., Garlind, A., Strandberg, B., Svensson, A.-L., Soreq, H., et al. (2002). Sustained cholinesterase inhibition in AD patients receiving rivastigmine for 12 months. *Neurology, 59,* 563-572.

Darvesh, S., Walsh, R., & Martin, E. (2007). Homocysteine thiolactone and human cholinesterases. *Cellular and Molecular Neurobiology, 27*(1), 33-48.

De Bree, A., Verschuren, W. M., Blom, H. J., & Kromhout, D. (2001). Alcohol consumption and plasma homocysteine: what's brewing? *International Journal of Epidemiology,* 30(3), 626-627.

De Lau, L. M. L., Schipper, C. M. A., Hofman, A., Koudstaal, P. J., & Breteler, M. M. B. (2005). Prognosis of Parkinson disease: risk of dementia and mortality: the Rotterdam Study. *Archives of Neurology, 62*(8), 1265-1269.

Dubois, B., Pilon, B., Lhermitte, F., & Agid, Y. (1990). Cholinergic deficiency and frontal dysfunction in Parkinson's disease. *Annals of Neurology, 28*(2), 117-121.

Duthie, S. J., Whalley, L. J., Collins, A. R., Leaper, S., Berger, K., & Deary, I. J. (2002). Homocysteine, B vitamin status, and cognitive function in the elderly. *The American Journal of Clinical Nutrition,* 75(5), 908-913.

Ebmeier, K. P., Calder, S. A., Crawford, J. R., Stewart, L., Cochrane, R. H., & Besson, J. A. (1991). Dementia in idiopathic Parkinson's disease: prevalence and relationship with symptoms and signs of parkinsonism. *Psychological Medicine, 21*(1), 69-76.

Ebmeier, K. P., Calder, S. A., Crawford, J. R., Stewart, L., Besson, J. A., & Mutch, W. J. (1990). Clinical features predicting dementia in idiopathic Parkinson's disease: a follow-up study. *Neurology, 40*(8), 1222-1224.

Elias, P. K., Elias, M. F., D'Agostino, R. B., Cupples, L. A., Wilson, P. W., Silbershatz, H., & Wolf, P. A. (1997). NIDDM and blood pressure as risk factors for poor cognitive performance. The Framingham Study. *Diabetes Care, 20*(9), 1388-1395.

Elgh E, Domellöf M, Linder J, Edström M, Stenlund H & Forsgren L. (2009). Cognitive function in early Parkinson's disease: a population-based study. *European Journal of Neurology,* 16: 1278-1284.

Emre, M. (2003). Dementia associated with Parkinson's disease. *The Lancet Neurology,* 2(4), 229-237. doi:10.1016/S1474-4422(03)00351-X

Fahn, S., Marsden, C.D., Calne, D.B. and Goldstein, M. (eds) (1987). "Members of the UPDRS Development Committee. Unified Parkinson's Disease Rating Scale", *Recent Developments in Parkinson's Disease,* 11: pp. 153–163

Finkelstein, J. D. (1998). The metabolism of homocysteine: pathways and regulation. *European journal of pediatrics, 157 Suppl 2,* S40-4.

Gelb, D. J., Oliver, E., & Gilman, S. (1999). Diagnostic criteria for Parkinson disease. *Archives of Neurology, 56*(1), 33-39.

Gibb, W. R., & Lees, A. J. (1988). A comparison of clinical and pathological features of young- and old-onset Parkinson's disease. *Neurology, 38*(9), 1402-1406.

Gliebus, G., & Lippa, C. F. (2007). The influence of beta-blockers on delayed memory function in people with cognitive impairment. *American journal of Alzheimers disease and other dementias, 22*(1), 57-61.

Gibson, A., Woodside, J. V., Young, I. S., Sharpe, P. C., Mercer, C., Patterson, C. C., Mckinley, M. C., Kluijtmans, L.A.J., Whitehead, A.S. & Evans, A. (2008). Alcohol increases homocysteine and reduces B vitamin concentration in healthy male volunteers—a randomized, crossover intervention study. *QJM: An International Journal Of Medicine,* 101(11), 881-887.

Gorelick, P. B., Scuteri, A., Black, S. E., Decarli, C., Greenberg, S. M., Iadecola, C., Launer, L. J., et al. (2011). Vascular Contributions to Cognitive Impairment and Dementia: A Statement for Healthcare Professionals From the American Heart Association/American *Stroke* Association. Stroke, STR.0b013e3182299496-. doi:10.1161/STR.0b013e3182299496

Hassin-Baer, S., Cohen, O., Vakil, E., Sela, B.-A., Nitsan, Z., Schwartz, R., Chapman, J., et al. (2006). Plasma homocysteine levels and Parkinson disease: disease progression, carotid intima-media thickness and neuropsychiatric complications. *Clinical neuropharmacology*, *29*(6), 305-11. doi:10.1097/01.WNF.0000236763.16032.60

Haugarvoll, K., Aarsland, D., Wentzel-Larsen, T., & Larsen, J. P. (2005). The influence of cerebrovascular risk factors on incident dementia in patients with Parkinson's disease. *Acta Neurologica Scandinavica*, *112*(6), 386-90. doi:10.1111/j.1600-0404.2005.00389.x

Hauser, R.A. (2010). Movement and Neurodegenerative Diseases: Parkinson's Disease, In: *Medscape reference*, accessed 14-07-2011, Available from: http://emedicine.medscape.com/article/1151267-overview

Hill, R. D. (1989). Residual effects of cigarette smoking on cognitive performance in normal aging. *Psychology and Aging*, *4*(2), 251-254.

Herishanu YO, Medvedovski M, Goldsmith JR & Kordysh E (2001). A case-control study of Parkinson's disease in urban population of southern Israel. *Canadian Journal of Neurological Sciences*, *28*, 144-147.

Hoehn, M. M., & Yahr, M. D. (1967). Parkinsonism: onset, progression and mortality. *Neurology*, *17*(2), 427-442.

Hughes, A. J., Daniel, S. E., Kilford, L., & Lees, A. J. (1992). Accuracy of clinical diagnosis of idiopathic Parkinson's disease: a clinico-pathological study of 100 cases. *Journal of Neurology*, *55*(3), 181-184. doi:10.1136/jnnp.55.3.181

Hughes, T. A., Ross, H. F., Musa, S., Bhattacherjee, S., Nathan, R. N., Mindham, R. H., & Spokes, E. G. (2000). A 10-year study of the incidence of and factors predicting dementia in Parkinson's disease. *Neurology*, *54*(8), 1596-1602.

Janvin, C. C., Aarsland, D., & Larsen, J. P. (2005). Cognitive predictors of dementia in Parkinson's disease: a community-based 4-year longitudinal study. *Journal of Geriatric Psychiatry and Neurology*, *18*(3), 149-154.

Jellinger K. (2011). Synuclein deposition and non-motor symptoms in Parkinson's disease. *Journal of the Neurological Sciences*, doi: 10.1016/j.jns2011.04.012

Jellinger, K. (2003). Prevalence of cerebrovascular lesions in Parkinson's disease. A postmortem study. *Acta Neuropathologica*, *105*(5), 415-9. doi:10.1007/s00401-003-0676-3

Jessup, M., Abraham, W. T., Casey, D. E., Feldman, A. M., Francis, G. S., Ganiats, T. G., Konstam, M. A., Mancini, D.M., Rahko, P.S., Silver, M.A., Stevenson, L.W., Yancy, C.W. (2009). 2009 focused update: ACCF/AHA Guidelines for the Diagnosis and Management of Heart Failure in Adults: a report of the American College of Cardiology Foundation/American Heart Association Task Force on Practice Guidelines: developed in collaboration with the International Society for Heart and Lung Transplantation. *Circulation*, 119(14), 1977-2016.

Kalmijn, S., Van Boxtel, M. P. J., Verschuren, M. W. M., Jolles, J., & Launer, L. J. (2002). Cigarette smoking and alcohol consumption in relation to cognitive performance in middle age. *American Journal of Epidemiology*, *156*(10), 936-944.

Kandiah, N., Narasimhalu, K., Lau, P.-N., Seah, S.-H., Au, W. L., & Tan, L. C. S. (2009). Cognitive decline in early Parkinson's disease. *Movement Disorders*, *24*(4), 605-8. doi:10.1002/mds.22384

Kelton, M. C., Kahn, H. J., Conrath, C. L., & Newhouse, P. A. (2000). The effects of nicotine on Parkinson's disease. *Brain and Cognition*, *43*(1-3), 274-282.

Kleykamp, B. A., Griffiths, R. R., & Mintzer, M. Z. (2010). Dose effects of triazolam and alcohol on cognitive performance in healthy volunteers. *Experimental and Clinical Psychopharmacology*, *18*(1), 1-16.

Korczyn, A. D. (2010). Vascular contribution to dementia in Parkinson's disease. *Neurodegenerative Diseases*, *7*(1-3), 127-130.

Kuhn W, Hummel T, Woitalla D & Muller T. (2001) Plasma homocysteine and MTHFR C677T genotype in levodopa-treated patients with PD. *Neurology*; 56 (2), 281-282.

Kuhn, W., Roebroek, R., Blom, H., Van Oppenraaij, D., & Müller, T. (1998). Hyperhomocysteinaemia in Parkinson's disease. *Journal of Neurology*, *245*(12), 811-812.

Lane, R. M., Potkin, S. G., & Enz, A. (2006). Targeting acetylcholinesterase and butyrylcholinesterase in dementia. *The International Journal of Neuropsychopharmacology*, 9(1), 101-124.

Larsen, J. P., Dupont, E., & Tandberg, E. (1994). Clinical diagnosis of Parkinson's disease. Proposal of diagnostic subgroups classified at different levels of confidence. *Acta Neurologica Scandinavica*, *89*(4), 242–251.

Levy, G., Tang, M.-xin, Cote, L. J., Louis, E. D., Alfaro, B., Mejia, H., Stern, Y., et al. (2002). Do Risk Factors for Alzheimer ' s Disease Predict Dementia in Parkinson ' s Disease ? An Exploratory Study. *Movement Disorders*, *17*(2), 250-257. doi:10.1002/mds.10086

Lezak, M.D., Howieson, D.B. & Loring, D.W. (2004). *Neuropsychological assessment* (4th edition), Oxford University Press, New York.

Litvinenko, I.V., Odinak, M.M, Pozdnyakov, A.V., Mogilnaya, V.I., Shatova, A.V. (2005). Plasma homocysteine level correlate with white matter brain lesions and cognitive impairment in Parkinson's disease. *European Journal of Neurology*, 12 (suppl 12), S100

Locascio, J. J., Corkin, S., & Growdon, J. H. (2003). Relation between clinical characteristics of Parkinson's disease and cognitive decline. *Journal of Clinical and Experimental Neuropsychology*, *25*(1), 94-109. doi:10.1076/jcen.25.1.94.13624

Luchsinger, J. A., Reitz, C., Honig, L. S., Tang, M. X., Shea, S., & Mayeux, R. (2005). Aggregation of vascular risk factors and risk of incident Alzheimer disease. *Neurology*, *65*(4), 545-551.

Marder, K., Flood, P., Cote, L., & Mayeux, R. (1990). A pilot study of risk factors for dementia in Parkinson's disease. *Movement Disorders*, *5*(2), 156-161.

Matteau, E., Dupré, N., & Simard, M. (2010). Idiopathic Parkinson's disease with and without Vascular Risk Factors: A Clinical Database Study. *The Journal US-China Medical Science*, 7, 15-18.

Mattson, M. P., & Shea, T. B. (2003). Folate and homocysteine metabolism in neural plasticity and neurodegenerative disorders. *Trends in Neurosciences*, *26*(3), 137-146.

Megnien, J. L., Gariepy, J., Saudubray, J. M., Nuoffer, J. M., Denarie, N., Levenson, J., & Simon, A. (1998). Evidence of carotid artery wall hypertrophy in homozygous homocystinuria. *Circulation*, 98(21), 2276-2281.

Menendez, M., Ribacoba, R., Jimenez, G., Virgili, J.R., Huerta, C. & de la Vega, V. (2007). Dementia and hyperhomocysteinemia in Parkinson's disease. *Movement Disorders*, 22 (suppl 16), S186

Miyake, Y., Tanaka, K., Fukushima, W., Sasaki, S., Kiyohara, C., Tsuboi, Y., Yamada, T. (2010). Case-control study of risk of Parkinson's disease in relation to hypertension, hypercholesterolemia, and diabetes in Japan. *Journal of the Neurological Sciences*, *293*(1-2), 82-6. doi:10.1016/j.jns.2010.03.002

Morris, M. S., Jacques, P. F., Rosenberg, I. H., & Selhub, J. (2001). Hyperhomocysteinemia associated with poor recall in the third National Health and Nutrition Examination Survey. 73(5), 927-933.

Movement Disorder Society Task Force on Rating Scales for Parkinson's Disease (2003). State of the Art Review The Unified Parkinson' s Disease Rating Scale (UPDRS): Status and Recommendations. *Society*, 18(7), 738 -750. doi:10.1002/mds.10473

Müller, T., Woitalla, D., Fowler, B., & Kuhn, W. (2002). 3-OMD and homocysteine plasma levels in parkinsonian patients. *Journal of neural transmission 1996, 109*(2), 175-179.

Müller, T., Woitalla, D., Hauptmann, B., Fowler, B., & Kuhn, W. (2001). Decrease of methionine and S-adenosylmethionine and increase of homocysteine in treated patients with Parkinson's disease. *Neuroscience letters, 308*(1), 54–56. doi:10.1016/S0304-3940(01)01972-3

Müller, T., Werne, B., Fowler, B., & Kuhn, W. (1999). Nigral endothelial dysfunction, homocysteine, and Parkinson's disease. *Lancet, 354*, 126-127.

Muslimovic, D., Post, B., Speelman, J. D., & Schmand, B. (2005). Cognitive profile of patients with newly diagnosed Parkinson disease. *Neurology, 65*(8), 1239-45. doi:10.1212/01.wnl.0000180516.69442.95

Nakaso, J., Yasui, K., Kowa, H., Kitayama, M., Takeshima, T. & Nakashima, K. (2006). Hyperhomocysteinemia: a predictive parameter for disease progression due to non-motor complications in Parkinson's disease. *Movement Disorders*, 2006, 21 (suppl 15), S488-489

Nakaso, K., Yasui, K., Kowa, H., Kusumi, M., Ueda, K., Yoshimoto, Y., Takeshima, T., et al. (2003). Hypertrophy of IMC of carotid artery in Parkinson's disease is associated with L-DOPA, homocysteine, and MTHFR genotype. *Journal of the Neurological Sciences*, 207(1-2), 19-23.

National Collaborating Centre for Chronic Conditions (2006). *Atrial fibrillation: National clinical guideline for management in primary and secondary care*. Royal College of Physicians. London, 2006 , accessed 01-08-2011, Available from: http://www.nice.org.uk/nicemedia/live/10982/30055/30055.pdf

Nobili F, Morbelli S, Arnaldi D, Ferrara M, Campus C, Brugnolo A et al. Radionuclide brain imaging correlates of cognitive impairment in Parkinson's disease (PD). *Journal of the Neurological Sciences*, doi: 10.1016/j.jns.2011.06.053

O'Suilleabhain, P. E., Oberle, R., Bartis, C., Dewey, R. B., Bottiglieri, T., & Diaz-Arrastia, R. (2006). Clinical course in Parkinson's disease with elevated homocysteine. *Parkinsonism & related disorders, 12*(2), 103-7. doi:10.1016/j.parkreldis.2005.10.002

O'Suilleabhain, P. E., Sung, V., Hernandez, C., Lacritz, L., Dewey, R. B., Bottiglieri, T., & Diaz-Arrastia, R. (2004). Elevated plasma homocysteine level in patients with Parkinson disease: motor, affective, and cognitive associations. *Archives of Neurology, 61*(6), 865-8. doi:10.1001/archneur.61.6.865

Ozer, F., Meral, H., Hanoglu, L., Aydemir, T., Yilsen, M., Cetin, S., Ozturk, O., et al. (2006). Plasma homocysteine levels in patients treated with levodopa: motor and cognitive associations. *Neurological Research, 28*, 853-858.

Papapetropoulos, S., Villar, J. M., & Mash, D. C. (2006). Is ischemic cerebrovascular disease a risk factor for dementia in patients with Parkinson's disease? *Acta Neurologica Scandinavica*, 113, 353-354.

Papapetropoulos, S., Ellul, J., Argyriou, a a, Talelli, P., Chroni, E., & Papapetropoulos, T. (2004). The effect of vascular disease on late onset Parkinson's disease. *European Journal of Neurology, 11*(4), 231-5. doi:10.1046/j.1468-1331.2003.00748.x

Parain, K., Hapdey, C., Rousselet, E., Marchand, V., Dumery, B., & Hirsch, E. C. (2003). Cigarette smoke and nicotine protect dopaminergic neurons against the 1-methyl-4-phenyl-1,2,3,6-tetrahydropyridine Parkinsonian toxin. *Brain Research, 984*(1-2), 224-232.

Park, H. J., Lee, P. H., Ahn, Y. W., Choi, Y. J., Lee, G., Lee, D.-Y., Chung, E. S., et al. (2007). Neuroprotective effect of nicotine on dopaminergic neurons by anti-inflammatory action. *European Journal of Neuroscience, 26*(1), 79-89.

Paul, R. H., Brickman, A. M., Cohen, R. A., Williams, L. M., Niaura, R., Pogun, S., Clark, C. R., et al. (2006). Cognitive status of young and older cigarette smokers: data from the international brain database. *Journal of clinical neuroscience, 13*(4), 457-465.

Perry, E. K., Morris, C. M., Court, J. A., Ceng, A., Fairbairn, A. F., McKeith, I. G., Irving, D., et al. (1995). Alteration in nicotine binding sites in Parkinson's disease, Lewy body dementia and Alzheimer's disease: possible index of early neuropathology. *Neuroscience, 64*(2), 385-395.

Petersen, R. C. (2004). Mild cognitive impairment as a diagnostic entity. *Journal of Internal Medicine, 256*(3), 183-94. doi:10.1111/j.1365-2796.2004.01388.x

Ravaglia, G., Forti, P., Maioli, F., Martelli, M., Servadei, L., Brunetti, N., Pantieri, G., et al. (2006). Conversion of mild cognitive impairment to dementia: predictive role of mild cognitive impairment subtypes and vascular risk factors. *Dementia and geriatric cognitive disorders, 21*(1), 51-8. doi:10.1159/000089515

Razani J, Boone K, Lesser I & Weiss D. (2004). Effects of cigarette smoking history on cognitive functioning in healthy older adults. *American Journal of Geriatric Psychiatry, 12,* 404-411.

Rektor, I., Goldemund, D., Sheardová, K., Rektorová, I., Michálková, Z., & Dufek, M. (2009). Vascular pathology in patients with idiopathic Parkinson's disease. *Parkinsonism & related disorders, 15*(1), 24-9. doi:10.1016/j.parkreldis.2008.02.007

Religa, D., Czyzewski, K., Styczynska, M., Peplonska, B., Lokk, J., Chodakowska-Zebrowska, M., Stepien, K., et al. (2006). Hyperhomocysteinemia and methylenetetrahydrofolate reductase polymorphism in patients with Parkinson's disease. *Neuroscience letters, 404*(1-2), 56-60. doi:10.1016/j.neulet.2006.05.040

Reutens, S., & Sachdev, P. (2002). Homocysteine in neuropsychiatric disorders of the elderly. *International Journal of Geriatric Psychiatry, 17*(9), 859-864.

Ritz, B., Ascherio, A., Checkoway, H., Marder, K. S., Nelson, L. M., Rocca, W. A., Ross, G. W., et al. (2007). Pooled analysis of tobacco use and risk of Parkinson disease. *Archives of Neurology, 64*(7), 990-7. doi:10.1001/archneur.64.7.990

Rodriguez-Oroz, M. C., Lage, P. M., Sanchez-Mut, J., Lamet, I., Pagonabarraga, J., Toledo, J. B., García-Garcia, D., et al. (2009). Homocysteine and cognitive impairment in Parkinson's disease: a biochemical, neuroimaging, and genetic study. *Movement Disorders, 24*(10), 1437-44. doi:10.1002/mds.22522

Rogers, J. D., Sanchez-Saffon, A., Frol, A. B., & Diaz-Arrastia, R. (2003). Elevated plasma homocysteine levels in patients treated with levodopa: association with vascular disease. *Archives of Neurology, 60*(1), 59-64.

Román, G. C., Tatemichi, T. K., Erkinjuntti, T., Cummings, J. L., Masdeu, J. C., Garcia, J. H., Amaducci, L., et al. (1993). Vascular dementia: diagnostic criteria for research studies. Report of the NINDS-AIREN International Workshop. *Neurology, 43*(2), 250-260.

Sachdev, P. S. (2005). Homocysteine and brain atrophy. *Progress in Neuropsychopharmacology & Biological Psychiatry,* 29(7), 1152-1161.

Schinka, J. A., Vanderploeg, R. D., Rogish, M., Graves, A. B., Mortimer, J. A., & Ordoric, P. I. (2002). Effects of the use of alcohol and cigarettes on cognition in elderly adults. *Journal of the International Neuropsychological Society, 8*(6), 811-818.

Scigliano, G., Musicco, M., Soliveri, P., Piccolo, I., Ronchetti, G., & Girotti, F. (2006). Reduced risk factors for vascular disorders in Parkinson disease patients: a case-control study. *Stroke: A Journal of Cerebral Circulation, 37*(5), 1184-1188.

Schulz, J. B., Lindenau, J., Seyfried, J., & Dichgans, J. (2000). Glutathione, oxidative stress and neurodegeneration. *European Journal of Biochemistry*, 267(16), 4904-4911.

Shibata, M., Morita, Y., Shimizu, T., Takahashi, K., & Suzuki, N. (2009). Cardiac parasympathetic dysfunction concurrent with cardiac sympathetic denervation in Parkinson's disease. *Journal of the Neurological Sciences, 276*(1-2), 79-83.

Shin, H.& Sohn, Y.H. (2006). Role of homocysteine in developing cognitive dysfunction in Parkinson disease; comparison with Alzheimer disease. *Movement Disorders*, 21 (suppl 15), S470

Shindo, K., Watanabe, H., Tanaka, H., Ohashi, K., Nagasaka, T., Tsunoda, S., & Shiozawa, Z. (2003). Age and duration related changes in muscle sympathetic nerve activity in Parkinson's disease. *Journal of Neurology, Neurosurgery & Psychiatry, 74*(10), 1407-1411.

Skoog I. (1994). Risk factors for vascular dementia: a review. *Dementia*, 5(3-4), 137-144.

Slawek, Wieczorek, D., Derejko, M., Dubaniewicz, M., Brockhuis, B., Sitek, E., Wilczewska, L., et al. (2008). The influence of vascular risk factors and white matter hyperintensities on the degree of cognitive impairment in Parkinson ' s disease. *Neurologia I Neurochirurgia Polska*, 505-512.

Sponne, I., Fifre, A., Koziel, V., Oster, T., Olivier, J.-L., & Pillot, T. (2004). Membrane cholesterol interferes with neuronal apoptosis induced by soluble oligomers but not fibrils of amyloid-beta peptide. *The FASEB Journal*, 18(7), 836-838.

Stathis, P., Kiebardis, A., Kiosterakis, G., Bournousozis, N., Karakis, P., Fytou-Pallikari, A., Kalkani, E. & Maltezou, M. (2006). Serum homocysteine concentrations and cognitive decline in Parkinson's disease patient: a controlled study. *Movement Disorders*, 21 (Suppl 15), S488-489

Stanger, O., Herrmann, W., Pietrzik, K., Fowler, B., Geisel, J., Dierkes, J., & Weger, M. (2003). DACH-LIGA homocystein (german, austrian and swiss homocysteine society): consensus paper on the rational clinical use of homocysteine, folic acid and B-vitamins in cardiovascular and thrombotic diseases: guidelines and recommendations. *Clinical chemistry and laboratory medicine*, 41(11), 1392–1403. doi:10.1515/CCLM.2003.214

Stegmayr, B., & Asplund, K. (1995). Diabetes as a risk factor for stroke. A population perspective. *Diabetologia, 38*(9), 1061-1068.

Stewart, R., & Liolitsa, D. (1999). Type 2 diabetes mellitus, cognitive impairment and dementia. *Diabetic Medicine*,16, 93-112.

Swan, G. E., & Lessov-Schlaggar, C. N. (2007). The effects of tobacco smoke and nicotine on cognition and the brain. *Neuropsychology Review, 17*(3), 259-73. doi:10.1007/s11065-007-9035-9

Tanaka, K., Mizukawa, K., Ogawa, N., & Mori, A. (1995). Post-ischemic administration of the acetylcholinesterase inhibitor ENA-713 prevents delayed neuronal death in the gerbil hippocampus. *Neurochemical Research*, 20(6), 663-667.

Tatemichi, T. K., Desmond, D. W., Paik, M., Figueroa, M., Gropen, T. I., Stern, Y., Sano, M., et al. (1993). Clinical determinants of dementia related to stroke. *Annals of Neurology, 33*(6), 568-575.

Todorović, Z., Dzoljić, E., Novaković, I., Mirković, D., Stojanović, R., Nesić, Z., Krajinović, M., et al. (2006). Homocysteine serum levels and MTHFR C677T genotype in patients with Parkinson's disease, with and without levodopa therapy. *Journal of the Neurological Sciences*, 248(1-2), 56-61. doi:10.1016/j.jns.2006.05.040

Tyas, S. L., White, L. R., Petrovitch, H., Ross, G. W., Foley, D. J.,Heimovitz, H. K. & Launer, L.J. (2003). Midlife smoking and late life dementia: The Honolulu Asia Aging Study. *Neurobiology of Aging*, 24, 589–596.

Uc, E. Y., McDermott, M. P., Marder, K. S., Anderson, S. W., Litvan, I., Como, P. G., Auinger, P., et al. (2009). Incidence of and risk factors for cognitive impairment in an early Parkinson disease clinical trial cohort. *Neurology*, *73*(18), 1469-1477.

Wald, D. S., Law, M., & Morris, J. K. (2002). Homocysteine and cardiovascular disease: evidence on causality from a meta-analysis. *British Medical Journal*, *325*(7374), 1202.

Weisskopf, M. G., Grodstein, F., & Ascherio, A. (2007). Smoking and cognitive function in Parkinson's disease. *Movement Disorders*, *22*(5), 660-5. doi:10.1002/mds.21373

Wiederkehr S, Laurin D, Simard M, Verreault R & Lindsay J. (2009). Vascular Risk Factors and Cognitive Functions in Nondemented Elderly Individuals. *Journal of Geriatric Psychiatry and Neurology*; 22(3): 196-206.

Williams-Gray, C. H., Foltynie, T., Brayne, C. E. G., Robbins, T. W., & Barker, R. A. (2007). Evolution of cognitive dysfunction in an incident Parkinson's disease cohort. *Brain*, *130*(Pt 7), 1787-1798.

Yan, S. D., Stern, D., & Schmidt, A. M. (1997). What's the RAGE? The receptor for advanced glycation end products (RAGE) and the dark side of glucose. *European Journal of Clinical Investigation*, *27*(3), 179-181.

Yasui, K., Kowa, H., Nakaso, K., Takeshima, T., & Nakashima, K. (2000). Plasma homocysteine and MTHFR C677T genotype in levodopa-treated patients with PD. *Neurology*, *55*(3), 437-440.

Ylikoski, R., Ylikoski, A., Raininko, R., Keskivaara, P., Sulkava, R., Tilvis, R., & Erkinjuntti, T. (2000). Cardiovascular diseases, health status, brain imaging findings and neuropsychological functioning in neurologically healthy elderly individuals. *Archives of Gerontology and Geriatrics*, *30*(2), 115-130.

Zgaljardic, D. J., Borod, J. C., Foldi, N. S., & Mattis, P. (2003). A review of the cognitive and behavioral sequelae of Parkinson's disease: relationship to frontostriatal circuitry. *Cognitive and behavioral neurology*, 16(4), 193-210.

Zoccolella, S., Lamberti, S. V., Iliceto, G., Santamato, A., Lamberti, P., & Logroscino, G. (2010). Hyperhomocysteinemia in L-dopa treated patients with Parkinson's disease: potential implications in cognitive dysfunction and dementia? *Current Medicinal Chemistry*, *17*(28), 3253-3261.

Zoccolella, S., dell' Aquila, C., Abruzzese, G., Antonini, A., Bonuccelli, U., Canesi, M., Cristina, S., et al. (2009). Hyperhomocysteinemia in levodopa-treated patients with Parkinson's disease dementia. *Movement Disorders*, *24*(7), 1028-33. doi:10.1002/mds.22511

Zoccolella, S., Lamberti, P., Iliceto, G., Diroma, C., Armenise, E., Defazio, G., Lamberti, S. V., et al. (2005). Plasma homocysteine levels in L-dopa-treated Parkinson's disease patients with cognitive dysfunctions. *Clinical chemistry and laboratory medicine : CCLM / FESCC*, *43*(10), 1107-10. doi:10.1515/CCLM.2005.193

Permissions

The contributors of this book come from diverse backgrounds, making this book a truly international effort. This book will bring forth new frontiers with its revolutionizing research information and detailed analysis of the nascent developments around the world.

We would like to thank L. Miguel Martins and Samantha H. Y. Loh, for lending their expertise to make the book truly unique. They have played a crucial role in the development of this book. Without their invaluable contribution this book wouldn't have been possible. They have made vital efforts to compile up to date information on the varied aspects of this subject to make this book a valuable addition to the collection of many professionals and students.

This book was conceptualized with the vision of imparting up-to-date information and advanced data in this field. To ensure the same, a matchless editorial board was set up. Every individual on the board went through rigorous rounds of assessment to prove their worth. After which they invested a large part of their time researching and compiling the most relevant data for our readers. Conferences and sessions were held from time to time between the editorial board and the contributing authors to present the data in the most comprehensible form. The editorial team has worked tirelessly to provide valuable and valid information to help people across the globe.

Every chapter published in this book has been scrutinized by our experts. Their significance has been extensively debated. The topics covered herein carry significant findings which will fuel the growth of the discipline. They may even be implemented as practical applications or may be referred to as a beginning point for another development.

The editorial board has been involved in producing this book since its inception. They have spent rigorous hours researching and exploring the diverse topics which have resulted in the successful publishing of this book. They have passed on their knowledge of decades through this book. To expedite this challenging task, the publisher supported the team at every step. A small team of assistant editors was also appointed to further simplify the editing procedure and attain best results for the readers.

Our editorial team has been hand-picked from every corner of the world. Their multi-ethnicity adds dynamic inputs to the discussions which result in innovative outcomes. These outcomes are then further discussed with the researchers and contributors who give their valuable feedback and opinion regarding the same. The feedback is then collaborated with the researches and they are edited in a comprehensive manner to aid the understanding of the subject.

Apart from the editorial board, the designing team has also invested a significant amount of their time in understanding the subject and creating the most relevant covers. They scrutinized every image to scout for the most suitable representation of the subject and create an appropriate cover for the book.

The publishing team has been involved in this book since its early stages. They were actively engaged in every process, be it collecting the data, connecting with the contributors or procuring relevant information. The team has been an ardent support to the editorial, designing and production team. Their endless efforts to recruit the best for this project, has resulted in the accomplishment of this book. They are a veteran in the field of academics and their pool of knowledge is as vast as their experience in printing. Their expertise and guidance has proved useful at every step. Their uncompromising quality standards have made this book an exceptional effort. Their encouragement from time to time has been an inspiration for everyone.

The publisher and the editorial board hope that this book will prove to be a valuable piece of knowledge for researchers, students, practitioners and scholars across the globe.

List of Contributors

Tatsuro Koike, Kazuhiko Suzuki and Tomohiro Kawahata
Hokkaido University Graduate School of Life Science, Sapporo, Japan

Maria Śmialowska and Helena Domin
Institute of Pharmacology, Department of Neurobiology, Polish Academy of Sciences, Krakow, Poland

V. Chandana Epa
CSIRO Materials Science & Engineering, Preventative Health Flagship and the CRC for Mental Health,
Parkville, Victoria, Australia

Junye Miao and Rongqiao He
State Key Laboratory of Brain and Cognitive Sciences, Institute of Biophysics, Chinese Academy of Sciences, Beijing, China

Ahmad Al Mutairy
University of Dammam, Saudi Arabia

Khalaf Al Moutaery, Abdulrahman Al Asmari, Mohammed Arshaduddin and Mohammad Tariq
Riyadh Military Hospital, Riyadh, Saudi Arabia

Ana C. Costa, L. Miguel Martins and Samantha H. Y. Loh
Cell Death Regulation Laboratory, MRC Toxicology Unit, Leicester, UK

Carla Caruso, Lila Carniglia, Daniela Durand, Teresa N. Scimonelli and Mercedes Lasaga
Research Institute for Reproduction, School of Medicine, University of Buenos Aires, IFEC-CONICET Department of Pharmacology, School of Chemistry, National University of Córdoba, Córdoba, Argentina

Zachary M. Harris and Jacob A. Sloane
Beth Israel Deaconess Medical Center, Harvard Medical School, USA

Said Ramdane
Private Office of Neurology, Algerian Society of Neurology, Algeria

Michael A. Myre
Center for Human Genetic Research, Dept. of Neurology, Massachusetts General Hospital, Boston, Massachusetts, USA

Sónia Costa, Raquel Tojal and Ana Valverde
Neurology Department, Hospital Professor Dr. Fernando Fonseca EPE, Amadora, Portugal

Gian Luigi Lenzi and Marta Altieri
Clinica Neurologica A, Department of Neurology and Psichiatry, Italy

Giorgio De Benedetto
Department of Cardiovascular, Respiratory, Nephrological and Geriatric Sciences, "Sapienza" University, Rome, Italy

Sellama Nadifi and Khalil Hamzi
Laboratory of Genetics and Molecular Pathology, Faculty of Medicine and Pharmacy, University Hassan II Casablanca, Morocco

Maxime Doiron and Martine Simard
École de Psychologie, Université Laval & Centre de Recherche Université Laval-Robert Giffard, Québec, Canada